IMMUNOTOXICOLOGY

DEVELOPMENTS IN HEMATOLOGY AND IMMUNOLOGY

Lijnen, H.R., Collen, D. and Verstraete, M., eds: Synthetic Substrates in Clinical Blood Coagulation Assays. 1980. ISBN 90-247-2409-0

Smit Sibinga, C.Th., Das, P.C. and Forfar, J.O., eds: Paediatrics and Blood Transfusion. 1982. ISBN 90-247-2619-0

Fabris, N., ed: Immunology and Ageing. 1982. ISBN 90-247-2640-9

Hornstra, G.: Dietary Fats, Prostanoids and Arterial Thrombosis. 1982. ISBN 90-247-2667-0

Smit Sibinga, C.Th., Das, P.C. and Loghem, van J.J., eds: Blood Transfusion and Problems of Bleeding. 1982. ISBN 90-247-3058-9

Dormandy, J., ed: Red Cell Deformability and Filterability. 1983. ISBN 0-89838-578-4

Smit Sibinga, C.Th., Das, P.C. and Taswell, H.F., eds: Quality Assurance in Blood Banking and Its Clinical Impact. 1984. ISBN 0-89838-618-7

Besselaar, A.M.H.P. van den, Gralnick, H.R. and Lewis, S.M., eds: Thromboplastin Calibration and Oral Anticoagulant Control. 1984. ISBN 0-89838-637-3

Fondu, P. and Thijs, O., eds: Haemostatic Failure in Liver Disease. 1984. ISBN 0-89838-640-3

Smit Sibinga, C.Th., Das, P.C. and Opelz, G., eds: Transplantation and Blood Transfusion. 1984. ISBN 0-89838-686-1

Schmid-Schönbein, H., Wurzinger, L.J. and Zimmerman, R.E., eds: Enzyme Activation in Blood-Perfused Artificial Organs. 1985. ISBN 0-89838-704-3

Dormandy, J., ed: Blood Filtration and Blood Cell Deformability. 1985. ISBN 0-89838-714-0

Smit Sibinga, C.Th., Das, P.C. and Seidl, S., eds: Plasma Fractionation and Blood Transfusion. 1985. ISBN 0-89838-761-2

Dawids, S. and Bantjes, A., eds: Blood Compatible Materials and their Testing. 1986. ISBN 0-89838-813-9

Smit Sibinga, C.Th., Das, P.C. and Greenwalt, T.J., eds: Future Developments in Blood Banking. 1986. ISBN 0-89838-824-4

Berlin, A, Dean, J, Draper, M.H., Smith, E.M.B., Spreafico, F., eds: Immunotoxicology. 1987. ISBN 0-89838-843-0

UNEP, ILO, WHO INTERNATIONAL PROGRAMME
ON CHEMICAL SAFETY (IPCS)

COMMISSION OF THE EUROPEAN COMMUNITIES

with the support of the United States Environmental Protection Agency
National Institute of Environmental Health Sciences and the participation
of the International Society of Immunopharmacology

Immunotoxicology

Proceedings of the International Seminar on the Immunological System as a Target
for Toxic Damage – Present Status, Open Problems and Future Perspectives

edited by

A. BERLIN
Commission of the European Communities, Health and Safety Directorate,
Luxembourg

J. DEAN
Chemical Industry Institute of Toxicology, Research Triangle Park, North
Carolina, U.S.A.

M.H. DRAPER
International Programme on Chemical Safety, World Health Organization,
Geneva, Switzerland

E.M.B. SMITH
International Programme on Chemical Safety, World Health Organization,
Geneva, Switzerland

F. SPREAFICO
Institute of Pharmacological Research "Mario Negri", Milan, Italy

1987 **MARTINUS NIJHOFF PUBLISHERS**
a member of the KLUWER ACADEMIC PUBLISHERS GROUP
DORDRECHT / BOSTON / LANCASTER
for
THE COMMISSION OF THE EUROPEAN COMMUNITIES
and UNEP, ILO, WHO INTERNATIONAL PROGRAMME
ON CHEMICAL SAFETY

IV

Distributors

for the United States and Canada: Kluwer Academic Publishers, P.O. Box 358, Accord Station, Hingham, MA 02018-0358, USA
for the UK and Ireland: Kluwer Academic Publishers, MTP Press Limited, Falcon House, Queen Square, Lancaster LA1 1RN, UK
for all other countries: Kluwer Academic Publishers Group, Distribution Center, P.O. Box 322, 3300 AH Dordrecht, The Netherlands

Library of Congress Cataloging in Publication Data

```
International Seminar on the Immunological System as
   a Target for Toxic Damage (1984 : Commission of the
   European Communities)
   Immunotoxicology : papers presented at the Interna-
tional Seminar on the Immunological System as a Target
for Toxic Damage.

   (Developments in hematology and immunology ; 16)
   1. Immunotoxicology--Congresses.  I. Berlin, A.
II. Title.  III. Series.
RC582.17.I57 1984     616.97        86-23690
```

ISBN-13:978-94-010-8414-7   e-ISBN-13:978-94-009-4307-0
DOI: 10.1007/978-94-009-4307-0

EUR 10041 EN
IPCS Joint Seminar 10
Book information

Publication arranged by: Commission of the European Communities, Direc-
torate-General Telecommunications, Information Industries and Innovation,
Luxembourg

Copyright/legal notice

The authors alone are responsible for the views expressed in the signed articles in this publication. None of the organizers of the symposium nor any person acting on their behalf is responsible for the use which might be made of the following information.

TABLE OF CONTENTS

VIII

The International Seminar on the Immunological System as a Target for Toxic Damage was held at The Commission of the European Communities (CEC) in Luxembourg on 6-9 November 1984. It was organized by the CEC and the International Programme on Chemical Safety of UNEP/ILO/WHO with the support of the U.S. Environmental Protection Agency and the National Institute of Environmental Health Sciences - USA and with the participation of the International Society of Immunophar-macology. These bodies are actively concerned with the scientific and applied aspects of immunotoxicology. The Seminar consisted of thirty-four invited papers and three major panel discussions covering current and future test strategies for the screening of immunotoxic substances, hypersensitivity and the health implications of immunotoxico-logical problems. It was attended by more than 200 scien-tists from 27 countries representing all the Member States of the European Economic Community and the six Regions of the World Health Organization. These scientists represented many different disciplines and interests.

The Seminar's principal objectives were:

- a review of recent advances in knowledge concerning the structure, function and dysfunction of the immunological system;

- a review of the effects of xenobiotics on the immune system in animals and humans;

- an examination of the human health implications of immunotoxicity;

- discussion and critical analysis of the procedures for the assessment of immunological damage, a discussion of needs for the further development of laboratory and epidemiological methods and their validation, and a consideration of current test strategies.

For the purposes of the Seminar, Immunotoxicology was defined as the discipline concerned with the study of the events that can lead to undesired effects as a result of interaction of xenobiotics (of whatever origin and nature) with the immune system. These undesired events may result as a consequence of 1) a direct and/or indirect action of the xenobiotic (and/or its biotransformation product) on the immune system; or, 2) an immunologically-based host response to the compound and/or its metabolite(s), or host antigens modified by the compound or its metabolite(s).

This Seminar was aimed at providing clear indications to responsible international and national organizations of desireable further activities in the field of immunotoxicology.

X

The immune system as a potential target for foreign chemicals
has received relatively little consideration in the past.
However it can not only be affected immediately and
preferentially, but injury of other organs or a general
deterioration of health can also bring about alterations in
function. In turn, a specific lesion of the immune system
can likewise lead to the damage of organs even to the extent
of compromising the general well-being of the entire
organism. In addition, chemically induced tissue damage can,
under certain circumstances, trigger a specific response in
the immune system, leading to a subsequent pathological state
that is far more serious than the original toxic lesion.
Thus immunotoxicology must always be viewed in a wider
content because of its possible implications for other
apparent organ specific toxicologies.

Many people have assisted in the work associated with the
Seminar, quite apart from the actual contributors, and we are
grateful to them all for a most successful Seminar which
brought together an impressive interdisciplinary spectrum of
knowledge. Special tribute must be paid to H. Amos, G.Bekesi,
D. Gardner, J. Graham, L. Moustafa, M. Th. Van der Venne
and J. Vos. In addition we are particularly grateful for the
work of H. F. Koelbl in the preparation of the text for
publication at short notice.

Dr. E. Bennett   Dr. M. Mercier
Director   Manager
Health and Safety Directorate   International Programme on
Commission of the European   Chemical Safety
Communities   World Health Organization

SYNOPSIS, CONCLUSIONS & RECOMMENDATIONS.

The current concepts of T and B cell circuits, their tinteractions in the regulation of immunoresponsiveness, and their role in the maintenance of health were presented. Attention was particularly focussed on newer, detailed models of cellular interactions and control mechanisms. These models provide a basis for elucidating immunoregulatory aspects of cellular interactions required for antigen recognition, antigen processing and presentation, the generation of cellular and humoral effector functions and production of lymphokines.

A serious consequence of dysregulation of these networks could be the development of autoimmunity which could follow from an involvement of cellular or humoral components or both. Selective influences of chemicals upon the different types of cells involved in down-regulatory circuits could result in a wide spectrum of autoimmune diseases ranging from autoimmune collagen vascular diseases to hypoplastic bone marrow syndromes. Another possibility is that a suppression of non-specific cell mediated immunity (CMI) and specific mechanisms of resistance for example, antibody production, could result in an increased susceptibility to infections, and possibly malignancies. For instance, a poor antibody response may favour the persistence of ciculating antigens and the generation of immune complexes with pathologic consequence. In this way exposure to chemicals could directly influence the immunopathology of an infectious disease.

The relationship between the immune system and cancer is complex and unclear. However, it is known that immunogenicity of tumour cells is essential to the development of strong cell-mediated anti-tumour responses. The in vivo evidence for tumour immunogenicity comes from observations of transplant rejection in immunized animals, of concomitant immunity (i.e. rejection of secondary tumour in animals bearing a primary tumour of the same type) and from lymphoid cell transfer experiments. In vitro evidence can be demonstrated in both humans and rodents for tumour immunogenicity by the presence of antibody and lymphocyte reactivity to tumour cells. Immunogenecity of experimental tumours, and possibly of human tumours, is a function of both the inducing agent (e.g. chemical, UV light and virus) and of immune selection which may occur during the early phase of tumour development.

In humans, the immunogenicity of spontaneous tumours and the precise role of anti-tumour immunity are as yet uncertain. Based on current knowledge the effector cells most likely responsible for limiting tumour development in humans are cytotoxic T-lymphocytes, natural killer cells and cytotoxic macrophages. The role of suppressor and enhancer feedback mechanisms in this process has yet to be fully elucidated. Evidence for the in vivo immunogenicity of at least some human tumours includes observations of occasional spontaneous rejection of established tumours, the occurence of an in-

creased frequency of spontaneous tumours in immunodeficient or immunosuppressed individuals, and histological evidence of immunologic activity in lymph nodes draining tumour sites. Serological responses to some human tumours, for example melanoma, has provided a rationale for developing human monoclonal antibodies as therapeutic agents. Cell-mediated immune reactivity, such as a proliferative, cytotoxic or lymphokine response, has been observed to autologous tumours in cancer patients. Furthermore positive reactivity to autologous tumour material has been shown to correlate with a favourable prognosis. Since certain chemicals are known to modulate potential anti-tumour effector mechanisms, this is an important aspect calling for further detailed investigation.

1. IMMUNE DYSFUNCTION AND DISEASE

The study and treatment of congenital immunodeficiencies in man has developed greatly over the last two decades and has resulted in a great increase in the understanding of immunological mechanisms. The development of more sensitive immunological assays and their application to a growing number of conditions have revealed that primary immunodeficiencies in man are more frequent than originally thought. Deficiencies have been dicovered in the lymphocyte systems, the phagocytic system, as well as genetic defects of complement components. Defects in the adaptative immune responses have been assessed in patients, and these have correlated well with the associated clinical picture.

Chemically induced immune defects can occur at any stage in life. However, there is evidence that the newborn and the senescent may be more susceptible to chemically induced immunological injury. There is also the possibility of damage in utero, particularly during immune organogenesis.

The identification of the apparently new infectious phenomenon of the acquired immunodeficiency syndrom (AIDS) in 1981 and its subsequent alarming spread, greatly heightened general interest in the immune system and its importance for general health. This syndrome is associated with the occurrence of infection with opportunistic pathogenic microbial agents (most notably Pneumocystis carinii), and the appearance of a characteristic type of neoplasm, Kaposi's sarcoma. AIDS is a devastating disease with an extremely high mortality rate, which approaches 100% for those cases reported prior to 1982. Although there is no single immune abnormality that is diagnostic for AIDS, depression in the absolute numbers of peripheral blood T-lymphocytes with the helper/inducer phenotype appears to occur in virtually all cases of AIDS, resulting in a lowering of the normal ratio of T-helper and T-suppressor lymphocytes. A putative etiological agent for this syndrome is a retrovirus, human T-cell leukemia virus III (HTLV-III) or lymphadenopathy associated virus (LAV). These viruses have been isolated from T-helper cells and are cytopathic for this subset of lymphocytes.

Besides the occurrence of immunodepression in certain congenital or acquired immunodeficiency disorders, immunosuppression may be iatrogenically induced either deliberately, as in
the management of organ transplant recipients, or patients
with autoimmune or collagen-vascular diseases, or obtained as
a side effect of treatment of cancer with cytotoxic drugs
and/or radiotherapy. These various states of immunodepression may be complicated not only by an increased incidence of
infections but also with increased incidence of certain kinds
of tumours. A study of organ transplant recipients showed
that certain malignancies were observed with remarkable
frequency, notably Kaposi's sarcoma, lymphomas, skin cancer
and some carcinomas notably those of the cervix, vulva, lung,
colon and breast. The incidence of Kaposi's sarcoma was
400-500 fold higher than expected, non-Hodgkin's lymphoma was
increased 28-49 fold and certain types of skin cancer were
7-21 times above those seen in the control populations.

The recognition that immunosuppression is associated with an
increased incidence of certain tumours emphasizes the importance of the immune system in host defences against
neoplasia. It is noteworthy that diverse states of immunodeficiency have an incrased incidence of tumours arising from
the immune cells themselves, namely lymphomas. If Kaposi's
sarcoma is a variety of lymphoreticular tumour, the situation
becomes even more intriguing. Thus studies of the various
groups of immunosuppressed patients, including those with and
without cancers, could provide clues to the etiology of the
neoplasms. This could shed light on the causes of similar
malignancies seen in the general popoulation, and on the role
of the immune system in the control of cancer.

2. IMMUNOTOXICOLOGY: HISTOPHATHOLOGY, IN VIVO AND IN VITRO MODELS, MOLECULAR MECHANISMS

The rationale for morphological examination of the lyumphoid
system was presented and discussed on the basis of evidence
that chemically induced immune alterations may become manifest as qualitative or quantitative changes in the histology
of lymphoid organs. This is similar to the situation in
humoral, cellular or combined immunodeficiency diseases in
man, that also have their characteristic pathomorphology.
The detection of these changes using routing histopathology
of lymphoid organs, based on haematoxylin and eosin staining
of formalin fixed and paraffin embedded tissues, has been
shown in many studies to be useful. Special techniques, such
as enzyme histochemistry, immunocytochemistry and electron
microscopy, can give important information about the nature
of the chemically-induced lesions in the lymphoid system. In
particular, recent progress in the development of immunoperoxidase techniques and the availability of monoclonal antibodies has enabled the identification of a number of lymphoid
subpopulations in tissue sections. Chemicals causing immune
suppression, immune stimulation or autoimmune alterations
have been identified by these morphological procedures.
Morphological and functional assays have been developed to
assess the following aspects of the immune system: host

resistance, cell-mediated immunity, humoral immunity, macro-phage function as well as general immunopathology.

A promising approach for elucidating mechanisms of hypersen-sitivity and autoimmunity is the popliteal lymph node (PLN) assay in rodents. This compares the reactivity of one popliteal lymph node following footpad injection of a test substance with the contralateral (control) PLN. Diphenylhy-dantoin (DPH) and some other drugs that have been associated with the induction of a variety of immunological diseases reminiscent of graft-versus-host diseases were tested in this assay to determine whether the processes involved in graft-versus-host reactivity and sensitization to DPH are identical. The results suggest the feasibility of this type of approach in elucidating mechanisms of hypersensitivity and autoreactivity, and may allow prediction of immunomodulatory compounds. The relationship of information obtained in these models to the actual occurrence of autoreactivity in the animal awaits further investigation and will be a prerequi-site in substantiating the usefulness of this approach.

Although many aspects of the immune system have been studied from a toxicological viewpoint there are a number of impor-tant areas that have received little attention, although they are clearly of importance. One of these is the gut-associated lymphoid tissue (GALT) which could be a unique and significant target for immunotoxic chemicals, particular-ly as there is some evidence that Peyers-patch-like lymphoid tissue in the lower gut may be the mammalian equivalent of the avian bursa of Fabricius. Since the oral route is one of the most important modes of entry for the long term low level exposures to chemicals, much more needs to be known about the processes of uptake of toxic chemicals across the gut epithe-lium and their possible toxic interactions with local lympho-id tissue. Such interactions could cause an interference in B cell production or function as well as IgA production and secretion.

Some progress has been made in the understanding of cellular and molecular mechanisms of immunotoxicity by extensive studies, both in vitro and in vivo, on the actions of speci-fic molecules such as 2,3,7,8-tetrachlorodibenzo-p-dioxin (TCDD) and 7,12-dimethylbenz(a)anthracene (DMBA). TCDD has been taken as a model for the halogenated aromatic compounds (dibenzo-p-dioxins and related compounds) that have been shown in recent years to be highly toxic for animals, but less so for man. Studies in animals have revealed that TCDD is a potent and specific immunosuppressive agent that can act at low doses on a variety of immune mechanisms including tactivation of suppressor cells. Furthermore its activity has been demonstrated to depend on the genetic backround of the test animal.

It is of note that the immune effects induced by 2,3,7,8-tetrachlorodibenzofurans and dibenzofuran analogues of TCDD are comparable to those found with TCDD, although the number of studies with these compounds are limited. Despite *the evidence that these compounds affect the immune system in animals there is, as yet, no conclusive evidence that these compounds are immunologically active in humans at the reported exposure levels. However, recent studies indicate that the immune system was compromised in patients poisoned in 1979 in Taiwan by the consumption of rice oil contaminated with chlorinated biphenyls and dibenzofurans.*

It appears that TCDD and isosteric analgues act through a common receptor (Ah) to produce characteristic patterns of toxic and biochemical responses, including epidermal hyperkeratinization and thymic atrophy. An in vitro model for thymic atrophy has been developed that is based on the cultivation of thymic epithelial (TE) cells, under conditions that select against thymic fibroblasts and macrophages, and on cocultivation of thymocytes on syngeneic TE monolayers. It was suggested that the thymic atrophy induced by TCDD is brought about by an alteration of the patterns of differentiation in the TE target cells, mediated at least in part by the Ah receptor. It was assumed that during the process of TCDD-induced differentiation, TE cells lose the ability to support thymocyte maturation. Impaired thymocyte maturation and proliferation may lead to the depletion of cortical thymocytes characteristic of TCDD-induced thymic atrophy. However the extraordinary potency of TCDD as a tumour promotor in animals and the evidence that T-lymphocyte cytotoxic effector cells are one of the major cell types participating in immune surveillance against neoplasms, suggest that modulation of T-lymphocyte maturation (and differentiation) by the Ah receptor may be one of the mechanisms associated with the carcinogenic potential of TCDD. Despite these findings in animals, there have been no reports of any such adverse effects of TCDD on the human immune system.

Benzidine is another example of a chemical used as a model compound. This chemical is a known human bladder carcinogen, and there is evidence in animals of immunosuppressive effects. In mice immune suppression occurred even at dose levels which were below those shown to induce neoplasms. The down-regulation in immunity caused by benzidine may be explained by the quantitive changes in arachidonic acid conversion products via oxidative metabolism.

Studies with polycyclic aromatic hydrocarbons (PAHs) have shown that, in general, carcinogenic PAH's are highly suppressive for humoral immunity and cell-mediated immunity, while their non-carcinogenic congeners are not. Suppression of various immune parameters following in vivo PAH exposure correlated with increased susceptibility to challenge with infectious agents and transplantable tumours. In vitro studies with the model PAH, 7,12-dimethylbenz(a)anthracence (DMBA) have suggested that PAH-induced suppression of immunity may be due, at least in part, to a selective alteration in the function of T-helper cells, specifically their production of the lymphokine IL-2.

Collaborative programmes have been undertaken to develop and validate batteries of test procedures based on models, such as have been mentioned, that could serve as an initial screening procedure for the assessment of the immunotoxicological potential of certain types of chemicals. Preliminary results have been encouraging and in particular a correlation was observed between changes in certain in vitro functional parameters and host susceptibility.

3. **INTERACTIONS OF** *SPECIFIC XENOBIOTICS WITH THE* **IMMUNE SYSTEM.**

There is a wide range of xenobiotics to which man is exposed in the workplace or in the environment and which might interact with the immune system. In addition some therapeutic substances are now known to possess unwanted immunomodulatory activities. The interaction of toxic chemicals with man or animals is dependent not only on chemical structure and exposure factors but also on age (particularly the neonatal period and old age) and nutritional status. The influence of these latter factors is essentially to produce in effect, an increase in exposure at the cellular level and thus increase the possibility of damage. As the cellular elements of the immune system are designed to interact with foreign elements, they are theoretically always in the front line as far as exposure to chemicals is concerned; thus, the immune system in the very young, the old and the malnourished could be at greater risk.

The changes in the immune system that have been observed so far to vary with age and nutrition were confined mostly to T cells. Thus thymic atrophy has been observed in the elderly and malnourished. However, the implication for health of these changes is not as yet understood. This emphasizes the need for immunotoxicological studies in laboratory animals of different ages and immunological status.

Sulphur dioxide and oxides of nitrogen. Over the past 20 years, laboratory studies in animals on the effect of common and widespread air pollutants such as SO_2 and NOx have shown conclusively that these agents increase susceptibility to respiratory infections. Interference with humoral and cell-mediated immunity in the lung are dependent on the concentration of the agent and the duration of exposure. However, such studies as have been published to date can be criticized because the conditions of the experiments still fall far short of those that are found in actual exposure situations. Thus at present it is not possible to assess with any confidence the immunotoxicity of common air pollutants to humans.

Asbestos. However there is one specific agent, asbestos, where inhalation exposure produces toxicity, immunomodulation and malignancy in humans. Recent studies have revealed two different mechanisms of macrophage plasma membrane changes following inhalation exposure to asbestos. These are associated with concomitant alterations in T-cell/macrophage interactions may which result in an imbalance in immune response. However, the relationship between these observed alterations in immune homeostasis and the symptoms of fibrosis and malignancy seen in humans with asbestosis remains to be elucidated. So far it has been established on the basis of clinical studies that asbestos exposure can result in immunological diseases with the development of non-organ specific autoantibodies. Dysfunctions were found in the activity of natural killer cells and T-lymphocytes as well as in humoral immunity. Patients with defective cellular immunity were observed to have a poor prognosis; the greater the defect the worse the prognosis. Defects in cellular immune function appear to precede the development of malignancy although no simple cause-effect relationship could be demonstrated. Similarities have been found in the immunological status of asbestos workers and their wives. For example, the percentage of subjects with a positive tuberculin response among control men was 10,2%, among their wives 11,9%, while among male asbestos workers it was 32,3%, and among their wives 31,8%.

Metals and metalic compounds. Because of their widespread use much attention has been given to the possibility of immunomodulation by metals. Only recently, however, have attempts been made to delineate the mechanisms responsible for the effects observed.

Dialkyltins. Certain dialkytin compounds induce a selective thymic atrophy which has been attributed to a direct effect of the compound on the thymus. A selective antiproliferative effect was observed on thymocytes in animal experiments both after in vivo and in vitro exposures, possibly as a result of an interaction of the chemical with membrane and/or cytoplasmic thiol (SH) groups. Dialkyltin reacts readily with SH-groups and the induced disturbances in biological functions, both after in vivo and in vitro exposure, can be restored or even prevented by addition of dithiol compounds. The dialkyltin effects on the ketoacid dehydrogenase system are also thought to be caused by dithiol interactions; however, the effects observed in vitro on thymocyte energy metabolism do not appear to be involved in the observed antiproliferative effects. The question of organ distribution of the dialkyltin compounds versus that of reactive thiol groups on target cells remains to be answered.

Mercury. The development of autoimmune diseases through modulation of T- and B- cell function by the interaction of mercury with cellular thiols has been studied extensively. It has been shown that $HgCl_2$ is a potent agent for inducing autoimmunity in rabbits, rats and mice. The resultant disease process includes autoimmune glomerulonephritis (all 3 species), lymphadenopathy together with the formation of antinuclear antibodies, and markedly enhanced serum IgE levels. In the rat, there are striking genetic differences in the susceptibility to mercury-induced immunotoxicity due to allelic differences at 2 or 3 loci, one of them being the MHC locus. Dosages that affect a susceptible strain were completely ineffective in a resistant strain. The genetic susceptibility for the production of autoantibodies to the

glomerular basement membrane and the development of glomerulonephritis is not expressed in the kidney but in the lymphoid tissue. In a susceptible strain of rats, injection of
either HgCl₂ or syngeneic lymphocytes preincubated with HgCl₂
in vitro induced popliteal lymph node (PLN) enlargement,
whereas no PLN enlargement was found in the resistant strain.
This and other observations suggest that a cellular mechanism
akin to the one operating in the graft-versus-host reaction
(GVHR) underlies the mercury-induced autoimmunity.

For some metals there is good experimental evidence to
suggest that a compromised immune system may underlie some of
the morbidity associated with exposure. Detailed clinical
studies should eventually ascertain the importance of the
immunotoxicological element in exposed subjects.

Polybrominated bibphenyls (PBBs). An immunotoxic syndrome
has been decribed following the accidental exposure of
Michigan farm residents to PBBs in 1973-1976. Dairy products
containing PBBs and contaminated meat were widely consumed
and subsequently PBBs were found in the serum and adipose
tissue of residents. The immunological changes observed
included: abnormal lymphocyte function, abnormal lymphocyte
surface markers and increased levels of IgG, IgA and C3. An
increased incidence of neoplasia was found among PBB exposed
residents examined between 1977 and 1982 with immune
dysfunction. In those with normal immunological status the
tumour incidence was 0,5% while in the group with confirmed
immune dysfunctions the incidence was 10,7%. In an occupational and age matched control the tumour incidence was 0,7%.

Contaminated cooking oil. The recent Spanish cooking oil
accident with its disasterous clinical sequele serves as a
reminder of the potential for large scale human exposure to
immunotoxic agents. The Spanish oil syndrome was characterized by an early and transient depression in T-suppressor
cell, evidence of cellular hyperactivity and the development
of antibodies. The similarity of this syndrome in its later
developments to certain autoimmune connective tissue diseases
and to chronic graft-versus-host disease (GVHD) make it
highly likely that an immunotoxic reaction had occurred.

4.   HYPERSENSITIVITY: BASIC CONCEPTS AND CLINICAL MANIFES-
      TATIONS RESULTING FROM EXPOSURE TO CHEMICALS.

Hypersensitivity is a manifestation of chemically induced
immunotoxicities that is a major area of clinical concern.
One of the commonest problems encountered at the clinic is
contact sensitization. In studying contact sensitivity it is
not only neccessary to identify the host factors that determine the magnitude of the response to contact sensitizers,
but also the particular chemical properties that confer the
ability to interact with host cells in a manner that elicits
contact sensitivity. Neither of these aspects are well
understood and until this information is available it will be
difficult to develop better strategies for identifying such
chemicals or predicting the sensitizing potential of new
chemicals.

Studies in experimental animals have shown that a variety of immunological factors are involved in determining the development of contact sensitivity. One of the first factors is the activation of antigen-presenting cells, usually of macrophage origin. The presence of Class II major histocompatibility products on the surface of these cells and the production of interleukin 1 are key requirements for these activated cells to stimulate other lymphocytes. Various substances may stimulate antigen presenting cells to produce interleukin 1, but it is not known whether chemically reactive contact sensitizers also have this capacity. The second factor in the immune response is the production of mediators such as interleukin 2 by activated lymphocytes. Disturbances in the production and/or responsiveness to these molecules can have profound consequences on the physiology of the immune response. A third factor controlling the immune response in hypersensitivity is the presence of various suppressor and possibly contra suppressor cell circuits. Finally, genetic factors, in particular the immune response (Ir) genes which code for class II antigens, influence the possibility of inducing hypersensitivity.

Pseudoallergy may be defined as a type of reaction similar to the allergic reaction but which does not involve the interaction of antigen and antibody or specifically sensitized immune cells. The classical immediate type allergic reaction is mainly caused by the binding of allergen and specific IgE on the mast cell, followed by the activation of the cell and the secretion of various mediators. However, the mast cell can be activated by mechanisms other than antigen-IgE interaction. For instance, dextran can directly activate mast cells from some rat strains. The clinical hypersensitivity reactions to dextran are probably due to the formation of antigen-antibody complexes and the activation of complement. The activation of complement via the alternative pathway and the formation of the anaphylatoxines C3a and C5a can also result in the activation of mast cells. In vitro experiments suggest that this mechanism may be involved in the reaction to radiographic contrast material. Several peptides are also capable of directly activating mast cells and such a mechanism may explain, for example, the adverse reactions to the ACTH (1-24) peptide. Here a common structural feature is a cationic head separated from a hydrophobic tail by a suitable number of inserted amino acid residues. It may therefore be possible to predict the likelihood of pseudo-allergic reactions of this type on the basis of chemical structure.

Drug hypersensitivity is well known but there are still many problems in understanding the mechanisms involved in some clinical adverse effects. A persistent problem is that of establishing a causal relationship between particular adverse clinical effect and a measured immune response, for example an antibody response. The "idiosyncratic" nature and possible low incidence of these hypersensitivity reactions to a given chemical may make them difficult to predict from animal studies and from the limited human exposures during premarke-

ting trials. Covert allergens in the environment, such as
those in toiletries and cosmetics, represent a significant
immunotix challenge to man. The role of ear-percing and
sleeper rings in initiating nickel sensitivity is well known,
and is an example of the need for more effective action in
reducing exposure and thus limiting the widespread morbidity
due to acknowledged sensitizers.

5. HEALTH IMPLICATIONS OF IMMUNOTOXIC EFFECTS

The health implications of immune dysfunctions are increased
risk of infectious diseases, development of neoplasia,
autoimmune disorders and allergies.

The "uniqueness" of the immune system relates to its extreme
complexity and the widespread dispersion of its cellular
constituents. In the organs of the body, such as the heart,
liver or kidney, the functioning cells are in a fixed relationship to each other and the functional reserve can be
related to relatively easily determined cell parameters (eg.
cell number). A toxic chemical compromises a certain fraction of the reserve and the clinical significance of such
damage is related to the size of the reserve and of the time
interval between reduction of function and the necessity for
an effective physiological response. However, when it comes
to an assessment of altered function in the immune system,
consideretion has to be given to the various subsets of
effector and regulatory cells which may exhibit different
sensitivities to therapeutic or toxic agents, and, as a
result, the activity of the immune system may be modified
both as to the kind of response as well as its magnitude.

A seemingly toxic effect of an agent on a particular immune
response may not necessarily lead to a detectable clinical
manifestation. This may be because the immune system has,
for this mechanism, a considerable amount of reserve, as well
as, a capacity to recover from insult by a rapid regeneration
of that particular cell population. Thus a particular effect
on the immune system observed in animals and judged to be
toxic may not have such significance when seen in humans.
The long term consequences of immunotoxicity in humans are
likely to be those involving autoimmunity and cancer. Such a
view is supported by the incidence of certain types of cancer
following immunosuppression in patients with organ
transplants. However carcinogenesis is a complex matter and
is likely to involve direct genetic effects such as those
affecting proto-oncogene or oncogene expression and the
function of differentiation factors; immunosuppression may
thus be considered as having primarily a facilitating effect
in the development of a cancer caused by other mechanisms.
However investigations into these aspects have produced
conflicting results. Thus there is a need for more basic
research and for the development of more appropriate animal
models in this important area. It needs to be recognized
that many of the components of the immune system are, as yet,
poorly defined and in consequence the study of their complicated interactions is greatly hampered.

Even though important information can be derived from in vitro studies, the integrated nature of the immune system and its fundamental importance in bodily defense means that crucial information can only come from whole animal studies. Despite the difficulties in the extrapolation of data from animal experimentation to man, the limited availability of clinical and epidemiological studies mean that much of the information necessary for regulatory decisions will have to be derived from animal studies. A particularly important aspect of animal experimentation is the discovery and use of animal strains with defined genetic susceptibilities. Some of these can mimic human disease especially those occurring in sensitive or suceptible sub-groups of the human population (e.g. mice that are susceptible to lupus-like conditions).

6. TEST STRATEGIES FOR THE SCREENING OF CHEMICALS FOR IMMUNOTOXIC PROPERTIES

The actions of chemicals on the immune system can result in either immunostimulation or immunosuppression. A number of theoretical and practical issues should be considered in the design of test strategies. These include: time-response and dose-response relationships, toxicokinetics, determination of direct versus indirect actions on the immune system, and the biologic relevance of in vitro tests to the actions of a given agent in vivo. The basic questions that need to be answered are: 1) whether the xenobiotic alters immune function, 2) if it does, what is the concentration and length of exposure required to produce a response and 3) does the response lead to further activation of immune mechanisms with subsequent adverse effects (e.g. autoimmune activity).

A comprehensive strategy for the assessment of immune functions would ideally involve an approach in which a flexible battery of assays is used, taking into account the initial effect observed as well as the nature and intended use of the chemical. Suspicion of potential immunotoxic potential detected in classical toxicology studies can be confirmed or characterized using appropriate methods selected from a battery of validated assays. A number of methods for assessing chemically-induced modulation of immune function in laboratory animals have been described. However, there is an urgent need for a considerable research effort to expand knowledge of the mechanisms of chemically induced immune alterations at both the cellular and molecular level. With such a foundation new and more effective test procedures could be developed and subjected to an international validation process.

At present inbred murine strains are the species of choice for studies on the immune system and for associated metabolic studies because of the availability of extensive genetic data, the availability of host resistance models and the similarity of the murine immune system to that of man. Rats, the mainstay of classical toxicological testing, unfortunately have no such extensive genetic or immunological data base. Primates can also be used to assess immune dysfunction but as the data base is even smaller they cannot at present be considered suitable for assy procedures. Overall there is thus a need to develop well-defined in vitro models employing human and other animal lymphoid tissue that can be correlated with established in vivo responses in a variety of animals. Studies in a given animal should include in vivo, ex vivo and in vitro techniques.

Much more effort should be directed to studies in humans despite the limitations and difficulties of such research. Studies involving post-exposure surveillance could be considered in those cases in which animal data or theoretical considerations gave rise to the suspicion that some sort of immunological change could occur.

Although the reality of chemical interference with major aspects immune functions has good experimental support there is no agreement on the significance, or even existence, of minor forms of immune dysfunction. In medical practice little attention is paid to lesser degrees of ill health, and priority is naturally given to life threatening diseases and many distressing conditions with immunological involvement receive scant attention. There is an urgent need to sharpen clinical appraisals so that the criteria for an accurate diagnosis of immunologically-mediated reactions can be established and subsequently allevated.

It is likely that within a few years a consensus will be reached on the need for a more precise investigation of immunotoxic reactions in man, although the operational and technical problems are formidable. There is concern that perception of the problems could lead to regulatory actions that may not be justified by the level of scientific knowledge. Already the question has been raised concerning the need for generating data specifically relevant to immune function during toxicity testing or drug safety clearance programmes in animals. Proponents of this view believe that specific tests for immunotoxicity should be introduced into animal toxicological testing schemes, perhaps on a tiered system. If some problems were indicated by such tests, more detailed studies would be called for, comprising an analysis of interaction with immunological systems at the cellular level. Others argue that a more classical toxicological approach of the kind currently employed is sufficient, and that any significant adverse effect on immunological systems will be identified by appropriate haematological and histopathological studies. Only if changes are seen should specific investigations be undertaken. however the latter approach may not possess adequate sensitivity while the former is compromised by lack of standardization and reproducibility of the test systems and by doubts concerning the relevance of the findings to clinical medicine.

Regarding that part of immunotoxicology concerned with the adverse immunological events of immunotherapeutics, the conclusion was that these agents present novel problems with respect to safety evaluation. These problems are derived from the large heterogeneity, and species-specificity of these agents. Furthermore, the biological activitu of manu such compounds, and possible adverse effects, may be influenced by the immune status of the host and by the conditions of treatment used. Although a degree of standard animal toxicological testing appears to be necessary for such agents prior to their human use, the conclusion was that flexibility in the utilization of classical preclinical toxicology is essential to avoid performing unnecessary studies. Thus, the objective should be integration of an intelligent use of classical toxicology and the search for immunopathologies induced by immunoactive therapies, taking into consideration the characteristics of the individual agents.

In the area of hypersensitivity there appears to be a widespread belief that current testing procedures for the prediction of hypersensitivity reactions are largely satisfactory. Although present animal models have been reasonably successful there is room for improvement particularly in relation to:

- the elimination of false positives

- the development and validation of other in vitro models

- the development of predictive toxicology based on molecular structure and metabolism

- improvements in the area of risk assessment.

In particular, the problem of animal testing, frequently using guineapigs, for delayed contact hypersensitivity remains controversial. There is evidence, based on experience with many sensitizing agents, that topical administration and intradermal injections may be less predictive compared to applications under occlusive dressing. This latter approach, however, demands carefully chosen experimental conditions, the use of appropriate concentrations of the test substances and a correct interpretation of the data.

Human patch testing involves consideration of the physiological state of the skin along with the nature and use of the chemicals involved. In some instances, testing is necessary at concentrations in excess of the normal application (e.g. cosmetics) because people often apply cosmetics liberally to skin blemishes and abrasions. This increases the effective dose particularly if there is altered skin permeability. Extensive efforts are being made to standardize the patch test, thus providing a much needed lead for others to follow in the development of human assays for hypersensitivity of immunotoxicity. Confounding factors include cross reactivity of certain non-sensitizing compounds and their possible interaction with microorganisms unique to certain test animals and man. Interpretation of such equivocal responses in guinea-pigs can be assisted by in vitro assays of cellular responses in exposed humans and other animals. It should be noted that if a low molecular weight chemical is to initiate a specific antibody response it must be able to form stable covalent bonds with host proteins. The presence of such a property in a chemical should thus raise suspicions about its hypersensitivity potential.

Human clinical research on the vulnerability of certain individuals could provide extremely valuable information. For example provocative challenges, including aerochamber exposure, can yield valuable information by observation of a single or dual drop in FEV_1 and/or PEFR and/or a late cough/febrile response. This can assist in identifying the causative factors and mechanisms. There is also a major concern regarding airway responses to chemicals. In the sensitized asthmatic, these are characterized by an early (15 min) and late (3-6 hours) reduction in lung function, which is associated with a non-selective increase in bronchial hyperactivity. Many mediators have been identified that are believed to be associated with cellular functions in the alveolar region.

7. CONCLUSIONS AND RECOMMENDATIONS

The following main conclusions and recommendations emerged from the Seminar:

Definition and domain of immunotoxicology

1. Immunotoxicology is defined as the discipline concerned with the study of the events that can lead to undesired effects as a result of interaction of xenobiotics with the immune system. These undesired events may result as a consequence of: 1) a direct and/or indirect action of the xenobiotic (and/or its biotransformation product) on the immune system; or, 2) an immunologically-based host response to the compound and/or its metabolite(s), or host antigens modified by the compound or its metabolite(s).

2. Immunotoxicology is an important and rapidly developing discipline that has not yet received adequate recognition in scientific, medical and public health circles. The number of individuals adequately trained in immunotoxicology is relatively small and centres with the expertise and facilities necessary to perform immunotoxicological investigations, and to train personnel in this discipline, are limited in number and unevenly distributed throughout the world.

Public health significance of immunotoxicology

3. Many xenobiotics, in common use, are known to produce different kinds of hypersensitivity responses. The frequency of such pathologies and their importance in terms of human morbidity is now well established, but not widely appreciated. Thus priority action should be taken by public health bodies to control unnecessary exposure to chemicals with known propensities to induce manifestations of hypersensitivity.

4. There is increasing evidence that a large number of xenobiotics may directly alter immune function in the absence of any direct damage to other body systems. Given the absolutely crucial role of the immune system in the maintenance of host integrity and the requirement for continuing

cell renewal, proliferation and differenciation it is understandable that xenobiotic-induced immune dysfunctions can ultimately bring about severe and diverse health effects ranging from autoimmune diseases to possible influences on the incidences of cancer. In view of the wide distribution of chemicals in the environment, and the belief that current knowledge about adverse health effects resulting from immunotoxic xenobiotics may represent only the " tip of the iceberg", the possibility that exposure to such substances may play a greater role in disease causation than previously suspected should be investigated as a matter of priority.

5.   It is important to recognize that in individuals with compromised immunity such as in malnutrition, infancy and old age there could be a greater susceptibility to immunotoxicants.

Immunotoxicity testing

6.   Considering the complexity of the immune system and the variety of adverse effects that may be induced by immunotoxicants, the current testing of chemicals and drugs for immunotoxic potential leaves much to be desired. However it should not be overlooked that a careful analysis of lymphoid organs for alterations in weight, morphology, cellularity and cellular function can provide valuable information about immunotoxicity. Although some testing approaches show promise for the identification of at least some types of potential immunotoxicants, there is still a need for considerable improvement.

In particular there is a need for work in the following areas:

-   a better understanding and improvement of the predictive value of current immunotoxicological tests particularly those that are concerned with immune function and host resistance assays;

-   the development and validation of new assay systems including in vitro tests;

-   the development of a system of international validation so that testing capabilities throughout the world can be improved.

7.   In view of the rapid development of knowledge that can be expected in the subjects of immunology and genetics, and in consequence, a deeper understanding of the ways that immune mechanisms can be altered, it essential that there should be a flexible approach to the testing of chemicals for immunotoxic potential.

8.   Regulatory bodies undertaking the issuing or revision of guidelines for immunotoxicity testing should note that much more effort should be devoted to the development and validation of immune function assays. Even in the area of hyper-

sensitivity where a number of tests are currently widely utilized there is a recognized need for improvement.

Research and development needs in immunotoxicology

9.   There is a considerable lack of knowledge regarding the mechanisms by which chemicals can interfere with immune functions. In view of the increasing knowledge about the large number and diversity of severe diseases that can arise from immune dysfunction a better understanding of the mechanisms of immunotoxicity at a cellular and molecular level is a major research priority.

10.   More research is also required at various levels in the general area of immunotoxicity testing. In view of the health implications of immunotoxicity and in the objective of obtaining improved means for both identifying potential immunotoxic xenobiotics and for scientifically evaluating the health hazards of events observed, research directed at the refinement of existing methodologies and the development of newer methodologies which might advance immunotoxicology risk assessment should be encouraged as a priority.

11.   The following are considered to be specific areas for research:

1) development of specific and more sophisticated animal modes;

2) studies of toxicokinetics and dose-response relation ships;

3) studies of the relationship between, and importance of, local versus systemic immune responses following exposure; and,

4) the correlation of health parameters to human exposure situations coupled with the development of clinical procedures for quantifying the signs and symptoms associated with lesser degrees of ill health such as rashes, respiratory problems and gastrointestinal upsets.

Data base development

12.   The multidisciplinary nature of immunotoxicological research raises problems concerning the communication between scientists in the various fields. There is also the problem of useful data generated in a research context being readily available to health professions and regulatory adminis- trators. The development of an integrated and evaluated data base should be considered as a valuable facility not only for the dissemination of data but also as a way of identifying areas where additional investigation is required.

Immunotoxicology as a discipline and its training/education needs

13. A wider application of recently developed immunological techniques could greatly improve the sensitivity and specificity of many toxicological methods. Increased use should be made of immunological techniques and reagents such us monoclonal antibodies and immunoperoxidase histochemistry in toxicology. Training in immunological techniques should be encouraged among toxicologists and support be given to programmes aimed at the refinement or development of novel immunological techniques or reagents that would be beneficial to toxicology.

14. In view of the basic and applied research needed in this discipline, as well as of the wide number of xenobiotics that appear to have the potential to interfere with the functions of the immune system, it was recommended that suitable training programmes in immunotoxicology be developed. It is particularly important that training in toxicology itself should include immunotoxicology.

15. Because of the serious health implications of immunotoxicity, attention should be given to ways of promoting a greater awareness among clinicians and occupational physicians of the possibility that xenobiotics, of many different types, can produce immune alterations which may have undesirable health consequences. Suitable time should be devoted to such aspects in undergraduate and post-graduate medical teaching curricula.

A TOXICOLOGIST'S VIEW OF IMMUNOTOXICOLOGY

L.C. Zbinden

Federal Institute of Technology,
ETH University of Zurich, Switzerland

1. GENERAL CONCEPTS.

Whenever awareness about a new area of concern in toxicology
reaches a critical level, national and international public
health authorities request the immediate development of
testing procedures with which large numbers of established and
new chemicals can be evaluated. Previous experience in the
areas of teratogenicity, carcinogenicity, mutagenicity and
others has shown that toxicologists respond enthusiastically
to such demands. Unfortunately, in their eagerness to test as
many chemicals as possible, scientists often do not spend
sufficient time studying the theoretical basis and medical
relevance of their experimental models. Moreover, classical
concepts of toxicology, e.g. the compulsory use of
excessively high doses, are uncritically applied in the newly
developed tests.

As soon as enough data are generated with a few arbitrarily
selected reference compounds, expert committees convene in an
effort to assure international harmonization of testing
requirements. This inconsiderate preference of testing over a
more scientific and analytical investigation of the problems
involved and all their ramifications inevitably results in an
accumulation of data often difficult to comprehend, let alone
be extrapolated to man. Other experts must then be called in
to assess the assay procedures and to judge the relevance of
the data generated.

It is indisputable that immunotoxicology is on the verge of
becoming an important public health issue. The first
regulatory requests for immunotoxicological testing have
already emerged (Petricciani, 1983). Thus, it is high time to
consider the scientific and medical aspects of the problem, to
ask a number of pertinent questions, and to formulate some
hypotheses, before opening the flood-gates for a boundless
testing activity.

For the toxicologist, the immune system is one of many
potential targets of foreign chemicals. In some cases, it is
affected immediately and preferentially, whereas under
different conditions, the changes are secondary to injury of
other organs or to a general deterioration of health. In
turn, a specific lesion of the immune system may lead to the
damage of organs and will often compromise the general
well-being of the organism. In addition, tissue damage can,
under special circumstances, trigger a specific response in
the immune system, leading to a pathological state that is far
more serious than the original toxic lesion. Thus, it is
unrealistic to treat immunotoxicology as a speciality of its
own: instead, it must always be viewed in light of its close
interrelationship with all other branches of toxicology.

2. CHEMICAL SUBSTANCES

Since the compounds that alter the immmune system can, depending on the circumstances of use, be considered immunotherapeutics or immunotoxins, it is perhaps more expedient to label them as "immunomodulators" (IM). This neutral term is all the more appropriate because it also describes the biphasic responses that are a trait particular of the immune system. Another even more general term for theses agents is "biological response modifiers" (BRM).

The chemical substances of interest in immunotoxicology are of a very diverse nature. They may first be divided into two groups: "intentional IM", i.e. substances developed for therapeutic inhibition or stimulation of specific immune responses, and "inadvertent IM", i.e. drugs and environmental chemicals whose effects on the immunological processes are unwanted and often undesirable. Among this latter group are immunomodulating contaminants, which have become particularly important as potentially sensitizing impurities in products manufactured by recombinant DNA and other biotechnologies (D'Agnolo, 1983).

Both groups of IM include a large variety of organic and inorganic small molecules, but a distinct and very peculiar group of immunomodulating chemicals are large molecules, often of biological origin: e.g. peptides, polysaccharides and proteins of greatly varying complexities. Among these, specific products of immunocompetent cells, e.g. immunoglobulins, lymphokines including interferons, thymosin etc., demand particular attention, since they are administered to humans by the parenteral route. The same is true for tissue extracts, peptide hormones and enzymes injected for therapeutic purposes. In order to judge these substances appropriately, it is of great importance to know whether they are of human origin or derived from another organism, mammalian, submammalian, microorganism or plant. But even when the substance is identical to that present in the human organism, it is essential to ascertain that not only the primary, but also the secondary and tertiary structures of the molecule are unaltered. Thus, exact identification and specification of the test substances submitted for study are as important for immunotoxicology as they are for all other branches of toxicology.

3. TOXICOLOGICAL TARGETS

In toxicology two working concepts can be distinguished: in the conventional approach, the experiment comes first. A standard test or battery of tests is performed, and the types and degrees of hazards for humans are subsequently estimated from the results obtained. In contrast, in the "pharmacological approach to toxicology," the potential targets of toxicity are identified first. The criteria for a relevant effect are then established, usually based on experience with reference substances, and the experimental model best suited to assess the pertinent toxicological

response is selected (Zbinden et al., 1984). In both
instances, toxicologists should have a good idea about the
nature and the symptomatology of the human diseases induced by
the chemicals with which the toxicological experiments are
conducted.

As far as immunotoxicology is concerned, the clinical
syndromes resulting from inhibition or overstimulation of the
most important immune mechanisms by foreign chemicals are
sufficiently defined. These syndromes include
immunodeficiency due to the destruction or functional
inhibition of lymphoreticular organs and the consequences,
i.e. reduced resistance against infections and possibly also
facilitation of tumor growth. In addition, there are various
forms of humoral and cellular hypersensitivity reactions,
including cutaneous and systemic anaphylaxis, organ-directed
allergies such as hemolytic anemia and allergic myocarditis,
the Arthus reaction, serum sickness, glomerulonephritis, graft
rejection and autoimmune diseases (Sharma, 1981a). However,
these phenomena represent merely the extreme manifestations of
immunotoxicological insults. It is probable that a large
number of far more subtle effects also modulate the immune
mechanisms, be it for example through influences on the
proliferation, differentiation, function and survival of
various immunocompetent cells and through alterations of their
surface receptors and biosynthetic capabilities. IM may also
act on the supply and function of components of the complement
system, on the activities of reticuloendothelial elements, the
motility and function of macrophages, etc. Changes of this
kind are known to occur in many experimental studies, but
their relevance is difficult to assess, and it is not possible
to establish a logical connection between them and clinically
well-defined disease states. For example, the H receptor
blocker cimetidine was shown to affect T cell function,
including suppression of natural killer cell activity. The
clinical meaning of these findings is not known
(Ruiz-Arguelles et al., 1982). If immunotoxicological
experiments are to become part of routine studies in the
safety evaluation of chemicals, it will be necessary to make
an effort to better define the toxicological targets, i.e. to
describe in detail changes of the immune system which should
be recognized and measured in experimental procedures.

4. TESTING STRATEGIES.

The complexities of the immune regulatory mechanisms and the
great variety of chemical substances that must be considered
make it unlikely that a single protocol can be devised which
would cover all aspects of immunotoxicology. As far as the
inadvertent IM are concerned, the major problem lies with
their large number. In fact, just about all chemicals must,
until proven otherwise, be considered potential inadvertent
IM. It follows that the first task of the toxicologist is
that of a preliminary assessment of the test compounds. This
should permit the identification of those substances that
represent a significant hazard and would, unless permanently
discarded, require more detailed analysis. For this purpose,

it is necessary to use highly sensitive screening tests that do not need to be very discriminative but that should cover the foremost areas of concern, i.e. humoral and tissue hypersensitivity, autoimmune responses and immunosuppression. For large molecules, including immunomodulating contaminants, this screening should be slanted towards hypersensitivity reactions, whereas with small molecules the whole spectrum of immunotoxicology should be covered equally. In order to avoid unneccessary work, the expected route of human exposure should be taken into account. For example, compounds applied to the skin should be tested primarily for local sensitization and chemicals taken by the oral route need not necessarily be examined for their sensitizing properties by the parenteral route.

For intentional IM a more sophisticated approach can be used. The main purpose of the studies is not the determination of immunomodulating properties, since these are already established, but the tests should be aimed at evaluating risk under the proposed conditions of use. Therefore, the toxicological investigation will not be concerned so much with inherent immunopharmacological properties, but will explore the potential, undesirable consequences of the immunotherapy. This will include the problems of resistance against infections, tumor promotion and stimulation of autoimmune processes, and also , naturally, the questions of allergies against the IM and the counterreactions occurring in the destabilized immune system.

5. SELECTION OF TEST PROCEDURES.

Experimental immunology has available a large variety of in vitro and in vivo tests with which the number, the integrity and the biological activities of immunocompetent cells can be assessed and concentrations of the products synthetized by them can be measured. Moreover, there are many different models with which the rate of immunological reactions and the development of immunological diseases can be studied (Street, 1981, Koller and Vos, 1981). Toxicologists are tempted to dip into this treasure chest quite indiscriminately and perform as many tests as they possibly can. But such an unstructured and vague procedure is not only problematic from the scientific point of view, but also most wasteful, as it is sure to lead to a mass of redundant information.

A more satisfactory and cost-effective solution is provided by a hierarchical approach. This involves the use of a set of basic tests covering the main areas of immunotoxicology. Secondary tests are performed when it is desirable to further characterize an observed effect.

Immunologists and toxicologists differ somewhat in their views about the structure of such a testing system. Immunologists, quite understandably, prefer their own models and like to work with their favorite species, mouse and guinea pig, for which many of the necessary analytical reagents are available and the most responsive strains of laboratory animals have been

identified. In order to make their tests more meaningful,
immunologists also like to experiment with special subjects,
e.g. newborn and immunodepressed animals and strains
genetically preconditioned to develop autoimmune diseases such
as the NZB mouse (Falchetti et al., 1983).

Toxicologists, on the other hand, prefer to use the young
adult or at most weanling, randomly-bred dogs and rats with
which the majority of conventional toxicological tests are
performed. And whenever possible, they like to do
immunotoxicological tests on the animals included in regular
toxicity studies.

There are advantages and disadvantages to both approaches. In
practice a combination of the two is likely to become the
generally accepted solution, with more emphasis on standard
toxicological methods for small molecular inadvertent IM, and
a more detailed immunopharmacological analysis for the
intentional IM and all other compounds likely to induce
hypersensistivity reactions. However, it must be noted that
certain immunotoxicological investigations just cannot be done
within standard toxicological studies as the protocols do not
permit the introduction of new variables. Thus, it is
impossible to investigate the development of an allergy and
the rise of immunoglobulin concentrations as a response to a
challenge with a reference antigen or with co-administration
of Freund's adjuvant. Other popular immunological tests,
including the induction of plaque-forming cells in spleen and
lymph nodes in response to antigens, allograft rejection,
graft versus host activity, delayed hypersensitivity to
tuberculin, survivival of transplanted tumor cells, clearance
of intravenously injected colloidal particles, resistance
against an experimental infection or response to an injection
of endotoxin are also excluded for the same reasons. On the
other hand, to use animals from routine toxicity experiments
for immunological investigations not only saves many animal
lives, but often permits a meaningful correlation between the
immunotoxicological effects and the changes in other organ
systems.

6. TOXICOLOGICAL PROCEDURES, POSSIBILITIES AND OPEN QUESTIONS.

It is not the purpose of this introductory paper to suggest a
scheme for the immunotoxicological assesssment of IM. Such
proposals have already beean published (Vos. 1977, Ovtcharov
et al., 1980, Falchetti et al., 1983, Renoux, 1983) and others
are presented in this volume. There are also sound proposals
for the analysis of potentially immunomodulating contaminants
of products obtained by recombinant DNA technology (Johnson,
1982). In this paper some remarks about the current attitudes
of toxicologists towards immunotoxicology and about the needs
for futher research will be made.

In the toxicological reports on most new drugs, pesticides,
consumer products, industrial chemicals and environmental
pollutants, the potential immunotoxicological effects are

rarely even mentioned. Notable exceptions are in reports on chemicals that are either applied to or likely to come into accidental contact with the skin. There are excellent animal models for the detection of the local sensitizing properties of such compounds. These test models have become part of the toxicological routine (Andersen, 1983, Maurer, 1983). However, in most other areas of safety evaluation, the approach to testing of the immune system is haphazard or, as for example in teratogenicity studies, practically non/existent. Only when indisputable evidence for involvement of the immune system is present, as illustrated by the extreme atrophy of the lymphatic organs in 2,3,7,8-tetrachlorodibenzo-p-dioxin (TCDD)-treated animals (Vos et al., 1973), are the toxicologists sufficiently concerned to initiate systematic investigations.

The example of TCDD also shows how many different and rather complex immunological test methods have been applied to further characterize an effect discovered in a relatively simple animal experiment. It is interesting to note that the assumption, formulated on the basis of the orginal toxicological observation, that TCDD is a potent immunosuppressant acting preferentially on the T-cell system, has essentially been confirmed by more sophisticated immunopharmacological analysis (Vos, 1977, Sharma, 1981b). This experience should inspire toxicologists with courage to investigate immunotoxicological phenomena within their own spere of activities.

In Table 1, investigations of the structural integrity and function of the immune system suitable for incorporation in standard, repeated-dose toxicity and teratogenicity studies are listed. Some are already part of the current routine and othes might be easily included. But for some of the tests, the necessary reagents and techniques must still be developed. A glance at this table shows that the targets of many of the procedures overlap. Thus, it is not necessary to use all of the techniques in every toxicological test.

However, not enough experience is available to determine which of the measurements are the most sensitive and reproducible ones. Systematic studies using suitable reference agents are needed to settle this question.

Additional problems are created by the rigid testing protocols of routine toxicology. For example, in all toxicological experiments, it is required to include groups of animals exposed to doses that cause target organ toxicity or discernible deterioration of general health, or both. Experience shows that in these animals the lymphoreticular sytem is often atrophic. It has been established that a variety of immunological functions are also often affected. In such instances, it is necessary to decide whether these changes are relevant immunotoxicological manifestations, or merely the non-specific consequence of general toxicity, or qualitative or quantitative malnutrition. This often requires special studies,

TABLE 1

POSSIBLE TEST FOR THE EVALUATION OF THE IMMUNE SYSTEM IN ROUTINE
TOXICITY STUDIES

Measurements	Time	Target
Weight of lymphatic organs	T	general
Total cell count of lymphatic organs	T	general
Total cell count of bone marrow	T	general
Histopathology lymphatic organs, bone marrow	T	general
Peripheral lymphocyte count	C	general
Total serum globulins	C	humoral
Concentration of immunoglobulins	C	humoral
Antibody-forming cells in lymphatic tissue	T	humoral
Lymphocyte response to B cell mitogens	C	humoral
Percentage of B lymphocytes	C	humoral
B-lymphocyte markers	C	humoral
Passive cutaneous anaphylaxis (a)	C	humoral
Circulating immune complexes	C	humoral, autoimmunity
Complement, total and fractions (b)	C	humoral
Presence of plasma cells in lymphatic organs	T	humoral
Lymphocyte response to T cell mitogens	C	cell-mediated
Percentage of T lymphosytes	C	cell-mediated
Subpopulations of T lymphocytes (c)	C	cell-mediated
Histamine release from isolated lung fragments upon antigen challenge	T	humoral (c)
Antinuclear antibodies	C	autoimmunity
Peripheral monocyte count	C	macrophage system
Phagocytic activity of macrophages	T	macrophage system

T = terminal (at autopsy). C = current (before, during, after
treatment). (a) = feasible, but cumbersome in dogs. (b) = reagents
not available for dogs. (c) = reagents not yet available for dogs,
not widely available commercialy for rats. (d) = mediated by mast
cells, but a measure for anaphylactic, humoral immune response, due
to IgE or IgE-like amtibodies.

including experiments with adrenalectomized animals (Vos,
1977).

Another difficulty is created by the protocol requirement to
obtain blood samples and sacrifice the animals at predeter-
mined time points. These often do not coincide with the
moment at which a particular immunotoxicological effect is at
its peak. In repeated-dose experiments, it is possible that a
change may disappear after a certain time, even though administration of the test compound continues. For example, in
rats treated with the interferon inducer tilorone, a marked
and short-lived lymphocytopenia occurred, but only after the

first few doses. Soon after the first dose, many abnormal
mononuclear cells appeared in the peripheral blood, but their
number gradually decreased during continued treatment, and
lymphocyte depletion in T-cell dependent areas of the lymph
nodes, which was also present in the early phase, disappeared
(Zbinden and Emch, 1972, Levine et al., 1974). Based on this
and similar observations, it is suggested that measurements
aimed at assessing the immune system in toxicological studies
be made not only during and at the end of treatment, but also
after the first or the first few doses. This may necessitate
the addition of more treatment groups to those required by the
standard protocol, but it is likely to provide much relevant
information, part of which might not otherwise be obtainable.

Finally, the problem of species and strain selection must be
mentioned. In routine toxicology it is advantageous to use,
whenever possible, the same randomly-bred strain of animals.
For the study of immunotoxicological problems, on the other
hand, the selection of a specifically sensitive strain of
animals for a particular test procedure has proven to be of
critical importance (Morin and Chedid, 1983).

7. STANDARD TOXICOLOGY WITH IM.

Another difficult question is whether or not standard safety
studies including single- and repeated-dose toxicity, reproductive toxicity, mutagenicity and carcinogenicity experiments
should be done with IM. Furthermore, if such tests are deemed
desirable, what protocols should be used and how should the
results be interpreted and extrapolated to man? With small
molecular IM devoid of intrinsic sensitizing properties
standard safety tests are certainly justified and can, in most
cases, be done according to conventional protocols. However,
in evaluating the results, the immunological properties must
be kept in mind, and changes related to immunomodulating
characteristics must be recognized as such and weighed
accordingly. Moreover, the fact that an immunomodulating
effect may be reversed at high doses should also be considered
(Morin and Chedid, 1983).

The problems encountered in toxicological experiments with
potentially or definitely sensitizing IM have been discussed
by Petricciani (1983). There is, in principle, no question
that such compounds could possess undesirable toxicological
properties that are unrelated to their primary immunomodulating activities. However, the question arises of whether such
qualities would be recognized in animal experiments that are
complicated by sensitizing effects of the test compound. At
this time it is not possible to give a definite answer.
However, it is possible that useful safety data can be
obtained from such studies, at least with some of the
compounds. Thus, an attempt should be made to conduct at
least some relatively short-term, repeated dose toxicity
experiments, and, if no anaphylactic responses or organ
lesions clearly related to hypersensitivity occur, long-term
and reproductive toxicity experiments should also be
considered. At the same time, research aimed at a better

knowledge of the relevance of such animal models should be undertaken, in particular with regard to an understanding of the toxicological characteristics of smaller peptides, both of human and non-human origin.

An important aspect of such studies is the detection of potentially relevant interactions of immunomodulating substances with other regulatory systems. Of particular interest are influences on the function of the hypophy-seal-adrenal axis which are evident from observations such as the immunomodulating effects of glucocorticoids and the corticotropin-releasing activity of thymosin (Healy et al. 1983). Another potentially important interaction is signalled by the finding of endorphin-like activity of interferons (Morin and Chedid, 1983). Toxicologial studies of IM should, therefore, also include appropriate investigations of the endocrine system, e.g. determinations of plasma corticosteroid, corticotropin and growth hormone concen trations and a detailed pathomorphological evaluation of endocrine and hormone-dependent organs (Vos, 1977).

Finally, efforts should also be undertaken to mobilize forces in clinical and pathology laboratories for the purpose of detecting immunotoxicological characteristics of test compounds. For exemple, immunohistochemistry can be used for the demonstration of immune complexes in critical targets such as the glomeruli of the kidney, and there are good laboratory methods for identifying antinuclear antibodies (Balazs and Robinson, 1983). Electrocardiography has been applied to demonstrate the development allergic myocarditis in rabbits sensitized by horse serum (Bickel, 1960). A particularly attractive and relevant area of research is the role of IM in the growth, promotion and metastasis formation of tumors and oncogene expression. In this area toxicologists now have at their disposal several elegant in vitro and in vivo models which could be used, perhaps in a somewhat modified form, to assess the co-carcinogenic properties of IM.

REFERENCES

Andersen, K.E., 1983. *Predictive skin and mucosa testing methods. In Allergic Responses and Hypersensitivities Induced by Chemicals, Health Aspects of Chemical Safety, Interim Document 12, World Health Organization, Regional Office for Europe, Copenhagen, pp 243-275.*

Balazs, T. & Robinson, C.J.G., 1983. *Procainamide/induced antinuclear antibodpes in beagle dogs. Toxicol. Appl. Pharmacol.* 71, 299-302.

Bickel, G., 1960 *Allergie et myocarde. Schweiz. med. Wchschr.* 90, 912-921.

D'Agnolo G., 1983 *The control of drugs obtained by recombinant DNA and other biotechnologies. In current Problems in Drug Toxicology. Eds G.Zbinden, F. Cohadon, J.Y.Detaille & G.Mazue. John Libbey Eurotext: Paris & London. pp 241-247.*

Falchetti, R., Silvestri, S., Battaglia, A., & Caprino, L., 1983. *Toxicological evaluation of immunomodulating drugs. In Current Problems in Drug Toxcology. Eds. G.Zbinden, F.Cohadon, J.Y.Detaille & G. Mazue. John Libbey Eurotext: Paris & London, pp 248-263.*

Healy, D.L., Hodgen, G.D., Schulte, H.M., Chrousos, G.P., Loriaux, D.L., Hall, N.R. & Goldstein, A.L., 1983. *The thymus-adrenal connection: thymosin has coricotropin-releasing activity in primates. Science* 222, 1353-1355.

Johnson, I.S., 1982. *Authenticity and purity of human insulin (recombinant DNA). Diabetic Care, 5, Suppl. 2, 4-12.*

Koller, L.D. & Vos, J.G., 1981 *Immunologic effects of metals. In Immunologic Considerations in Toxicology, Vol. 1. Ed. R.P. Sharma. CRC Press, Inc.: Boca Raton FL, pp 67-78.*

Levine, S., Gibson, J.P., & Megel, H., 1974. *Selective depletion of thyumus dependent areas in lymphoid tissue by tilorone. Proc. Soc. Exp. Biol. Med.* 146, 245-248.

Maurer, T. 1983. *Contact and photocontact allergens. A manual of predictive test methods. Marcel Dekker Inc. New York, Basel.*

Morin, A. & Chedid, L., 1983. *Apport de l'immunopharmacologie dans l'evaluation toxicologique des immunomodulants. In Current Problems in Drug Toxicology. G. Zbinden, F. Cohadon, J.Y. Detaille & G. Mazue, Eds. John Libbey Eurotext: Paris & London, pp 294-302.*

Ovtcharov, R., Guentcheva, G., & Michailova, S., 1980. Some approaches to experimental testing of drugs for immunotoxicity. Arch. Toxicol., Suppl. 4 ,, 120/131.

Petricciani, J.C., 1983. An overview of safety and regulatory aspects of the new biotechnology. Regulatory Toxicol. Pharmacol. 3, 428-433.

Renoux G., 1983. Les exigences de l'evaluation immunopharma-cologique d'un medicament. In Current Problems in Drug Toxicology. G. Zbinden, F. Cohadon, J.Y. Detaille & G. Mazue, eds. John Libbey Eurotext: Paris & London, pp 310-314.

Ruiz-Arguelles, A, Seroogy, K.B., & Ritts, R.R.Jr. 1982. In vitro effect of cimetidine on human cell-mediated cytotoxicity. 1. Inhibition of natural killer cell activity. Cellular Immunol. 62, 1-12.

Sharma, R.P.(a), 1981. Tissue and cell injury in immune mechanisms. In Immunologic Considerations in Toxicology, Vol. 1, R.P. Sharma ed., CRC Press, Inc. Boca Raton, FL, pp 37-44.

Sharma, R.P.(b), 1981. Effects of Tetrachlorodibenzo-p-di oxin (TCDD) on immunologic systems. In Immunologic considerations in Toxicology, Vol. 1, R.P. Sharma, ed., CRC Press Inc. Boca Raton FL, pp 89-102.

Street, J.S.c., 1981. Pesticides and the immune system. In Immunologic Considerations in Toxicology, Vol. 1, R.P. Sharma, ed., CRC Press, Inc. Boca Raton FL, pp 45-66.

Vos, J.G., 1977. Immmune supression as related to toxicology. CRC Crit. Rev. Toxicol. 5, 67-101.

Vos, J.G., Moore, J.A., & Zinkl, J.G., 1973. Effect of 2,2,7,8-tetrachlorodibenzo-p-dioxin on the immune system of laboratory Environmental Health Perspectives, Experi-mental Issue 5, 149-162.

Zbinden, G. & Emchp, E., 1972. Effect of tilorone HCl, an oral interferon inducer, on leukopoiesis in rats. Acta Haematol. 47, 49-58.

Zbinden, G., Elsner, J., & Boelsterli U., 1984. Toxicological Screening,Regulatory Toxicol. Phatmacol. In press.

THE CELLS OF THE IMMUNE SYSTEM, AN UPDATE ON THEIR INTERACTIONS AND SIGNALS

L. Adorini

Laboratorio di Patologia, ENEA-CRE,
Rome, Italy.

INTRODUCTION

The definition of the two major compartments of lymphocytes, T and B cells, followed by the detailed analysis of immunoregulatory cell interactions, has permitted an identification of the very precise and sophsticated mechanisms which modulate and control the interaction, of every cellular and soluble component of the immune system. Basically it is possible to distinguish four different types of cellular interactions in the immune response (Fig. 1). In the case of macrophage-T cell interaction antigen is processed by macrophages and selected epitopes are presented, associated with self-MHC molecules to T cells (associated recognition). Linked recognition refers to the necessity for two functionally distinct cells to recognize antigenic determinants on the same molecule in order for an effective cellular interaction to occur. Typically, linked recognition occurs between carrier-specific T cells and hapten-specific B cells and is mediated by an hapten-carrier conjugate antigen bridge. This type of interaction is restricted by MHC molecules since carrier-specific T cells are activated only when antigen is presented in association with self MHC on antigen-presenting cells and they can interact only with B cells sharing the same MHC I-region haplotype as that of antigen-presenting cells. In the case of polyclonal interaction the initial step is also dependent on MHC-restricted antigenic stimulation but the interaction does not require an antigen bridge and takes place via non-specific mediators (lymphokines), provided that hapten and carrier determinants, although unlinked, are present. Idiotype-anti-idiotype interaction occurs when a cell type recognizes on its partner immunoglobulin determinants; idiotypes, allotypes, or isotypes. B and possibly T cells specific for idiotypic determinants form the basis for the network concept of immune regulation.

The two major immunoregulatory cell types are helper and suppressor T cells and we shall examine briefly their interactions and signals.

HELPER T CELLS

The differentiation of B cells into antibody-forming cells requires the cooperation of specific helper T cells which may be mediated by different mechanisms of cellular interactions. The antigen-bridge model postulates that a close physical proximity of hapten-primed B cells and carrier-primed T cells is the mandatory requisite for effective cellular interaction whereas in the case of polyclonal B cell activation stimulation of B cells by the appropriate antigen (hapten conjugated to a carrier molecule different from that recognized by T cells) causes the expression on the B cell surface of membrane receptors for T cell and macrophage-derived lymphokines. These two helper mechanisms usually operate simultaneously and synergistically and are mediated by two distinct types of carrier-specific helper T cells denominated Th1 and Th2 (1). Th1 are carrier-specific helper cells that require linked recognition to activate, in a MHC-restricted fashion, B cells. Th1 and Th2 can be separated by nylon-wool adherence and although both cell subsets could independently help B cells, the addition of a small number of cells from one fraction to the other demonstrates a marked synergism in the induction of antibody response. Th2 cells, the nylon-adherent subset, were found to provide unrestricted help to B cells stimulated with hapten conjugate to a different carrier (polyclonal activation) and to express determinants coded for in the I-J region of the H-2 complex.

Besides carrier-specific helper T cells, a third subset of T cell has been described, able to cooperate with B cells by directly recognizing isotypic allotypic or idiotypic structures of B cell surface immunoglobulins (2). This helper T cell type may possess a dual specificity for both the antigen and the antigen receptor (idiotype) and could thus represent the counterpart of carrier-specific helper cells (3).

Interactions have been described not only between Th1 and Th2 cells but also between carrier-specific and idiotype-specific helper T cells. For example, in the hen egg-white lysozyme (HEL) system two distinct peptides derived from the HEL molecule, the N-terminal C-terminal peptide (N-C) and the L11 peptide, include epitopes that, in genetically non responder strains (H-2^b and H-2^s), preferentially stimulate suppressor and helper T cells, respectively. In genetically responder mice both peptides induce predominantly helper T cells (4). The HEL-specific antibodies are mostly directed against determinants included in the N-C region of the molecule and are characterized by a major cross-reactive idiotype (IdX). HEL-specific and IdX-specific helper T cells can be separated by absorption on HEL and IdX-coated plates and the coculture of these two helper T cell subsets reconstitutes the antibody response to HEL (5). These results imply that optimal B cell activation requires both idiotypic complementarity and antigen-mediated linked recognition. It is not known whether these two signals reach the same B cell simultaneously or sequentially nor whether the same or different B cell clones are activated by the two helper T cell types.

SUPPRESSOR T CELLS

Supression of the immune response is mediated by a complex series of cellular interactions involving different cell types and in a suppressive circuit it is usually possible to identify inducer, transducer (amplifier) and effector T cells. Besides suppressor cells specific for antigen epitopes, the counterpart of carrier-specific helper T cells, idiotype, allotype and isotype-specific suppressor cells have been described. A unifying consensus model of the suppressive pathway has not yet been delineated, given the complexity of suppressive circuits, and we shall briefly outline some well-defined systems of immunosuppression.

Benacerraf, Dorf, Greene and co-workers have proposed a model, based on the analysis of anti-azobenzene arsonate (ABA) and anti-4-hydroxy-3-nitrophenyl acetyl (NP) responses, involving the sequential activation of three cell types, denominated Ts1, Ts2 and Ts3 (6). In this case (Fig. 2) I-J$^+$ macrophages present antigen, in the context of I-J molecules to pre-Ts1 cells driving them to differentiate into Ts1 cells. These idiotype-positive, antigen-specific, Lyt1$^+$, I-J$^+$ cells produce a soluble factor, TsF1, which induces the differentiation of pre-Ts2 cells to Ts2. The TsF1-pre-Ts2 cell interaction is antigen-specific and is restricted by genes mapping in the Igh-1 locus, associated to the immunoglobulin heavy chain (V_H) locus and in some cases also by genes mapping in the I-J region of the H-2 complex. Ts2 cells, specific for idiotype rather than antigen, produce a factor, TsF2, which activates antigen-specific and idiotype-positive Ts3 effector cells. Ts3 cells suppress T helper cells by releasing both specific and non-specific factors.

Gershon and co-workers (7) have proposed a model of cellular interaction, based on the analysis of suppression of the primary anti-SRBC antibody response, involving also three different Ts cell types: inducer (Tsi), acceptor or trans-ducer (Tsa) and effector (Tse) (Fig. 3). Antigen first activates Lyt1$^+$, Qa-1$^+$, I-J$^+$ Tsi cells. These cells are analogous to helper T cells but they are programmed to acti-vate Tsa cells to differentiate into Tse cells via an antigen-specific, I-J$^+$ factor, TsiF. Induction of Tse by TsiF is restricted by Igh-1 genes but not by MHC genes. Tse cells inhibit antigen-specific T helper cells by releasing an antigen-specific, H-2 restricted, I-J- TseF. This factor may also inhibit Tsi cells, thus generating a feedback suppression loop. Besides this feedback suppression loop Gershon's model describes a second regulatory mechanism denominated contrasup-pressor circuit. Contrasuppressor T cells (Tcs) are organized in a circuit in which Lyt 2$^+$, I-J$^+$ effector cells (Tcse) are induced via Tcsa by Tcsi, and act by rendering helper T cells resistant to the suppressive activity mediated by TseF.

In the suppressive circuit described by Tada and co-workers (Fig. 4) Tsi cells release TsiF which can suppress directly Th2 cells or amplify the suppressive effect via the sequential activation of Tsa and Tse which release TseF inhibiting Th1 cells (1).

THE IDIOTYPIC NETWORK

The term idiotype was originally coined to designate unique antigenic determinants present on immunoglobulin molecules of a certain animal responding to a given antigen. However, the discovery of extensive idiotypic cross-reaction has rendered the original definition obsolete and idiotypes are currently defined as antigenic determinants present in the immunoglobulin chain variable domains. The concept of the immune system as a functional idiotypic network stemmed from a theory proposed by Jerne (8) to explain the observation that a given idiotype may be associated with combining sites specific for different antigens and that the same antigenic specificty may be associated with different idiotypes. The fundamental idea of the network theory is that each combining site not only recognizes antigenic determinants but it is also recognized by anti-idiotypic determinants within the same immune system. The basic features of Jerne's network are illustrated in Fig. 5. The induction of the first set of idiotypes (1) is stimulated by an antigenic epitope (E) on an immunogenic molecule. A second, idiotypically complementary set (2) is activated when a certain threshold level is reached and will induce suppressive or enhancing events. In addition, two other cell types were postulated: the "internal image" set (3) bearing idiotypic determinants recognized by the first set, and thus similar to the antigenic epitope and the "parallel" set (4) with the same idiotypic determinants as (1) but with different antigenic specificity. This network theory created a speculative framework of a radically different nature, not only of the regulation of the immune system, but of the immune system itself. This becomes an antigen-independent, self-regulated network of interactions in which all the components are in mutual equilibrium receiving positive and negative signals from within the system. Antigen introduction perturbs the network, and its effects reverberate through the entire system, until a new stable state is reached.

Thus, the basic requirement for an idiotypic network encompassing all the lymphocytes in the immune system is the mutual recognition of idiotypes and anti-idiotypes by T and B cells. This requirement is clearly fulfilled by B cells whereas T cells have not been found to express mRNA species able to hybridize with B cell idiotypic probes in the same antigenic system, casting some doubts on the strict idiotypic relatedness between T and B cells. However, the structure of T and B cell receptors for antigen is very similar and somme type of idiotypic connectance may indeed take place. Again, in the lysosyme system a model has been proposed relating idiotypic and antigenic specificity of helper T cells, suppressor T cells and B cells induced by HEL (9). A minimal network model implicating four different lymphocytes bearing complementary receptors is shown in Fig. 6. HEL immunization of B10 (H-2b) non responder mice induces suppressor T cells specific for the N-C region of the HEL molecule. These supressor T cells would interact via idiotypic complementarity with an IdX-specific helper T cell, or through antigen-bridge with carrier-specific helper T cells. As already mentioned plate absorption experiments have demonstrated that IdX-positive, N-C-specific B cells are optimally stimulated by two different signals one coming from anti-idiotype positive helper T cells (idiotypic complementarity) and the other from carrier (L_{II})-reactive helper T cells (antigen-bridge). Thus, the antibody specificity in the response to HEL is restricted antigenically and idiotypically. Likewise, suppressor T cells raised in a non-responder mouse strain show a remarkably similar restriction to this same determinant. The presence of the same antigenic and idiotypic determinants on these two cell populations ensures communication between suppressor T cells and B cells via helper T cells, with complementary idiotypic and epitopic receptors. Thus, the two major specific communication systems among lymphocytes engaged in the antibody response, antigen-bridge and idiotypic complementarity, have been integrated in a regulatory circuit.

In conclusion, a possible scenario of antigen-triggered interactions in the regulation of the immune response may comprise three distinct events:

1. before antigen. The system is in equilibrium through a subtreshold level of mutually inhibitory complementary cell interactions.

2. antigen enters. After a degree of macrophage processing antigenic epitopes are complexed to class II MHC molecules, the Ir gene products, and presented to helper or suppressor T cells. Intercellular communications can then take place among T cells over a bridge of native antigen or via idiotypic complementarity, either directly or mediated by the release of antigen-specific and non-specific products. Accordingly, clonally restricted B cells will be stimulated to proliferate and differentiate into antibody-forming cells by both antigen-specific and non-specific signals. The immunodominance of certain epitopes, presumably the resultant of macrophage presentation and repertoire availability, will also influence the relative preponderance of helper or suppressor T cells in the circuits. In this way antigen sets the framework in which the idiotypic network will operate to attain a new level of homeostasis.

3. antigen is eliminated. After having conditioned the system into certain options, the antigen looses its primary, steering, regulatory function. The long-term, overall regulation of the system is then mainly sustained by a self-contained, self-limited, "closed" idiotypic network.

LYMPHOKINES

A series of non-specific signals amplifies the antigen-specific response from the clonal level to the effector cell population by promoting the proliferation and differentiation of cells involved in the immune response.

Proteins able to transmit non-specific proliferation and differentiation signals are collectively termed lymphokines and some of them have been characterized in considerable detail and are now available as recombinant DNA products. The rapid progress in the functional and structural characterization of lymphokines has been considerably increased by the availability of cell lines secreting, constitutively or after mitogen induction, high concentration of lymphokines and by the utilization, as target cells, of cell lines acutely dependent for their proliferation on the presence of a particular lymphokine (10).

The most important and best characterzed lymhokines are:

1. <u>Interleukin 1 (IL-1)</u>, a family of proteins (m.w.12-16,000) produced by macrophages and several other cell types which induce IL-2 production by T cells. IL-1 is also a co-inducer of B cell activation.

2. <u>Interleukin 2 (IL-2)</u>. This protein (m.w. 16,000 in humans, (ca 22,000) in mice) promotes the growth of T cells. Antigen, presented by macrophages in association with MHC products, transmits a primary activation signal to antigen-specific T cells. Simultaneously, macrophage-derived IL-1 induces the differentiation of activated T cells into IL-2 producing cells. IL-2 produced by these cells induce in other T cells the expression of IL-2 receptors and therefore the ability to proliferate in response to IL-2. This indicates that antigen per se does not induce proliferation, which is exclusively IL-2-dependent, and that the IL-2-driven T cell proliferation is non-specific since it will expand any activated T cell clone.

3. <u>Gamma interferon (IFN-ɣ)</u>. Immune or gamma IFN (m.w. ca 18,000) is produced by activated T cells and amplifies the response of cytotoxic T cells, natural killer (NK) cells and helper T cells.

4. <u>Colony stimulating factor (CSF)</u>. This lymhokine (m.w. 30,000) is produced by T cells and acts on macrophages by increasing IL-1 production.

5. <u>Interleukin 3 (IL-3)</u>. This protein (m.w. 41,000) is released by activated T cells and it promotes the differentiation and the proliferation of immature T cells and of cells of the macrophage/monocyte lineage.

6. <u>B cell growth factor (BCGF)</u>. At least two distinct BCGFs have been identified, produced by T

cell lines after mitogen induction. BCGF activity, the B cell counterpart of IL-2, is restricted to the promotion of B cell proliferation and it does not induce B cell differentiation.

7. B cell diffferentiation factor (BCDF). The differentiation of B cells towards antibody-forming cells requires a class of lymphokines designated B cell differentiation factors. At least two such factors have been identified, one leading preferentially to the secretion of IgM and another to the secretion of IgG.

8. T cell preplacing factor (TRF). This lymphokine is produced by Lyt 1^+ T cells in a macrophage and antigen-dependent induction process and is maximally active on B cells when added late in culture. TRF is therefore thought to provide a terminal signal to antigen-stimulated proliferating B cells to differentiate into antibody-secreting plasma cells.

The lymphokine-mediated immunoregulatory events are summarized in fig. 7. Macrophages and T cells interact synergistically in a cyclic amplification loop in which T cells produce CSF that stimulates macrophages to produce IL-1. IL-1 gives also a positive signal to antigen-stimulated T cells which produce IL-2 and IL-3 proliferative and differentiation signals for T cells. T cells also produce BCGF, BCDF and TRF lymphokines necessary for expansion and differentiation of antigen-specific B cell clones. All these T cell-derived lymphokines are not produced by discrete T cell subsets but, apparently, any Lyt 1^+ cell is potentially able to secrete all T-cell lymphokines. The growing interest in lymphokine research derives, in large part, from its relevant clinical implications since several immunological defects or dysregulations appear to be at the level of lymphokine production and/or lymphokine receptor expression. The reconstitution of the immunodeficient individual by administration of exogenous lymphokines or by pharmacological agents that are able to regulate endogenous production will certainly have an important influence in treatment and biotechnological research.

ASSOCIATE RECOGNITION   LINKED RECOGNITION

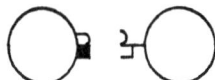   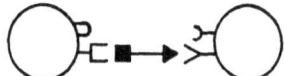

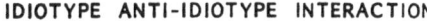

POLYCLONAL INTERACTION   IDIOTYPE ANTI-IDIOTYPE INTERACTION

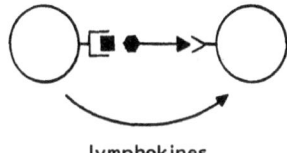   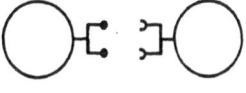

lymphokines

Fig.1.   Cellular interactions in the immune response.   Key to symbols: □ MHC determinant; ■ and ♠ carrier determinants; → haptenic determinants; ● idiotypic determinant.

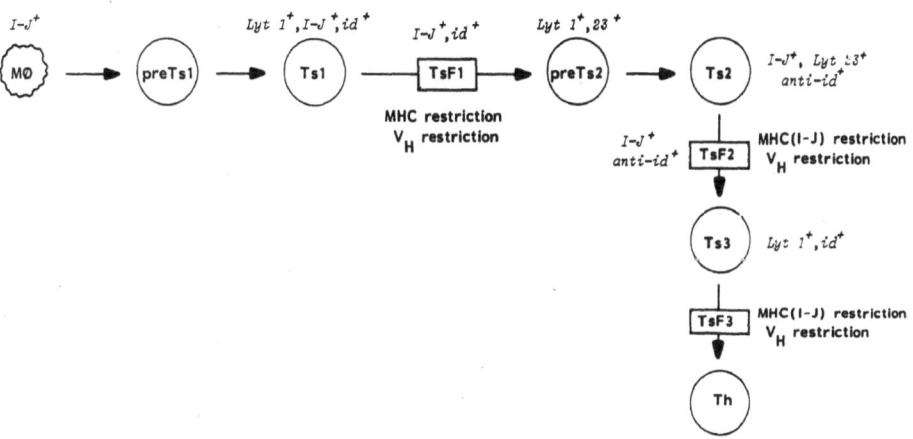

Fig.   2.   Sequential activation of suppressor T cells according to Benacerraf and colleagues (6).

20

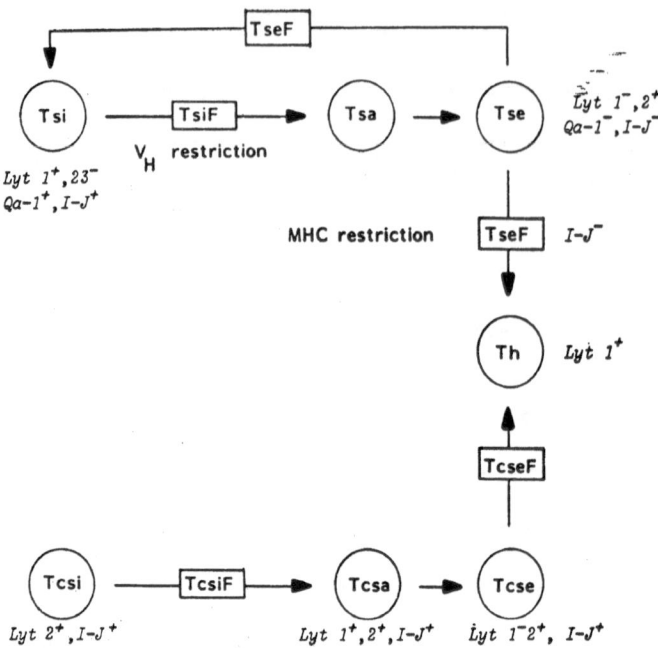

Fig. 3. Suppressor and contrasuppressor circuits according to Gershon and colleagues (7).

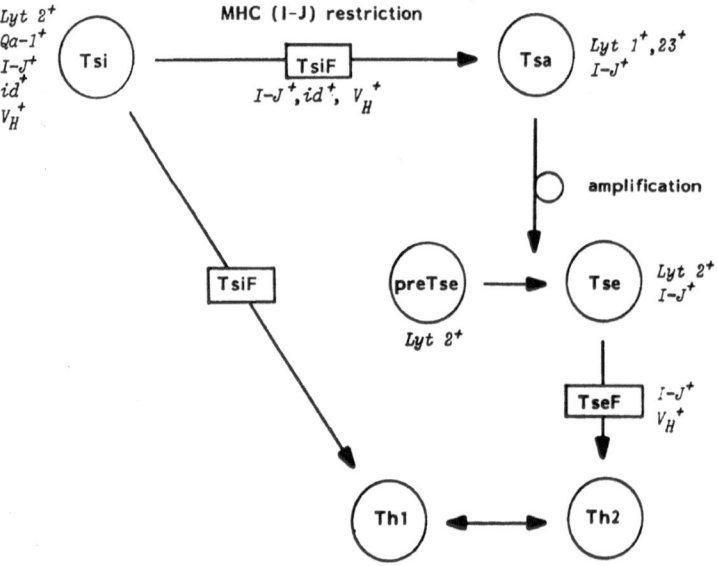

Fig. 4. Immunosuppressive circuits according to Tada and colleagues (1).

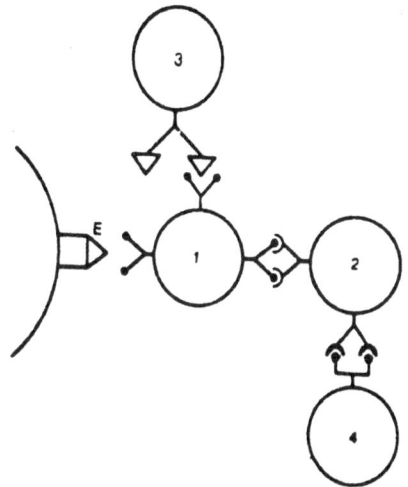

Fig. 5. Schematic representation of Jerne's idiotypic network. E = antigenic epitope on an immunogenic molecule. 1 = epitope recognizing set; 2 = anti-idiotypic set; 3 = "internal image" set; 4 = non antigen specific parallel set.

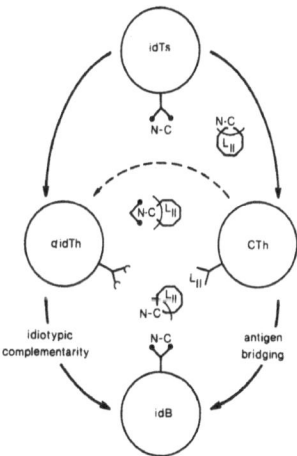

Fig. 6. Cellular specificities and a possible network of interactions in the response to HEL. The octagon represents the HEL molecule, operationally divided into hapten (N-C) and carrier (L$_{II}$) specific determinants. Optimal activation of idiotypic positive, hapten specific B cells (idB) is achieved through interaction with idiotype specific helper T cells (αidTh) and carrier specific helper T cells (CTh). A possible interaction between these two types of helper T cells is suggested by the broken arrow indicating presentation of idiotypic determinants by carrier specific helper cells to idiotype specific helper cells. Idiotype positive, hapten specific suppressor T cells (idTs) could interact via idiotypic complementarity with idiotype specific helper T cells, or via antigen bridge with carrier specific helper T cells.

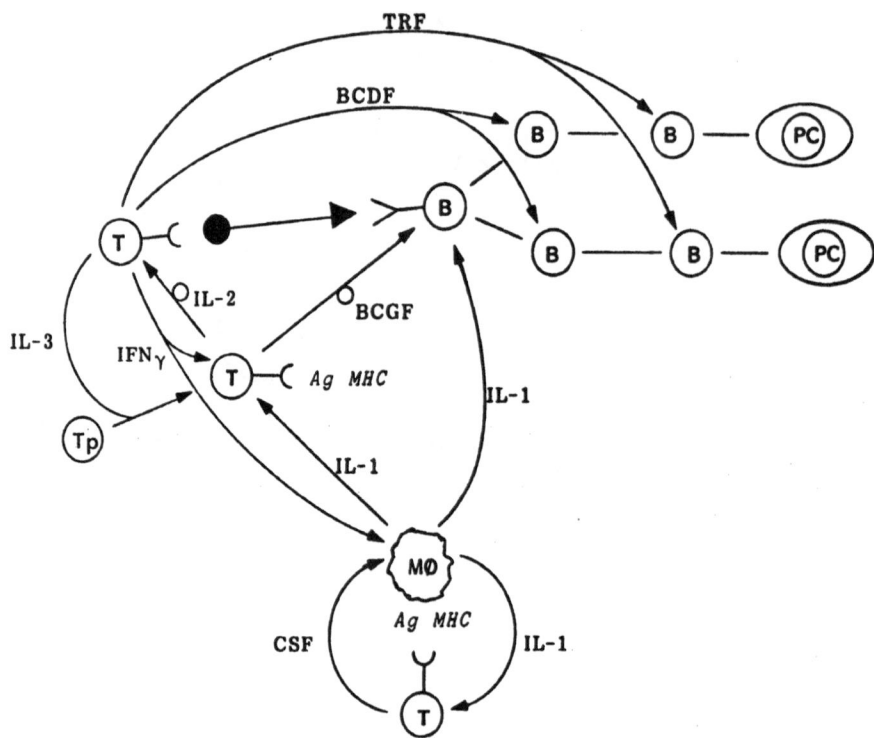

Fig.7. The lymphokine cascade.

REFERENCES

1. Tada, T., 1984. Help, suppression and specific factors. In: Fundamental Immunology, W.E. Paul, ed., Raven Press, New York, p. 481.

2. Janeway, C.A., Bert, D.L., & Shen, F.W., 1980. Cell cooperation during in vivo anti-hapten antibody response. V. Two synergistic Ly 1+23- helper cells with distinct specificities. Eur. J. Immunol. 10: 231.

3. Bottomly, K., & Mosier, D.E., 1981. Antigen-specific helper T cells required for dominant idiotype expression are not H-2 restricted. J. Exp. Med. 154: 4112.

4. Adorini, L., Harvey, M.A., Miller, A. & Sercarz, E.E., 1979. Fine specificity of regulatory T cells. II. Suppressor and helper T cells are induced by different regions of hen egg-white lysozyme in a genetically non responder mouse strain. J. Exp. Med. 150: 293.

5. Adorini, L., Harvey, M.A., & Sercarz, E.E., 1979. The fine specificity of regulatory T cells. IV. Idiotypic complementarity and antigen-bridging interactions in the anti-lysozyme response. Eur. J. Immunol. 9:906.

6. Benacerraf, B., Greene, M.I., Sy, M-S & Dorf, M.E., 1982. Suppressor T cell circuits. Ann. N.Y. Acad. Sci. 392: 300.

7. Flood, P.M., Gershon, R.K., & Green, D.R., 1984. Information transfer between T cell sets: I-J+ molecules that direct immunoregulatory signals. In: Progress in Immunology V, Y. Yamamura & T. Tada, eds., Academic Press, New York. p. 567.

8. Jerne, N.K., 1974. Towards a network theory of the immune system. Ann. Immunol. (Inst. Pasteur) 125C: 373.

9. Adorini, L., Harvey, M.A., & Sercarz, E.E., 1980. The antigen bridge and idiotypic interactions as parallel communication systems. In: Strategies of Immune Regulation, E.E. Sercarz & A. Cunningham, eds., Academic Press, New York. p. 483.

10. Moller, G., 1982. (ed) Interleukins and lymphocyte activation. Immunol. Rev. 63.

RELATIONSHIP BETWEEN THE IMMUNE SYSTEM AND CANCER

R.W. Baldwin

Cancer Research Campaign Laboratories
Nottingham, United Kingdom

1. INTRODUCTION.

The notion that malignant cells may be subject to control by
the immunological network of the host has been established
conclusively by showing that the adoptive immune system can
respond to experimentally induced animal tumours (1, 2).   In
these systems it has been shown that immunodepression leads to
enhanced growth of tumors and/or to increased metastatic
spread (3).   Conversely, there is considerable evidence to
show that immunotherapeutic manipulation can be used to
suppress growth of local and/or metastatic tumors(4).   The
relevance of the findings with primary and syngeneically
transplanted rodent tumors to human cancer remains unresolved.
This is principally because of the lack of appropriate methods
for defining human tumour antigens and detecting specific
immune responses to them in cancer patients.   Contemporary
studies on tumor cell-lymphocyte interactions will probbably
provide a more acceptable approach to this problem.

In addition to the putative specific rejection responses,
natural resistance involving macrophages and natural killer
(NK) cells can exert a significant anti-tumour response.
Natural cytotoxicity mediated by populations of non-specifically sensitized lymphocytes, (including NK cells) has
attracted considerable interest since they may be viewed as a
first line of defence against nascent tumors and may also be
cytotoxic for blood-borne tumour cells so limiting metastatic
spread (5, 6).   NK cell mediated cytotoxic reactions have been
demonstrated against animal and human tumors and numerous
agents, particularly interferon, can augment NK activity
suggesting that this host effector cell may be manipulated
therapeutically (7).

2. SPECIFIC IMMUNE RECOGNITION OF MALIGNANT CELLS.

For a tumour to generate specifically sensitized T lymphocytes
(as well as initiate antibody production) it must express
antigens which are immunogenic in the host. This requirement
is fulfilled by many experimental animal tumours induced by
chemical carcinogens or oncogenic viruses (1,2).   Tumours
induced by DNA- or RNA- containing viruses may express an
array of plasma membrane associated cellular antigens (8).
This is reflected in the specificity of the immunity induced
against these types of tumours which is 'virus related',
although not due simply to host recognition of viral antigens
associated with virus-induced tumours.   These characteristics
basically differentiate virus-induced tumours from those
induced by chemical carcinogens where tumour-associated
antigens exhibit a high degree of polymorphism so that tumours
appear to express individually-distinct antigens (2).

Tumour rejection antigens on animal tumours have been demonstrated by showing that some form of immunization, e.g.
implantation of attenuated tumour cells, suppresses tumour
growth. This approach is not permissible in human cancer and
investigations have largely had to be limited to in vitro
assays for cell mediated and/or antibody responses.

The original evidence cited in identifying cell mediated
responses to human tumour associated antigens was derived
primarily from studies showing that peripheral blood lymphocytes from patients were cytotoxic when tested in vitro against
tumour cells derived from the lymphocyte donor, or from other
patients with tumours of the same histological type (9).
These studies are not now viewed as acceptable since the in
vitro cytotoxicity test measures responses mediated by naturally cytotoxic (NK cells) as well as T lymphocytes which may
have been stimulated following recognition of tumour antigen.

Other tests for detecting T lymphocyte responses to human
tumours have been introduced including leucocyte migration
inhibition and leucocyte adherence inhibition assays, but none
have found widespread acceptance (10). There is growing
evidence, however, that T lymphocyte recognition of human
tumour associated antigens can be demonstrated using in vitro
sensitization procedures involving culture of peripheral blood
lymphocytes, and in some cases tumour-infiltrating
lymphocytes, with autologous tumour cells, i.e. mixed
lymphocyte-tumour cell culture, MLTC (11-14). MLTC has been
used to generate sensitized lymphocytes following stimulation
with autologous tumour cells derived from sarcomas (11),
malignant melanoma (12) and carcinomas of the lung (13) and
colon and breast (14). The reactivities of the sensitized
effector cells have been demonstrated using both proliferative
and cytotoxicity assays. Important questions are raised by
the autologous MLTC studies particularly with respect to the
nature of the 'auto/recognitive' antigen on malignant cells,
and further advances in this approach are anticipated following recent developments in procedures for the in vitro maintenance and expansion of T lymphocyte populations in media
containing T cell growth factors, such as interleukin-2,
(IL-2) (15). The generation of cloned lines of
tumour-reactive T lymphocytes in IL-2-containing media is a
major advance making it possible to delineate patterns of
anti-tumour reactivity at the clonal level (13, 14). There
are already reports, for example, of the generation of T cell
clones showing reactivity for melanoma cells used for autologous MLCT stimulation, which do not react with autologous
fibroblasts or mitogen-stimulated lymphoblasts (13). Also, in
another example, an HLA-restricted T cell line has been
produced whose cells are cytotoxic for the autologous human T
cell leukaemia/lymphoma/virus associate T cell lymphoma (16).
There are still technical problems with respect to the design
of culture conditions for maintaining long term growth of T
cell clones. In addition, the characteristics of lymphocyte
populations may undergo change in long term culture so complicating identification of the tumour cell component responsible
for T lymphocyte sensitization in patients. This is illustrated by recent studies on 'activated lymphocyte killer cells'

derived from malignant melanoma-infiltrating lymphocytes by
culture in T cell growth factor (17). These effector cells
initially showed restricted cytotoxicity for the autologous
tumour, but on continuous culture acquired cytoxicity for both
melanoma and non-melanoma derived target cells.

Effector Cells in Tumour Rejection.

A role for specifically sensitized T lymphocytes in tumour
rejection was originally deduced from studies with rodent
tumours showing that immunity could not be induced in T cell
deprived hosts, e.g. congenitally athymic mice. Adoptive
transfer experiments have also demonstrated the requirement
for specifically sensitiyed T lymphocytes in tumour rejection.
But the role of cytotoxic T cells in tumour rejection is
currently undergoing a re-appraisal (18). For example, the
non cytotoxic Ly1+ subset of T cells is required for effective
control of murine tumours (19) and cells in this subset are
also effective in chemoimmunotherapy of the Friend virus
induced leukaemia (20). A similar pattern is emerging with
respect to rat tumours where a non-cytotoxic T cell subset
(defined by monoclonal antibody W3/25) derived from
tumour-immunized donors adoptively transfer immunity to
virusand chemically-induced tumours (21). The precise function of the non-cytotoxic T cell populations in eliciting
tumour rejection is not clear, but one view is that they
collaborate, through factor production, with non-T cells
including macrophages and NK cells (18). For example, the
W3/25 T subset of rat T cells which can adoptively transfer
immunity, produces IL-2 on antigen stimulation (22) and
augments NK activity (23).

Supression of Tumour Immunity

Immunogenic tumours usually grow progressively when transplanted into normal immunocompetent recipients, whereas
pre-immunization, e.g. with radiation-attenuated tumour
cells, confers effective immunity to a subsequent tumour
challenge. This suggests that a developing tumour may
'escape' host immunosurveillance in a positive manner and a
number of pathways have been proposed (1, 24,25). 'Blocking
factors' such as circulating tumour antigen or immune complexes have been postulated to be involved, but the generation
of suppressor T cells (Ts) is probably the most important
pathway leading to abrogation of tumour immunity (24, 26).
The powerful influence of Ts lymphocytes is illustrated by
studies on UV-induced murine tumours which are highly immunogenic but are prevented from being rejected by impairment of
rejection responses through the production of suppressor cells
(27). The 'down-regulation' of tumour immunity by Ts lymphocytes is further illustrated by experiments showing that
rejection of a highly immunogenic murine fibrosarcoma, following adoptive transfer of spleen cells from tumour immune mice,
was abrogated by the simultaneous transfer of tumour-bearer
spleen cells (28).

3. NATURAL KILLER CELLS.

The role of natural killer cells in host resistance against malignant cells is being investigated in some considerable detail since these effector cells are present in most individuals (5) and they can be rapidly activated by agents such as Interferon (IFN). Also NK activation does not require prior host sensitization, as is the case with specific lymphocyte responses to antigenic stimuli, and so they may be viewed as a primitive type of host defence. Indeed the concept of NK cells functioning as a first line of defence against nascent malignant cells is seen as but one facet of a host surveillance system which provides a means for the destruction of infectious agents, especially virus-infected cells, and NK cells may even be involved in allograft rejection (29).

Human natural killer cells belong to a morphologically distinct lymphocytic population identified as large granular lymphocytes, LGL (30). But this cell population is quite heterogeneous with respect to markers which can be defined by monoclonal antibodies such as HNK-1 (31) and VEP13 (32). It has been shown for example, that a population of HNK-1+ cells lacks NK activity and this illustrates the need for more precise typing of human NK cells. Clinical studies of NK cells have been concerned largely with identifying activities of various tissue compartments, including tumours and tumour-draining lymph nodes (33, 34) and also how these can be augmented by various agents including interferon (7). The general conclusion is that solid tumours as well as malignant effusions are generally deficient in infiltrating NK cells (33). The reasons for this are complex, but one factor appears to be active suppression by tumour infiltrating cells characterized by adherent properties (35).

NK Cells in Tumour Rejection.

Much of the evidence supporting the view that NK cells modulate tumour growth in vivo has been derived from investigations correlating tissue and blood NK cell levels with growth of rodent tumours (5,6,29). More direct evidence that NK cells modulate tumour growth in vivo has been derived from experiments showing that their depletion leads to a diminished capacity for controlling tumours and also abrogates the therapeutic response induced by NK-activating agents. Murine NK cells express a neutral ganglioside (asialo-GM1 ganglio-N-tetraosylceramide) and removal of cells by treatment with rabbit anti-asialo GM1 and complement abrogates NK cell activity. Furthermore injection of this antiserum into mice markedly increased the tumorigenicity of one variant of the murine L5178Y lymphoma (cl. 27V-IC-2) selected for NK sensitivity but had no effect upon an NK-resistant subline (cl.27AV) (36). Elimination of intravenously injected murine lymphoma (YAC) cells, labelled with ^{125}I- iododeoxyuridine (^{125}I- dUrd) has also been used to assess the in vivo role of NK cells in tumour removal (37). This technique has been extended to show that the in vivo clearance of radioisotope labelled lymphoma cells was reduced some 30-fold following treatment of mice with anti-asialo GM1 antiserum (38). Similarly mouse antisera directed against NK cell determinants (anti-NK1) has been used to deplete NK activity in vivo and concomitantly there was a reduction in the ability of treated mice to eliminate intravenously injected 125 I-dUrd-labelled lymphoma cells (39).

Murine NK cells have been established in vitro and cloned as permanent cell lines so providing invaluable reagents for elucidating the role of NK cells in tumour rejection. This approach is typified by studies in which the effect of cloned NK cells was assayed in a model system in which the development of melanoma B16 lung colonies following intravenous inoculation of tumour cells was assessed in mice rendered NK-deficient by Cyclophosphamide (Cy) treatment (40). Injection of cloned NK cells 3 hours before intravenous injection of tumour cells produced a 50 to 85% reduction in lung tumour colonies compared with control (Cy-treated) mice using an NK-sensitive melanoma line. In contrast, injection of cell line-derived lymphoid cells lacking NK activity did not influence pulmonary tumour colonies.

Adoptive transfer of cloned NK cells was also able to inhibit the development of radiation-induced leukaemia (40). In this model, 70 to 90% of C57BL/6 mice receiving four weekly doses of low dose γ -irradiation from 4 weeks of age, develop lethal thymic leukaemia 3 to 5 months after the final irradiation. Injection of cloned NK cells immediately after the final irradiation was most effective in suppressing leukaemia development whereas later treatment (2 to 3 months after irradiation) was not effective. This type of split-dose irradiation results in marked depression of NK activity and the experiments suggest that the adoptive transfer of cloned NK cells may effect the elimination of nascent leukaemogenic cells so providing resistance to the development of radiation-induced leukaemia.

IMMUNOCOMPETENCE AND CANCER

Experimental animal tumours

It is well established that immunosuppression induced in several ways leads to increased incidences in experimental animal tumours and in some cases metastatic spread (4,41). This is well illustrated by early studies showing that selective immunosuppression with anti-lymphocyte antibodies enhances responses to oncogenic viruses. The influence of immunosuppression in chemical carcinogenesis is less clear and the situation here is complicated by more recent findings indicating that immunosuppression can be manipulated so as to remove cell suppression and so enhances tumour immunity (42).

Human cancer

The influence of immunosuppression on human cancer has been examined particularly with respect to immunosuppressive therapies (43). There is, for example, considerable data indicating increased cancer incidences in organ transplant recipients receiving immunosuppressive therapy.

The related question of the significance of immunocompetence in cancer patients with respect to prognosis is still unclear. Several investigations have established that patients with solid tumours, except where widespread dissemination is present, do not have gross defects in immune function. For example, trials with breast cancer patients and age-matched healthy controls revealed no major change in immunocompetence as assessed by tests for peripheral blood T and B lymphocyte levels and monocyte counts. T lymphocyte subset analysis using monoclonal antibodies indicated that the relative numers of cells with helper or suppressor phenotype were similar in both groups.

Finally functional tests including con A- and PHA-induced lymphocyte blastogenesis responses were not depressed, except in stage IV disease (44). From these tests it was concluded that immuno-competence was not impaired at the time of diagnosis. In contradistinction to this report, other groups have reported defects in immune function in cancer patients which have been considered to be prognostic. This is illustrated by one trial in which depressed PHA-induced lympho-proliferative responses were seen at relapse following surgical resection in lung cancer (46). Also, the capacity to generate autologous tumour cell induced lymphocyte responses has been reported to correlate with tumour-free period and survival time in patientys with lung cancer or sarcomas. More precise methods are required for elucidating the pathways leading to immunosuppression in patients with recurrent or metastatic disease. It is know for example, that peripheral blood lymphocytes from patients with metastatic cancer show a decreased capacity to produce interleukin-2 which is required for regulation of cellular immunity (47). The related question as to the cause of the immunodepression in patients with recurrent or metastatic disease is also highly pertinent especially if such changes are not observed in early disease.

CONCLUSIONS

1. Growth of malignant cells can be suppressed by host responses. This involves, in varying degrees, activated T cells, macrophages and natural killer cells.

2. Immunosuppression by extrinsic agents enhances growth of both animal and human cancers.

3. Cancer patients may or may not be immunosuppressed in the early stages of disease. Where metastatic cancer has developed, frequency of immunosuppression is much greater. it is not known, however, if the immunosuppression contributes to metastatic spread or is a consequence of this.

30

REFERENCES

1. BALDWIN, R.W. (1983). Specific antitumor immunity and its role in host resistance to tumors. In: R.B. Herberman (ed), Basic and Clinical Tumor Immunology. pp. 107-128.

2. BALDWIN, R.W. & PRICE, M.R. (1982). Neoantigen expression in chemical carcinogenesis. In: F.F. Becker (ed), Cancer: A comprehensive treatise. I. Etiology: Chemical and physical carcinogenesis. pp 507-548.

3. FROST, P. & KERBEL, R.S (1983). Immunology of metastasis: can the immune response cope with disseminated tumor? Cancer Metastasis Reviews, 2, 239-256.

4. PIMM, M.V. & BALDWIN, R.W. (1978). Immunology and immunotherapy of Experimental and Clinical Metastases. In: R.W. Baldwin (ed), Secondary Spread of Cancer, Academic Press, London. pp. 163-209.

5. HERBERMA N, R.B. (Ed). (1982). NK Cells and Other Natural Effector Cells. Academic Press, N.Y. pp. 1-1608.

6. HANNA, N. (1982). Role of natural killer cells in control of cancer metastasis. Cancer Metastasis Reviews, 1/1, 45-64.

7. BALDWIN, R.W. (1983). Immunotherapy of cancer. In: H.M. Pinedo, Cancer Chemotherapy, Annual 5, pp. 193-216.

8. KURTH, R., FENYO, E.M. KLEIN, E. & ESSEX, M. (1979). Cell-surface antigens induced by RNA tumour viruses. Nature, 279, 197-201.

9. EMBLETON, M.J. & BALDWIN, R.W. (1979). Asessment of cell mediated immunity to human tumor associated antigens. International Reviews of Experimental Pathology, 17, 49-95.

10. HERBERMAN, R.B. (Ed). Compendium of Assays for Immunodiagnosis of Human Cancer.- Developments in Cancer Research, Vol.1., Publishers, Elsevier/North Holland.

11. VANKY, F., WILLEMS, A., KREICBERGS, T., APARISI, M., ANDREEN L-A., BROSTROM, U., NILSONNE, U., KLEIN, E., & KLEIN, G. (1983). Correlation between lymphocyte-mediated auto-tumor reactivities and clinical course. I. Evaluation of 46 patients with sarcoma. Cancer Immunology, Immunotherapy, 16, 11-16.

12. DE VRIES, J.E., SPITS, H. (1984). Cloned human cyto-
    toxic T lymphocyte (CTL) lines reactive with autologous
    melanoma cells. I. In vitro generation, isolation, and
    anlaysis to phenotype and specificity. J. of
    Immunology, 132, 510-519.

13. VANKY, F., PETERFFY, A., BOOK, K., WILLEMS, J., KLEIN,
    E., & klein, G. (1983). Correlation between
    lymphocyte-mediated auto-tumor reactivities and the
    clinical course. II. Evaluation of 69 patients with
    lung carcinoma. Cancer Immunology Immunotherapy, 16,
    17/22.

14. VOSE, B.M. & WHITE, W. (1983). Tumour-reactive lympho-
    cytes stimulated in mixed lymphocyte and tumour culture.
    Cancer Immunology, Immunotherapy, 15, 227-236.

15. MOELLER, G. (Ed). Interleukins and lymphocyte
    activation. Immunological Reviews, 63, 5-209.

16. MITSUYA, H., MATIS, L.A., MEGSON, M., BUNN, P.A., MURRAY,
    C., MANN, D.L., GALLO, R.C. & BRODER, S. (1983).
    Generation of an HLA-restricted cytotoxic T cell line
    reactive against cultured tumor cells from a patient
    infected with human T cell leukemia/lymphoma virus.
    Journal of Experimental Medicine, 158, 994-999.d

17. BURNS, G.F., GOOD, M.F., RIGLAR, C., BARTLETT, P.F.,
    CRAPPER, R.M., MacKAY, I.R. (1984). Activated lympho-
    cyte killer cells derived from melanoma tissue or peri-
    pheral blood. Clinical Experimental Immunology - in
    press.

18. ROBINS, R.A. & BALDWIN, R.W. (1983). Role of T lympho-
    cyte subsets in tumor rejection: Implication for develo-
    ping biological response modifiers and monitoring
    tumor-host interactions during tumor development. J. of
    Biological Response Modifiers, 2: 101-109.

19. BHAN, A.K., PERRY, L.L., CANTOR, H., McCLUSKEY, R.T.
    BENACERRAF, B., GREENE, M.I. (1981). The role of T cell
    sets in the rejection of a methylcholanthrene induced
    sarcoma (S1509a) in syngeneic mice. American Journal of
    Pathology, 102, 20-27.

20. GREENBERG, P.D., CHEEVER, M.A. & FEFER, A. (1981).
    Eradication of disseminated murine leukemia by chemo-
    immunotherapy with cyclophosphamide and adoptively
    transferred immune Lyt 1+2- lymphocytes. J. Experimen-
    tal Medicine, 154/3, 952-963.

21. FERNANDEZ-CRUZ, E., GILMAN, S.C. & FELDMAN, J.D.
    (1982). Immunotherapy of a chemically-induced sarcoma in
    rats: characterization of the effector T cell subset and
    nature of suppression. J. Immunology, 128/3, 1112-1117.

22. CANTRELL, Doreen A, ROBINS, R.A. & BALDWIN, R.W. (1982). Rat lymphocyte subsets: Cellular requirements for the generation of T-cell growth factor. Cellular Immunology, 70, 367-372.

23. BRITTEN, Veronica, ROBINS, R.A. & BALDWIN, R.W. (1984). in vitro activation of natural killer-like cytotoxicity by specifically in vivo primed T-helper lymphocytes in the rat. immunology - in press.

24. NORTH, R.J., DYE, E.S., MILLS, C.D. & CHANDLER, J.P. (1982). Modulation of antitumor immunity: immunobiological approaches. Springer Seminars in Immunopathology, 5/2, 193-220.

25. HELLSTROM, K.E. HELLSTROM, I. & NELSON, K. (1983). Antigen-specific suppressor ("Blocking") factors in tumor immunity. In: A. Nowotny (ed). Biomembranes 11, Plenum Press N.Y. pp. 365-388.

26. NAOR, D. (1979). Suppressor cells: permitted or promotors of malignancy. Advances in Cancer Research 29, 45-125.

27. KRIPKE, M.L. (1976). Antigenicity of murine skin tumors induced by ultraviolet light. J. National Cancer Inst., 53, 1333-1336.

28. BERENDT, M.J. & NORTH, R.J. (1980). T cell mediated suppression of anti-tumor immunity. An explanation of progressive growth of an immunogenic tumor. Journal of Experimental Medicine, 151, 69-80.

29. HERBERMAN, R.B. (1982). Immunoregulation and natural killer cells., Molecular Immunology, 19/10, 1313-1321.

30. OLDHAM, R.K. (1983). Natural killer cell: Artifact to reality: An odyssey in biology. Cancer Metastasis Reviews, 2, 323-

31. ABO, T., MILLER, C.A., CARTLAND, G.L. & BALCH, C.M. (1983). Differentiation stages of human natural killer cells in lymphoid tissues from fetal to adult life. Journal of Experimental Medicine, 157, 273-284.

32. RUMPOLD , H., KRAFT, D., OBEXER, G., BOCK, G. & GEBHART, W. (1982). A monoclonal antibody against a surface antigen shared by human large granular lymphocytes and granulocytes. Journal of Immunology, 129, 1458-1464.

33. INTRONA, M. & MANTOVANI, A (1983). Natural killer cells in human solid tumors. In: Fidler, I.J. (ed). Cancer Metastasis Reviews, Vol. 2, pp 337-350. Martinus Nijhoff (Publishers).

34. KIMBER, I., MOORE, M., HOWELL, A., WILKINSON, M.J.S. (1983). Native and inducible levels of natural cytotoxicity in lymph nodes draining mammary carcinoma. Cancer Immunology, Immunotherapy, 15, 32-38.

35. UCHIDA, A., COLOT, M. & MICKSCHE, M. (1984). Suppres-
     sion of natural killer cell activity by adherent effusion
     cells of cancer patients. Suppression of motility,
     binding capacity and lethal hit of NK cells. British
     Journal of Cancer, 49, 17-23.

36. KAWASE, I., URDAL, D.L.,BROOKS , C.G. & and HENNEY, C.S.
     (1982). Selective depletion of NK cell activity in vivo
     and its effect on the growth of NK-sensitive and
     NK-resistant tumor cell variants. International Journal
     of Cancer, 29/5, 567-574.

37. GORELIK, E. & HERBERMAN, R.B. (1981). Radioisotope
     assay for evaluation of in vivo natural cell-mediated
     resistance of mice to local transplantation of tumor
     cells. International Journal of Cancer, 27/1, 709-720.

38. WILTROUT, R.H., GORELIK, E., BRUNDA, M.J., HOLDEN, H.T.
     & HERBERMAN, R.B. (1983). Assessment of in vivo natural
     antitumor resistance and lymphocyte migration in mice:
     comparison of 125 I-Iododeoxyruidine with 111
     Indium-Oxine and 51 Chromium as cell labels. Cancer
     Immunology, Immunotherapy, 14/3, 172-179.

39. POLLACK, Sylvia B. & HALLENBECK, Linda A. (1982). In
     vivo reduction of NK activity with anti-NK serum: Direct
     evaluation of NK cells in tumor clearance. International
     Journal of Cancer, 29/3, 203-207.

40. WARNER, J.F. & DENNERT, G. (1982). Effects of a cloned
     cell line with NK activity on bone marrow transplants,
     tumour delopment and metastasis in vivo. Nature, 300,
     31-34.

41. BALDWIN, R.W. (1973). Immunological aspects of
     carcinogenesis. Advances in Cancer Research, 18,1-

42. NORTH, R.J. (1982). Cyclophosphamide-facilitated
     adoptive immunotherapy of an established tumor depends on
     elimination of tumor-induced suppressor T cells. Journal
     of Experimental Medicine, 155/4, 1063-1074.

43. KINLEN, L.J. (1982). Immunosuppressive therapy and
     cancer. In: Israel Penn (Ed), Cancer Surveys, vol.1,
     No.4, pp. 565-583

44. LUDWIG, C., HARTMANN, D., LANDMANN, R., WESP, W.,
     ROSENFELDER, G. & OBRECHT, J.P. (1983). Immunocompe-
     tence in patients with early breast cancer. 2nd European
     Conference on Clinical Oncology, p. 170.

45. BRAUN, D.P., NISIUS, S., HOLLINSHEAD, A., HARRIS, J.E.
     (1983). Serial immune testing in surgically resected
     cancer patients. Cancer Immunolgy, Immunotherapy, 15/2,
     114-120.

34

46. *NAKAYAMA, E., ASANO, S., TAKUWA, N., YOKOTA, J. & MIWA, S. (1983). Decreased TCGF activity in the culture medium of PHA stimulated peripheral mononuclear cells from patients with metastatic cancer. Clinical and Experimental Immunology, 51, 511-516.*

THE IMMUNE SYSTEM AND INFECTIONS

P. Lambert

Hospital Cantonal, Universitaire Geneva,
Geneva, Switzerland

1. INTRODUCTION

Although a particular emphasis has often been given to other aspects immunology, a protective role against infections remains the major function of the immune system.

It is now obvious that different effector mechanisms, directly dependant on the modalities of antigen presentation, can be involved in different infectious diseases. Thus, with bacteria and some viruses, antibodies able to interact with complement and leucocytes are especially important. In other infections various cellular mechanisms are responsible for protection. Therefor, the influence of "immunotoxic" substances on immunity to infections should be considered in the context of the effector mechanisms involved.

2. T-CELL MEDIATED IMMUNE RESPONSES IN INFECTIOUS DISEASES.

Immunity to many infectious agents appears to involve the participation of specific T-cell immunity. In vitro, the main effector mechanisms are : (a) lysis of infected target cell expressing recognizable surface antigenic determinants ; (b) release of lymphokines acting on macrophages and other leucocytes ; (c) release of immune interferon acting on both leucocytes and tissue parenchymal cells (1).

It was often assumed that different T-cell sub-sets were involved in the expression of cytotoxic activity and in lymphokine mediated reactions. At the clonal level, this distinction between T-cells expressing different effector functions is not always clear-cut. Differences in effector functions may sometimes reflect differences in the receptor specificity of T-cell (e.g. recognition via class I or class II MHC antigens in association with antigens of the infectious agent) rather than physiological differences between T-cell subsets (2).

The relevance of these effector mechanisms to in vivo immunity and recovery from infectious diseases often remains to be clearly established. There is evidence that class I restricted virus-specific T cell are involved in recovery from certain acute virus infections. These cell population express specific antiviral cytotoxic activity in vitro. It is suggested that the same phenomenon occurs in vivo. Recently, adoptively transfered T cell clones with in vitro demonstrated cytotoxic activity were shown to exert a killing effect on virus infected cells in vivo (e.g. influenza virus, MSV) (3,4). Their in vivo effects probably reflect the killing of virus-infected target cells during the eclipse phase of the infection. However, other mechanisms such as lymphokine production, may be operative in vivo. In models using a facultative intracellular bacterium (L. monocytogenes) it has been shown that class II restricted T cell population release lymphokines after triggering with a specific antigen ; these mediators have been shown to activate macrophage and to increase their bacteriacidal activity (5).

In the majority of intracellular infections, the final destructive event may also depend on the activity of non-specific cells. Two major effector mechanisms can be identified : intracellular killing by phagocytic cells (e.g. in mycobacterial or toxoplasmal infection) and extracellular cytotoxicity, mediated for example by macrophage or by "natural killer" cells (6). A further possible role for the lymphokine system is the activation and recruitment of non-specific effector cells. A striking example is the enhancement of natural killer activity by interferon.

Functionnally different T cell subpopulation may be induced under different immunizing conditions. For example, live virus may in many instances induce a potent cytotoxic T cell response in parallel with delayed-type hypersensitivity and helper T cell activation, whereas antigenic viral components fail to induce cytotoxic T cells but can induce DTH T cells and helper cells. The difference may be qualitative since inactivated non-fusing virus, in general, does not prime for cytotoxic T effector cells restricted by class I antigens of the MHC, whereas inactivated fusing viruses do (3).

The finding that DTH reflects a T cell response, but not necessarily protection against reinfection, emphasiwes that DTH may not be a reliable indicator of protection. For example, killed L. monocytogenes induces DTH but no protection in mice, whereas hamsters that have recovered from Leishmania enriettii are resistant to challenge with this organism but show no detectable cutaneous DTH to Leishmania antigen. Similarly, leishmania-specific T cells with helper activity can induce a DTH reaction in Leishmania infected mice, but, paradoxically, this leads to an increased local proliferation of parasites within macrophages (7).

3. ANTIBODY-MEDIATED IMMUNE RESPONSES.

It has long been clear that, in many infectious diseases, circulating antibody is the major protective mechanism, e.g. in responses to encapsulated bacteri, toxoids, and enteroviruses. Especially important is the capacity of an immunized individual to give a better response to subsequent exposure to the parasite, i.e. to develop immulogical memory. All responses probably represent a balance between stimulation and suppression, the latter being particularly potent where self antigens or antigens closely resembling self are concerned : some meningococcal polysaccharides may fall into this category.

Current knowledge of effector mechanisms suggests the desirability of producing antibody isotypes that interact with the complement system or with leucocytes, e.g. in man IgG1 and IgG3, In certain situations, the production of secretory IgA, or IgE antibodies, may be beneficial whereas in other situations these classes of antibody may have deleterious effects. Little is known about the exact mechanisms that govern the control of the expression of different antibody isotypes. There is some evidence that a distinct subpopulation of T helper cells controls the formation of IgE antibodies. The same may be true for other isotypes. Many antibody responses are controlled by suppressor mechanisms, which may be antigen-specific or nonspecific. Some appear to be mediated by antibodies and T cells, others by activated macrophages or by humoral mediators such as prostaglandins or interferon. These may be involved in the regulation of isotype expression.

The induction of appropriate antibodies depends on factors related to the antigen (e.g. nature and amount of antigens, route of presentation to the host, adjuvant effects, presence of corresponding antibodies) as well as on factors related to the host (e.g. age, genetic constitution, nutritional status, concomitant infections). For example, meningococcal polysaccharides with MW under 120,000 are poorly immunogenic and at low doses may induce a tolerant state. Antibody production against such polysaccharides will be inhibited by the presence of cross-reacting antibodies and will also be very poor in young children. The induction of IgA deserves special attention in view of its importance in mucosal immunity. However, the production of specific IgA can be detrimental (e.g., meningococcal disease) (8). The induction of IgE appears now to be of particular relevance to the development of protective responses against metazoan parasites (e.g. schistosomiasis) (9).

4. PROTECTION AND IMMUNOPATHOLOGY

The pathological expression of infections can be directly influenced by the immune response of the host. Immune protection against viruses and other intracellular parasites may be mediated, at least partially, by host cell destruction. Thus the clinical outcome of an infection may be determined by the balance between viral cytopathogenicity and the competing T cell-mediated destruction of host cells. This balance between protective and harmful T cell effects may be influenced by viral parameters on the one hand, or host factors on the other. Immunization of the host can modulate this balance in either direction. In extreme cases full or partial protection can be accompanied by severe immunopathology.

Immunopathology can also result from an impaired immune response. Thus, a poor antibody response may favor the persistance of circulating antigens and the generation of immune complexes. Similarly, immune complexes involving low avidity antibodies tend to persist and be pathogenic. a low responsiveness to viruses or parasites of low cytopathogenicity can also favor the development of chronic imnmunnopathologically mediated diseases (10).

REFERENCES

1. *Immunological recognition and effector mechanisms in infectious diseases. Ed, G, Torrgiani and R. Bell, Schwabe and Co., Basel, 1981.*

2. *Zinkernagel, R.M. Experiments and speculation on antiviral specificity of T and B cells. Immunol, Rev. 58, 131-155, 1981.*

3. *Ada, G.L., N.K. Mac and C. Sweet. The regulation of influenza virus infection. In : "Progress in Immunology V", pp. 1295-1304, ed. Y. Yamamura and T. Tada, Academic Press Japan, Inc., 1983.*

4. *Engers, H.D., T. Lahaye, G.D. Sorenson, A.L. Glasebrook, C. Horvath, K.T. Brunner. Functional activity in vivo of effector T cells populations II anti-tumor activity exhibited by syngeneic anti-MoMULV-specific cytolytic T cell clones. J. Immunol. 133, 1664-1670, 1984.*

5. *Zinkernagel, R.M., A. Althage, B. Adler, R.V. Blanden, W.F. Davidson, U. Kees, M.B.C. Dunlop and D.C. Shreffler. H-2 restriction of cell-mediated immunity to an intracellular bacterium. Effector T cells are specific for Listeria antigen in association with H-2I region coded self-markers. J. Exp. Med. 145, 1353-1367, 1977*

6. *Eugui, E.M. and A.C. Allison. Activation of natural killer cells and its possible role inm immunity to intracellular parosites. In : "Immunological recognition and effector mechanisms in infectious diseases", ed. G. Torrigiani and R. Bell, Schwabe and Co., Basel, 161-188, 1981.*

7. *Titus, R.G., G.C. Lima, H.D. Engers, J.A. Louis. Exacerbation of murine cutaneous leishmaniasis by adoptive transfer of parosite-specific helper T cell populations capable of mediating leishmania major-specific delayed-type hypersensitivity. J. Immunol. 133, 1594-1600, 1984.*

8. *Griffiss, J.McL. Bactericidal activity of meningococcal antisera. Blocking by IgA of lytic antibody in human convalescent sera. J. Immunol. 114, 1779-1784, 1975.*

9. *Capron, A., J.P. Dessaint, M. Capron, M. Joseph. Effector mechanisms against schistosomes. Progress in Immunology V, ed. Y. Tamamura and T. Tada, Academic Press Japan, Inc. 1305-1316, 1983.*

10. *Zinkernagel, R.M. Protection and damage by immunity to intracellular parasites. Int. J. Microbiol. 1, 85-90, 1983.*

MECHANISMS OF AUTOIMMUNITY

Helga Gleichmann & Ernst Gleichmann

Diabetes-Research Institute and Medical Institute
of Environmental Hygien at the University of Duesseldorf
Duesseldorf, F.R.G.

INTRODUCTION

The immune system is highly specialized in recognizing and responding to foreign elements invading from the outside world while no apparent immune reactions develop towards self-constituents. Originally, it had been proposed that this state of self-tolerance was achieved by deletion of selfreactive clones during ontogeny and autoimmunity resulted from the effect of "forbidden clones" (1). From more recent experimental scrutiny, however, we know that potentially autoreactive lymphocytes do exist in the intact, healthy immune system. Normally, however, these cells are controlled by mechanisms precluding their reactivity or, at least, precluding the development of harmful autoimmunity.

The existence of autoreactive lymphocytes has been been established in the case of B cells (2-8). At least three different pathways, all of which involve T helper (T^H) cells, can lead to activation of the autoreactive B cells and thus cause the formation of autoantibodies (Fig. 1). the designation autoantibody is an unambiguous one where a serological reactivity to veritable autoantigens has been established, e.g. andibodies reacting with acetylcholine receptors in myasthenia gravis, with basement membrane structures in Goodpasture's syndrome, and so forth. Further examples of such genuine autoantibodies are listed in the uppr part of Table 1. Other immunological diseases are also mediated by antibodies, but the antibodies react to foreign determinants attached to self-constituents. An example for this is the autoimmune hemolytic anemia resulting from antibodies directed to penicillin, or the pesticide dieldrinm attached to human red blood cells (Table 1, A II). Thus, although these antibodies are deleterious for selfconstituents, such as erythrocytes, they are not, by definition, autoantibodies. Yet another example of an antibody-mediated immunological disease in which a self-constituent is damaged is glomerulonephritis resulting from deposition in the kidney of immune complexes which contain foreign material, such as microbial antigens, combined with the corresponding antibody. Thus, in this type of immunological diseases the relevant antigens are foreign, but self-constituents, such as erythroocytes and glomeruli, are damaged as innocent bystanders of specific antibody reaction.

To induce an antibody response to most antigens, cooperation between specific T^H cells and B-cells is required; this is especially so for the generation of antibodies possessing high affinity and belonging to the IgG class. During their cooperation the T^H cell responds to the so-called carrier portion of the antigen while the B cell responds to the so-called haptenic portion. A requirement for effective cooperation is that both the carrier and hapten determinants are on the same molecule so that a carrier-hapten bridge betweeen the specific T^H and B cell is formed. To relate this to autoimmunity one must realize that normal subjects have B cells that can respond to many self-antigens once they receive T-cell help. However, the control mechanisms that prevent autoreactive T^H cells from being activated are much tighter. Hence, because the required T^H cells are normally unresponsive, no proliferation of and antibody production by the autoreactive B cells can occur. The T-cell bypass concept, developed by Allison et al. (5), describes a detour around this restriction leading to stimulation of specific T^H cells, but not by self-antigen. Instead, the T^H cells participating in certain cases of autoantibody formation respond to foreign determinants introduced into the body. Thereby the T-cell help required by B cells is provided and autoantibody formation triggered.

Two variants of the T-cell bypass concept have been proposed (5). In the fiirst one (Fig. 1.A), the foreign determinant F occurs on a particular self-antigen S_F. Hence, a carrier-hapten bridge between the carier-reactive T^H and the autoreactive B cell is formed. Experimental examples of this pathway are the formation of anti-thyroglobulin autoantibodies following injection into mice of heterologous thyroglobulin (16) or of anti-erythrocyte autoantibodies following injection of rat erythrocytes (17). Generallly speaking, the antigenic material injected in these experiments contains two kinds of antigenic determinants. One kind is truly foreign because it consists of determinants characteristic of the heterologous donor. the other kind consists of determinants shared by both the donor and the host. These determinants are thus self-antigens occurring on host thyroglobulin and erythrocytes, respectively. The new, heterologous, antigenic determinants will stimulate T^H cells so that B cells, with receptors for self-determinants on the injected antigen, will receive help and produce autoantibody. This mechanism requires that the T^H and the B cell be contiguous and, thus, that the self-component be physically linked to the foreign component stimulating T^H cells. Only those of the autoreactive B cells are activated which are linked to the activated T^H cell by the carrier-hapten bridge. Thus, the specificity of the resulting autoantibodies is confined to those determinants occurring on the altered self-antigen S_F (Fig. 1.A).

In the second variant of the T-cell bypass concept the foreign antigenic determinant F is not confined to a particular self-antigen, but is part of the immune system itself in that it occurs on B cells (Fig. 1.B). An experimental example of this is the lupus-like autoimmuniity induced by systemic graft-versus-host reaction (GVHR). Clinical examples of this pathway to autoantibody formation probably include infections with lymphotropic viruses, such as the Epstein-Barr virus, and cases of drug-induced systemic lupus erythematosus (SLE) (see below). As shown in Fig. 1.B, T^H cells react to the foreign determinant and thus provide help to all B cell <u>irrespective</u>

of the immunological specificity of the latter. Therefore, as will be specified in detail below, several clones of autoreactive B cells, each possessing receptors for a different self-antigen, can be activated. Thus, the specificity of the resulting autoantibodies is a different and more heterogeneous one than that of the autoantibodies generated by the carrier-hapten bridge.

In a third condition allowing for autoantibody formation (Fig. 1.C) both the B and the T$_H$ cell are truly autoreactive. The recent experimental evidence supporting that possibility has been obtained from deliberate autoimmunization of normal animals and subsequent analysis of their T cells proliferating in response to the respective self-antigen (6,10). Furthermore, in human patients with spontaneously occurring myasthenia gravis T cells proliferating in vitro in response to acetylcholine receptor have been identified (11). Whether such proliferating autoreactive T cells can, indeed, react as T^H cells, as we assume in Fig. 1.C, has not yet been formally established, however. the experimental evidence indicates that, in normal animals, these autoreactive T cells are under tight control by specific T suppressor (T^S) cells (10).

As is the case with antibody-mediated immunological diseases, cell-mediated immunological lesions can likewise be divided into those caused by truly autoreactive T cells and those caused by T cells responding to foreign agents attached to self-constituents (Table 1.B). Evidence for the existence of truly autoreactive T cells has been provided by recent animal experiments from the group of Irun Cohen (10). They showed that T cells generated by autoimmunization to antigens, such as basic protein of myelin and thyroglobulin, were able to induce experimental allergic encephalomyelitis and thyroiditis, respectively, when transferred to normal, otherwise untreated, syngeneic recipients. That cell-mediated immunological lesions can develop as a result of T cell reactivity to foreign antigens associated with self-components is indicated by a large body of experimental and clinical evidence. Examples of this kind of cell-mediated immunological lesions are the contact dermatitis caused by gold salts or nickel, but many other examples, involving different tissues and different etiologic agents exist. Yet another example of an immunological lesion mediated by T cells is provided by cases of aplastic anaemia where a patient's T lymphocytes suppress the growth of erythroid and myeloid colonies in vitro (18, 19). Here, the eliciting antigen, if present at all, is unknown.

The present paper focuses first on the well-defined cellular pathogenesis of a spectrum of immunological diseases which can be induced by T lymphocytes in genetically normal mice undergoing systemic GVHR. In this model T lymphocytes respond to allogeneic structures of the major histocompatibity complex (MHC), i.e. H-2. The last part of the paper deals with the possible pathogenic mechanism(s) of GVHR-like immunological disorders which arise after exposure to foreign compounds and might be due to GVH-like reactions of T lymphocytes towards self-structures rendered non-self by the etiologic agent.

GRAFT-VERSUS-HOST REACTION (GVHR)

Experimental design

GVHR can be induced by injection of parental strain lymphocytes into adult, otherwise untreated F_1 hybrid recipients. For genetic reasons, the grafted cells are tolerated and not rejected by the semiallogeneic F_1 host. The injected T lymphocytes, however, recognize alloantigens which the F_1 host has inherited from the other parental strain (Fig. 2). these alloreactive donor T lymphocytes mediate the development of various immunological lesions. For the induction of immunological diseases by GVHR two conditions are required. 1) alloreactive T lymphocytes have to be present in the inoculum, and 2) a histoincompatibility has to be present in the F_1 recipient in order to activate the donor T lymphocytes. In non-irradiated F_1 mice, the histoincompatibility has to be provided by the recipient's H-2 complex.

Spectrum of GVHR-Induced Immunological Disorders

Fig. 3A shows the spectrum of pathological symptoms which can be induced by GVHR. the majority of these alterations have been observed as sequelae of GVHR in both man (20-21) and laboratory animals (21-23). Two basic forms of GVHR-induced pathological lesions have been distinguished. One form is characterized by stimulatory pathological symptoms, as shown on the left hand side of Fig. 3A. These symptoms include a persistent lymphoid hyperplasia of mainly B lymphocytes resulting in hyper- γ -globulinaemia and the formation of autoantibodies characteristic of SLE, such as antibodies against nuclear antigens (ANA), double-stranded DNA (dsDNA), erythrocytes, and thymocytes (3, 24-29). In addition, stimulatory GVH symptoms include a severe immune complex glomerulonephritis (ICGN) in which antibodies agains ANA and envelope antigens of murine leukemia virus (MuLV) are involved (30). This ICGN may be accompanied by deposition of immunoglobulin along the basement membrane of skin (4). These SLE-like GVH symptoms may occur together with symptoms characteristic of other collagen vascular diseases including arthritis (24, 31, 32) arthritis (32), Sjùgren- and scleroderma-like lesions, and liver changes resembling sclerosing cholangitis (31, 32). Usually, the stimulatory GVH symptoms present themselves as chronic GVH disease (GVHD).

The other basic form of GVHR-induced lesions is characterized by suppressive (hypoplastic) pathological symptoms (see right side of Fig. 3A) which clinically manifest themselves as an acute GVHR. The suppressive GVH symptoms consist of a severe hypoplasia of the lympho-hemopoietic compartment leading to aplastic anaemia and hypo- -gammaglobulinaemia (27-29, 33, 34). The microbiological status of the recipients has an influence on whether or not this form of GVHR will terminate at lethal GVH disease.

Subsets of Alloreactive T Lymphocytes Induce Either Stimulatory or Suppressive GVHR Syndromes

Several experimental approaches have been taken to analyze if functionally different subsets of alloreactive donor T cells are activated in the F_1 recipient undergoing different forms of GVHD. One approach was to separate the donor T cells into Lyt subsets before transferring them into F_1 recipients. In a second approach unseparated T cells were injected into F_1 recipients differing only at class I and/or II H-2 antigens (26, 27). In addition, in vitro studies were performed to dissect the cellular and immunogenetic requirements of allohelp and allosuppression (35). Based on the results of thesse experiments a general concept of the cellular pathogenesis of GVHR-induced diseases has been elaborated, as illustrated in Fig. 3B.

Thus, when the donor's Lyt 1+2- T-helper (T^H) cells (28) are activated by class-II MHC structures of the F_1 recipient persistent lymphoid hyperplasia and SLE-like GVHD developed (26, 27). Whether these class-II-reactive donor T cells also trigger the GVH-associated malignant lymphomas (23, 36) and symptoms of collagen vascular disease, such as arthritis, Sjùgren- and scleroderma-like disease, has not yet been established.

The cellular interactions leading to suppressive pathological GVH symptoms are more complex. Optimal induction of the suppressive GVH symptoms required non-Lyt-separated donor T cells (28) and incompatibility in the F_1 recipients at both class I and class II MHC structures (27). In such parent F_1 combinations there is a sequential alloactivation, first of donor T_H cells and then T-allosuppressor/killer ($T^{S/K}$) cells that cause the suppressive pathological symptoms (Fig. 3B; 27, 29, 33). Thus, after a brief initial activation of Lyt 1^+2^- donor T^H cells, which results in a transient lymphostimulation and B-cell activation in the first week of GVHR, class I-specific Lyt 2^+ donor $T^{S/K}$ cells are induced (29, 34, 37). The detection of these F_1-reactive $T^{S/K}$ effector cells in GVHR, mice was strictly confined, both in time and in the parent F1 combinations being compared, to mice exhibiting the suppressive pathological symptoms (27, 29, 34). This established that F1-reactive donor $T^{S/K}$ cells are the effector cells causing the hypoplastic GVHR syndrome (Fig. 3A).

Mechanism of Autoantibody Formation During GVHR

There is general agreement that potentially autoreactive B lymphocytes exist in healthy individuals, including genetically normal F_1 mice (50). Although normally silent these F1 B cells are able to secrete IgC autoantibodies upon adequate activation. During GVHR such an activation is delivered by the donor's alloreactive T^H cells. Host (F1)-derived T cells, in contrast, counteract autoimmunization by the GVHR and are thus not required for the activation of those autoreactive B cells (3, 30). The mechanism underlying the GVHR-induced autoimmunization most likely is abnormal T-B-cell cooperation. During normal T-B-cell cooperation for antibody production both TH and B cells react to antigenic sites <u>on the same molecule</u> (Fig. 4A). A stable carrier-hapten bridge is formed between the two specific cells. the haptenic part of the immunogen is recognized by the B cell and delivers signal 1, whereas the carrier part is recognized by the TH cell. The TH cell secretzes helper factor(s), here designated signal 2 (38). Macrophages participate in this activation process as antigen-presenting cells.

During <u>abnormal</u> T-B-cell cooperation F_1B cells receive signal 1 by specific antigen, or hapten, and signal 2, i.e. help, by alloreactive T^H cells of the parental donor strain (5, 38, 39; Fig. 4B). The T^H cells are Lyt 1^+2^- cells recognizing allogeneic class-II MHC antigens (35). Antibodies resulting from abnormal T-B-cells cooperation <u>in vivo</u> belong mainly to the IgG class (39, 40) and have high <u>affinity</u> (42).

The first investigations of abnormal T-B-cell cooperation during GVHR were performed with <u>non</u>-self compounds as antigen such as sheep red blood cells (SRBC), or haptens such as trinitrophenyl (TNP) and dinitrophenyl (DNP), coupled to special carrier molecules. These studies demonstrated that a positive allogeneic effect, i.e. a maximally enhanced IgG antibody response, induced by alloreactive T^H cells (39, 40) only occured if the foreign antigen was present at the onset of GVHR, thus providing signal 1 to the F1B cells (255, 40, 42-48). Hence, in addition to signal 2 (allohelp), signal 1 (provided by epitopes on the antigen) is required for abnormal T-B-cell cooperation to become optimally effective.

During GVHR, alloreactive donor T^H cells provide signal 2, or help, to the F_1B cells. This type of help is undiscriminatory because all F_1B cells are semiallogeneic and can thus receive allohelp (Fig. 4B). Nevertheless, the resulting B-cell stimulation is a highly selective one. The reason for this is that the mere presence of a self-antigen is not enough to provide an adequate signal 1 to the corresponding autoreactive B cell. Apparently, only those kinds of self-antigen depicted in fig. 4B 3 and 4 seem to supply an effective signal 1. By this reasoning we try to explain the observation that auto-antibody formation in SLE-like GVHD fails to be a random polyclonal event (9, 16).

GVHR-LIKE IMMUNOLOGICAL DISORDERS INDUCED BY MODIFIED SELF

Concept of Pathogenesis

The basic principles established for T cell alloreactivity, as operating in GVHR, might also operate in the cellular pathoge-nesis of GVHR-like disease developing after exposure to an etiologic agent. GVHR-like cellular interactions may be stimulated in autologous or syngeneic systems provided cell-surface determinants of lymphohemopoietic B cells and/or antigen-presenting cells were modified by a give etiologic agent. These "altered-self" structures might trigger reac-tions by autologous T cells comparable to the reactions of parental strain T cells toward the allogeneic structures on F_1 recipient cells (Fig. 5).

Thus, autologous or syngeneic T$_H$ cells may be preferentially activated if a foreign antigen X is recognized in association with class II MHC determinants (39, 49, 50). In contrast, T$^{K/S}$ cells may be preferentially activated if the same foreign antigen X is recognized in association with class I MHC determinants (51). Thus, depending on the T cell subpopulation activated, stimulatory or suppressive pathological symptoms amy develop, as shown in Fig. 3A. Certain drugs and viruses such as Epstein Barr, cytomegalo and rubella virus, are suspected to create such non-self structures because they have been found to be associated with various GVHR-like diseases in man.

Drugs Known to Induce GVHR-like Diseases

An array of drugs have been reported to precipitate in some patients symptoms out of the broad spectrum of GVHR-like pathological symptoms shown in Fig. 3A. For example, the anticonvulsant drug diphenylhydantoin (DPH) has been reported to cause hyper- μ -globulinaemia, drug-induced SLE, arthritis, dermatitis, toxic epidermal necrolysis, B-cell lymphomas, aplastic anemia and hypo- μ globulinaemia (23, 52, 53). Furthermore, lymphadenopathy, features of drug-induced SLE, or thrombocytopenia and granulocytopenia developed during therapy of rheumatoid arthritis with D-penicillamine (54) or captopril, an anti-hypertensive drug inhibiting angiotensin-I-converting enzyme (55). Hydralazine, another antihypertensive drug also causes drug- induced SLE (56).

Studies on the Pathogenic Mechanism of Drug-Induced GVHR-Like Symptoms

The popliteal lymph node (PLN) assay, an established method for measuring local GVH and HVG reactivity, was used to explore the immunological effects of sensitizing drugs in vivo. It was found that subcutaneous injection of DPH, D-penicillamine, or captotril into the hind foot pad of mice resulted in a significant dose-dependent enlargement of the draining popliteal lymph node. T lymphocytes were required for triggering this drug-induced enlargement. Congenitally athymic nu/nu recipients, i.e. T cell-deprived mice, failed to react to the inoculation of these drugs, whereas their +/nu counterparts readily did so (57, and H.G., unpublished results). Although T cells were required for the DPH-induced PLN enlargement the majority of the proliferating cells in the PLN were non-T cells (57, 58). These observations exclude that the PLN reactions were caused by a direct mitogenic effect of DPH on B lymphocytes. Furthermore, neither DPH, nor D-penicillamine or captopril exerted non-specific mitogenic or comitogenic effects on lymphocytes in vivo and in vitro (58, 59, 60 and H.G. unpublished results). Subcutaneous injection of phenobarbital, a drug that is pharmacologically and chemically related to DPH, but does not cause GVHR-like side-effects, failed to induce PLN enlargement (58).

Additional studies with DPH reveled that subcutaneous inoculation of DPH induced a more than 100-fold increase of IgG-secreting cells in the draining PLN as compared to the uninjected controlateral PLN (58). Syngeneic spleen cells

which had been penetrated with DPH in vitro also induced
significant PLN enlargement. The specificity of the
DPH-induced antibodies remains to be tested. It is unlikely,
that these antibodies are directed agains the small haptenic
compound DPH. This assumption is consistent with the finding
that DPH-specific antibodies were only rarely seen in patients
sensitized to the drug (59, 61). A DPH-specific lymphoproliferation in vitro was demonstrated in several patients sensitized to the drug (53, 60).

The data on DPH is consistent with the concept that the parent
molecule, or its metabolites, can render membrane structures
of potentially stimulatory cells, such as dendritic cells and
B lymphocytes, "non-self". T lymphocytes would then recognize
these altered membrane determinants in conjunction with
autologous MHC structures and respond in a GVHR-like manner,
resulting in the development of the respective immunological
lesions.

The proposed immunopathogenesis induced by an etiologic agent
may also be relevant for the mechanism of mercury chloride
($HgCl_2$)-induced lesions in rats (62-63). Autoimmune
glomerulonephritis, splenomegaly, antinuclear and anti-DNA
antibodies were observed in $HgCl_2$-susceptible strains, but not
in strains carrying other MHC haplotypes. $HgCl_2$-induced
B-cell activation was observed, both in vivo and in vitro,
only in the susceptible strain. Interestingly, the B-cell
activation in vitro was T-cell-dependent (62).

No PLN enlargement was found in several mouse strains which
had been treated with hydralazine or methyldopa, drugs that
are well known to induce SLE and autoimmune hemolytic anemia,
respectively (64, 65). The pathogenetic mechanism(s) by which
these drugs induce the immunological injuries remain to be
evaluated.

Interestingly, in man, a high association has been reported
between certain genetic factors and several etiologic agents
causing GVHR-like symptoms (Table 2). There is a preponderance of both HLA-DR4 positivity and slow acetylation in
patients with hydralazine-induced SLE (56). Moreover, significant association has been found between gold- or
D-penicillanine- induced glomerular nephropathy and HLA-DR3
and B8 (66), between vinylchloride-induced severe
scleroderma-like lesions and DR5 (67), and between DR3 and DR4
and SLE-like autoantibodies after ingestion of the Spanish
toxic oil (68). DPH-induced IgA-deficiency is associated with
HLA-2 (69).

CONCLUSION

The genetic and cellular requirements for induction by GVHR of
a broad spectrum of immunological disorders on the one hand
and the GVHR-like features induced by DPH (57, 58) and HgCl2
(62, 63) on the other hand are considered relevant for the
pathogenesis that may underly some of the human GVHR-like
diseases associated with certain HLA alleles. A give etiolo-

gic agent is assumed to induce an antigenic site X on cell-surface determinants ("altered-self"). In a susceptible individual autologous T lymphocytes lmight recognize and respond to these antigenic sites akin to the way parental strain T lymphocytes recognize and respond to semiallogeneic MHC structures of F_1 cells in the GVHR model (Fig. 3, 9). Thus, T^H cells are preferentially by activated if the antigenic site X is mainly associated or seen together with class-II HLA structures. In contrast, $T^{K/S}$ cells are preferentially activated if the antigenic site X is mainly associated or seen together with class-I HLA structures. Correspondingly, immunological disorders consisting of stimulatory or suppressive GVHR-like symptoms would ensue as illustrated in Fig. 3. Certainly, a number of other immunological and non-immunological factors such as lymphokines, sex hormones, and metabolic pathways of the etiologic agent, also contribute to the complex processes eventually resulting in immunopathological lesions. Therefore, in most cases the induction of disease by an etiologic agent depends on the presence of susceptibility alleles at a number of different genetic loci. Assessment of the pathogenic pathways by which identified etiologic agents induce immunological diseases should increase our knowledge of the etiopathology of the same diseases developing spontaneously. These investigations may help to elaborate methods to eventually prevent and/or cure those diseases.

Table 1. Classification of some immunological reactions leading to
pathological symptoms

A. Antibody-mediated pathological symptoms

I. Genuine autoantibodies

Organ-specific self-antigens involved	Resulting diseases
Erythrocytes	Autoimmune hemolytic anemia
Granulocytes	Autoimmne granulocytopenia
Thrombocytes	Autoimmune thrombocytopenia
Glomerular basement membrane	Goodpasture's syndrome
Acetylcholine receptor	Myasthenia gravis
Insulin receptor	Some cases of insulin-resistant diabetes
Intrinsic factor	Pernicious anemia
Thyroglobulin	Autoimmune thyroiditis
Other hormones	Autoimmune endocrinopathies
Intercellular antigens in the epidermis	Pemphigus

Ubiquitous self-antigens	
Double-stranded DNA	Systemic lupus erythematosus (SLE
Single-stranded DNA and other nuclear antigens	SLE and other collagen vascular diseases
Various cytoplasmic and cell--membrane antigens, such as cardiolipin	SLE and other collagen vascular diseases

II. Antibodies to drugs or
environmental agents bound to
self-antigens

drugs, such as penicillin	Immune hemolytic anemia
"	Immune granulocytopenia
"	Immune thrombocytopenia
"	Serum sickness
"	Anaphylaxis
Pesticide (dieldrin) (14)[a]	Immune hemolytic anemia

B. Cell-mediated pathological lesions

I. Cell-mediated immunity
to self-antigens

T-cell line specific for basic protein of myelin (10)	Experimental allergic encephalomyelitis
T-cell line specific for cross-reacting antigen on Mycobact. tuberculosis and rat joints (10)	Experimental arthritis

II. Cell-mediated immunity to drugs
    or environmental agents attached
    to self-antigens

Various drugs including   Contact dermatitis
    local anaesthetics,   and/or fixed drug
    penicillins, sulfonamides   eruptions
Heavy metals, such as gold salts,   Contact dermatitis and/or
    nickel, mercurials   fixed drug eruptions
Pesticides (15)   Contact dermatitis

---

a
   Selected references only are given.

Table 2. Selected reports on HLA associations with induced autoimmune phenomena

Symptoms	Induced By	HLA Association	References
Drug-induced SLE	Hydralazine	DR4	56
Nephropathy	D-Penicillamine	DR3 and B8	66
Nephropathy	Aurothiomalate	DR3 and B8	66
Selective IgA deficiency	Diphenylhydantoin	A2	69
Various autoantibodies	Spanish toxic oil	DR3, DR4	68
Severe scleroderma like-lesions	Vinyl-chloride	DR5	67

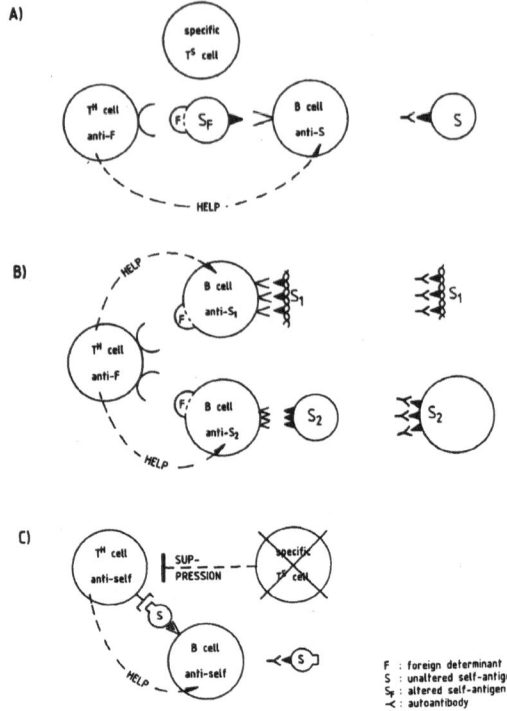

Fig. 1 Depicting three different pathways leading to autoantibody formation. A common feature of all three possibilities is that normally occurring autoreactive B cells are stimulated to antibody formation by the combined action of 1) their recognition of epitopes characteristic of self-antigen and 2) the activation of T helper (T^H) cells. A common feature of (A) and (B) is that foreign antigenic determinants (F) have been introduced into the syste. Hence, the T^H cell cooperating with the autoreactive B cells react, not with native self antigen, but with foreign determinant F. In C), by contrast, foreign determinants are lacking and both the B cell and the T^H cell are autoreactive.

In A), the foreign determinant F is located on the same molecule or cell as the unaltered self-epitope to which the autoreactive B cell reacts.

In B), the foreign determinant F is physically separate from the unaltered self-antigen S to which the B cell reacts. As a result of this, only those of the autoreactive B cells are activated that react to self-antigens possessing repeating identical epitopes (9). This possibility is elaborated in greater detail below (cf. Fig. 4B).

In C), it is assumed that autoreactive T^H and B cells can cooperate because of a failure of normally occurring specific T suppressor (T^S) cells. Experimental evidence for this pathway stems from the establishment in vitro of autoreactive T-cell lines obtained from either animals (10) or patients with myastehia gravis (11).

As in any other immunological reaction, the reactivity of the TH cells involved in autoantibody formation may be counteracted by specific TS cells. Direct evidence for this is strongest in the experiments underlying pathway (A) and (C). The fine specificity of such T^S cells is not depicted, however, because there are several possibilities for it: (1) the T^S cell may have an anti-idiotypic receptor for the idiotype, i.e. the antigen recognition structure, on the T^H cell (12), (2) both the TS and the TH cell may have an identical receptor and thus compete for the epitopes on the antigen, or (3) the T^S and T^H cell may recognize different epitopes on a given antigen (reviewed in 13).

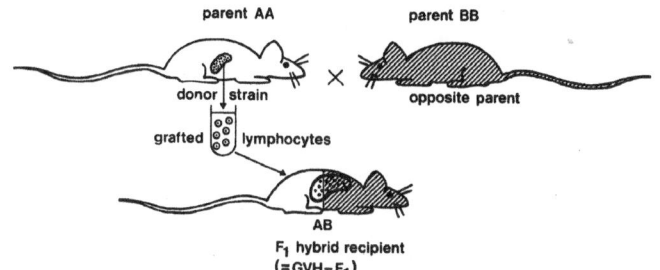

Fig.   2 Induction of GVHR in F_1 mice. Parental strain T lymphocytes, injected into F_1 recipients, react to MHC-incompatible structures derived from the opposite parent.

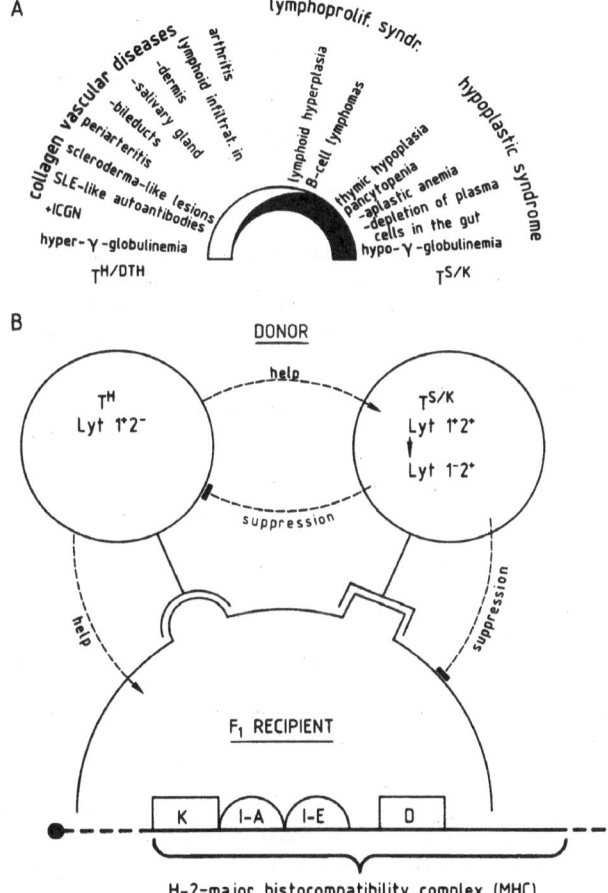

Fig.   3 Spectrum and concept of cellular pathogenesis of immunological disorders resulting from GVHR in F_1 mice

A.   Spectrum of pathological lesions that may develop in GVH F_1 mice **B**. Concept of the basic cellular and MHC requirements for induction of stimulatory (left) and suppressive (right) GVHR lesions, respectively. the F_1 cell depicted at the bottom represents a stimulator/target cell situated at various anatomical sites, such as lympho-hemopoietic tissue, endothelium, synovia, skin, salivary gland, bile ducts, gut and lungs.

52

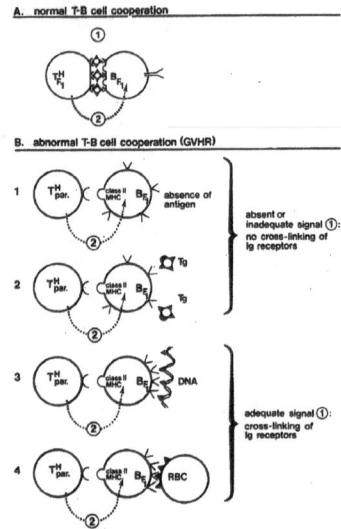

Fig. 4 Hypothesis showing essential differences between normal and abnormal T-B-cell cooperation in order to explain the special autoantibody formation seen in SLE-like GVHD. All B cells depicted here are unprimed; hence, their average receptor affinity is low and stable binding of the epitopes on the antigen is crucial.

A. In normal T-B-cell cooperation the B and the T^H cells react to antigenic sites on the same molecule, thus a stable carrier-hapten bridge between the two specific cells is formed. The haptenic part of the immunogen is recognized by the B cell resulting in signal 1 to the B cell (29); the carrier part of the immunogen is recognized by the T^H cells which secrete helper factor(s), here designated signal 2 (29). Macrophages also participate in normal T-B cooperation, but are not depicted here.

B. In abnormal T-B-cell cooperation the alloreactive T^H cell reacts to a molecule, i.e. alloantigen, which is physically separate from the molecule the B cell reacts to. This alloreaction provides help, or signal 2, to all F_1 B cells irrespective of their antibody specificity. Other than in normal T-B-cell cooperation, there is no T^H cell that focuses the epitopes to the B cell. Hence the B cell has to interact with the hapten all by itself. For an effective signal 1, multipoint binding between the epitopes on the hapten and the B cell is required.

1) If there is no hapten, no signal 1 is delivered and the B cell cannot be triggered into optimal proliferation and IgG production.

2) Antigen is a globular protein, such as autologous thyroglobulin (Tg); whose epitopes can only bind in a monovalent fashion to the Ig receptors of the B cell. Monovalent binding is ineffective, because it is of low avidity and does not cross-link the Ig receptors.

3) and 4) Antigen possesses repeating identical epitopes located on either a rigid backbone, such as DNA, or a cell surface; in addition, epitopes may be electrically charged. This allows for multipoint high avidity binding to and cross-linking of the Ig receptor and thus provides an adequate signal 1. B cells are direven into clonal proliferation and maximal IgG secretion.

The difference between 1) and 2) on the one hand and 3) and 4) on the other hand accounts for the phenomenon of selective IgG (auto)antibody formation found in SLE-like GVHD where autoantibodies to DNA and cell-surface epitopes, but not to globular protein antigens, such as Tg, are formed.

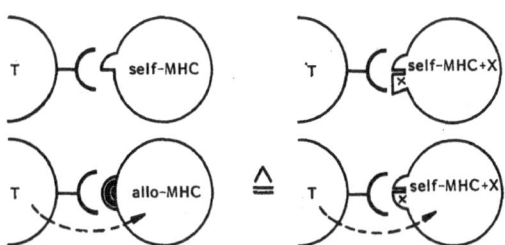

Fig. 5 Simplified scheme of T-cell reactions towards MHC structures

<u>A</u>.   The T cell has a receptor for recognition of unaltered self-MHC structures. However, the T cell remains inactive because the avidity of this interaction is too low.

<u>B</u>.   Here, the T cell also remains inactive because the complex formed between self-MHC and the antigenic site X does not fit its receptor.

<u>C</u>.   The T cell is activated by specific recognition of allogeneic MHC structures, as in GVHR.

<u>D</u>.   The T cell is activated because the complex formed between self MHC and the antigenic site X fits its receptor. This situation is virtually identical with the T cell alloreactivity shown in C.

REFERENCES

1. Burnet, F.M., 1959, In: The Clonal Selection Theory of Acquired Immunity. Vanderbilt University Press, Nashville, Tennessee.

2. Fialkow, P.J., Gilchrist, C. & Allison, A.C., 1973, Autoimmunity in chronic graft-versus-host disease. Clini. Exp, Immunol. 13, 479-486.

3. Gleichmann, E. & Gleichmann, H., 1976, Diseases caused by reactions of T-lymphocytes to incompatible structures of the major histocompatibility complex: I. Autoimmune hemolytic anemia, Eur. J. Immunol. 6, 899-906.

4. Elven, E.H. van, Agterberg, J. Sadal, S., & Gleichmann, E., 1981, Diseases caused by reaction of T lymphocytes to incompatible structures of the major histocompatibility complex: II. Autoantibodies deposited along the basement membrane of skin and their relationship to immune-complex glomerulonephritis. J. Immunol. 126, 1684-1691.

5. Allison, A.C., Denman, A.M. & Barnes, R.D., 1971, Hypothesis. Cooperating and controlling functions of thymus-derived lymphocytes in relation to autoimmunity. Lancet 2, 135-140.

6. Rose, N.R., Kong, Y,M,, Okayasu, I., Giraldo, A.A., Beisel, K. & Sundick, R.S., 1981, T-cell regulation in autoimmune thyroiditis. Immunol. Rev. 55, 299-314.

7. Fournie, G.J., Lambert, P.H. & Miescher, P.A., 1974, Release of DNA in circulating blood and induction of anti-DNA antibodies after injection of bacterial lipopolysaccharides. J. Exp. Med. 140, 1189-1206.

8. Fernandez, C. Hammerstroem, L., Moeller, G., Primi, D. & Smith, C.J.E., 1979, Immunological tolerance affects only a subpopulation of the antigen-specific B lymphocytes: evidence against clonal deletion as the mechanism of tolerance induction. Immumol. rev. 43, 3-41.

9. Gleichmann, E., Pals, S.T., Rolonk, A.G., Radaszkiewicz, T. & Gleichmann, H., 1984, Graft-versus-host reactions: clues to the etiopathology of a broad spectrum of immunological diseases, Immunology Today, 5, in press.

10. Cohen, I.R., Ben-Nun, A., Holoshitz, J., Maron, R. & Zerubavel, R., 1983, Vaccination against autoimmune T lymphocytes. Immunology Today, 4, 227-230.

11. Hohlfeld, R., Toyka, K.V., Heininger, K., Grosse-Wilde, H. & Kalies, I. 1984, Autoimmune human T-lymphocytes specific for acetylcholine receptor are restricted to HLA-DR and inhibited by anti-DR antibodies. Nature 310, 244-246.

12. Bona, C. & Paul, W.E., 1979, Cellular basis of regula-
    tion of expression of idiotype. I. T-suppressor cells
    specific for MOPC 460 idiotype regulate the expression of
    cells secreting anti-TNP bearing 460 idiotype. J. Exp.
    Med., 149, 592-600.

13. Koelsch, E., 1984, interaction of suppressor & helper
    antigenic determinants in the dominance of either tolera-
    nce or immunity (editorial). Scand. J. Immunol. 19,
    387-393.

14. Hamilton, H.E., Morgan, D.P. & Simmons, A. (1978), A
    pesticide (dieldrin)-induced immunohemolytic anemia.
    Environ. Research, 17, 155-164.

15. Ercegovich, C.D., 1973, Relationship of pesticides to
    immune responses. Fed. Proc. 32, 2010-2016.

16. Weigle, W.O., 1980, Analysis of autoimmunity through
    experimental models of thyroiditis and allergic
    encephalomyelitis. Adv. Immunol. 30, 159-275.

17. Cox, K.O., & Howles, A., 1981, Induction and regulation
    of autoimmune hemolytic anemia in mice. Immunol. Rev.
    55, 31-51.

18. Bacigalupo, A., Podesta, M., Van Lint, M.T., Vimercati,
    R., Cerri, R, Rossi, E., Risso, M., Carella, A., Santim,
    G., Damasio, E., Giordano, D. and Marmont, A.A., 1981.
    Severe aplastic anemia: correlation of in vitro tests
    with clinical response to immunosuppression in 20
    patients. Brit. J. Haematol. 47, 423-432.

19. Torok-Storb, B.J., Sieff, C., Storb, R., Adamson, J. &
    Thomas E.D., 1980, In vitro tests for distinguishing
    possible immune-mediated aplastic anemia from
    transfusion-induced sensitization. Blood 55, 211-215.

20. Hansen, J.A., Woodruff, J.M. & Good, R.A., 1981, The
    graft-versus-host reaction in man. Genetics clinical
    features and immunopathology. In: Comprehensive
    Immunology. Safai, B. Good, R.A.(eds.) New York, Plenum
    Press 7, 229-257.

21. Brill, H. & Benner, R.. 1982. Cell-mediated immunity
    to histocompatibility antigens. CRC Crit. Rev. Lab.
    Sci. (in press).

22. Beschorner, W.E., P.J. Tutschka & G.W. Santos, 1982.
    Chronic graft versus-host disease in the rate rediation
    chimera. Transplantation 33 393-399.

23. Gleichemann, H. & Wilke, W., 1976, Autoimmunization and
    lymphomagenesis in parent F1 combinations differing at
    the major histocompatibility complex: model for sponta-
    neous disease caused by altered self-Antigens?
    Transplant. Rev. 31, 156-224.

56

24. Gleichmann, E., van Elven, E.H., van der Veen, J.P.W., 1982, A systemic lupus erythematosus (SLE)-like disease in mice induced by abnormal T-B-cell cooperation. Preferential formation of autoantibodies characteristic of SLE. Eur. J. Immunmol. 12, 152-158.

25. van Rappard-van der Veen, F.M., Kiesel, U, Poels, L. Schuler. W., Melief, C.J.M., Landegent, J. & Gleichmann, E., 1984, Further evidence against random polyclonal antibody formation in mice with lupus-like graft-versus host disease. J. Immunol. 132, 1814-1820.

26. van Rappard-van der Venn, F.M., Rolink, A.G., & Gleichmann, E., 1982, Diseases caused by reactions of T lymphocytes towards incompatible structures of the major histocompatibility complex. VI. Autoantibodies characteristic of systemic lupus erythematosus induced by abnormal T-B-cell cooperation across I-E. J. Exp. Med. 155, 1555-1560.

27. Rolink, A.G., Pals, S.T. & Gleichmann, E., 1983, Allosuppressor- and allohelper-T cells in acute and chronic graft-versus-host disease. II. F1 recipients carrying mutations at H-2K and/or I-A J. Exp. Med. 157, 755-771.

28 Rolink, A.G. & Gleichmann, E., 1983, Allosuppressor and allohelper-T cells in acute and chronic graft-versus-host disease. III. Different Lyt subsets of donor T cells induce different pathological symptoms. J. Exp. Med. 158, 546-558.

29. Pals, S.T., Radaszkiewicz, T. & Gleichmann, E., 1984, Allosuppressorand allohelper-T cells in acute and chronic graft-versus-host disease. IV. Activation of donor allosuppressor cells is confined to acute GVHD. J. Immunol. 132, 1669-1678.

30. Rolink, A.G., Gleichmann, H. & Gleichmann, E., 1983, Diseases caused by reactions of T lymphocytes to incompatible structures of the major histocompatibility complex. VII Immune-complex glomerulonephritis. J. Immunol. 130, 209-215.

31. van Rappard-van der Veen, F.M., Radaszkiewicz, T., Terraneo, L. & Gleichmann, E., 1983, Attempts at standardization of lupus-like graft-versus-host disease: Inadvertent repopulation by DBA/2 spleen cells of H-2-different non-irradiated F1 mice. J. Immunol. 130, 2693-2701.

32. Pals, S.T., Radaszkiewicz, T., Roozendaal, L. & Gleichmann, E., 1984, Chronic progressive polyarthritis and other symptoms of collagen vascular disease induced by graft-versus-host reaction. J. Immunol., (in press).

33. Rolink, A.G., Radaszkiewicz, T., Pals, S.T., van der Meer, . & Gleichmann, E., 1982, Allosuppressor- and allohelper-T cells in acute and chronic graft-versus-host disease. I. Alloreactive suppressor cells rather than killer T cells appear to be the decisive effector cells in lethal graft-versus-host disease. J. Exp. Med. 155, 1501-1522.

34. Pals, S.T., Gleichmann, H. & Gleichmann, E., 1984, Allosuppressor- and allohelper-T cells in acute and chronic graft-versus-host disease. V. F1 mice with secondary chronic GVHD contain F1-reactive allohelper but no allosuppressor T cells. J. Exp. Med. 159, 508-523.

35. Rolink, A.G., van der Meer, W.G.K., Melief, C.J.M. & Gleichmann, E., 1983, Intra-H-2 requirements for the induction of maximal positive and negative allogeneic effects in vitro. Eur. J. Immunol. 13, 191-197.

36. Pals, S.T., Zijlstra, M., Radaszkiewicz, T., Cuypers, T., Schoenmakers, H.J., Melief, C.J.M., Berns, A. & Gleichmann, E., 1984, Immunological induction of malignant lymphoma: graft-versus-host reaction-induced-B-cell lymphomas contain reintegrations of several types of murine leukemia virus sequences. (submitted for publication)

37. Hurtenbach, U. & Shearer, G.M., 1983, Analysis of murine T-lymphocyte markers during the early phases of GVH-associated suppression of cytotoxic T-lymphocytes response. J. Immunol. 13, 1561-1566.

38. Bretscher, P., 1973, Hypothesis: a model for generalised autoimmunity. Cell Immunol. 6, 1-11.

39. Katz, D.H., 1977, Lymphocyte differentiation, recognition and regulation. Nez York, Academic Press Inc., 410-482.

40. Ordal, J.C. & Grumet, F.C., 1972, Genetic control of the immune response.The effect of graft-versus-host reaction on the antibody response to poly-L(Tyr, Glu)-poly-D, L-Ala-poly-L-Lys in nonresponder mice. J. Exp. Med. 136, 1195-1206.

41. Elfenbein, G.J., Green, I. & Paul, W.E., 1973, The allogeneic effect: increased affinity of serum antibody produced during a secondary response. Eur. J. Immunol. 3, 640-644.

42. McCullagh, P.J., 1972, The abrogation of immunological tolerance by means of allogeneic confrontation. Transplant. Rev. 12, 180-207.

43. Feldmann, M. & Basten, A. , 1972, Cell interactions in the immune response in vitro. IV. Comparison of the effects of antigen-specific and allogeneic thymus-derived cell-factors. J. Exp. Med. 136, 722-736.

44. Hamilton, J.A. & Miller, J.F.A.P., 1973, Induction of a primary antihapten response in vivo by a GVHR. J. Exp. Med. **138**, 1009-1014.

45. Klaus, G.G.B. & McMichael, A.J., 1974, Immunological properties of haptens coupled to thymus-independent carrier molecules. II. The influence of the GVHR on primary antibody responses to hapten-coupled polysaccharides and proteins. Eur. J. Immunol. **4**, 505-511.

46. Osborne, D.P. & Katz, D.H., 1973, The allogeneic effect in inbred mice. III. Unique antigenic structural requirements in the expression of the phenomenon on unprimed cell populations in vivo. J. Exp. Med. **137**, 991-1008.

47. Golding, H. & Rittenberg, M.B., 1982, In vitro and in vivo allogeneic effects: differential modulation of B-cell subpopulations. J. Immunol. **128**, 1625-1629.

48. Golding, H. & Rittenberg, M.B., 1982, In vivo allogeneic effects: shift in the isotype profile of primary TI-2 responses in mice undergoing graft-vs-host reaction. J. Immunol. **129**, 1878-1882.

49. Kindred, B. & Shreffler, D.C., 1972, H-2 dependence of cooperation between T and B cells in vivo. J. Immunol. **109**, 940-943.

50. Benacerraf, B. & Germain, R.N., 1978, The immune response genes of the major histocompatibility complex. Immunol. Rev. **38**, 70-119.

51. Zinkernagel, R.M. & Doherty, P.C., 1975, H-2 compatibility requirement for T-cell-mediated lysis of target cells infected with lymphocytic choriomeningitis virus. Different cytotoxic T-cell specificaties are associated with structures coded for in H-2K or H-2D. J. Exp. Med. **141**, 1427-1436.

52. Shelby, H.J. Rothman, S.J. & Buckley, R.H., 1980, Phenytoin hypersensitivity. J. Allergy Clin. Immunol. **66**, 166-172.

53. Rosenthal, C.J., Noguera, C.A., Coppola, A. & Kapelner, S.N., 1982, Pseudolymphoma with mycosis fungoides manifestations, hyperresponsiveness to diphenylhydantoin, and lymphocyte disregulation. Cancer **49**, 2305-2314.

54. Jaffe, I.A., 1979, Penicillamine in rheumatoid arthritis: clinical pharmacology and biochemical properties. Scand. J. Rheumatol. (Suppl.) **28**, 58-64.

55. Editorial. Captopril: benefits and risks in severe hypertension. Lancet **2**, 129-130.

56. Batchelor, J.R., Welsh, K.I., Mansilla-Tinoco, R., Dollery, C.T., Hughes, G.R.V., Bernstein, R., Ryan, P., Maish, P.F., Aber, G.M., Bing, R.F. & Russel, G.I., 1980, Hydralazine-induced systemic lupus erythematosus: influence of HLA-DR and sex on susceptibility. Lancet 1, 1107-1109.

57. Gleichmann, H., 1981, Studies on the mechanism of drug sensitization: T cell-dependent popliteal lymph node reaction to diphenylhydantoin. Clin. Immunopathol. 18, 203-211.

58. Gleichmann, H., Pals, S.T. & Radaskiewicz, T., 1983, T cell-dependent B-cell proliferation and activation induced by administration of the drug diphenylhydantoin to mice. Hematol. Oncology 1, 165-176.

59. Holland, P. and Mauer, A., 1965, Drug-induced in vitro stimulation of peripheral lymphocytes. Lancet 1, 1368-1369.

60. Schoepf, E., Schultz, K.H., Kessler, R., Taugner, M. & Braun, W., 1975, Allergologische Untersuchungen beim Lyell-Syndrome. Z. Hautkr. 50, 865-873.

61. Hyman, L.R., Ballow, M. & Knieser, M.R., 1978, Diphenyl-hydantoin interstitial nephritis: roles of cellular and humoral immunologic injury. J. Pediatr. 92, 915-920.

62. Druet, P., Sapin, C. Druet, E. & Hirsch, F., 1983, Genetic control of mercury-induced immune response in the rat. In: Nephrotoxic Mechanisms of Drugs and Environmental Toxins. (Ed. G.A. Porter), Plenum Medical Book Company, New York/London, 425-435.

63. Weening, J., Hoedemaker, P.J. & Bakker, W.W., 1981, Immunoregulation and anti-nuclear antibodies in mercury-induced glomerulopathy in the rat. 45, 64-71.

64. Perry, H.M., 1981, Possible mechanisms of the hydralazine-related lupus-like syndrome. Arthritis Rheum. 24, 1093-1104.

65. Worlledge, S.M., 1973, Immune drug-induced hemolytic anemias. Sem. Hematol. 10, 327-344.

66. Wooley, P.H., Griffen, J., Panayi, G.S., Batchelor, J.R., Welsh, K.I. & Gibson, T.H., 1980, HLA-DR antigens and toxic reaction to sodium aurothiomalate and D-penicillamine in patients with rheumatoid arthritis. N. Engl. J. Med. 303, 300-302.

67. Black, C.M., Walker, A.E. & Catoggio, L.J., 1983, Genetic susceptibility to scleroderma-like syndrome induced by vinyl chloride. Lancet 1, 53-55.

68. Vicario, J.L., Serrano-Rios, M., San Andres, F. & Arnaiz-Villena, A., 1982, HLA-DR3, DR4 increase in chronic stage of Spanish oil disease. Lancet 1, 276.

69. *Shakir, R.A., Behan, P.O., Dick, H. & Lambie, D.G., 1978, Metabolism of immunoglobulin A, Lymphocyte function, and histocompatibility antigens in patients on anticonvulsants. J. Neurol. Neurosurg. Psychiatry. <u>41</u>, 307-311. IMMUNOGL*

PRIMARY IMMUNODEFICIENCIES

J.L. Touraine

INSERMU-80, Hospital E. Herriot Pavillon P,
Lyon, France

"To be able to correct by means of organ, cellular and molecular engineering the defects that characterize patients with primary immunodeficiency diseases, and to prevent in this way the infectious and malignant diseases that destroy them, is to provide substantial witness that the new knowledge of immunobiology has pragmatic value". R.A. Good & F.H. Bach (1974).

INTRODUCTION

The new medical field devoted to the study and treatment of primary immunodeficiencies has developed tremendously over the last two decades. After the initial description of severe combined immunodeficiency diseases (1) and agammaglobulinemia (2) in the early 50's, these and other immunodeficiency diseases have created much interest in the scientific and medical communities. Simultaneous studies from the clinical side and in the laboratory have led to rapid advances. The finding of new defects has more than once revealed the existence of a particular cell, or a particular differentiation stage or a particular molecule. Animal models have been developed, lending themselves to more complete investigations and wider therapeutic trials.

Classification of primary immunodeficiencies has progressed with the development of more refined immunological investigations (3,4).

PREDOMINANTLY ANTIBODY DEFECTS

1. X-linked agammaglobulinemia

The Bruton-type agammaglobulinemia is transmitted by the X chromosome, on a recessive mode, and therefore is only seen in boys (frequency of the order of 1 in 100,00). It results from an instrinsic defect in the B-cell line with a lack of differentiation between the pre-B-cell and the B-cell stages. The cell-mediated immunity is normal.

The disease appears early in life, usually before two years of age. Infections are vey frequent, especially with obligatory extracellular parasitic organisms. The most frequent pathogens in these patients are pneumococcus, streptococcus, meningococcus, staphylococcus, pseudomonas, hemophilus influenzae. Respiratory infections are frequent, resulting in bronchectasias. In addition, infections of the meninges, ears, sinuses, skin and conjunctivae may be found. There is also an increased frequency of septicemia and gastroenteritis (intestinal infections with bacteria or parasites, especially giardia lamblia). Viral infections are usually not more frequent or severe than in normal subjects, with the exception of viral hepatitis which has a poorer prognosis. Other complications observed with an increased frequency include auto-immune manifestations (rheumatoid type of polyarthritis), leukemias and allergic manifestations. The serum levels of IgM, IgG, IgA, IgD and IgE are extremely low. The level of secretory IgA is also low. Allo-hemaglutinins are virtually absent. The antibody response is extremely low. B-cells and plasma cells are absent from the the blood, the bone marrow, the lymphoid organs. No lymphoid follicles are observed by histological examination of lymph nodes. By contrast, T-lymphocytes, thymus, delayed - type hypersensitivity, in vitro tests for cell-mediated immunity are normal. Treatments is by the intramuscular or intravenous administration of gammaglobulins (mainly IgG). The doses given and the frequency of injections or infusions may vary but it is necessary to maintain a permanent level of serum IgG above 2.5 g/l. Recent studies have suggested that an even more significant improvement can be obtained when the level is permanently in the normal range, i.e. above 7.5 g/l. Manifestations of intolerance can occur but they are less frequent and severe with the most recent preparations and with a slow administration. In addition to immunoglobulin therapy, the patient should receive antibiotics for each infectious episode, with special attention to the development of bronchiectasis.

2. Common variable hypogammaglobulinemia

This group of diseases is very heterogeneous. It includes congenital and acquired immunodeficiencies revealed at the age of 2-3 years or later on in life. The immunodeficiency is less pure than in X-linked agammaglobulinemia but the frequency is higher. The predominant defect may reside in the B-cells or in the helper T-cells. In still other cases activated suppressor T-cells are believed to play a role in the pathogenesis. A possible association with a malignant hemopathy should always be looked for.

3. Isolated IgA deficiency

This is one of the most frequent immunodeficiency (more than one out of one thousand individuals). The diagnosis can be certain after the age of 3 years only. Sometimes a partial deletion of chromosome 18 can be observed. The immunoglobulin defect may be asymptomatic or can be associated with infections, especially respiratory and intestinal infections. It has been suggested that patients with clinical symptoms are especially those with an associated defect of IgG sub-classes (5).

4. Agammaglobulinemia and thymoma

5. X-linked hypogammaglobulinemia with growth hormone defi- ciency

6. Autosomal recessive agammaglobulinemia

7. IgG and IgA deficiency with increased IgM (and IgD)

8. Selective deficiency of IgM

9. Selective deficiency of IgG

lo. Kappa chain deficiency

11. Antibody deficiency with normal or hypergammaglobinemia

12. Transcobalamin-2 deficiency

13. Agammaglobulinemia associated with EBV infection (with a genetic predisposition).

14. Transient hypogammaglobulinemia of infancy

PREDOMINATION CELL-MEDIATED IMMUNITY DEFECTS

1. Di George syndrome (6). This syndrome is characterized by a congenital absence of thymus and parathyroids, associeted with cardio-vascular abnormalities and facial malformations. These abnormalities are due to an embryopathy resulting in the lack of development of the third and the fourth pouch/arch. In a few cases, the disease is observed in infants of alcoholic mothers with zinc deficiency or in infants with partial deletion of chromosome 22. In rare cases, several children of the same family present with the disease. In most cases the disease is sporadic and suggests an embryopathy of an unknown origin.

Hypoparathyroidism results in hypocalcemia and convulsions. The thymic defect results in infections with facultative intracellular parasitic organisms early in life. These organisms include salmonella, brucella, listeria monocytogenes, tubercle bacillus, BCG, pneumocystis carinii, mycobacterium leprae, toxoplasma gondii, candida, and all viruses. Vaccinations with live viruses are contra-indicated as they may result in severe infections. Blood transfusions are also contra-indicated as they can induce a graft-versus-host reaction if blood has not been irradiated.

The thymus is lacking and is not seen on x-rays. Lymphopenia is sometimes found. T-lymphocytes are in reduced number. Lymphocytes are very few in the deep cortex of lymph nodes. T-lymphocytes do not proliferate in response to phytomitogens. Immunoglobulin levels are normal. Antibody production is only partially reduced toward thymus dependent antigens. T lymphocyte precursors in the bone marrow are normal. Thymic factors in the serum are extremely low. More frequent than the complete form of the disease are the partial Di George syndromes with an incomplete defect of cell-mediated immunity. The treatment for the most severe forms of the Di George syndrome includes a fetal thymus transplant, in addition to cardiac surgery if necessary, and to the correction of hypocalcemia. In the partial forms of the Di George syndrome, repeated injections of thymic factors can result in a sufficient restoration of cell-mediated immunity.

2. The Hong and Good syndrome. This syndrome results from an hypoplasia of the thymus and the thyroid (lack of development of the second and the third pouch/arch).

3. The Nezelof syndrome (7) can either be classified as a cell mediated defect or as a combined immunodeficiency despite the fact that immuno- globulins are quantitatively normal.

COMBINED IMMUNODEFICIENCY DISEASES

1. Severe combined immunodeficiency (SCID) with adenosine deamimnase (ADA) deficiency (8). This autosomal recessive disease is due to the effect on T-cells, and less importantly on B-cells, of toxic metabolites due to the enzyme deficiency. Heterozygotic levels of ADA are found in the parents's serum. Severe infections with either intracellular or extracellular organisms develop, usually after the second month of age. The severity of such infections can result in death usually during the first two years of age. Pulmonary and intestinal infections are especially severe. Vaccination with live vaccine or transfusion of any blood product which has not been irradiated are absolutely contra-indicated.

Lymphopenia is frequent, T-cell numbers are low and those present are not functional. B-cells are usually decreased and, before immunological reconstitution, they do not differentiate into immunoglobulin-secreting plasma cells. Antibodies are extremely low. Most lymphoid organs are severely hypoplastic. The patients can be isolated in sterile "bubbles". The most efficient treatment is bone marrow transplantation from an HLAS-identical family donor. In the lack of such a donor the patients can be treated with fetal liver and thymus transplantation. Repeated red cell transfusions can lead to a partial and transient improvement. Reconstitution of the T-cell compartment by means of bone marrow transplantation gives a possibility for the patients' own B-cells to differentiate into plasma cells.

The full immunological reconstitution and the good health of the patients many years after such a transplantation demonstrate that ADA deficiency has no severe consequences on the other cells of the body.

2. "Bare lymphocyte syndrome" (9). This combined immunodeficiency results from the lack of expression of HLA antigens at the surface of cells of hematopoietic origin, especially lymphocytes. This disease has demonstrated the crucial role of HLA antigens in the development of a normal immunity. It

has also revealed the existence of genes, outside the major histocompatibility complex of chromosome 6, controlling the expression of HLA determinants. Two forms of the syndrome have been observed : type I, with a lack of expression of class I HLA antigens, and type II, with a lack of expression of class II HLA antigens. In both cases a combined immunodeficiency results from the immunogenetic defect but type I has more severe clinical manifestations.

3. SCID in the context of reticular dysgenesis

4. SCID with low T-cell and B-cell numbers

5. SCID with low T-cell and normal B-cell numbers

6. Combined immunodeficiency with predominant T-cell defect

7. Purine nucleoside phosphorylase deficiency

8. Nezelof syndrome or thymic dysplasia with normal immunoglobulins

9. Incomplete immunodeficiencies

a) Wiskott-Aldrich syndrome (10). The disease is transmitted by the X chromosome on a recessive mode. It is revealed during early childhood by hemorrhages due to thrombopenia and thrombopathia. In addition chronic eczema develops, with infectious manifestations (bacterial, viral or fungal infections). IgM are usually decreased while IgA, IgG and IgE are normal or increased. Antibody production is low. B-lymphocytes and plasma cells are found in normal numbers. T-cells are progressively decreased in numbers and functions.

b) Ataxia-telangiectasia (11). This autosomal recessive disease is revealed during early childhood. It associates a cerebellum-type ataxia, conjunctival and cutaneous telangiectasia, gonad dysgenesis, sometimes a peripheral neuropathy and an immune deficiency accompanied by infectious manifestations, in particular bacterial infections of the respiratory tract leading to bronchiectasis. It frequently results in death before adulthood, due to infections or, in more than 10% of cases, to malignancies (12). IgM is frequently increased (monomers). IgG, IgE are often decreased. T-lymphocyte numbers and functions progressively decrease with age.

The treatment of combined immunodeficiencies varies with the type of disease and the availability of an HLA-identical family donor. Many of the diseases can be cured or significantly improved with a bone marrow transplant from an HLA identical family donor. In 65% of cases, however, such a compatible donor is not found. Mismatched bone marrow transplantation can be undertaken but it bears a high risk of graft-versus-host reaction, despite methods used to remove T-cells from the transplanted bone marrow. In all cases, except for the complete SCID, a conditioning of the recipient is necessary. Patients with SCID, lacking a perfectly matched bone marrow donor can be completely cured by the transplant of a fetal liver and thymus from a 8 to 12 week fetus. Despite HLA-mismatch, such a transplant can result in a complete immune reconstitution (13).

There are a number of other lymphocyte deficiencies which still remain difficult to classify. Several isolated T-cell deficiencies of various types are among this group. Another example of important immunodeficiency awaiting for a better pathophysiological understanding is the hyper-IgE syndrome (14); these patients have atopic eczema, recurrent infections leading to abscesses, and an increased level of serum IgE.

DEFECT OF PHAGOCYTOSIS, BACTERICIDIA OR COMPLEMENT COMPONENTS

In addition to neutropenia of different types and origins, a number of diseases involve phagocytic cells.

Chronic granulomatous disease (15) is associated with a variety of enzyme deficiencies responsible for diminished functions of PMNs and macrophages. It is frequently trans-mitted with the X chromosome but there are some disorders transmitted by autosomes. Infections occur due to staphylo-cocci, fungi and Gram-negative micro-organisms. These infec-tions are found in the liver, lungs, lymph nodes and skin. Bactericidia is very significantly decreased and the reduction of the nitro-blue of tetrazolium (NBT) is abnormal. NAD(P)H oxidase actividy is very low in most patients; Bone marrow transplantation from an HLA-identical family donor has some-times resulted in cure of the disease but the infectious risk in the post-transplant period is high.

The Chediak-Higashi syndrome associates abnormalities of PMNs, monocytes and macrophages on the one hand, and a lack of natural killer cell activity on the other hand.

Complement defects have been described for most of the known components. Sometimes they are asymptomatic. In many other cases, there are responsible for an increased incidence of infections, nephropathies, especially glomerulopathies, lupus-type syndromes and angioneurotic oedema. A few patients have been improved by transfusions of plasma or plasma components.

This relatively short paper on primary immunodeficiencies cannot pretend to be exhaustive and it has left aside several diseases. The purpose was mainly to indicate that any young patient developing infections of a particular type, if severe or frequent should be investigated with a pathophysiological mind in order to ascertain if it is one of the large group discussed above. This approach results not only in a better understanding of the disease process but also in an improve-ment of therapeutic possibilities.

Finally, informations derived from the studies of such patients are also applicable to the understanding of the many and frequent secondary immunodeficiencies which are described in another paper.

REFERENCES

1. GLANZMANN E. and RINIKER P. 1950 Essentielle lymphocytophtise. Ein neues Krankheitsbild aus der S°uglingspathologie. Ann. Paediat. (Basel) 175, 1-32.

2. BRUTON O.C. 1952 Agammaglobulinemia. Pediatrics, 9, 722.

3. TOURAINE J.L. 1975 Les deficits immunitaires. Lyon Med. 233, 1223-1237.

4. Meeting Report 1983 : Primary Immunodeficiency Diseases. Report prepared for the WHO by a scientific group on immunodeficiency Clin. Immunol. Immunopathol., 28, 450-475.

5. OXELIUS V.A., LAURELL A.B., LINDQUIST B., GOLEBIOWSKA H., AXELSON U., BJOERKANDER J., HANSON L.A. 1981 IgG subclasses in selective IgA deficiency. N. Engl. J. Med. 304, 1476-1477.

6. DI GEORGE A.M., 1968 Congenital absence of the thymus and its immunologic consequences: concurrence with congenital hypoparathyroidism. In: Immunologic Deficiency Diseases in Man. D. Bergsma and R.A. Good (Ed), 116. The National Foundation New York.

7. NEZELOF C., JAMMET M.L., LORTHOLARY P. LABRUNE B. and LAMY M. 1964. L'hypoplasie hereditaire du thymus : sa place et sa responsabilite dans une observation d'aplasie lymphocytaire normoplasmocytaire et normoglobulinemique du nourrisson. Arch. Franc. Pediat. 21, 897-920.

8. PICKERING R.J., POLLARA B. and MEUWISSEN H.J. 1974 Meeting report Workshop on severe combined immunological deficiency disease and adenosine deaminase deficiency. Clin. Immunol. Immunopathol. 3, 301-303.

9. TOURAINE J.L. 1981 The Bare Lymphocyte Syndrome: Report on the Registry. Lancet, 1, 319-321.

10. COOPER M.D., CHASE H.P., LOWMAN J.T., KRIVIT W. and GOOD R.A. 1968 Immunologic Deficiency Diseases in Man. D. Bergsma and R.A. Goo (Ed), 378, The National Foundation. New York.

11. PETERSON R.D.A. and GOOD R.A. 1968 Ataxia telangiectasia. In : Immunologic Deficiency Diseases in Man. D. Bergsma and R.A. Good (Ed), 370, The National Foundation, New York.

12. SPECTOR B.D., PERRY III G.S., KERSEY J.H. 1978 Genetically determined immunodeficiency diseases (GDID) and malignancy : report from the Immunodeficiency- Cancer Registry. Clin. Immunol. Immunopathol., 11, 12-29.

68

13. *TOURAINE J.L. 1983 Bone marrow and fetal liver trans-plantation in immunodeficiencies and inborn errors of metabolism : lack of significant restriction of T-cell function in long-term chimeras despite HLA-mismatch. Immunol. Rev.* 71, 103-121.

14. *BUCKLEY R.K. 1980 Immunologic studies in 21 patients with the Hyper IgE syndrome. In: Primary Immunodeficiencies, M. Seligmann and W.H. Hitzig (Ed.)* 495, *Elsevier, Amsterdam.*

15. *HOLMES B., PAGE A.R., WINDHORST D.B., QUIE P.G., WHITE J.G. and GOOD R.A. 1968 Fatal granulomatous disease : A genetic defect of phagocytic function. In : Immuno-logic Deficiency Diseases in Man, D. Bergsma and R.A. Good (Ed),* 443, *The National Foundation, New York.*

THE NEOPLASTIC CONSEQUENCES OF IMMUNODEPRESSION

I. Penn

Department of Surgery,
University of Cincinnati Medical Center,
U.S.A.

INTRODUCTION

Immunodepression may be iatrogenically induced either, deliberately, as in the management of organ transplant recipients or patients with auto-immune or collagen-vascular diseases, or inadvertently, as a side effect of treatment of cancer with cytotoxic drugs and/or radiotherapy (Hanto et al 1983; Kinlen et al 1979; Kinlen 1982; Penn 1978 a and b; Penn 1981; Penn 1982; Penn 1984; Sieber 1975). Immunodepression may also occur spontaneously in certain congenital immunodeficiency disorders (Filipovich et al 1980; Filipovich et al 1984) and it may be acquired as in the Acquired Immunodeficiency Syndrome (AIDS) (Friedman-Kien et all 1982; Ziegler et all 1984). These various states of immunodepression are characterized by defects in cellular or humoral immunity or by both. They are complicated by an increased incidence of infections and of cancer. In this report we shall consider the various types of malignancies that occur in different immunodeficient states.

CANCERS IN ORGAN TRANSPLANT RECIPIENTS

Organ transplant recipients are given immunosuppressive therapy for many months or years to prevent or treat rejection of the organ (Penn 1978 a and b; Penn 1981; Penn 1982; Penn 1984). Most patients have been treated with a combination of Azathioprine and Prednisone. Other commonly used medications include antilymphocyte or antithymocyte globulin (ALG or ATG), Cyclophosphamide, and recently, Cyclosporine, and OKT$_3$ and other anti-T cell monoclonal antibodies. Other immunosuppressive measures used in some patients are splenectomy, thoracic duct fistula and local irradiation of the graft. In bone marrow transplantation the immunosuppressive regimen is different. The patients are given a large dose of cyclosphosphamide or total body irradiation to "condition" them to accept the graft, and then are given relatively small doses of immunosuppressive drugs for several months to prevent graft versus host disease.

From 1968 till May, 1984, the Cincinnati (formerly Denver) Transplant Tumor Registry (CTTR) received information on 2,063 types of cancer that arose in 1,934 organ transplant recipients, (Penn 1978 a and b; Penn 1981: Penn 1982: Penn 1984). The patients included 1,882 who received kidney, 35 heart, 6 liver, 6 bone marrow, 3 pancreas, and 2 combined heart and lung transplants. The tumors commonly seen in the general population including carcinomas of the lung, prostate, colon and rectum, female brreast, and invasive carcinoma of the uterine cervix were not increased in incidence in transplant recipients. Instead certain neoplasms were observed with remarkable frequency. Skin and lip cancers were commonly seen, but the incidence varied with the amount of exposure to sunshine. In areas where exposure was limited. there was a 4 to 7 fold increase, but in regions with high sunshine exposure there was an almost 21 fold increase above the already high incidence seen in the local control population (Penn 1981; Penn 1982; Penn 1984). In two epidemiologic studies the incidence of non-Hodgkin's lymphomas was found to be 28 to 49 fold above that observed in the age-matched population (Kinlen et al 1979; Kinlen 1982). In situ carcinomas of the uterine cervix showed a 14 fold increase over controls (Porreco et al 1975). Non-melanoma skin cancers and in situ carcinomas of the uterine cervix are excluded from most cancer statistics. If we omit them from the CTTR data several other tumors then show striking increase in incidence. Kaposi's sarcoma makes up 4.8% of neo-plasms in the CTTR, in comparison with its incidence in the general population in the United States before the AIDS epidemic started, when it made up only 0.02 to 0.07% of all malignanciens (Penn 1981; Penn 1982; Penn 1984). The high incidence of Kaposi's sarcoma in this worldwide collection of patients is comparable to that seen in areas of the world where it occurs with greatest frequency, namely in the black population of the rain forest area of Africa, where it makes up 3 to 9% of all cancers. These findings are in keeping with a study showing that the incidence of Kaposi's sarcoma in renal transplant recipients is increased 400-500 fold over that seen in a control population of the same ethnic origin (Harwood et al 1979). Carcinomas of the vulva and perineum make up 3.9% of tumors in the CTTR, a much higher figure than is prevalent in the general population (Penn 1981; Penn 1982; Penn 1984). There were also small increases in the incidence of leukemia, carcinomas of the kidney, and carcinomas of the liver and biliary passages (Penn 1984).

As the length of follow-up of organ transplant recipients has increased it has become evident that certain tumors appear at fairly distinct time intervals after transplantation. Compared with other known oncogenic stimuli in man, which often take 15 to 20 years or more before they produce obvious tumors, malignancies appear a relatively short time after transplantation (Penn 1978 a and b; Penn 1981; Penn 1982; Penn 1984). First to appear is Kaposi's sarcoma at an average of 20 (range 2 1/2 to 225 1/2) months after transplantation. Next are the lymphomas which appear at an average of 30 (range 1 to 153 1/2) months after transplantation. Other cancers (excluding carcinomas of the vulva and perineum) appear at an average of 60 (range 1 to 206) months following transplantation. The tumors that are diagnosed at the longest time after transplantation are those of the vulva and perineum which appear at an average of 90 (range 20 to 215) months.

The incidence of neoplasms increases with the length of
follow-up after transplantation (Penn 1978 a and b; Penn
1981; Penn 1982; Penn 1984). Of 418 renal transplant
patients who survived at least one year 26% had tumors; at 10
years 14 of 30 survivors (47%) were so afflicted (Sheil et al
1981). Similarly, the actuarial risk of developing cancer in
124 cardiac transplant recipients, was 2.7+ 1.9% at one year
and 25.6+ 11.0% at 5 years. These statistics emphasize the
need to follow transplant patients indefinitely (Penn 1981;
Penn 1982; Penn 1984).

The malignancies affected a relative young group of patients
whose average age at the time of transplantation was 40 years
(range 7 months to 70 years). Forty-nine percent were under
the age of 40 years at the time of transplantation.
Sixty-four percent of patients were male and 36% female, in
keeping with the 2:1 ratio of male to female patients who
undergo renal transplantation.

Skin and Lip Cancers

The most common tumors arose in the skin and lips and made up
789 of 2063 (38%) types of cancer reported (Penn 1978 a and b;
Penn 1981; Penn 1982; Penn 1984). Their incidence increased
with the length of follow-up after transplantation. In an
Australian study skin malignancies occured in 8% of patients
who survived at least one year after transplantation, but the
neoplasms affected 17% of those who survived four years or
longer (Penn 1981; Penn 1982; Penn 1984). In addition, 28%
of the four-year survivors had premalignant keratoses.

The skin cancers in transplant patients showed several unusual
features in comparison with those seen in the general
population (Penn 1978 a and b; Penn 1981; Penn 1982; Penn
1984; Sheil et al 1981). Basal cell carcinomas outnumber
squamous cell carcinomas in the general population, but this
relationship was reversed in transplant recipients in whom
squamous cell carcinomas made up 52% and basal cell carcinomas
28%. Another 13% were made up of both types of neoplasms.
Another difference was the youth of the transplant patients,
whose average age was 30 years younger than those with similar
lesions in the community at large. In addition, multiple
tumors were present in at least 346 of 789 transplant
recipients (44%), an incidence in this worldwide colleciton of
patients comparable to that seen only in the areas of high
sunshine exposure. Several individuals each had more than 50
skin cancers. Malignant melanomas made up 5% of the skin
cancers in this series compared with an incidence of 2.7% in
the generral population of the United States.

Most skin neoplasms were of low-grade malignancy but a
significant proportion were very aggressive (Penn 1981; Penn
1982; Penn 1984). Lymph node metastases occurred in 58
patients (7%), 48 of whom had sguamous cell carcinomas, 8 of
whom had malignant melanomas and 2 of whom had Merkel's cell
tumors. Of the squamous cell carcinomas that involved lymph
nodes, 34 involved the skin only, 7 involved the lips only,
and 7 were cases with skin and lip involvement but in 4 of

these instances the metastases probably arose from the skin
lesions. Metastases caused the deaths of 46 patients with
skin cancer (6%), 30 with squamous cell carcinomas, 14 with
malignant melanomas and 2 with Merkel's cell tumors. Of the
fatalities caused by squamous cell carcinomas, 22 were caused
by lesions arising in the skin, 3 by lesions from the lips and
5 from lesions involving the lips and skin, but the skin
lesions apparently were responsible for the fatal metastases
in 3 of the patients. These findings are consistent with a
more than 10 fold increased mortality from squamous cell
carcinomas in Australian renal transplant recipients (Kinlen
et al 1979). The behavior of skin cancers in the present
series is in sharp contrast with the pattern seen in the
general population, in whom they account for only 1 to 2% of
all cancer deaths, the great majority of which are caused by
malignant melanoma (Penn 1981; Penn 1982; Penn 1984).

Lymphomas

Lymphomas in transplant patients show several unusual features
when compared with their behavior in the general population
(Kinlen 1982; Penn 1978 a and b; Penn 1981; Penn 1982;
Penn 1984). They comprise 3 to 4% of all tumors seen in the
community at large, but made up 289 of 2,063 tumors (14%) in
the CTTR data base. If we exclude non-melanoma skin cancers
and in situ carcinomas of the uterine cervix, the corrected
incidence rises to 20%. Ideally we should classify lymphomas
according to the cell of origin such as T cell, B cell, null
cell, etc. In the present series 37 lymphomas and 7
lymphoproliferations, which were suspected to be lymphomas,
arose from B cells. In several other lymphomas the cells did
not demonstrate cellular immunoglobulin and could not be
characterized further. Thus far, only 2 T cell tumors have
been reported, including one case of mycosis fungoides. Some
investigators describe a spectrum of lesions in transplant
patients ranging from infectious mononucleosis-like polyclonal
B cell proliferations at the one extreme, to frank monoclonal B cell lymphomas at the other (Hanto et al 1983). In
between there is a stage where some polyclonal B cell proliferations undergo a clonal cytogenetic alteration leading to
malignant transformation and the emergence of monoclonal B
cell lymphomas.

An unusual feature of the lymphomas is the rarity of Hodgkin's
disease (Penn 1978 a and b; Penn 1981; Penn 1982; Penn
1984). There were only 11 cases among 289 patients (4%) with
lymphomas. This contrasts with its incidence in the general
population where it comprises 18% of all lymphomas. If we
exclude the 11 patients with Hodgkin's disease and another 6
with myelomas (plasma cell lymphomas), we are left with 272
patients with non-Hodgkin's lymphomas. By far the most common
tumor in these patients was reticulum cell sarcoma which
occurred 63%. The non-Hodgkin's lymphomas were markedly
different from those in the general population in several
respects. Extranodal involvement occurred in from 24 to 48%
of patients in the general population. In the present study,
the distribution of the lymphomas was not known in 2 patients,

but of the remaining 270 extranodal disease occurred in 208 (77%). Most of the 62 patients with nodal involvement had widespread disease involving mainly the liver, lungs, spleen, bone marrow, renal allograft and brain. In the 208 recipients with extranodal disease a single organ was affected in 142 (68%). The single organ most frequently involved was the central nervous system which was affected in 80 of 142 patients (56%). Overall 101 of the 270 patients (37%) had central nervous system involvement. Patients with meningeal involvement were not included in these statistics. Lesions of the central nervous system almost always occurred in the brain but rarely involved the spinal cord. The brain lesions frequently had a multicentric distribution. The remarkably high incidence of brain involvement contrasts with a 1% incidence of focal cerebral involvement by non-Hodgkin's lymphomas in a series of 1,039 patients in the general population (meningeal involvement occurred in 3.7%) (Penn 1981; Penn 1982; Penn 1984). Another striking feature in the 270 recipients was the frequency of lymphomatous involvement of the allograft which occurred in 43 recipients (16%), 38 renal, 2 cardiac, 2 pancreatic and 1 hepatic (Penn 1981; Penn 1982; Penn 1984). An additional unusual manifestation of the lymphomas was that the tumor presented in the soft tissues at the sites of injection of antilymphocyte or antithymocyte globulin in at least 4 patients.

Kaposi's Sarcoma

There were 69 patients with this disorder, 46 males and 23 females. The 2:1 male to female ratio is the same as that seen in transplant patients having other malignancies, but is much less than the 9:1 to 15:1 ratio seen with Kaposi's sarcoma in the general population. Six of the 69 patients (9%) had other neoplasms, an incidence similar to that seen in the community at large. Fifty of the 69 patients (72%) had "benign" Kaposi's sarcoma involving the skin, conjunctiva or oropharyngolaryngeal mucosa, and 19 (28%) had the "malignant" variety with involvement of the internal organs. Of the 50 patients with "benign" disease 26 (52%) had complete remissions following treatment. Five of these 26 remissions (19%) occurred when the only treatment consisted of a drastic reduction of immunosuppressive therapy (Penn 1981; Penn 1982; Penn 1984). The other remissions followed surgery, radiotherapy or chemotherapy. In the malignant group 3 patients (16%) had complete remissions after chemotherapy or radiotherapy together with alteration of immunosuppressive therapy.

Carcinomas of the Uterus

Carcinomas of the cervix occurred in 131 of the 702 women in this series (19%). In situ lesions made up at least 79% of the cases. This neoplasm is probably more common than is realized. It is therefore, advisable that all post-adolescent female patients undergo pelvic examinations and cervical smears on a regular basis. Carcinomas of the body of the uterus are uncommon. Perhaps this is because most transplant patients are young whereas this tumor occurs mainly in post-menopausal women.

Carcinomas of the Vulva and Perineum

Carcinomas of the vulva, perineum, scrotum, penis, peri-anal skin and anus occurred in 56 patients, 41 female and 15 male. Compared with the general population the patients were surprisingly young. The average age of the females at the time of transplantation was 29 (range 15-55) years and of the males 37 (range 25-51) years. In females there was sometimes a "field effect" with involvement by cancer of the vulva and vagina and/or cervix of the uterus. A prior history of condyloma acuminatum or herpes genitalis suggests an etiologic role by oncogenic viruses in these immunosuppressed patients (Penn 1982; Penn 1984).

CANCERS IN NONTRANSPLANT PATIENTS RECEIVING IMMUNOSUPPRESSIVE THERAPY

Immunosuppressive drug therapy has been used to suppress immunity or inflammatory responses in a large number of auto-immune disorders, collagen-vascular diseases, and disorders of obscure etiology (Kahn et al 1979; Kinlen et al 1979; Penn 1978 a and b; Penn 1981; Penn 1982; Penn 1984). The dosage was usually smaller and the duration of treatment shorter than is used in treating cancer or in the management of organ transplant recipients. Malignancies have developed in these patients, but it is difficult to determine their exact frequency as some auto-immune disorders are, per se, associated with an increased incidence of neoplasms. By personal communication and a review of the literature, the author has collected data on 149 cancers that developed in 143 patients who were treated for the disorders mentioned above (Penn 1978 a and b; Penn 1981; Penn 1982; Penn 1984). Thirty percent of the malignancies were leukemias and 20% were lymphomas, the majority of which were reticulum cell sarcomas. In addition, there were at least 16 case reports of Kaposi's sarcoma. Several studies demonstrate an increased incidence of neo-plasm following immunosuppressive therapy for the disorders mentioned above.

Fifteen of 1,853 patients (0.85%) with rheumatoid arthritis, treated mainly with Chlorambucil or Cyclophosphamide, developed actue leukemia (Kahn et al 1979). The cancer was not observed in patients treated for less than 6 monts, or in those who received a total dose of less than 1 gm of Chlorambucil of 50 gm of Cyclophosphamide. In addition, 4 of 35 patients (11.4%) treated with Chlorambucil for severe psoriatic arthropathy developed acute leukemia. In another series 1,349 patients were given Azathioprine, Cyclophosphamide or Chlorambucil for at least 3 months as treatment for the disorders mentioned above (Kinlen et al 1979). The types of tumors that subsequently developed were similar to those seen in transplant patients. There was an increased incidence of NHL (4 cases observed compared with 0.34 expected), squamous cell carcinoma of the skin (2 observed against 0.38 expected), bladder cancer (4 observed against 1.00 expected), and other tumors (29 observed compared with 20.74 expected) (Kinlen et al 1979; Penn 1984). In another study of 54 patients treated with Cyclophosphamide for systemic lupus erythematosus or theumatoid arthritis, 2 cases of bladder cancer were observed, compared with 0.02 expected (Penn 1984).

SECOND TUMORS IN PATIENTS RECEIVING CHEMOTHERAPY FOR CANCER

Most cancer chemotherapeutic agents have immnosuppressive side effects (Harris et al 1976; Penn 1978 a and b; Penn 1981; Penn 1982; Penn 1984). In consequence patients are prone to infectious complications and, paradoxically, new malignancies. While the latter probably result from direct oncogenic or cooncogenic effects of the treatments used, we cannot exclude immunosuppression as a possible etiologic factor.

The most common new cancers were acute leukemias, lymphomas, and carcinomas of the urinnary bladder (Penn 1978 a and b; Penn 1981; Penn 1982; Penn 1984). Most leukemias were preceded by a period of therapy-induced marrow depression and by a pre-leukemic phase. The mean interval from diagnosis of the primary neoplasm to development of acute leukemia was 4 to 6 years. In some instances leukemias appeared after chemotherapy had been discontinued for some months or even years.

In several reports the incidence of acute myeloid leukemia in treated Hodgkin's disease was 0.9% to 2% (Coleman et al 1982; International Agency for Research on Cancer 1981; Rosner et al 1982; Sieber 1975). The risk of developing acute myeloid leukemia was increased 5 to 75 fold. In treated multiple myeloma the incidence of this type of leukemia was 0.6% to 7.0% and the risk was increased 100 fold (Penn 1982; Penn 1984; Rosner, et al 1982; Sieber 1975). Patients treated with Chlorambucil for polycythemia rubra vera had a 2.3 times higher incidence of acute leukemia compared with individuals treated with P^{32} and a 13 times greater incidence than persons treated by phlebotomy (Penn 1982; Penn 1984). An increased frequency of acute myeloid leukemia has also been noted in treated non-Hodgkin's lymphoma, acute lymphoblastic leukemia, and chronic lymphocytic leukemia (Penn 1982; Penn 1984; Rosner et al 1982). Three of 13 patients given adjuvant chemotherapy with Chlorambucil for breast cancer developed acute leukemia (Penn 1982; Penn 1984; Rosner et al 1982). In another study 4 of 1,460 breast cancer patients treated with Cyclophosphamide developed acute leukemia (Portugal et al 1979). The incidence of acute leukemia in treated ovarian cancer was 0.2% to 1.4% (Reimer et al 1977). The risk increased 21 to 26 fold within 2 years of treatment, but rose to 66 to 170 fold in patients who survived more than 2 years. We may raise the question whether the development of acute leukemia in the above diseases represents part of the natural history of the original cancers in patients who were kept alive sufficiently long by chemotherapy or by chemotherapy combined with radiotherapy. This viewpoint is strengthened by the occasional simultaneous appearance of leukemia in untreated patients with Hodgkin's disease or multiple myeloma (Rosner et al 1982). However, as acute myeloid leukemia was rarely seen in patients with these two diseases before the era of intensive therapy it seems highly likely that the patient's treatment played a major role in the development of the hematologic malignancy. This conclusion is strengthened by an increase in the incidence of acute leukemia following chemotherapy of ovarian cancer, a disease in which leukemia is not considered to be part of the natural history (Penn 1982; Penn 1984; Reimer et al 1977; Rosner et al 1982).

There are conflicting opinions about the incidence of non-Hodgkin's lymphoma following the treatment of Hodgkin's disease (Coleman et al 1982; Penn 1984). In 1,222 patients with Hodgkin's disease treated with chemotherapy, radiotherapy or combined modality therapy the actuarial risk at 10 years for the development of subsequent second neoplasms was 9.9%. Leukemias made up 3.5%, lymphomas 0.5% and solid tumors 5.9%. The latent period from Hodgkin's disease to the development of second lymphomas was as long as 15.5 years. In another study of 579 patients treated with Hodgkin's disease 6 subsequently development non-Hodgkin's lymphomas. The actuarial risk of developing the second tumor was approximately 4.5% at 10 years. In these two series the development of non-Hodgkin's lymphomas appears to be related to the potentially carcinogenic treatments that were used. However, in another series of 51 Hodgkin's disease patients, 5 developed non-Hodgkin's lymphomas 4 to 11 years after the onset of Hodgkin's disease, but 4 of the 5 had received no treatment, and the investigators concluded that, in some patients with the lymphocytic Predominance Nodular variety of Hodgkin's disease, the disorder may spontaneously evolve into a more malignant non-Hodgkin's lymphoma (Penn 1984).

A variety of other second tumors have been reported following the treatment of various primary cancers (Coleman et al 1982; Penn 1984; Rosner et al 1982). Most common were carcinomas of the bladder, Kaposi's sarcoma, carcinomas of the lung, skin, breast, colon, pancreas and soft tissue sarcomas. However, most reports are of isolated cases or small numbers of a particular neoplasms and estimations of relative risk are not available. However, special mention should be made of the development of cancer of the urinary bladder following cytotoxic therapy (Penn 1984). Of 83 cases of second tumors following Cyclophosphamide therapy for cancer 17 were bladder neoplasms. Another alkylating agent, Chlornaphazine, is metabolized to yield B-naphthylamine, which is known to be a carcinogen in the human bladder. Since several vesical carcinomas developed in patients following its administration Chlornaphazine was withdrawn from clinical use.

NEOPLASMS IN CONGENITAL IMMUNODEFICIENCY DISORDERS

At least 14 types of naturally occurring immunodeficiency states have been identified (Filipovich et al 1980; Filipovich 1984). Up till 1984, the Immunodeficiency Cancer

Registry, at the University of Minnesota, has accumulated data on 385 patients. Several disorders account for most patients with neoplasms, namely, ataxia-telangiectasa with 130 cancer cases, common variable immunodeficiency disease with 88 cancer cases, Wiskott-Aldrich syndrome with 62 cancer cases, and severe combined immunodeficiency disease with 24 cancer cases. Sixty-six percent of patients were under the age of 20 years. Males out-numbered females in a ratio of 2:1 largely because several disorders were X-linked recessive syndromes.

The types of tumors seen differed significantly from those observed in the general population (Filipovich et al 1980; Filipovich et al 1984). Most neoplasms common to the general childhood population, i.e., nervous system neoplasms, rhabdomyosarcoma, Wilm's tumor, Ewing's sarcoma and retinoblastoma have rarely been reported in immunodeficient children. Instead the most common malignancies were non-Hodgkin's lymphomas (44%), carcinomas (23%), leukemias (15%) and Hodgkin's disease (7%). the non-Hodgkin's lymphomas had several features in common with those seen in transplant patients. The most frequent lymphoma was reticulum cell sarcoma which comprised 42% of cases. Those malignancies studied by modern immunologic techniques were of B cell origin. A spectrum of lesions ranging from B cell hyperplasias to frank lymphomas was seen. The brain was a frequent primary tumor site. For example, in Wiskott-Aldrich syndrome brain involvement by non-Hodgkin's lymphoma occurred in 31% of patients. Lymph node and gastro-intestinal tract involvement were also frequent.

Carcinomas of the stomach were the most common epithelial neoplasms reported to the Immunodeficiency Cancer Registry (22/55, 45%) (Filipovich et al 1980; Filipovich et al 1984; Penn 1984). Of these 27% arose in patients with combined variable immunodeficiency disease at a median age of 54 (range 15 to 67) years. The high incidence of gastric carcinoma is in contrast with the distribution of gasto-intestinal malignancies in the general population where colonic neoplasms occur much more frequently than gastric cancers.

Leukemia occurred in 15% of patients compared with a 3% inciddence in the general population (Filipovich et al 1984). A notable finding was the occurrence of acute lymphocytic leukemia before or after the diagnosis in non-Hodgkin's lymphoma in several groups of patients.

NEOPLASMS IN THE ACQUIRED IMMUNODEFICIENCY SYNDROME (AIDS)

This syndrome consists of profound and perhaps irreversible abnormalities in cellular immune function associated with opportunistic infections and aggressive neoplasms (Friedman-Kien et al 1982; Penn 1984; Ziegler et al 1984). AIDS occurs in socially, ethnically and genetically diverse hosts. The major group affected consists of homosexual men, particularly those with numerous, anonymous sexual contacts. Others include intravenous drug abusers, hemophiliac patients, recipients of random blood transfusions, female sexual partners of persons with the syndrome, and prisoners. Up to 6% do not fall into any known category. The cause of the immuno suppression is not known. Many investigators believe that it is caused by an infectious agent. Potential culprits are Cytomegalovirus, Epstein-Barr virus, Hepatitis B virus, Human T cell leukemia virus, lymphadenopathy associated virus. African swine fever virus, and a fungus which releases a Cyclosporine-like immunosupppressive product. At present most suspicion focuses on the human T-cell leukemia virus and the lymphadenopathy associated virus.

The predominant malignancy seen in AIDS is Kaposi's sarcoma (Friedman-Kien et al 1982; Penn 1984). Much less commonly lymphomas have been observed and epithelial neoplasms have been reported rarely. It is not clear why only homosexual men have a higher incidence of Kaposi's sarcoma and non-Hodgkin's lymphoma in comparison with other AIDS risk groups. Of 3,308 patients with AIDS, 858 had Kaposi's sarcoma without pneumocystis carinii pneumonia and another 225 had both disorders. Thus a total of 1,083 patients (33%) had Kaposi's sarcoma. The risk of development of Kaposi's sarcoma in AIDS patients is approximately 100 times greater than that for the general population. This malignancy involves the skin in the majority of patients, but the cutaneous lesions frequently look different from those seen in patients with Kaposi's sarcoma in the general population and are frequently overlooked or misdiagnosed. More than half the patients with skin involvement have one or more lesions in the gastro-intestinal tract. These are best diagnosed by upper and lower gastro-intestinal endoscopy.

Kaposi's sarcoma in AIDS frequently involves lymph nodes. Other less commonly affected sites are the mucous membranes of the mouth and pharynx, the liver, spleen, lungs, conjunctiva, brain, testis, pancreas, aorta, and heart. In AIDS patients Kaposi's sarcoma may occur in virtually any organ. Kaposi's sarcoma in AIDS differs from that seen in transplant patients in whom lymph node involvement is rare, visceral disease is less common, and fatalities from the malignancy are less frequent (Penn 1984). In addition, the immunosuppression in transplant patients can be reduced or totally stopped with the possibility of subsequent regression of the s=disease whereas, in AIDS persistence of immunodeficiency is a major feature (Penn 1984).

Thus far non-Hodgkin's lymphomas have been reported in 90 homosexual men, most of whom had AIDS or the generalized lymphadenopathy syndrome which is regarded as a prodromata of AIDS (Ziegler et al 1984). Their median age was 37 years, similar to that of AIDS patients in general. The non-Hodgkin's lymphomas showed many features resembling those seen in transplant and naturally occurring immunodeficiency patients (Penn 1984; Ziegler et al 1984). The histologic subtypes and malignant cell pheno-types were consistent with a B cell origin, although one neoplasm had T cell characteristics. Serial pathologic studies of lymph nodes from some patients with the generalized lymphadenopathy syndrome showed gradations from B cell proliferations to lymphomas. Nearly all patients had extranodal disease. Thirty-eight of 88 patients (432%) had central nervous system involvement, with a brain mass in 21, meningeal involvement in 14, cranial or peripheral nerve involvement in 5, and paraspinal lesions in 5. The bone marrow was affected in 30 patients.

Unusual sites of lymphomas, possibly related to the route of sexual intercourse involved, were intraoral lymphomas in 4, and anorectal lymphomas in 3. Cancers of the mouth and anorectum have been reported in young homosexual men (Li et al 1982; Loazada et al 1982; Penn 1984). The location of the lesions may be related to the route used for sexual relations, and to preceding infections in these areas, including herpes simplex, condyloma acuminatum, and other infections.

CAUSES OF CANCER

This is discussed in detail elswhere (Filipovich et al 1984; Harris 1976 ; International Agency for Research on Cancer 1981; Penn 1978 a and b; Penn 1982; Penn 1984; Sieber 1975; Ziegler et al 1984). The neoplasms probably arise from a complex interplay of multiple factors including depression of immunity, liberation or activation of oncogenic viruses, oncogenic or co-oncogenic effects of the immunosuppressive agents or other treatments given to the patient, and variations in individual susceptibility to carcinogenic stimuli.

SUMMARY AND CONCLUSIONS

The discovery that immunosuppression is associated with an increased incidence of certain tumors emphasizes the importance of the immune system in host defenses against neoplasia. It is curious that the diverse states of immunodeficiency described above have in common an increased incidence of tumors arising from the immune cells themselves, namely lymphomas. If Kaposi's sarcoma is a variety of lymphoreticular tumor, as some investigators believe, the situation becomes even more intriguing.

We should try to use immunosuppressive therapy as little as possible. In auto-immune and other disorders such treatment should be reserved for severe cases that fail to respond to other forms of therapy. However, immunosuppressive therapy is essential for the survival and function of organ transplants. Attempts are being made to replace the present blunderbus attack on the immune system with more specific methods of control of certain elements of the immune system. Ultimately, it is hoped to develop methods of immune unresponsiveness directed specifically, and only, at the foreign antigens of the transplanted organ. In the field of cytotoxic therapy attempts are being made to develop less immunosuppressive and less carcinogenic forms of treatment.

We need to study various groups of immunosuppressed patients,

including those with and without cancers, to obtain clues to
the etiology of the neoplasms. This information may shed
light on the causes of similar malignancies seen in the
general population, and on the role of the immune system in
the control of cancer. Hopefully such knowledge may provide
immunological methods for the prevention and cure of cancer.

ACKNOWLEDGEMENT

The author wishes to thank numerous colleagues, working in
transplant and cancer therapy centers throughout the world,
who have generously contributed data concerning their patients
to the Cincinnatiu Transplant Tumor Registry.

REFERENCES

Coleman, C.N., Kaplan, H.S., Cox, R., Varghese, A.,
    Butterfield, P. and Rosenburg, S.A. 1982. Leukemias,
    non-Hodgkin's lymphomas and solid tumours in patients
    treated for Hodgkin's disesase. Cancer Surveys 1:
    733-744.

Filipovich, A.H., Spector, B.D., Kersey, J., Fraumeni, J.,
    Schottenfeld, D., Stolley, P.D. (1980):
    Immunodeficiency in humans as a risk factor in the
    development of malignancy. Preventive Med. 9: 252-259

Filipovicph,A.H., Zerbe, D., Spector, B.D., Kersey, J.H.
    (1984): Lymphomas in persons with naturally occurring
    immunodeficiency disorders; in, Pathogenesis of
    Leukemias and Lymphomas: Environnemtal Influences
    (McGrath, I.T., O'Connor, G.T., Ramot, B., eds.) pp.
    225-234, (Raven Press, New York).

Friedman-Kien, A.E., Laubenstein, L.J., Rubinstein, P.,
    Buimovici-Klein, E., Marmor, M., Stahl, R., Spigland, I.,
    Kim, K.S., Zolla-Pazner, S. (1982): Disseminated
    Kaposi's sarcoma in homosexual men. Ann. Int. Med.
    96: 693-700.

Hanto, D.W., Gajl-Peczalska, K.J., Frizzera, G., Arthur, D.C.,
    Balfour, H.H. (Jr.), McClain, K., Simmons, R.L.,
    Najarian, J.S. (1983): Ebstein-Barr virus (EBV) induced
    polyclonal B-cell lympho-proliferative diseases occurring
    after renal transplantation. Clinical, pathologic, and
    virologic findings and implications for therapy. Ann.
    Surg. 193: 356-369.

Harris, C.C. (1976): The carcinogenicity of anticancer
    drugs: A hazard in man. Cancer 37: 1014-1023.

Harris, J., Sengar, D., Stewart, T., and Hyslop, D. (1976):
    The effect of immunosuppressive chemotherapy on immune
    function in patients with malignant disease. Cancer 37:
    1058-1069.

Harwood, A.R., Osaba, D., Hofstader, S.L., Goldstein, M.B., Cardella, C.J., Holecek, M.J., Kunynetz, R., and Giammarco, R.A. (1979): Kaposi's sarcoma in recipients of renal transplants. Amer. J. Med. 67: 759-765.

IARC monographs on evaluation of the carcinogenic risk of chemicals to humans. Some antineoplastic and immunosuppressive agents. Lyon, France: WHO International Agency for Research on Cancer (1981) 26: 1-411.

Kahn, M.F., Arlet, J., Bloch-Michel, H., Caroit, M., Chaouat, Y., and Renier, J.C. (1979): Leucemies aigues apres traitement par agents cytotoxique en rhumatologie. 19 observations chez 2006 patients. Nouvelle Presse Medical 8: 1393-1397.

Kinlen, L.J., Sheil, A.G.R., Peto, J., and Doll, R. (1979): Collaborative United Kingdom-Australasian study of cancer in patients treated with immunosuppressive drugs. British Medical Journal 2: 1461-1466.

Kinlen, L.J. (1982): Immunosuppressive therapy and cancer. Cancer Surveys 1: 565-583.

Li, F.P., Osborn, D., Cronin, C.M. (1982): Anorectal squamous carcinoma in two homosexual men. (Letter to the editor). Lancet 2: 391.

Lozada, F., Silvermann, S. (Jr), Conant, M. (1982): New outbreak of oral tumors, malignancies and infectious diseases strikes young male homosexuals. Calif. Dent. J. 10: 39-42.

Penn, I. (1978a): Malignancies associated with immunosuppressive or cytotoxic therapy. Surgery 83: 492-502.

Penn, I. (1978b): Tumors arising in organ transplant recipients, in Klein, G., and Weinhouse, S., (eds.): in Advances in Cancer Research. New York: Academic Press, vol. 28, pp. 31-61.

Penn, I. (1981): The price of immunotherapy. Cur. Prob. Surg. 18 (11): 682-751.

Penn, I. (1982): The occurrence of cancer in immune deficiencies. Cur. Prob. Cancer 6 (10): 1-64.

Penn,I. (1984): The occurrence of malignant tumors in immunosuppressed states. In Klein, E. (ed.) "Acquired Immunodeficiency Syndrome". Basel, Karger, In Press.

Porreco, R., Penn, I., Droegemueller, W., Greer, B., and Makowski, E. (1975): Gynecologic malignancies in immunosuppressed organ homograft recipients. Obstet. Gynec. 45: 359-364.

Portugal, M.A., Falkson, H.C., Stevens, K. and Falkson, G. (1979): Acute leukemia as a complication of long-term treatment of advanced breast cancer. Cancer Treatment Reports 63: 177-181.

Reimer, R.R., Hoover, R., Fraumeni, J.F. (Jr.), Young, R.C. (1977): Acute leukemia after alkylating-agent therapy for ovarian cancer. N. Eng. J. Med. 297: 177-181.

Rosner, R., Grunwald, H.W., and Zarrabi, H.M. (1982): Cancer after the use of alkylating and nonalkylating cytotoxic agents in man. Cancer Surveys 1: 599-612.

Sheil, A.G.R., Mahony, J.F., Horvath, J.S., Johnson, J.R., Tiller, D.J., Steward, J.H., and May, J. (1981): Cancer following successful cadaveric renal transplantation. Transplant. Proc. 13: 733-735.

Sieber, S.M. (1975): Cancer chemotherapeutic agents and carcinogenesis. Cancer Chemother. Rep. 59: 915-918.

Ziegler, J.L., Beckstead, J.A., Volberding. P.A., Abrams, D.I., Levine, A.M., Lukes, R.J., Gill, P.S., Burkes, R.L., Meyer, P.R., Metroka, C.E., Mouradian, J., Moore, E., Riggs, S.A., Butler, J.J., Cabanillas, F.C., Hersh, E., Newell, G.R., Laubenstein, L.J., Knowles, D., Odajnyk, C., Raphael, B., Koziner, B., Urmacher, C., Clarkson, B.d. (1984): Non-Hodgkin's lymphoma in 90 homosexual men: Relationship to generalized lymphadenopathy and Acquired Immunodeficiency Syndrome (AIDS). In press.

Because of space limitations the publications of numerous authors cannot be cited. Most can be found in the publications by Coleman, et al (1982), International Agency for Research on Cancer (1981), Kinlen, et al (1979), Kinlen, (1982), Penn (1978) a and b), Penn (1981), Penn (1982), Penn (1984), Rosner, et al (1982), Sieber (1975) and Ziegler, et al (1984).

IMMUNOLOGICAL ABNORMALITIES IN THE ACQUIRED IMMUNODEFICIENCY SYNDROME

A.H. Rook, J.F. Manischewitz, & A.S. Fauci

Division of Virology, Office of Biologics Research
and Review, Center for Drugs and Biologics,
Bethesda, U.S.A.

INTRODUCTION

Since June and July of 1981 when the Centers for Disease Control (CDC) initially reported the occurrence of 5 cases of Pneumocystis carinii pneumonia and 26 cases of Kaposi's sarcoma in previously well homosexual men (CDC, 1981), there has literally been an explosion in the numbers of new cases of this devastating syndrome that we now recognize as the acquired immunodeficiency syndrome or AIDS. By May 1984 more than 4,400 cases of AIDS, occurring in 46 states and the District of Columbia, had been reported to the CDC (CDC weekly surveillance report on AIDS). Moreover, at least 700 cases had been documented in at least 33 countries outside of the United States (CDC, unpublished statistics).

AIDS is characterized by a variety of disorders of both cellular and humoral immunity which render those afflicted susceptible to infection with a great number of opportunistic pathogenic microbial agents. In addition, the occurrence of one type of neoplasm, Kaposi's sarcoma, represents a particularly common feature of the syndrome. Thus, the current CDC definition of AIDS (Table 1) specifically includes the occurrence of an opportunistic infection or Kaposi's sarcoma which are indicative of a deficiency in cellular immunity in a previously healthy individual less than 60 years of age. The prior use of immunosuppressive drugs or the previous presence of an underlying malignancy known to be associated with an immunodeficiency state precludes one from making the diagnosis. The recent description of the human T-lymphotropic retrovirus, HTLV-III in the United States (Gallo et al., 1984) and the lymphadenopathy associated virus or LAV in France (Barre'-Sinoussi et al., 1983) which were isolated from a large number of individuals with AIDS, and which may be the putative causative agent(s) of the syndrome, will undoubtedly after our ability in the future to recognize individuals with the syndrome, and thus, will surely result in a modification of the current CDC working definition.

The most common initial manifestation of AIDS, which occurs in about 50% of patients, is infection with Pneumoncystis carinii (CDC weekly surveillance report on AIDS). Roughly one-quarter of the patients initially present with Kaposi's sarcoma alone, while 7% present with Kaposi's sarcoma and Pneumoncystis carinii pneumonia. The remaining 17% present with another

There are four major population groups affflicted with AIDS
(Table 3). Homosexual and bisexual men, particularly those
who are highly promiscuous, constitute the largest group,
accounting for 70% of all cases reported in the United States.
Intravenous drug abusers, predominantly those who practice
needle-sharing, account for another 17% of the cases. The
continued high frequency of cases in these two groups, as well
as a persistent increase in the numbers of cases occurring in
hemophiliacs and in recipients of blood transfusions, strongly
suggest that the putative causative agent is both blood-borne
and sexually transmissable.

The devastating nature of AIDS is reflected in the high
mortality rate for those with the syndrome. At the time of
this writing, the overall mortality for all cases in the
United States reported to the CDC is 44%. However, if one
examines the mortality rate for the cases reported to the CDC
prior to 1982, it approaches 100% (CDC weekly surveillance
report on AIDS). Moreover, in view of the absence of
documented cases of recovery from the syndrome, this disease
may prove to be ultimately fatal for all cases involved.

IMMUNOLOGIC ABNORMALITIES

At the initial clinical presentation, patients with AIDS
almost invariably manifest some in vitro disorder of cellular
immunity and many exhibit abnormal humoral immunity as well
(Fauci et al., 1984). Abnormalities of immune function that
have been previously reported to occur are shown in Table 4.
While all of these abnormalities, to a variable degree, have
been characteristically associated with AIDS, the spectrum of
these abnormalities and their severity depend upon the stage
of the disease for each individual. Moreover, there is no
single immune abnormality that is diagnostic for AIDS.
Nevertheless, one abnormality, specifically a depression in
the absolute numbers of peripheral blood T-lymphocytes which
bear the helper/inducer phenotype, appears to occur
in virtually all cases of AIDS. It is this depression in the
numbers of helper/inducer T-lymphocytes in relationship to the
numbers of so-called suppressor/cytotoxic T-lympocytes which
results in a lowering of the normal ratio (usually 1.5-2:1) of
T-helper to T-suppressor cells. Helper/inducer and
suppressor/cytotoxic cells can be identified by their
abilities to bind the monoclonal antibodies OKT4 or Leu-3 and
OKT8 or Leu-2, respectively.

Use of these monoclonal antibodies has made it possible to
define a variety of other clinical conditions which can result
in an alteration of the helper to suppressor cell ratios. It
is noteworthty that systemic viral infection is often accompanied by a depressed helper to suppressor ratio, although it
is usually due to an increase in the numbers of T8 or Leu-2
cells rather than a decrease in the numbers of T4 or Leu-3
cells, the latter being typical of AIDS. As an example, both

cytomegalovirus (CMV) (Carney et al., 1981) and Epstein-Barr virus (EBVV) (Reinherz et al., 1980) infections are associated with a depressed helper to suppressor T cell ratio, and in most cases, absolute numbers of T-helper cells are either normal or only slightly reduced, while T-suppressor/cytotoxic cells are usually dramatically increased. This observation is important since infection with CMV and EBV is exceedingly common among the leading risk group for the development of AIDS, homosexual men. Thus, when attempting to make the diagnosis of AIDS, it is helpful to know the absolute numbers of the different T-cell subsets in the peripheral blood rather than simply relying upon the ratio of T-helper to T-suppressor cells as a diagnostic index.

The precise relationship between the depression in the numbers of helper/inducer T lymphocytes to the other observed immuno-logic abnormalities in AIDS is presently unclear. However, many of the abnormalities do appear to result from deficient T-cell help, such as the inability to generate virus-specific or alloreactive cytotoxic T cells and the inability of T cells to provide help to B lymphocytes for the normal production of immunoglobulins.

An underlying cause for deficient T cell help may be deficient production of certain important immunoregulatory lymphokines such as interleukin 1 and 2 and interferon-gamma. Murray and colleagues (1984) have demonstrated that, in contrast to normal lymphocytes, lymphocytes from AIDS patients often fail to produce interferon-gamma in response to antigenic stimuli. Moreover, several groups have similarly demonstrated deficient IL-2 production by AIDS lymphocytes (Lane et al., 1984; Ciobanu et al., 1984). In preliminary studies, a factor in the serum of AIDS patients has been identified which inhibits the producction of interleukin-2 by normal lymphocytes (Siegel et al., 1984). This factor could contribute to the observed deficiency in interleukin-2 production by AIDS patients. These defects in lymphokine production are relevant to many of the immunologic abnormalities since a variety of in vitro immune functions can be restored to normal levels simply by addition of lymphokine containing media (Rook et al., 1983; Murray et al., 1984).

In this regard, since we have determined that active CMV infection can be documented in nearly all patients with AIDS (Faucci et al., 1984), we have focused attention in our laboratory on those immune responses which appear to be most important for recovery from CMV infection, specifically cytotoxic T cells and natural killer cells, and on means by which these immune responses can be augmented in vitro by the addition of lymhokines. In transplant patients, the ability to develop CMV-specific cytotoxic T cell responses and the level of natural killer cell activity during acute CMV infec-tion are crucial determinants of the outcome of infection (Rook et al., 1984; Quinnan et al., 1982). Patients who fail to develop a T-cell response and who have depressed natural killer cell activity almost invariably have severe or fatal infection. Thus, it is noteworthy that the vast majority of

AIDS patients studied by us have had absent CMV-specific cytotoxic T-cell responses despite active CMV infection and many exhibited deficient natural killer cell activity as well. Repeated testing over several months demonstrated that most patients experienced a progressive decline in their natural killer cell activity (Rook et al., submitted for publication). A high frequency of disseminated infection with CMV is observed among AIDS patients and a profound deficiency in T cell and natural killer cell activity probably accounts for their susceptibility to serious disease with this virus.

In an effort to find immunostimulatory agents that might reconstitute the deficient cytotoxic lymphocyte responses, AIDS lymphocytes were cultured in a variety of lymphokines. The depressed cytotoxic effector mechanisms were found to be refractory to the in vitro effects of either interferon- or interferon- (Figure 1). However, cultivation of AIDS patients lymphocytes in the presence of interleukin-2 consistently produced a marked enhancement of both CMV-specific cytotoxicity (Figure 2) and natural killer cell activity (Figure 3, Rook et al., 1983).In view of the potential importance of cytotoxic T cells and natural killer cells as important defense mechanisms against many microbial agents as well as in anti-tumor surveillance, these effects of interleukin-2 have important implications for the therapy of AIDS.

In addition to the profoundly disordered T-cell immunity observed in AIDS, monocyte function has recently been described to be abnormal (Smith et al., 1984). In response to a variety of chemotactic stimuli, including C5a and lymphocyte-derived chemotactic factor, monocyte chemotaxis of AIDS patients is significantly impaired in comparison to normal individuals. Further, monocyte cytotoxicity and the ability of monocytes to release interleukin-1 in response to lipopolysaccharide are depressed. Thus, deficient monocyte recruitment and function at sites of infection could contribute to the imparied granuloma formation in response to microorganisms such as M. avium intracellulare, and could lead to their dissemination which is so frequently observed in AIDS.

The recent description of decreased numbers of Ia-positive epidermal Langerhans' cells in the skin (Belsito et al., 1984) have suggested indirectly that the antigen presenting capacity of the immune system may also be disordered. Langerhans' cells are related to dendritic cells, the latter cell type being important for antigen presentation to helper T lymphocytes. An abnormality in antigen presentation could contribute to the observed in vitro abnormalities in T-cell function. In addition, since Langerhans' cells are the major antigen presenting cells in the skin, their dysfunction could contribute to the pathogenesis of Kaposi's sarcoma.

The original observations that most patients with AIDS had either elevated or normal serum levels of immunoglobulins initially led to the erroneous belief that B lymphocyte function was normal. However, the studies of Lane et al.

(1983) have demonstrated that the peripheral blood B lymphocytes of patients with AIDS are polyclonally activated and are
secreting abnormally large quantities of immunoglobulin. In
addition, sera from most AIDS patients contain immune
complexes. The polyclonal B lymphocytes activation can be
quantitated in vitro in a reserve hemolytic plaque-forming
cell assay (Figure 4). In addition to having increased levels
of spontaneous plaque forming cells in the peripheral blood,
the B lymphocytes of AIDS patients exhibit a decreased capacity to respond to activation signals, most likely due to the
in vivo state of activation. Since active EBV infection has
been documented to occur in virtually all AIDS patients
(Quinnan et al., 1984; Fauci et al., 1984), these findings of
abnormal B lymphocyte function may be due to activation and
transformation of peripheral blood B lymphocytes by EBV in the
absence of the normal regulatory T-lymphocyte influences.

Another common component of the abnormal B lymphocyte function
in AIDS is the inability to generate a de novo serologic
response to new protein antigens. Lane et al. (1983) demonstrated that AIDS patients were incapable of making serum
antibody to the potent protein immunogen keyhole limpet
hemocyanin. The failure to produce antibodies in response to
new antigenic stimuli may, thus, confound the ability to use
serologic tests for diagnostic purposes in this population of
patients.

In addition to the abnormalities of peripheral blood mononuclear cell function which encompasses T, B, and natural killer
lymphocytes and monocytes, many patients with AIDS exhibit
serologic markers of altered immune function. As mentioned
above, Siegel et al. (1984) have observed the presence of a
serum factor which inhibits the production of interleukin-2 by
normal peripheral blood lymphocytes. Other serum factors have
been recognized which are capable of supressing a variety of
in vitro immune responses of normal lymphocytes
(Cunningham-Rundles et al., 1983). Other abnormalities
include the presence of an acid-labile form of interferon (De Stefano et al., 1982), elevated thymosin
levels (Hersh et al., 1983) and the presence of lymphocyto-
toxic antibodies (Williams et al., 1984).

As mentioned above, the extent of the immunological abnormalities in an individual with AIDS is dependent upon the stage at
which the disease is diagnosed. What is clear is that
patients who present with Kaposi's sarcoma alone often have
fewer immune defects at the time of diagnosis than do patients
who initially present with life-threatening opportunistic
infections. Moreover, the degree of immune deficit at the
time of diagnosis may correlate with the overall prognosis for
survival. This is supported by the observation that patients
who initially present with Kaposi's sarcoma have a longer life
expectancy than those with opportunistic infections.

ISOLATION OF AN ETIOLOGICAL AGENT

Attempts to isolate a putative etiological agent for this syndrome have focused on infectious agents whose spread is consistent with the epidemiological distribution of this syndrome, specifically being sexually transmissable and blood-borne, and upon agents which have the capacity to induce aberrations of the helper T lymphocyte subpopulation. Microbial agents such as hepatitis B virus, EBV and CMV are all sexually transmissable, are all blood-borne and are all exceedingly common among the individuals in the leading risk groups for AIDS. In our studies at the National Institutes of Health, all of the initial 34 patients examined had evidence of active CMV infection documented either by virus isolation or the presence of IgM serum antibodies to CMV (Quinnan et al., 1984). Yet, other laboratories have not observed the same high frequency of CMV infection. The differences in the results may depend upon the rapidity with which clinical specimens are processed for virus culture, particulary since CMV is labile and virus titer decreases with passage of time. From our studies, it is nevertheless clear that CMV is a frequent cause of morbidity among AIDS patients. Moreover, at death, most AIDS patients have evidence of widely disseminated CMV infection (Macher et al., 1983).

In addition, because CMV possesses immunosuppressive potential, much attention has been given to this virus as a potential factor or co-factor in the pathogenesis of the immunological abnormalities in AIDS. Active CMV infection of normal individuals is associated with depressed lymphocyte responses to mitogens (Carney et al., 1981) and the depressed ability to release lymphokines, and, transplant patients with CMV infection experience a high frequency of secondary superinfections with other organisms (Rand et al., 1978). As mentioned above, active CMV infection is characteristically associated with a depression of the T-helper to T-suppressor ratio; however, this is due primarilt to an increase in OKT8 positive cells (suppressor/cytotoxic) while OKT4 positive cells (helper/inducer) are usually normal or only slightly decreased. At present, there is no good evidence to suggest that CMV can infect helper T lymphocytes or result in their depletion which is a characteristic of AIDS. Thus, while CMV infection occurs frequently in AIDS patients, is immunosuppressive and is a common cause of morbidity, there is currently no direct evidence to link CMV with the cause of AIDS.

From the outset, the human T cell leukemia (HTLV) family of retroviruses has been of interest in the study of AIDS, especially because they exhibit a particular predilection to infect and induce abnormalities in the OKT4 positive subset of T lymphocytes (Broder etal., 1984). HTLV-I and II have been associated with leukemias and lymphomas characterized by the proliferation of OKT4 positive cells. In certain parts of the world where HTLV-I is endemic, such as southern Japan and the Caribbean, as much as 15% of the population demonstrates serologic evidence of prior infection. In non-endemic areas including much of the United States, 1% or less of the population possess anti-HTLV serum antibodies, indicating a low frequency of infection.

In May 1983 Gelmann et al. reported the presence of integrated HTLV proviral genomic sequences in the DNA of lymphocytes from two of thirty-three AIDS patients studied. Gallo et
al. (1983) were able to recover a retrovirus, identified as
HTLV-I, from the T lymphocytes of one of the individuals. At
the same time, Barre'-Sinoussi and colleagues (1983) reported
the isolation of a new human retrovirus, that was distinct
from HTLV-I and II, from the lymph node cells of a homosexual
man with the chronic lymphadenopathy syndrome. Thus, it was
evident that infection with HTLV occurred with a greater
frequency among individuals with AIDS than in the general
population, and the observations of Barre'-Sinoussi and colleagues indicated that a new genetic varient of the HTLV famlily
might be associated with AIDS.

More recently Gallo et al. (1984) were also able to isolate a
new T-lymphotropic retrovirus (HTLV-III) from the lymphoctytes
of 26 of 72 AIDS patients and from 18 of 21 individuals with
chronic unexplained lymphadenopathy and leukopenia, characteristic of a pre-AIDS syndrome. In addition, most of the AIDS
sera tested in Gallo's laboratory have been found to contain
antibodies to HTLV-III, while large numbers of normal sera do
not. Similarly, LAV has been isolated with increasing frequency from patients with AIDS who are being studied by
Montagnier and colleagues in France. These studies provide
strong evidence for the association of HTLV-III and LAV with
AIDS. The precise relationship between HTLV-III and the
retrovirus isolated by Barre'-Sinoussi, now referred to as LAV
(lymphadenopathy associated virus), is unclear and remains to
be determined.

At present, HTLV-III and LAV have been isolated predominantly
from T lymphocytes with the helper/inducer phenotypes (OKT4,
Leu-3). Moreover, both HTLV-III and LAV are cytopathic for
this subset of T lymphocytes and can produce the in vitro
destruction of these cells. These observation are of interest
since one of the characteristic laboratory manifestations of
AIDS is the depletion of that T cell population. As mentioned
above, many of the immunologic abnormalities in AIDS appear to
result from a deficiency in T-Helper cell function which may
be due to HTLV-III infection of T-helper cells. Whether
abnormalities of monocyte, B-lymphocyte and natural killer
lymphocyte function arise secondarily as a result of HTLV-III
infection of T-helper cells, or result directly from infection
with an agent such as HTLV-III is an important question which
deserves future study.

90

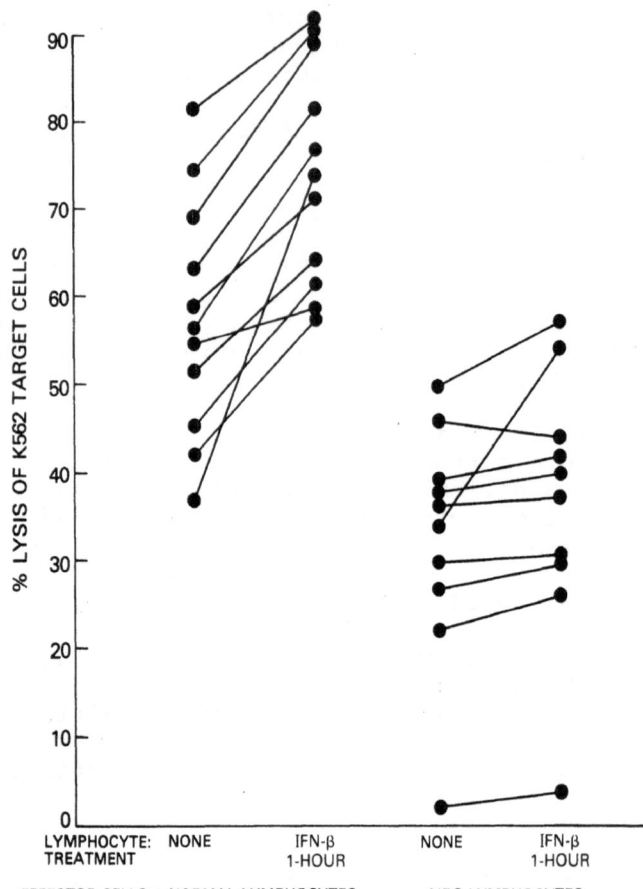

Figure 1. The effect of in vitro IFN-Beta on the NK cell activity of lymphocytes from normal subjects and AIDS patients in a standard 16 hour ^{51}Cr release assay using K562 cells as targets.

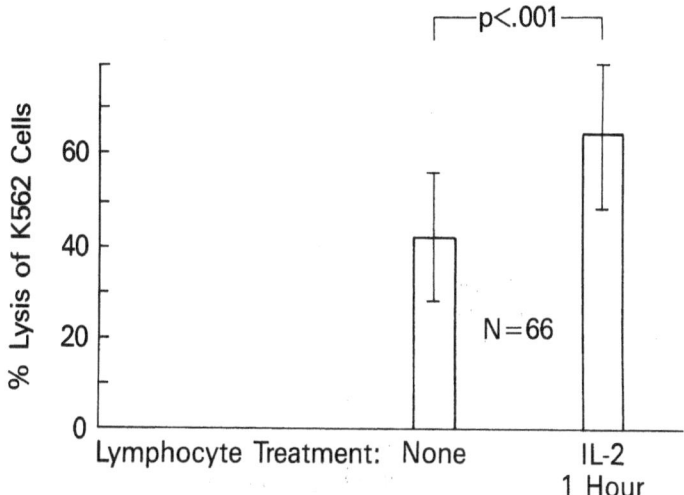

Figure 2. The effect of *in vitro* IL-2 on the CMV-specific cytotoxic lymphocyte activity of AIDS patients. Assays were 16 hour ^{51}Cr release employing pairs of CMV-infected and uninfected human diploid skin fibroblasts as targets. Each experiment had at least one pair of partially HLA-matched and one pair of HLA-mismatched targets for each group of effector PBL to determine if the response was HLA-restricted or non-HLA-restricted. The % CMV-specific lysis was calculated by subtracting % lysis uninfected fibroblasts from % lysis of CMV-infected fibroblasts.

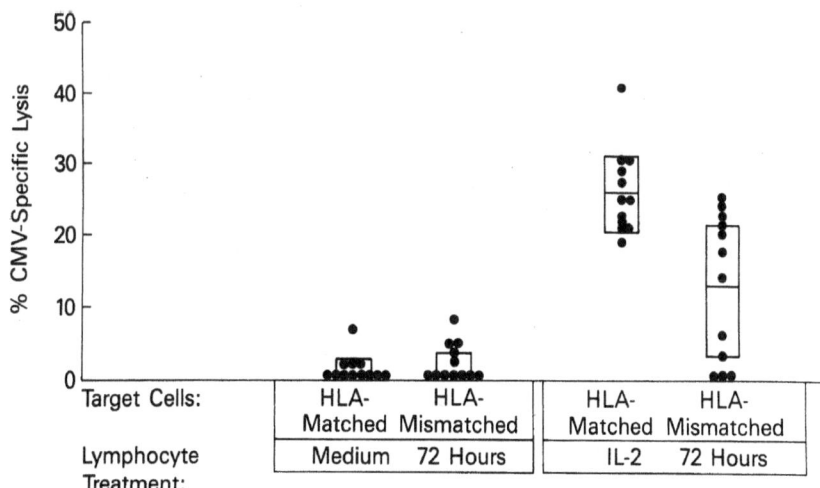

Figure 3. The effect of *in vitro* IL-2 on the NK cell activity of lymphocytes from AIDS patients. PBL were either untreated or cultured in IL-2 for 1 hour prior to assay.

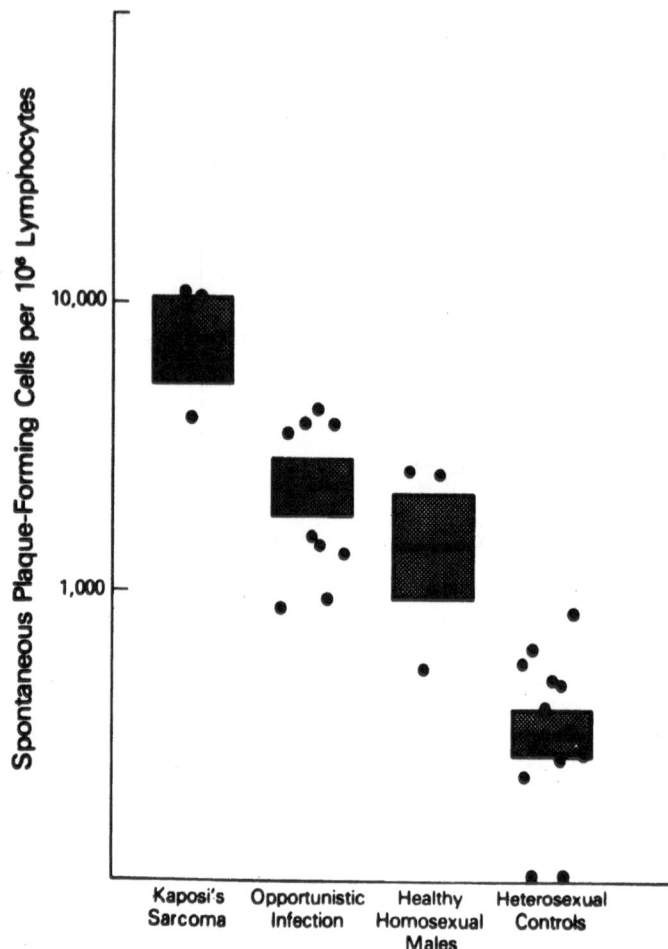

Figure 4. Enumeration of spontaneous plaque-forming cells in patients with Koposi's sarcoma, patients with opportunistic infections only, healthy homosexual men, and heterosexual controls. (From Lane et al.; reprinted by permission of the New England Journal of Medicine 309:453-458, 1983).

Table 1.   Centers for Disease Control Definition of the
Acquired Immunodeficiency Syndrome

Presence of reliably diagnosed disease at least moderately indicative of
underlying cellular immunodeficiency (Kaposi's sarcoma in a patient
under 60 years of age, Pneumocystis pneumonia, other opportunistic
infections).

Absence of known causes of underlying immunodeficiency and of any other
reduced resistance reported to be associated with the disease
(immunosuppressive therapy, lymphoreticular malignancy).

Table 2.   Opportunistic Infections Compatible with the CDC
Definition of the Acquired Immunodeficiency Syndrome

Protozoal and helminthic infections

Cryptosporidiosis, intestinal, causing diarrhea for more than one month
(on histologic study or stool microscopic study).

Pneumocystis carinii penumonia (on histologic study or microscopic study
of a "touch" preparation or bronchial washings).

Strongyloidosis, causing pneumonia, central nervous system infection, or
disseminated infection (on histologic study).

Toxoplasmosis, causing pneumonia or central nervous sytem infection (on
histologic study or microscopic study of a "touch" preparation).

Fungal infections

Candidiasis, causing esophagitis (on histologic study or microscopic
study of a "wet" preparation from the esophagus, or endoscopic findings
of white plaques on an erythematous mucosal base).
Cryptococcosis, causing central nervous system or disseminated infection
(on culture, antigen detection, histologic study, or India ink
preparation of cerebrospinal fluid).

Bacterial infections

"Atypical" mycobacteriosis (species other than tuberculosis or lepra),
causing disseminated infection (on culture).

Viral infections

Cytomegalovirus, causing pulmonary, gastrointestinal tract, or central
nervous system infection (on histologic study).

Herpes simplex virus, causing chronic mucocutaneous infection with
ulcers persisting more than one month, or pulmonary, gastrointestinal
tract, or disseminated infection (on culture, histologic study, or
cytologic study).

Progressive multifocal leukoencephalopathy (presumed to be caused by a
papovavirus) (on histologic study).

Table 3. Hierarchial Order of Acquired Immunodeficiency Syndrome
Risk Groups, May 1984*

	MALES		FEMALES		TOTAL	
	CASES	PERCENT OF MALES	CASES	Percent OF FEMALES	CASES	Percent OF TOTAL
Homosexual or Bisexual†	3071	77.0	0	0.0	3071	71.9
Intravenous Drug User	586	14.7	155	55.0	741	17.3
Haitian	146	3.7	27	9.6	173	4.1
Hemophiliac	30	0.8	0	0.0	30	0.7
None Apparent/Unknown	156	3.9	100	35.5	256	6.0
Total	3989	100.0	282	100.0	4271	100.0

*Data are courtesy of the Centers for Disease Control.

†The risk groups listed are hierarchically ordered; cases with multiple risk factors
are tabulated only in the risk group listed first.

Table 4. Abnormalities of Immune Function in Patients with AIDS

1. Lymphopenia--predominantly due to a selective defect in the
   helper/inducer subset (OKT4, Leu-3) of T-lymphocytes.

2. Abnormal _in vitro_ T-cell function

   A. Decreased blast transformation.
   B. Decreased antigen-specific cytotoxic T-cell function.
   C. Decreased alloreactivity.
   D. Decreased ability to provide help to B-lymphocytes.

3. Abnormal natural killer cell function.

   A. Decreased cytotoxicity.
   B. Refractoriness to _in vitro_ augmentation of cytotoxicity by
      interferons alpha and beta.

4. Abnormal monocyte function.

   A. Decreased chemotaxis.
   B. Decreased cytotoxicity.
   C. Decreased interleukin-1 release.

5. Polyclonal B-cell activation.

   A. Elevated levels of total serum immunoglobulins and circulating
      immune complexes.
   B. Inability to mount a de novo serologic response to a new
      antigen.
   C. Increased numbers of spontaneous immunoglobulin-secreting
      cells.
   D. Refractoriness to the normal _in vitro_ signals for B-cell
      activation.

6. Abnormal lymphokine production.

   A. Decreased antigen simulated interleukin-2 release _in vitro_.
   B. Decreased antigen stimulated interferon-gamma release _in vitro_.
   C. Decreased interleukin-1 release in response to
      lipopolysaccharide _in vitro_.
   D. Decreased virus induced interferon-alpha release _in vitro_.
   E. Abnormal presence of acid-labile interferon-alpha in the serum.

REFERENCES

Barre'-Sinoussi F, Chermann JC, Rey F, Nuyeyre MT, Chomaret S, Aruest J, Dauguet C, Axler-Blin C, Vezinet-Brun F, Rouzioux C, Royenbaum W, Montagnier L. (1983) Isolation of a T-Lymphotropic Retrovirus from a Patient at Risk for Acquired Immune Deficiency Syndrome (AIDS). Science 220:868-871.

Belsito DV, Sanchez MR, Baer RL, Valentine F, Thorbecke GJ. (1984) Reduced Langerhans' Cell Ia Antigen and ATPase Activity in Patients with the Acquired Immunodeficiency Syndrome. N. Engl. J. Med. 310:1279-82.

Broder S, Bunn PA, Jaffe ES, Blattner W, Gallo RC, Wong-Stoal F, Waldmoon TA, De Vita VT. (1984) T-Cell Lymphoproliferative Syndrome Associated with Human T-Cell Leukemia Lymphoma Virus. Ann Int. Med. 100:543-557.

Carney WP, Rubin RH, Hoffman RA, Hansen WP, Healey K, Hirsch MS. (1981) Analysis of T Lymphocyte Subsets in Cytomegalovirus Mononucleosis. J. Immunol. 126:2114-2116.

Centers for Disease Control. (1981) Kaposi's Sarcoma and Pneumocystis pneumonia Among Homosexual Men--New York City and California. MMWR 25:305-8.

Centers for Disease Control. (1981) Pneumocystis pneumonia-Los Angeles. MMWR 30:250-2.

Ciobanu N, Kruger G, Welte K, Safai B, Venuta S, Gold J, Feldman SP, Wong CY, Kozinger B, Moore MAS, Mertelsmann R. (1983). Defective T Cell Response to PHA and Mitogenic Monoclonal Antibodies in Male Homosexuals with Aids and Its In Vitro Correction by Interleukin-2. J. Clin. Immun. 3:332-340.

Cunningham-Rundles S, Michelis MA, Masur H. (1983) Serum Suppression of Lymphocyte Activation In Vitro in Acquired Immunodeficiency Disease. J. Clin. Immunol. 3:156-65.

DeStefano E, Friedman RM, Friedman-Kien AE, Goedert JJ, Henriksen D, Preble OT, Sonnenbend JA, Vilcek J. (1982) Acid-labile Human Leukocyte Interferon in Homosexual Men with Kaposi's Sarcoma and Lymphadenopathy. J. Infect. Dis. 146:451-455.

Fauci AS, Macher AM, Longo DL, Lane HC, Rook AH, Masur H, Gelmann EP. (1984) AIDS: Epidemiologic, Clinical, Immunologic, and Therapeutic Considerations. Ann Int. Med. 100:92-1o6.

Gallo RC, Sarin PS, Gelmann EP, Robert-Guroff M, Richardson E, Kalyanaraman VS, Mann D, Sidhu GD, Stahl RE, Zolla-Payner S, Leibowitch J, Popovic M. (1983) Isolation of Human T-Cell Leukemia Virus in AIDS. Science 220:865-868.

Gallo RC, Salahuddin SZ, Popovic M, Shearer GM, Kaplan M, Haynes BF, Palker TJ, Redfield R, Oleske J, Safai B, White G, Foster P. Markham PD. (1984) Frequent Detection and Isolation of Cytopathic Retroviruses (HTLV-III) from Patients with AIDS and at Risk for AIDS. Science 224:500-503.

Gelmann EP, Popvic M, Blayney D, Masur H, Sidhu G, Stahl Gallo RC. (1983) Proviral DNA of a Retrovirus, Human T-Cell Leukemia Virus, in Two Patients with AIDS. Science 220:862-865.

Hersh EM, Reuben JM, Rios A, Monsell PWA, Newell GR. (1983) Elevated Serum Thymosin Alpha1 Levels Associated with Evidence of Immune Dysregulation in Male Homosexuals with a History of Infectious Diseases or Kaposi's Sarcoma (Letter). N. Engl. J. Med. 308:45-6.

Lane HC, Masur H, Edgar LC, Whalen G, Rook AH, Fauci AS. (1983) Abnormalities of B-cell Activation and Immunoregulation in Patients with the Acquired Immunodeficiency Syndrome. N. Engl. J. Med. 309:453-8.

Lane HC, Masur H, Rook AH, Quinnan GV, Gelmann E, Steis R, Longo D, Palestine A, Macher A, Fauci AS. (1984) Treatment of Patients with the Acquired Immunodeficiency Syndrome with Interleukin-2 or Interferon-Gamma. Clin. Research 32:351A.

Macher AM, Reichert D, Straus S, Longo DL, Parillo J, Lane HC, Fauci AS, Rook AH, Manischewitz JF, Quinnan GV, Jr. (1983) Death in the AIDS Patient: Role of Cytomegalovirus. N. Engl. J. Med. 309:1454.

Murray HW, Rubin BY, Masur H, Roberts RB. (1984) Impaired Production of Lymphokines and Immune (Gamma) Interferon in the Acquired Immunodeficiency Syndrome. N. Engl. J. Med. 310:883-889.

Quinnan GV, Jr., Kirmani N, Rook AH, Manischewitz JF, Jackson L, Moreschi G, Santos GW, Saral R. Burns WH. (1982) Cytotoxic T Cells in Cytomegalovirus Infection: HLA-restricted T-lymphocyte and Non-T-lymphocyte Cytotoxic Responses Correlate with Recovery from Cytomegalovirus Infection in Bone-Marrow-Transplant Recipients. N.Engl. J. Med. 307:7-13.

Quinnan GV, Jr., Masur H, Rook AH, Armstrong G, Frederick WJR, Ames J, Epstein JS, Macher AM, Manischewitz JF, Jackson L, Smith HA, Parker M, Pearson GR, Parillo J, Straus S. (1984) Herpesvirus Infections in the Acquired Immunodeficiency Syndrome. JAMA (in press).

Raned KH, Pollard RB, Merigan TC. (1978) Increased Pulmonary Superinfections in Cardiac Transplant Recipients Undergoing Primary Cytomegalovirus Infection. N. Engl. J. Med. 298:951-53.

Reinherz El, O'Brien C, Rosenthal P, Schlossman SF. (1980) the Cellular Basis for Viral-Induced Immunodeficiency: Analysis by Monoclonal Antibodies. J. Immunol. 125: 1269-74.

Rook AH, Masur H, Lane HC, Frederick WJF, Kasahara T, Macher AM, Djeu JY, Manischewitz JF, Jackson L, Fauci AS, Quinnan GV, Jr. (1983) Interleukin-2 Enhances the Depressed Natural Killer Cell and Cytomegalovirus-Specific Cytotoxic Activities of Lympho-cytes from Patients with the Acquired Immunodeficiency Syndrome. J. Clin Invest. 72:398-493.

Rook AH, Quinnan GV, Jr., Frederick WJR, Manischewitz JF, Kirmani N, Dantzler T, Lee BB, Currier CB, Jr. (1984) Importance of Cytotoxic Lymphocytes During Cytomegalo-virus Infection of Renal Transplant Recipients. Am. J. Med. 76:385-392.

Selik RM, Haverkos HW, Curran JW. (1984) AIDS Trends in the United States, 1978-1982. Am. J. Med. 76:493-500.

Siegel JP, Djeu JY, Stocks NI, Masur H, Fauci AS, Lane HC, Gelmann EP, Quinnan GV, Jr. (1984) Serum from Patients with the Acquired Immunodeficiency Syndrome (AIDS) suppresses production of interleukin-2 by normal peri-pheral blood lymphocytes.Clin.Res.358A.

Smith PD, Ohura K, Masur H, Lane HC, Fauci AS, Wahl SM, (1984) Monocyte Function in the Acquired Immunodeficiency Syndrome. clin. Research 32:358A.

Williams RC, Masur H, Spira TJ. (1984) Lymphocyte Reactive Antibodies in Acquired Immune Deficiency Syndrome. J. Clin. Immun. 4:118-123.

MONITORING THE HUMAN IMMUNE SYSTEM

G. Riethmueller , H.W.L. Ziegler-Heitbrock & E.P. Rieber

Institute of immunology , universitùt,
Muenchen , F.R.G.

INTRODUCTION

The aim of this presentation is to discuss current changes taking place in the field of monitoring the human immune system (IS). The assessment of immune functions in a longitudinal fashion in individual patients has remained a cardinal problem for the clinical immunologist as well as for the neophyte immunopharmacologist. The difficulties for comparative, quantitative measurements arise from the peculiar nature of the immune response itself and our limited access to the active elements of this complex defence system.

In its functioning the IS cannot be compared with other adaptative organs. While the endocrine pancreas responds with insulin release in an almost identical fashion upon repeated glucose stimulation, an immune response based on activation, proliferation and differrentiation of unique cell clones is by itself a singular event. Probing the IS in vivo by introducing bona fide new antigens like the bacteriophage ∅x174 or a contact sensitizer like dinitrochlorobenzene (DNCB) gives valid information on immunological competence; it is, however, irreproducible, because the IS does not return to its original state. Thus, in this respect, probing the immune system resembles in some ways modern nuclear particle physics, where observation of an object interferes with its natural state. Apart from this rigorous reasoning, ethical considerations preclude monitoring of the IS by induction of primary immune responses against a series of new antigens in an individual patient.

Another special feature of the IS is its highly individualized "eigen"" activity which is reflected in the characteristic broad variation of immune responses in genetically identical individuals. If one takes the spleen cells of individual inbred mice belonging to one litter and kept under identical environmental conditions, performs a PHA stimulation in vitro and measures thymidine incorporation in triplicates after three days, a broad variation of thymidine uptake becomes notable. Thus, it can be understood why the simple in vitro lymphocyte activation assay has resisted the combined standardization efforts of innumerable national and international standardization committees.

Thus, to monitor the IS we have to define the problems arising from the peculiar individual nature of this complex system and to search for those accessible indicators which can give quantitative information on the various interactions the IS is undergoing with its own particular environment.

THE DYNAMIC "EIGEN" ACTIVITY OF THE IMMUNE SYSTEM AND THE VENOUS BLOOD SAMPLING BIAS

Early observation on natural antibodies, i.e. non-induced by exogenous agents, and the completeness of the immunological repertoire in germ-free animals delivered by cesarian section gave first indications that the IS develops and unfolds in complete isolation from the environment. Thus there is an astounding turnover of B and T cells going on without pertur-bations by the external environment, even in the adult organism. In rodents experimental data show that about one third of the blood lymphocytes have newly arrived from the regenerating tissue. The majority of newly formed lymphocytes transported by the blood are short-lived and rarely enter the recirculating pool. Exogenous perturbations of the IS, like primary of secondary immunization or viral infections, heavily influence the composition of the circulating blood lymphocytes. Moreover the turnover of lymphocytes and most probably that of immunoglobulins, as well, changes under various conditions and seems to be different in young and old organisms. Thus, it seems hazardous to base firm conclusion on an analysis of circulating lymphocytes representing less than 0.5 % of the total lymphocyte mass that is in a conti-nuous flux of changing proportions of subpopulations. Before entering a detailed discussion of in vitro testing the in vivo assays should be presented first.

DELAYED TYPE HYPERSENSITIVITY SKIN TEST

This procedure is a relatively simple test giving a reliable indication on the present state of an established cellular immunity. Antigens which typically give positive results in a majority of healthy adult individuals in Western Europe are streptokinase-streptodornase,PPD,candida,trychophyton mumpsan-tigen and tetanus.

Another procedure presently widely adopted in Europe uses Tetanus Toxoid, Diphteria Toxoid, Steptococci, Old-tuberculin, Candida, Trychophyton and Proteus furnished not as lyophilized antigens, but adsorbed to a multiple applicator (Multitest Merieux[R]). The source, nature and stability of antigens is crucial. The FDA Panel on Review of Skin Test Antigens found only 5 of 25 tested preparations to be reproducibly stable, safe and effective.

Pitfalls:

A reaction of immediate type hypersensitivity has to be distinguished from the typical delayed reaction which develops only after 12 h and gains its maximum between 24 and 48 h. Furthermore the test can be negative during acute viral infections (measles, mumps, influenza) and other generalized infections.

Interpretation

As to the interpretation of the reaction , a positive skin test against PPD for instance may represent residual cell-mediated immunity , while a de novo induction of a cellular immune reaction is no longer possible. On the other hand skin testing by itself may sensitize or boost an existing immunity. Thus the procedure as such is not suitable for monitoring on a repeat basis.

Induction of delayed hypersensitivity by contact sensitizers

Systemic sensitization to highly reactive compounds such as dinitro-chlorobenzene or dinitrofluorobenzene may be readily induced by direct application of the dissolved substances to the skin. As animal models have shown, peripheral sensitization is an important aspect of this test. For induction of a positive reaction the Langerhans cells of the epidermis as well as circulating T cells have to be functioning. Furthermore, a positive delayed-type hypersensitivity reaction depends on a functioning mast cell system with the whole armamentarium of vasoactive peptides and amines involved.

Induction of a primary humoral immune response

As stated in the introduction, a primary immune response is an unique event for the individual patient and not suited for monitoring. However, for certain diagnostic purposes immunization with a nonpathogenic bacteriophage ($\emptyset$x174) or with the immonogenic keyhole limpet haemaglutinin (KLH) may be highly informative, particularly when the kinetics of the response, the switch of IgM IgG antibodies and affinity of antibodies are considered.

APPROACHES TO IN VITRO MONITORING OF LEUKOCYTE FUNCTION

Lymphocytes

The genuine domain where monitoring of the IS seems to be most informative is the field of in vitro assays of lymphocyte functions. However, the recognition of the extreme heterogeneity of lymphocytes, the variation with time of the different circulating subpopulations puts a serious question mark behind most of the current tests performed according to generally accepted protocols; i.e. to a sample of blood mononuclear cells, add plant mitogen and measure thymidine uptake.

The above mentioned inability to define a reasonable normal range of the PHA response is clear evidence that this system cannot detect subtle quantitative changes in lymphocyte activation, and yet, the task of monitoring environmental toxic effects upon the IS makes it mandatory to detect subtle changes in the regulator and effector elements of the system. A further goal is to understand the significance of such changes for the overall defence capacity as well as the capability of self- non-self-discrimination. It is now clear that the extent of lymphocyte activation measured after stimulation of unseparated cell population is a function of the different regulatory elements present in the culture. Suppressor or helper T cells, B lymphocytes , natural killer cells, monocytes and various as yet undefined subpopulations are modifying the final outcome of the in vitro response. Thus one prerequisite for performing global lymphocyte activation tests with polyclonal activators is to define with a much detail as possible the composition of the population of lymphocytes to be activated. Monoclonal antibodies to various differentiation antigens are the tools of choice for defining distinct lymphocyte populations. While it is common practice to distinguish major subsets of lymphocytes by single markers, additional important information can be drawn from multiple parameter analysis, where expression of several function-associated markers can give further resolution.

The detection of the Interleukin-2 receptor by a specific monoclonal antibody is a good example of such an analysis. We have to be aware, however, that the Interleukin-2 receptor shows transient expression and may be present on B cells as well as monocytes.Since expression of Interleukin-2 receptor requires immune stimulation of T cells, additional information is gained when a simultaneous T4 or T8 determination reveals which subpopulation is being stimulated. Such an analysis requires directly labelled monoclonal reagents and is performed most easily with a flow-through-cytophotometer (FACS, EPICS) Class II antigens of MHC may serve as another class of activation signs for T cells. Again it will be useful in the future to know which subpopulations are expressing gene locus specific DR, DQ or DP molecules.

Evidence is presently emerging that the appearance of cellular subpopulations characterized by unexpected simultaneous expression of two markers may serve as indicators of certain functional states of the IS. Thus, T8+Leu7+double marker cells are distinctly increased in several immunodeficiency syndromes and have been found in haemophiliac patients exhibiting inverted T4/T8 ratios (1).

Considering the continuous flux of T cells from generating organs - even in adults - the emergence of a distinct T4+T8+double marker subset in the circulation may reflect a peculiar renewal situation or increased turnover. So far the clinical or functional significance of the appearance of such small populations is unknown. In addition little or no information at all is available as to how the various smaller subsets modify an overall mitogen induced proliferation. Also the attempt is warranted to correlate both doseand time-response kinetics of mitogen- or antigen-stimulated cultures with the relative proportions of quiescent of activated subpopulations present at the onset of cultivation.

Instead of measuring polyclonal activation by mitogens, activation of subclasses can be obtained by subclass specific monoclonals. Thus, the response of T4+ and T8+-subclasses can be separately measured by stimulating with the corresponding monoclonal antibody specific for T3. It is foreseeable that plant mitogens will be replaced by monoclonal antibodies, however, the requirements of accessory cells in antibody induced stimulation is even more critical than with plant mitogens.

Monitoring monocyte/macrophage function

Monocytes/macrophages carry out important modulatory functions in the immune response. Antigen presentation is one of the most important ones, however, the details of antigen processing required for effective presentation are still unknown. Handling of monocytes for in vitro assays is critical, since mere adherence of the cells suffices to induce activation. The measurement of stimulated release of various mediators such as prostaglandins and interleukins is fraught with such in vitro induced artefacts. A particular activity of monocytes is their cytotoxicity against other cells. Recent technical advances have made it possible to shorten the assay times considerably. A survey of available monocyte cytotoxicity test shows that most of the current tests require incubation periods of more than 24 h. We have been able to develop a cytotoxicity test which in addition of being of short duration is specific for monocytes (2). The xenogeneic target cell Wehi 164 pretreated with Actinomycin D is resistant to lysis by natural killer cells, thus monocyte cytotoxicity can be assessed without troublesome purification steps entailing uncontrolled activation of cells.

B Lymphocytes

Heterogeneity of B lymphocytes is a widely discussed subject in immunology. Thus far no clear phenotypic distinction of B memory lymphocytes has been possible. B lymphocytes comprise only a minor portion of total circulating lymphocytes. Mouse data indicates that , B lymphocytes subpopulations revealing particular markers (PanT) may be predictive for certain autoimmune or neoplastic disorders. The reverse hemolytic plaque test seems to be a sufficiently sensitive method to detect circulating Ig secreting B cells which seem to indicate the polyclonal activation of the sessile B cell compartment.

CONCLUDING REMARKS

Monitoring the human immune system has remained a formidable task for the clinician. The individual fluctuating "eigen" activity of the immune system seems to be responsible for the broad variation characteristic for the specific immune respnse. In contrast to other adaptive systems the specific immune response is not characterized by the production and secretion of homogeneous factors like hormones or enzymes but shows a wide variation of unique responding cells and reactive molecules. Monitoring of the human IS has the big handicap that circulating leukocytes are the only accessible elements of the system. Though in vivo tests are available by which a true primary immune response can be measured such tests are not feasible for a continuous monitoring. Because of the heterogeneity of circulating cells a finely tuned marker analysis is a crucial requirement for adequate functional tests. Particular emphasis should be placed on multiple parameter analysis employing function associated markers and/or markers for developmental stages. In man, turnover studies of subpopulations are required . At the same time the regulatory activity in such subsets has to be determined. Production of nonspecific factors, as well as the response to such factors, should be considered in further monitoring attempts. In order to circumvent ambiguities resulting from polyclonal stimulation with plant mitogens, the use of subpopulation specific monoclonal antibodies is recommended. Such antibodies have to be carefully selected, because of requirements imposed by the particular recognized epitope as well as by Fc receptor restrictions that are important for obtaining optimal accessory cell support.

Monocyte cytotoxicity testing may now be more practical and meaningful, because of available short term assays avoiding troublesome purification steps. It has become clear that a new era of immune monitoring is about to unfold. The new technologies utilizing monoclonal antibodies as structural and functional probes will enable us to look more precisely at these circulating mononuclear cells , which in themselves represent only a small fraction of the total immune system. They also offer the possibility of measuring lymphokine factors and differentiation factors like thymic hormones which are present at very low concentrations in the circulating blood.

REFERENCES

1. ZIEGLER, H.W.L. et al., 1985, Clin.exp. Immunol., <u>61</u>, 633-641

2. ZIEGLER, H.W.L. & RIETHMUELLER, G., 1984, INCI, <u>72</u>, 23-29

IMMUNORESTORATION IN SECONDARY IMMUNODEFICIENCY

J.W. Hadden

Immunopharmacology Program, University of S.Florida,
College of Medicine,
Tampa, U.S.A.

INTRODUCTION

Twenty years ago, the study of immunodeficiency concentrated on congenital, primary immunodeficiency in which a cell population or molecule was genetically absent or dysfunctional. Secondary immunodeficiency was restricted to immunosuppressive treatment for organ transplantation and autoimmune diseases, to lymphoid malignancies such as Hodgkins disease, and to cytotoxic anticancer therapy. With the advent of appropriate immunodiagnostic tests to assess the number and function of the various components of the immune system and other bulwarks of natural bodily defenses, our understanding of· secondary immuno-deficiency began to grow, and now twenty years later we have a more comprehensive and explicit view of the extent of immunodeficiency.

Most seconday immune deficiencies involve defects more in cellular than humoral responses i.e., those mediated by T cells, macrophages, and natural killer (NK) cells, however, no modification of the system by xenobiotics, either by immuno-toxin or immunotherapeutic agent is completely selective for a single cell population and no defect involving one cell population is without compensatory or secondary changes in other cell populations. The study and attempted therapy of immunotoxicity is, therefore, by definition, extremely complex.

In this presentation, I will summarize the major areas of secondary immunodeficiency resulting from immunotoxic influences, I will not discuss secondary immunodeficiencies resulting from :(1) malnutritional (see Good, R.A., et al. (1982) for review);(2) aging, (see Makinodan, T., et al. (1976) for review), (3) acute and chronic infections with pathogens which produce immunosuppressive products (see Floersheim, G.L. (1979) for review) and (4) cancer in which immunosuppression results from malnutrition and products of both the tumor and the immune system (see Wanebo, H.J. (1978) for review). I will present certain immunosuppressive and anticancer drugs and environmental immunotoxicants and end with a discussion on the prospects for immunorestoration. Immunotoxicology, for this discussion will be simply defined as the harmful effects of xenobiotics and environmental agents on the immune system. Table I summarizes a number of drugs and chemicals for which sufficient information exists to classify them as immunotoxic. These agents are discussed in detail elsewhere (see Dean, J.H., et al. (1984); Gibson, G.G., et al., (1983) and the other appropriate chapters in this text).

Table 1. IMMUNOSUPPRESSIVE INFLUENCES

Immunoimpressive Drugs	Environmental Immunotoxicants

Azathioprine/6-mercaptopurine
Glucocorticosteroids
Other anticancer drugs
Prescription drugs
Abused drugs (ethanol
   cannabinoids, and opiates)
	Benzene
	Halogenated aromatic hydrocar-
	   bons (PCB's, PBB's and
	   dibenzodioxins)
	Polycyclic aromatic hydrocar-
	   bons
	Insecticides (organophosphates
	   and chlorines and carbonates)
	Metals (Pb, Ni, Cd, Hg)

IMMUNOSUPPRESSIVE DRUGS

Azathioprine/6-mercaptopurine (6MP) (see Spreafico, F., et al. (1977) Azathioprine is usually used in conjunction with glucocorticoid therapy for immunosuppressive therapy in organ transplantation and occasionally in autoimmune disorders. Azathioprine is a nitroimidazole modified 6MP designed to resist methylation. The immunosuppressive actions of Azathioprine and 6MP are similar and thought to be mediated by the metabolite thioinosinic acid. The immunosuppressive effects of Azathioprine are thought to derive from an action to inhibit DNA, RNA and protein synthesis by blocking de novo purine synthesis. In high doses Azathioprine inhibits erythropoiesis, myelopoiesis, and lymphopoiesis and is, therefore, suppressive of all aspects of the immune system. Primary immune response are more inhibited than secondary responses. At clinically employed doses, Azathioprine therapy in rodent and man is particularly suppressive for T cell-mediated responses. Interestingly, Azathioprine reversibly inhibits T lymphocyte function thus, T cell numbers are not reduced. The selectivity of the action of Azathioprine on T cells and its reversibility implies that more than an antimetabolic action may be involved. Bach and co-workers (Dardenne, M., et al., 1973) have presented data to indicate that Azathioprine preferentially binds and inactivates certain receptor sites on T lymphocytes. In the light of recent evidence that a purine is a component of transfer factor (Kirkpatrick, C.H. et al., 1981) and that inosine-like compounds induce T cell differentiation and modulate T cell function (Hadden, J.W., et al., 1984) it seems possible that Azathioprine and 6MP may bind and be antagonistic for a functionally important T cell purine receptor.

Glucocorticosteroids (see Parrillo, J.E. et al., 1979 for review) Despite many years of the use of steroids for both immunosuppressive and anti-inflammatory therapy, their precise mechanisms of action remain unclear. While steroids are lytic for T cells in murine species, in man, they are not. The transient lymphopenia which follows their administration to man has been shown to result from redistribution not destruction. Actions of glucocorticoids at therapeutic doses are more suppressive for T cells than B cells. Recent evidence (Benet, L.Z.; et al., 1983; Duncan, M.R., et al., 1982) indicates that effects of glucocorticoids to inhibit the triggering of T lymphocytes for DNA synthesis and lymphokine production (T cell and macrophage growth factors) are central to their suppressive action based on dose-response and immuno-pharmacokinetic criteria. Effects to suppress macrophage and natural killer cell function, particularly lymphokine-induced, are probably also important. Glucocorticoids, like Azathioprine, used therapeutically do not destroy cells and their effects are rapidly and completely reversed by disconti-nuance of therapy.

Cyclophosphamide Cyclophosphamide is a cycle-specific alkyla-ting agent with preferential effects on B lymphocytes and humoral immune response. In some cases low doses may augment cellular immune responses through action either on T-B cell interaction and/or on suppressor T cells. Therapeutically, it has been used in autoimmune disorders with somme efficacy. At high doses both B and T cells are destroyed; however, B cell numbers and function recover more slowly than those of T cells. While the immunosuppressive effects of this agent may persist following discontinuance of therapy, the relative sparing of plasma cell antibody responses makes secondary infection from humoral immunodeficiency rare. When it occurs, immunoglobulin therapy is corrective. Infection secondary to neutropenia is more common with cyclophosphamide especially with high doses used in cancers paricular lymphomas, leukemias and lymphosarcomas.

Cyclosporin A (2) The cyclosporins, are derived from fungi and are closed ring methylated amino acid structures. Clinical uses to date have been in the treatment of renal allograft rejection and graft-versus-host (GVH) disease following bone marrow transplantation. Cyclosporin A is preferentially suppressive for T cells and at low doses inhibits T lymphocyte proliferation, lymphokine production, and cytotoxic T cell generation. While also potentially hepatotoxic and nephrotoxic, it is not hematotoxic or myelotoxic.

CYTOTOXIC DRUGS USED IN CANCER

These drugs have been individually reviewed elsewhere (see Ehrke, M.J., et al., 1984 for review). Collectively, these drugs are cytolytic for a wide range of cell types and their actions to inhibit malignant cell growth is frequently compli-cated by their effect to inhibit normal cells particularly the processes of erythropoiesis and/or myelopoiesis. these side effects are usually the limiting factor to the use of maxi-mally tumoricidal doses. Their effects on the immune system are pleomorphic. Originally, these drugs were thought to be uniformly immunosuppressive; however, recent evidence (see Faanes, R.B., et al., 1980) indicates they may at times be immunorestorative by inhibiting tumor-induced immunosuppression. To the extent that they are immunosuppres-sive their effects are generally greater on cellular than humoral immune responses. In general their effects are reversible with discontinuance. The persistence of cancer frequently makes discontinuance impossible and severe immuno-suppression is common in cancer chemotherapy. More pre-clinical and clinical experimentation is needed to deter-mine how immunotherapy may be best employed to reverse their immunosuppressive effects and prevent tumor recurrence and infection (see Faanes, R.B., et al. 1980; Gillissen, G., 1982; Spreafico, f., et al., 1983 for review).

ENVIRONMENTAL IMMUNOTOXICANTS (see Gibson, G.G, et al. 1983; Goldstein, A.L., et al., 1982; Dean et al. in this text)

Benzene

Benzene exposure, particularly when severe is associated with suppression of all marrow-derived elements including erythocytes, neutrophils platelets, and lymphocytes (Dean, J.H., et al. 1984; Lange, A., et al., 1973; Smolik, R., et al., 1973; Wierda, D., et al., 1981) and in animals death usually results from overwhelming infection. In animals, experimental exposures have well documented the capacity of benzene and/or its metabolites to suppress marrow cellularity and function and have correlated dose-dependent lymphocyto-penia with impairments of both humoral and cellular immunity. Chronic exposure of humans to benzene has been associated with decreased levels of serum complement, IgA and IgG but not IgM. While these observations provide evidence that benzene is immunotoxic for man, the nature and magnitude of the defects remain to be clarified.

Halogenated Aromatic Hydrocarbons (Dean, J.H., et al., 1984; McConnel, E.E., et al., 1980; Nicholson, W.J., et al., 1979; Shigematsu, N., et al., 1978; Silkworth, J.B., et al., 1979; Thomas, P.J., et al., 1978; Vos, J.G. et al.,)

This family of chemicals are manufactured for industrial uses and are present as contaminants of other useful chemicals. As pollutants, their ubiquity and biological persistence make them of concern. In addition to their immunotoxicity most are teratogenic and carcinogenic. The relation of their immunoto-xicity and carcinogenicity remains to be determined.

Polychlorinated biphenyls (PCB's)

These compounds are used as heat transfer media and plastici-zers and have yielded widespread environmental contamination. The composition of PCB mixtures vary but it appears to be the content of dibenzofurans which determines toxicity. High doses of PCB's in animals induce atrophy of primary and secondary lymphoid organs and impair immunoglobulin synthesis, thus antibody production. Effects on cell-mediated immunity are variable and further studies are needed. PCB immunotoxi-city has been correlated in animals with increased susceptibi-lity and mortality to challenge with viruses, bacteria, or parasites. Decreased resistance to tumor challenge has also been reported: however, the latter data are conflicting,. Human exposures to PCB's through contamination of rice oil in Japan and China have resulted in chloracne, decreased serum Ig levels and impaired cell mediated immunity with decreased T cell numbers and function, in association with increased susceptibility to respiratory infection.

Polybrominated Biphenyls (PBB's)

Flame retardants (e.g., Firemaster BP-6 or FF-1) used in clothing manufacture contain mixtures of PBB's. In 1973 BP-6 was introduced into the food chain in Michigan when it was accidentally substituted for magnesium oxide as a food supplement for livestock. In affected cattle, sheep and chickens, runting, infection and death resulted in association with thymic atrophy and lymphoid depletion. Meat and dairy products subsequently ingested by the human population led to high levels of PBB's in serum and adipose tissue of local residents. Immunologic disturbances in these people included depressed T cell numbers, increased null cells, and increased Ig levels. This population is being monitored for late sequelae. Animals exposed to sublethal levels of PBB's show greater suppression of antibody responses than CMI responses. PBB-exposed mice fail to show decreased resistance to infectious challenges at doses comparable to those to which the Michigan subjects were exposed.

Dibenzodioxins (see Dean, J.H., et al., 1984; Faith, R.E., et al., 1980; Gibson, G.G., et al., 1983; Vos, J.G., et al., 1978)

Tetrachlorodibenzo-p-dioxin (TCDD) is a contaminant of the herbicide trichlorophenoxyacetic acid and the disinfectant hexachlorophene. Toxic responses to TCDD in animals include teratogenesis, wasting and thymic atrophy. Immunological studies have shown depressed antibody responses, cell mediated immnity and lymphoproliferative responses in association with increased susceptibility to pathogen and tumor challenge, particularly in neonates of exposed mothers. Considerable human exposure has resulted from industrial accidents and widespread use of Agent Orange as a defoliant in Vietnam; however, despite the presence of chloracne in some of the affected individuals, normal immune function was observed in the majority. Mild and transient abnormalities were found in some factory workers but a consistent and clear picture has not yet emerged. Studies are in progress to assess the impact, if any, of exposure of military personnel in Vietnam; however, the latency between exposure and study make it unlikely that significant results will be obtained.

Polycyclic Aromatic Hydrocarbons (PAH) (Dean, J.H., et al., 1984; Nicholson, W.J., et al., 1979; Zedeck, M.S., 1980)

These hydrocarbons are ubiquitous pollutants derived from fossil fuels. They consist of three or more fused benzene rings containing only hydrogen and carbon. Examples are methylcholanthrene, benzanthine, benzanthracine, and benzopyrine. As a group, they are generally carcinogenic. Experiments in animals have demonstrated that longlasting impairment of both humoral and cellular immunity are induced by a number of the compounds. Their immunosuppressive effects

correlates with their carcinogenicity. Their effects particularly on antibody producing cells, involve prolonged reduction
of cell number; however, their effects on T cells appear to
be less severe and less persistent. The impact of relatively
low but chronic levels of environmental PAH exposure in man
remain to be determined as far as immunosuppression is
concerned.

Insecticides (Dean, J.H., et al., 1984; Ercegovich, C.D.,
1973; Nicholson, W.J., et al., 1979)

Three clases of insecticides, the organophospates (e.g.
parathion), the carbonates (e.g. carbaryl) and the organo
chlorines (DDT) that have been in wide general use have been
studied for immunutoxicity. The organophosphates and chlorines at high, near lethal, levels have been shown to induce
impaired humoral and cellular immunity and resistance in
animal studies. As a class, their potential for human immunotoxicity is considered to be low; however, the long term
effects of environmental accumulation is difficult to assess.

Metals (Dean, J.H., et al., 1984; Nicholson, W.J., et al.,
1979 and Lawrence et al this volume)

Industrial exposure by inhalation or ingestion to a number of
metals such as lead, nickel, cadmium and mercury can lead to
morbidity and immunotoxic effects both in the lung and
systemically. The mechanism of their suppression may be
similar and only lead will be discussed here. Several studies
have indicated that significant lead exposure is associated
with impaired resistance to bacterial and viral challenge.
While substantial data indicate lead exposure can inhibit
antibody formation in vitro and in vivo, effects on cell
mediated immunity are less consistent. The effects of lead,
as with other metals, may result from its affinity for sulfhydryl groups. Sulfhydryl reagents, as well as metal chelators,
may represent the most specific therapy for toxic
accumulation. Human ingestion of leaded paint or exposure to
inhaled particulate lead has been related to increased susceptibility or severity of infection.

Drugs

Drugs used to treat non-immunologic diseases may produce
immunotoxic side effects unknown to us. Evidence is accumulating to indicate that B-lactam containing antibiotics,
diphenylhydantoin, and estrogens (particularly
diethylstilbestrol) may have significant immunosuppressive
effects (Sorrell, T., et al., 1975; Gillissen, G., 1982;
Luster, M.I., et al.., 1982). Since other drugs may be
immunotoxic in ways that have not yet been analyzed, more
information is needed to assess possible side effects of drugs
on the immune system. As with the use of steroids, a degree
of immunotoxicity does not constitute an absolute contraindi-
cation for clinical use; however, the possible effects of
drugs having immune side effects is important to understand
and monitor , particularly when they are used with intended
immunosuppressive therapy.

Abused Drugs (Dean, J.H., et al., 1984).

Cannabinoids, ethanol, and opiates have been shown directly and indirectly through abnormal life styles and malnutrition to contribute to impaired immune function and resistance.

THE PROSPECTS FOR IMMUNOTHERAPY

The foregoing, seen through the eyes other than those of the immuno-toxicologist, might imply that immunotoxic experiences are ubiquitous and that the predicted complications are infection, cancer, and ultimately, death. It is important to realize that few individuals are ever exposed to levels of any of the substances discussed which would clearly lead to morbidity let alone mortality. While the risk can not be ruled out, it is reassuring to learn that the human immune system has a number of levels of protection. First line bulwarks of natural defense mediated by granulocytes, macrophages, and natural killer cells alone and collectively offer considerable potential for defence (up to 75% ablation) before a common pathogen exposure becomes compromising. Similarly, both T and B cell immune systems have considerable reserve and marked impairment is necessary before diseas incidence or severity increases. For these reasons it is only with a potent irreversible immunotoxic experience or the compounding of multiple immunotoxic influences that intervention might be considered.

For many of the chemicals discussed, avoidance or removal of the toxin is all that is required. In situations like cancer and acquired immunodeficiency disease syndrome (AIDS), this is not possible. For these diseases immunotherapy has been under development to attempt to restore immune response to improve survival. The notion of treating a failing immune system is a relatively recent one. However, by nature of the same logic that we treat hypertensive cardiovascular disease to prevent cerebral vascular accidents, we may expect in the future to treat the failing immune system to prevent infection and cancer. Once the complications develop, such treatments have been shown to be less effective.

For many years we have successfully employed vaccines to prevent both viral and bacterial diseases. In those with congenital immune defects, gammaglobulin administration and bone marrow transplantation are proven modes of therapy. In secondary immunodeficiencies a number of experimental therapies are under development. For experimental immunoprophylactic therapy and immunotherapy we have available a number of biologicals and drugs with demonstrated effects to restore or enhance immune response , particularly of the cellular immune system. Their actions differ in terms of the target cells and functions involved and the therapeutic use of these agents in a complementary or even synergistic way can be envisioned (see Hadden, J.W., et al., 1983 for further discussion). the suggested use of combinations of agents may startle some, yet it is to be reminded that we treat congestive heart failure with a variety of agents designed to attack the problem from

different, complementary standpoints, and the same logic
applies to treatment of the immune system.

Clearly, before this will become a clinical reality, the
sciences of immunopharmacology and immunotoxicology will need
to continue to mature. The first criteria for such contemplated therapy will be: (1), the presence of safe, well characterized immunobiologicals and drugs which predictably modify
specific immune defects in a reproducible manner which can be
clinically monitored and (2) an immunotoxic/immunodeficiency
disease which is significant, not readily reversible and shown
to predispose to life threatening complications. Only in
circumstances meeting these criteria and following the appropriate animal experimentation would human trials under rigidly
controlled conditions be considered warranted. To provide a
background for such therapy, I will introduce briefly some of
the immunotherapeutic agents under development for use in
cancer and other immunodeficiencies. These agents have been
reviewed elsewhere in detail and the reader is referred to
these sources (Hadden, J.W., et al., 1983; Hadden, J.W.,
1983: Hersh, E.M., et al., 1981) for more information.

IMMUNOTHERAPY AGENTS

Biologicals (see Hadden, J.W., 1983) (Table II)

Table II. IMMUNORESTORATIVE AGENTS

Biologicals		Drugs
Thymic hormones	thymosis	Levamisole
	thympoietin	NPT 16416
	thymulin	DTC
	thymostimulin	Isoprinosine
	thymic humoral factor	NPT 15392
		Muramyl dipeptides
Lymphohokines	T cell growth factor	Azimexon
	macrophage growth factor	Bestatin
	macrophage activating	Tuftsin
	factor	Pyrimidinoles
	interferons	

Thymic Hormones. A number of hormones have been isolated from
the thymus and have been shown to induce the maturation of T
cell precursors and to promote the differentiated and proliferative functions of mature T cells (Goldstein, A.L., et al.,
1982; Schulof, R.S., et al., 1981). These hormone preparations include thymosin fraction V, thymosin α1, thymopoietin,
thymulin (previously facteur thymique serique), and thymic
humoral factor. Of these, thymosin α1, thymopoietin and
thymulin have been purified and synthesized chemically or by
genetic engineering techniques. With the exception of thymic
humoral factor each of these factors has been shown to be
present in thymic epithelial cells based on immunofluorescence
studies. The differential biological roles of these secretory
factors have not been fully established; however, they are
thought to regulate the progressive maturation of T cells and
to contribute through their heterogeneity to differential

regulation of various T cell functions. While their intrathymic role remains unclear, their presence in the circulation
and the correlation of their declining levels with increasing
age and with the development of various immune-based diseases
lends strong support to their role as hormonal regulators. In
a variety of circumstances in which animals have been rendered
thymus-deficient, (e.g., thymectomy), these hormone preparations have been show to restore, at least partially, defective
T cell function. Based upon this experimental rationale these
substances, have been employed clinically to treat both
primary and secondary immunodeficiency. The results to date
have been encouraging and while they are not specifically
indicated or licensed to treat any particular disease in the
United States, their consideration for use in treating the
deficits arising from thymus atrophy, as occurs in PBB, PAH,
and asbestos exposure, seems reasonable.

Lymphokines (Hadden, J.W., 1983). A large variety of T cell
produced soluble mediators termed lymphokines have been
described; however, space limitations do not allow an elaboration here. Perhaps the lymphokines most relevant to
consider in immunologic reconstitution of patients immunosuppressed by immotoxicants are T cell growth factor (TCGF),
macrophage growth/colony stimulating factor (MGF/CSF), and
interferon (IFN).

TCGF. T cell growth factor has an action to promote clonal
expansion of T lymphocytes by acting as a second signal in the
initation of proliferation and by perpetuating repeated
subsequent cell divisions. It also is an inducer of natural
killer (NK) cells and increases their cytocidal activity.
Recently, we have found it to be a promoter of differentiation
of immature intrathymic lymphocytes (Chen, S.S., et al., 1983)
and have suggested that in concert with thymic hormones it is
an essential factor in T lymphocyte maturation and exit from
the thymus to replenish the peripheral T cell pool. Defects
in TCGF production and action have been described in AIDS,
aging and autoimmune disorders. It seems logical to predict
that as chemically pure, genetically engineered TCGF becomes
available its therapeutic use in T cell lymphopenic disorders
with deficient delayed hypersensitivity will be attempted and
its use in conjunction with thymic hormones may yield synergistic reconstitution.

MGF/CSF. This factor (macrophage growth factor/colony stimulating factor) acts to promote monocyte/macrophage proliferation in the bone marrow and in the periphery (Hadden, J.W., et
al, 1981; Sadlik, J.R., et al., 1983). It is complemented in
its action by other CSF's which act on both granulocyte and
macrophage precursors. In addition, MGF/CSF has been described to activate macrophage bactericidal capacity (Hadden,
J.W., et al., 1981). While therapeutic application has not
been attempted in man, as purified molecular preparations
become available, their use to reconstitute the number and
function of these cell populations will be warranted. MGF/CSF
will be particularly useful to increase macrophage-mediated
resistance to facultative intracellular pathogens including
tubercle bacilli, leprosy bacilli, Salmonella and Brucella and

various viruses, fungi and parasites.

IFN. The interferons represent a group of antiviral proteins which inhibit the intracellular replication of viruses, inhibit both normal and malignant cell proliferation, and promote killer cell functions of T cells, macrophages and NK cells (Johnson, H.M., 1982). With quantities of IFN available, therapy of infections and tumours in both animals and humans has been attempted. It is apparent from these studies that pretreatment with interferon may prevent certain viral infections. To a lesser extent, treatment after the onset of infection may ameliorate the course of infection. Gamma or immune interferon is a lymphokine produced by T cells and although the most extensive clinical experience with interferons has involved alpha or leukocyte interferons, the therapeutic application of immune interferon would be calculated, based on animal experiments to be, more effective and perhaps less toxic than the interferons. Within the context of treatment of patients suffering from immunotoxicity, general application of IFN's would not be recommended since their antiproliferative effects may inhibit immune reconstitution. The most appropriate applications would be in specific infections, viral and otherwise, to which macrophage and NK cells are critical in resistance.

Immunotherapeutic Drugs.

Levamisole (Amery, W.K., 1979; Renoux, G., 1978; Symoens, J., et al., 1977). Levamisole (2,3,4,6-tetrahydro-6-phenyli-midazo (2,1-b) thiazole) was one of the first chemically-defined immunostimulants to be developed. Its immunopharmacology includes actions on lymphocytes, macrophages and granulocytes to modify their mobility, secretion and proliferation. It can enhance or suppress immunity depending on the dose and timing of administration. In vivo levamisole treatment augments cellular more than humoral immune response, and its effect on humoral immunity is probably dependent on its action on T cells and macrophages. Levamisole is an immunopotentiator in that demonstrable positive effects usually require the concomitant adminsitration of a primary stimulus such as antigen. The magnitude of its effects appears to be greater when the stimulus is suboptimal and when the responding immune system is suboptimal. For this latter characteristic, levamisole has been termed an "immunonormalizing" drug. In general, its action is weak and non-responder strains of mice and individual humans exist . For unknown reasons it has mild side effects of metallic taste, nervousness, nausea and vomiting . However, occasio-nally , more severe side effects such as dermatitis and agranulocytosis have occured , particularly in individuals with HLA B 27 and rheumatoid arthritis.

In murine and human tumor protocols in which the primary tumor was decreased by chemotherapy, radiation or surgery , subse-quent levamisole treatment has been shown to increase mean survival time and/or the number of individuals surviving. The effect when observed in humans with cancer has been a small increase (15%) in the number of patients remaining in remission following tumor reduction by other primary therapies. Clinical efficacy in rheumatoid arthritis comparable to penicillamine has also been reported. Reports of efficacy have appeared in such diverse disorders as chronic and recurrent viral infections, herpes, chronic and recurrent bacterial infections, aphthous stomatitis, erythema multiforme and lupus erythematosus. Each of these disorders is immune based and, almost without exception in each, immune disturbance has been demonstrated which can be interpeted as contributing to the pathogenesis. While the clinical applications can be justified and supported, the issues of less than moderate efficacy, prolonged periods to achieve a response, a certain non-responder frequency, and an inability to monitor effects of this drug on the immune system simply and consistently, have accounted for its slow acceptance. Within the context of immunorestoration, a number of reports support the ability of levamisole to increase defective delayed hypersensitivity. In an animal study (Burley-Rosset, M., et al., 1979), it reversed the effect of aging on the immune response and prevented the otherwise high incidence of spontaneous tumor development. Thus while active in the context of immunorestoration, toxicity and inconsistent efficacy make it not the first agent to consider.

Other sulfur-containing agents. NPT 16416. (7,8-dihydrothiazole-3,2,4-hypoxanthine) was synthesized by us to produce a nontoxic drug similar in structure and action to levamisole (Hadden, J.W., et al., 1982). NPT 16416 is less toxic than levamisole. It increases active rosetting of T lymphocytes and induces T cell differentiation in the Komuro and Boyse assay. Like levamisole, only small effects are observable on T cell lymphoproliferative responses; however, at higher doses B cell responses to endotoxin and pokeweed are augmented. In mice, T cell antibody responses are augmented by low doses of NPT 16416. The immunotherapeutic effects of this compound remain to be determined.

Sodium diethyldithiocarbamate (DTC) (Renoux, G., et al., 1981). DTC is a less toxic sulfur containing compound than levamisole. The cellular targets of action are presumed to be T cells based upon effects of DTC to induce T cell differentiation in vivo. Like levamisole, DTC induces in vivo a thymic hormone-like factor which is thought to derive from the liver rather than the thymus. Other actions remain to be investigated. DTC has been used safely as a treatment of human patients with metal poisoning. In addition to pharmacologic effects to protect animals against certain carcinogens and ionizing radiation, DTC increases both humoral and cellular immune responses. In vivo administration to humans has been demonstrated to restore T cell proliferative responses to mitogens and depressed T cell rosette forming cells, actions shared by the thymic hormones. The therapeutic effects of this compound remain to be determined.

Other sulfur-containing compounds (Hadden, J.W., et al., 1981) which may prove more useful than levamisole include thiabendazole, thiazolobenzimidazole (WY 18251-(3-(p-chlorophenyl (thiazole (3,2-a) benzimidazole-2-acetic acid), and cimetidine

(N"-cyano-N-methyl-N'-2 (-methylimidazole-4yl) methylthioe-thyl-guanidine).

Isoprinosine (Hadden, J.W., & Giner-Sorolla, A., 1981; Hadden, J.W. et al., 1981; Ginsberg, T., et al., 1982; Simon, L.N., et al., 1983). Isoprinosine (a complex of p-ace-toamidobenzoic acid, N,N-dimethylamino-2-propanol and inosine (3:3:1 molar ratio) has been developed as an antiviral agent. The components of isoprinosine form a complex by a variety of physico-chemical criteria and as a complex, it displays biological activities either not apparent or weakly so when the components are employed alone. Isoprinosine is virtually non-toxic , with only an increase in serum uric acid levels reported as a side effect. It has been applied worldwide to treat thousands of humans with viral or virus-related disorders. In carefully controlled studies, significant, mild to moderate efficacy to reduce symptoms and/or shorten disease period or recurrences have been reported in subacute sclero-sing panencephalitis (SSPE), and in herpes simplex type II, influenza and rhinovirus infections.

While direct antiviral activity might be involved to explain these clinical results, it seems much more likely that effects of this compound on the immune system make a more plausible explanation. The immunopharmacology of isoprinosine includes actions to induce T lymphoctyte differentiation in a way comparable to thymic hormones and to augment lymphocyte, macrophage, and NK cell functions in a potentiator mode of action. In general, the activity, of isoprinosine both in vitro and in vivo, has been more consistently reproducible and of greater magnitude than that of levamisole. While most of the clinical studies have been for viral infections, a consi-derable amount of data supports effects of isoprinosine to augment, in patients, virus-specific immune parameters, mitogen and lymphokine responses, active rosettes and skin test responses.

Isoprinosine has been shown to be active in murine systems to potentiate vaccine protection in L1210 leukemia, to potentiate interferon therapy in lethal virus and tumor challenges, and to reduce spontaneous tumor development in NZB mice with autoimmune disease. Isoprinosine therapy has promoted resto-ration of depressed immunologic responses in humans with cancer treated with radiation and decreased infections in chemotherapy-treated leukemia patients. Within the context of immunoprophylaxis two features of isoprinosine are particu-larly notable; the first is that it has been taken continu-ously for up to 13 years without significant side effects, and the second is that unlike other agents, it has not been shown to be immunosuppressive based either on dose or frequency of administration. These data , in addition to the animal studies, should justify the immunoprophylactic application of isoprinosine in immunosuppressed patients. Such trials are in progress for patients with the recently described acquired immunodeficiency syndrome (AIDS).

NPT 15392 (Hadden, J.W. & Giner-Sorolla, A., 1981; Simon, L.N., et al., 1983). A structurally similar compound, NPT

15392, (9-erythro-2-hydroxy-3-nonylhypoxanthine) shares each of the immunopharmacological activities of isoprinosine. Specifically, NPT 15392 at low doses induces T cell by Chedid and co-workers in France does not induce fever and shows both adjuvant and protective activity. The critical immunopharmacologic features of MDP action include promotion of macrophage activation for tumoricidal and bactericidal activity and for secretion of enzymes and monokines. The effect of MDP on the macrophage is a direct one not requiring lymphokine or other influence. In vitro studies indicate action of MDP on T helper and suppressor function and on B cell proliferation as well. The participation of monokines and other macrophage-derived mediators in these functions has not been completely ruled out. In vivo MDP can augment both humoral and cellular immunity. While the major focus on MDP has been on its use as an adjuvant in vaccines, its immunopharmacology strongly suggests useful applications in infections in which the macrophage plays a role in the resistance. Synergistic interactions with lymphokines have been described.

Azimexon (Chirigos, M.A., et al., 1982). Azimexon (BM12,531), 2-(2-cyanaziridinyl)-(1)-(2-carbamolyaziridinyl)-(1)-propane, is an orally active immunostimulant. Its immunopharmacology, from in vitro studies, includes direct action on both lymphocytes and macrophages. In vivo studies show that it augments cell-mediated immunity, T cell dependent humoral immunity, NK cell activity, and induces an expansion of the reticuloendothelial system with splenomegaly. It promotes leukocytosis and hastens recovery from leukopenia. In animals with cancer, the drug is more active in increasing survivan and longevity in adjuvant protocols with irradiaition and chemotherapy than is levamisole. In human patients, it increased a variety of depressed immune parameters. The only significant side effect known to date is a dose-related toxic hemolytic anemia which may limit clinical indications.

Bestatin (Umezawa, H., 1981). Bestatin (2S, 3R)-3-amino-2-hydroxy-4-phenylbutyryl-1-leucine) is a non-toxic, orally active immunostimulant extracted from Streptomyces olivoreticuli. The cellular targets of its action appear to be the macrophage, the bone marrow precursors for granulocytes, NK cells, and possibly T lymphocytes. In vivo injection of bestatin in mice increases DNA synthesis in the spleen, thymus, and bone marrow but not in other organs tested. In vivo treatment of mice is associated with increases in antibody production to sheep erythrocytes and delayed hypersensitivity to sheep erythocytes or oxazolone. It aslo acts to restore immune response in tumor-bearing or chemotherapy-treated mice. Some tumor growth inhibition was observed by bestatin treatment in animals bearing slow growing tumors and increased survival was observed following chemotherapy in L1210 leukemia or Erhlich's ascites tumor. Prophylactic therapy reversed immune senescence and inhibited spontaneous tumor development in aged mice. Human toxicity has been negligible and in some patients effects to increase NK cell activity and E rosette forming T cells have been observed.

Tuftsin (Najjar, V.A., et al., 1981; Nishioka, K., et al., 1981). Tuftsin (Thr-lys-Pro-Arg) represents residues 289-292 of the heavy chain of the gamma-globulin molecule. It is thought to be liberated by selective cleavage with tuftsin-endocarboxypeptidase. Tuftsin stimulates motility, phagocytosis, processing of antigen, and tumoricidal activity of macrophages. Tufsin also increases neutrophil chemotaxis, phagocytosis, and killing and, NK cell activity. As a biological peptide, it is without significant side effects. In vivo administration of tuftsin to mice induces macrophages activated for tumoricidal activity and increases both T cell-dependent or independent antibody production as well as antibody-dependent cytotoxicity. In murine tumor models, tuftsin prolonged survival in both L1210 leukemia and the Cloudman S-91 melanoma. In addition, immunoprophylactic therapy in aged mice reduced the incidence of spontaneous neoplasms.

Pyrimidinoles (Stringfellow, D., 1981). In general, interferon inducers have been limited in their development by their toxicity and the refractory state to interferon induction which follows their administration. Two compounds 2-amino-5-bromo-6-phenyl-4-pyrimidinol (ABPP) and 2-amino-5-iodo-6-phenyl-4-pyrimidinol (AIPP), both show antiviral and antitumor activity. While both activate macrophages and NK cells, only ABPP is an inducer of interferon. The mechanism of their effects on macrophages and NK cells remains, therefore, to be fully clarified. The comparative effects of AIPP to ABPP remain of great interest since it apparently has potent immunododulating effects without interferon induction as a side effect.

CONCLUSION

In general, these therapies have been remarkably safe in both animals and man. Those agents having the greatest clinical experience in man, (i.e., the various thymic hormone preparations, low dose interferon, isoprinosine, and levamisole) have been employed in literally tens of thousands of patients with negligible or minor side effects and no reported case of immunotoxicity that I am aware of.

Presuming therapy will be relatively safe, the efficacy of these therapies needs to be assessed. Based upon our experience with cancer and the initial therapeutic efforts in AIDS, none of these agents used alone offers hope of increasing survival by curing active, progressive disease. In these two circumstances and, as I predict the case will be with intense, irreversible immunotoxic exposure, a combination approach may be necessary (Hadden, J.W., 1983).

The relevance of the foregoing agents and strategies in application to the therapy of immunosuppression following immunotoxic exposure may ultimately be small in the sense that only excessive accidential exposures will prove sufficiently immunotoxic to justify experimental therapy. If, however, it turns out that the effects of many of these environmental chemicals to be carcinogenic depends not only on their capacity to be mutogenic but also the capacity to be immunosuppressive, immunoprophylaxis may be a meaningful approach in those exposed and identified to be immuno-suppressed in order to reverse the predisposition to cancer.

REFERENCES

1. Amery, W.K. (1979): Time in chemo-immunotherapy models: an absolute or a relative variable? Int. J. Immunopharmacol., 1: 65-68.

2. Borel, J.F. (1981): Cyclosporin-A - present experimental status.Transplantation Proceedings, Vol. XIII, No. 1: 344-348.

3. Bekesi, J.G., Holland, J.F., Anderson, H.A., Fischbein, A.S., Rom, W., Wolff, M.S., and Selikoff, I.J. (1978): Lymphocyte function of Michigan dairy farmers exposed to polybrominated biphenyl. Science, 199: 1207-1209.

4. Bekesi, J.G., Roboz, J.P., Solomon, S., Fischbein, A., and Selikoff, I.J. (1983): Altered immune function in Michigan residents exposed to polybrominated biphenyl. In: Immunotoxicology, edited by G.G. Gison, R. Hubbard and D.V. Parke, pp. 181-191. Academic Press, London.

5. Benet, L.Z., Tsang, S.Y., and Legler, U.F. (1983): Biotransformation of immunotherapeutic agents. In: Advances in Immunopharmacology 2, edited by J.W. Hadden, L. Chedid, P. Dukor, F. Spreafico and D. Willoughby, pp 17-22. Pergamon Press, Oxford.

6. Bruley-Rosset, M., Florentin, I., Kiger, N., Schulz, J., and Mathe, G. (1979): Restoration of impaired immune functions of aged animals by chronic bestatin treatment. Immunology, 38: 75-83.

7. Cerutti, I., Chaney, C., Schlumberger , J.F. (1978): Isoprinosine increases the antitumor action of interferon. Cancer Treatment Reports, 62: 1971-1976.

8. Chen, S.S., Tung, J.S., Gillis S., Good, R.A., and Hadden, J.W. (1983): Changes in surface antigens of immature thymocytes under the influence of T cell growth factor and thymic factors. Proc. Natl. Acad. Sci., 80; 5980-5984.

9. Chirigos, M.A., and Mastrangelo, M.J. (1982): Immuno-restoration by chemicals. In: Immunological Approaches to Cancer Therapeutics, edited by E. Mihich, pp 191-240. John Wiley and Sons, New York.

10. Dardenne, M., and Bach, J.-F. (1973): Studies on thymus products. Immunology, 25: 343-352.

11. Dean, J.H., Murray, M.J., and Ward, E.C. (1984): Toxic modifications of the immune system. In:Toxicology: The basic Science of Poisons, edited by Casarett and Doullis (in press).

12. DiLuzio, N.R., and Chihara, G. (1981): Polysaccharides and related substances I. In: Advances in Immunopharmacology, edited by J.W. Hadden, L. Chedid, P. Mullen and F. Spreafico, pp 477-490. Pergamon Press, Oxford.

13. Duncan, M.R., Sadlik, J.R., and Hadden, J.W. (1982): Glucocorticoid modulation of lymphokine-induced macrophage proliferation. Cell. Immunol., 67: 23-36.

14. Ehrke, M.J., and Mihich, E. (1984): Immunoregulation by chemotherapeutic agents. In: The Reticuloendothelial System: A comprehensive Treatise, vol. V, edited by J.W. Hadden and A. Szentivanyi (in press). Plenum Press, New York.

15. Ercegovich, C.D. (1973): Relationship of pesticides to immune responses. Fed. Proc., 32: 2010-2016.

16. Faanes, R.B., Merluzzi, V.J., Ralph, P., Williams, N., and Tarnowski, G.S. (1980): Restoration of tumor and drug-induced immune dysfunction. In: International Symposium on New Trends in Human Immunology and Cancer Immunotherapy, edited by B. Serrou and C. Rosenfeld, pp 953-964. Doin Editeurs, Paris.

17. Faith, R.E., Luster, M.I., and Vos, J.G. (1980): Effects on immunocompetence by chemicals of environmental concern. In: Reviews in Biochemical Toxicology, Vol. 2, edited by E. Hodgson et al., pp 173-212. Elsevier, New York.

18. Floersheim, G.L. (1979): Immunosuppressive effects of miscellaneous agents. In: Drugs and Immune Responsiveness, edited by J.L. Turk and D. Parker, pp 1-24. University Park Press, Baltimore.

19. Gibson, G.G., Hubbard, R., and Parke, D.V., editors (1983): Immunotoxicology, Academic Press, London.

20. Gillissen, G. (1982): Influence of cephalosporins on humoral immune response. In: The Influence of Antibiotics on the Host Parasite Relationship, edited by Eickenber. Hahn and Opferkuch, pp 5-11. Springer-verlag, New York.

21. Ginsberg, T., and Hadden, J.W. (1982): Immunopharmacology of methisoprinol. In: Frontiers in Immunomodulation, edited by H. Fudenberg and F. Ambrogi, (in press). Plenum Press, New York.

22. Goldstein, A.L., Low, T.L.K., Thurman, G.B., Zatz, M., Hall, N.R., McClure, J.E., Hu, S-K., and Schulof, R.S. (1982): Thymosins and other hormone-like factors of the thymus gland. In: Immunological Approaches to Cancer Therapeutics, edited by E. Mihich, pp 137-190. John Wiley and Sons, New York.

120

23. Good, RA., Martinez, C., and Gabrielsen, A.E. (1964): Clinical considerations of the thymus in immunobiology. In: The Thymus in Immunobiology, edited by R.A. Good and A.E. Gabrielsen, pp 3-48. Hoeber Medical Div., Harper & Row, New York.

24. Good, R.A., West, A., and Fernandes, G. (1982): Influences of mutrition on immunity. In: Immunological Approaches to Cancer Therapeutics, edited by E. Mihich, pp 487-504. Wiley-Interscience, New York.

25. Hadden, J.W., Cornaglia-Ferraris, P., and Coffey, R.G. (1984): Purine analogs as immunomodulators. In: Progress in Immunology IV, (in press). Academic Press, London.

26. Hadden, J.W. (1984): Perspectives on the immunotherapy of AIDS. N.Y. Acad. Sci., (in press).

27. Hadden, J.W. Chedid, L., Dukor, P., Spreafico, F., and Willoughby, D, editors (1983): Advances in Immunopharmacology 2. Pergamon Press, Oxford.

28. Hadden, J.W. (1983): Chemically defined immunotherapeutic agents. In: 13th International Cancer congress, Part E. Cancer Management, edited by E.a. Mirand, W.B. Hutchinson and E. Mihich, pp 273-286. Alan Liss Inc., New York.

29. Hadden, J.W. (1983): Immunotoxicology: the prospects for immunorestoration. In:Immunotxicology, edited by G.G.Gibson, R. Hubbard and D.V. Parke, pp 329-342. Academic Press, London.

30. Hadden, J.W., and Stewart, II, W.E. , editors (1981): The Lymphokines. Humana Press, New Jersey.

31. Hadden, J.W., Englard, A., Sadlik, J.R., and Hadden, E. (1981): Lymphokine - induced macrophage proliferation and activation. In: Lymphokine and Thymic Hormones, edited by A. Goldstein and M. Chirigos, pp 159-172. Raven Press, New York.

32. Hadden, J.W., Giner-Sorolla, A., Hadden, E., Ikehara, S., Pahwa, R., Coffey, R., Castellazzi, A-M., Jones, C., Maxwell, K., and Simon, L. (1982): NPT 16416: a levamisole-like purine with immunomodulatory effects. Int. J. Immunopharmacol., 4: 287.

33. Hadden, J.W., and Giner-sorolla, A. (1981): Isoprinosine and NPT 15392: modulators of lymphocyte and macrophage development and function. In: Augmenting Agents in Cancer Therapy, edited by E.M. Hersh, M.A. Chirigos and M.J. Mastrangelo, pp 497-522. Raven Press, New York.

34. *Hersh, E.M. (1983): Immunotherapy of human cancer: current status and prospects for future development. In:* Advances in Immunopharmacology 2, *edited by J.W. Hadden et al., pp 487-499. Pergamon Press, Oxford.*

35. *Hersh, E.M., Chirigos, M.A., and Mastrangelo, M.J., editors (1981):* Augmenting Agents in Cancer Therapy. *Raven Press, New York.*

36. *Johnson, H.M. (1982): Modulation of the immune response by interferons and their inducers. In:* Immunological Approaches to Cancer Therapeutics, *edited by E. Mihich, pp 241-256. John Wiley and Sons, New York.*

37. *Kirkpatrick, C.H., and Burger, D.R. (1981): Transfer factor: progress toward isolation and characterization. In:* The Lymphokines Biochemistry and Biological Activity, *edited by J.W. Hadden and W.E. Stewart, II, pp 261-274. Humana Press, New Jersey.*

38. *Lange, A., Smolik, R., Zatonski, W., and Szymanska, J. (1973): Serum immunoglobulin levels in workers exposed to benzene, toluene, and xylene.* Int. Arch. Arbeitsmed., *31: 37-44.*

39. *Lederer, E., and Chedid, L. (1982): Immunomodulation by synthetic muramyl peptides and trehalose diesters. In:* Immunological Approaches to Cancer Therapeutics, *edited by E. Mihich, pp 107-136. John Wiley and Sons, New York.*

40. *Loose, L.D., Silkworth, J.B., Pittman, K.A. Benitz, K.F., and Mueller, W. (1978): Impaired host resistance to endotoxin and malaria in polychlorinated biphenyl- and hexachlorobenzene-treated mice.* Infect. Immun., *20: 30-35.*

41. *Luster M.I., and Dean, J.H. (1982): Immunological hypersensitivity resulting from environmental or occupational exposure to chemicals: a state-of-the-art workshop summary.* Fundamental & Appl. Toxicol., *2: 327-330.*

42. *Luster, M.I., Boorman, G.A., Dean. J.H., Luebke, R.W., and Lawson, L.D. (1980b): The effect of adult exposure to diethylstilbestrol in the mouse. Alterations in immunological function.* J. Reticuloendoth. Soc., *28: 561-569.*

43. *Makinodan, T., and Yunis, E., editors (1976):* Immunology and Aging. *Plenum Press, new York.*

44. *McConnell, E.E. (1980): Acute and chronic toxicity, carcinogenesis, reproduction, teratogenesis, and mutagenesis in animals, pp 241-266. Elsevier/North Holland Biomedical Press, New York.*

122

45. Najjar, V.A., Chaudhuri, M.K., Konopinska, D., Bech, B.D., Layne, P.O., and Linehan, L. (1981): Tuftsin (Thr-Lys-Pro-Arg), a physiological activitor of phagocytic cells: a possible role in cancer suppression and therapy. In: Augmenting in Cancer Therapy, edited by E.M. Hersh, M.A. Chirigos and M.J. Mastrangelo, pp 459-478. Raven Press, New York.

46. Nicholson, W.J., and Moore, J.A. (1979): Health effects of halogenated aromatic hydrocarbons. Ann. N.Y. Acad. Sci., 320: 1-730.

47. Nishioka, K., Amoscato, A.A., and Babcock, G.F. (1981): Tuftsin: a hormone like tetrapeptide with antimicrobial and antitumor activities. Life Sci., 28: 1081-1090.

48. Parrillo, J.E., and Fauci, A.A. (1979): Mechanisms of glucocorticoid action on immune processes. Ann. Rev. Pharmacol. Toxicol., 19: 179-201.

49. Pompidou, A., Touraine, J.L., Simon-Lavoine, N., and Hadden, J.W. (1980): Immunomodulatory effects of cyclomunine in vitro. Int. J. Immunopharmacol., 2: 141-144.

50. Renoux, G. (1978): Modulation of immunity by levamisole. Pharmac. Ther., 2: 397-423.

51. Renoux, G., and Renoux, M. (1981): Immunologic activity of DTC: potential for cancer therapy. In: Augmenting Agents in Cancer Therapy, edited by E.M. Hersh, M.A. Chirigos and M.J. Mastrangelo, pp 427-440. Raven Press New York.

52. Sadlik, J.R., Hadden E.M., and Hadden, J.W. (1983): Lymphokine induced macrophage proliferation: purification and characterization of antigen induced MGF/CSF. In: Advances in Immunopharmacology 2, edited by J.W. Hadden, L. Chedid, P. Dukor, F. Spreafico and D. Willoughby, pp 221-227. Pergamon Press, Oxford.

53. Schulof, R.S., and Goldstein, A.L. (1981): Thymosins and other thymic hormones. In: The Lymphokines, edited by J.W. Hadden and W.E. Stewart, II, pp 397-442. Humana Press, New Jersey.

54. Shigematsu, N., Ishmaru, S., Saito, R., Ikeda, T. Matsuba, K., Sugiyamo, K., and Masuda, Y. (1978): Respiratory involvement in PCB poisoning. Environ. Res., 16: 92-100.

55. Silkworth, J.B., and Loose, L.D. (1979): PCB and HCB induced alteration of lymphocyte blastogenesis. Toxicol. Appl. Pharmacol., 49: 86.

56. Simon, L.N., Hoehler, F.K., McKenzie, D.T., and Hadden, J.W. (1983): Isoprinosine and NPT 15392: immunomodulation and cancer. In: Biological Response Modifiers in Human Oncology and Immunology, edited by T. Klein, S. Specter, H. Friedman and A. Szentivanyi, pp 241-259. Plenum Press, New York.

57. Smolik, R., Grzybek-Hryncewicz, K., Lange, A., and Antzatonski, W. (1973): Serum complement levels in workers exposed to benzene, toluene, and xylene. Int. Arch. Arbeitsmed., 31: 243-247.

58. Sorrell, T., and Forbes, I. (1975): Depression of immune competence by phenytoin and carbamazepine. Clin. Exp. Immunol. 20: 273-285.

59. Spreafico, F., and Anaclerio, A. (1977): Immunosuppressive agents. In: Immunopharmacology 3, edited by J.W. Hadden, R.G. Coffey and F. Spreafico, pp 245-278. Plenum Medical Book Compagny, New York.

60. Spreafico, F., Alberti, A., Allegrucci, M., Canegrati, A., Colotta, F., Luini, W., Merendino, A., Pasqualetto, E., Romano, M., Sirone, M., and Vecchi, A. (1983): On the mode of action of immunodepressive agents. In: Advances in Immunopharmacology 2, edited by J.W. Hadden et al., pp 745-752. Pergamon Press, Oxford.

61. Stringfellow, D. (1981): 6-aryl pyrimidinoles: interferon inducers-immunomodulators-antiviral and antineoplastic agents. In: Augmenting Agents in Cancer Therapy, edited By E. Hersh, M.A. Chirigos and M.J. Mastrangelo, pp 215-228. Raven Press, New York.

62. Symoens, J., and Rosenthal, M. (1977): Levamisole in the modulation of the immune response : the current experimental and clinical state. J. Reti. Endothel. Soc., 21: 175-221.

63. Thomas, P.J., and Hinsdill, R.D. (1978): Effect of polychlorinated biphenyls on the immune responses of Rhesus monkeys and mice. Toxicol. Appl. Pharmacol., 44: 41-52.

64. Umezawa, H., editor (1981): Small Molecular Immunomodifiers of Microbial Origin. Pergamon Press, Oxford.

65. Vos, J.G., Faith, R.E., and Luster, M.I. (1980): Immune alterations, pp 241-266. Elsevier/North Holland Biomedical Press, New York.

66. Vos, J.G., Kreeftenberg, J.G., Engel, H.W.B., Minderhoud, A., and VanNoorle Jansen, L.M. (1978): Studies on 2,3,7,8-tetrachlorodibenzo-p-dioxin-induced immune suppression and decreased resistance to infection: endotoxin hypersensitivity, serum zinc concentrations and effect of thymosin treatment. Toxicology, 9: 75-86.

124

67. Wanebo, H.J., Pinsky, C.M., Beattie, E.J., and Oettgen, H.F. (1978): *Immunocompetence testing in patients with one of the four common operable cancers - a review.* Clinical Bulletin, 8: 15-22.

68. Wierda, D., Irons, R.D., and Greenbe, W.F. (1981): *Immunotoxicity in C57BL/6 mice exposed to benzene and Aroclor 1254.* Toxicol. Appl. Pharmacol., 60t: 410-417.

69. Zedeck, M.S. (1980): *Plycyclic aromatic hydrocarbons, a review.* J. Environ. Pathol. Toxicol., 3: 537-567.

THE ROLE OF HISTOPATHOLOGY IN ASSESSMENT OF IMMUNOTOXICITY

J.G. Vos

National Institute of Public Health and Environmental Hygiene
Bilthoven, The Netherlands

INTRODUCTION

The lymphoid tissue can be structurally divided in to primary and secondary lymphoid organs or tissues. In the primary organs, the antigen-independent proliferation of lymphocytes takes place. Generation of T-lymphocytes from stem cells occurs in the thymus. In birds, the bursa of Fabricius has been shown to be the primary organ that supports extensive lymphopoiesis of B cells (the mammalian equivalent of the bursa of Fabricius may exist in different sites, e.g. the bone marrow or as suggested by Hall in this volume , in the lower gut) The secondary lymphoid tissue, in which the complex cellular interactions take place which form the basis of the immune response, includes the spleen, lymph nodes and the mucosa associated lymphoid tissues in the alimentary and respiratory tracts.

The rationale for morphologic examination of the lymphoid system in immunotoxicity testing rests in the belief that chemically-induced immune alterations may become manifest as qualitative or quantitative changes in the histology of lymphoid organs. This is similar to the situation in humoral, cellular or combined immunodeficiency diseases in man, in which a characteristic pathomorphology has been described (Heymet et al, 1977). For the detection of these changes routine histopathology has been shown in many studies to be valuable. For in depth investigation enzyme and immune histochemistry are proving their worth as powerfull tools.

In this paper, an outline is given of the architecture of the lymphoid tissue; various histological techniques are discussed; and examples are presented of chemicals that cause immune alterations as identified by these morphological procedures.

STRUCTURE OF LYMPHOID ORGANS

Thymus The thymus derives embryologically from the endoderm of the third and fourth branchial pouches, and reaches its maximum size during neonatal life, after which a gradual process of involution begins. Histologicaly, the thymus is a lymphoepithelial organ consisting of many lobules, each containing a cortex and medulla. Stem cells, which originate from the bone marrow, undergo extensive proliferation particularly in the periphery of the cortex. Lymphocytes (thymocytes) of varying size are closely packed in the cortex, together with epithelial cells and macrophages. Thymocytes migrate from the cortex, to the medulla where they further differentiate, before they migrate to the peripheral lymphoid

system of mature cells. Like the cortex, the medulla contains
many epithelial cells. Direct contact of thymocytes with the
epithelial cells,and/or thymic hormones produced by these
epithelial cells, are thought to be necessary for thymocytes
differentiation. Medullary epithelium is also organized into
Hassall's corpuscles the precise function of which is not
known.

Lymph nodes Lymph nodes are secondary lymphoid organs that
contain lymphocytes within a reticular stroma. They receive
lymph from a neighbouring region of the body by way of afferent lymphatics which enter the nodes at the subcapsular
sinus. Within the nodes, lymph flows through the superficial
and deep cortex and medullary sinuses towards the efferent
lymphatics.

In the node, there is compartmentation of B and T lymphocytes.
The superficial cortex contains follicular aggregations made
up predominantly of B cells. Following antigenic stimulation
primary follicles enlarge to secondary follicles having a
pale-staining central area of macrophages and proliferating
lymphocytes. In these so-called germinal centres
B-lymphocytes differentiate to plasma blasts, and become
antibody producing plasma cells in the medullary cords which
lie between the medullary sinuses. T lymphocytes are confined
to the interfollicular and deep cortical regions, referred to
as thymus-dependent or paracortical area. In nude (athymic)
mice and rats the thymus-dependent area is largely devoid of
lymphocytes. Following stimulation with an antigen that
evokes a T cell-mediated response, the paracortical area
enlarges with lymphoblasts becoming evident. The paracortical
area contains postcapillary venules lined by specialized high
endothelium through which circulating lymphocytes enter the
node. This is the main place where blood lymphocytes enter
the lymphatic circulation, enabling a continuous circulation
from blood to lymph and back to blood. Drainage of lymph
fluid by cannulation of the thoracic duct thus results in a
severe depletion of circulating lymphocytes and of the
thymus-dependent area.

Spleen The spleen is the largest lymphoid organ in the circulation which functions to clear particulate materials from the
blood by its abundant number of phagocytes and also concentra-
tes blood-born antigens. It is also the site of erythrocyte
storage and of removal of effete erythrocytes and leukocytes.
Histologically, the spleen is divided into the white pulp, the
major lymphoid mass surrounding small arteries and arterioles,
and the red pulp containing cellular cords with many macrophages and erythrocyte-filled venous sinuses. As in the lymphnodes , T and B cell areas are segregated. The diffuse
lymphoid tissue immediately surrounding the arteriole is
populated predominantly by recirculating small T cells, the
so-called periarteriolar lymphocyte sheath (PALS), which may
be functionally similar to the paracortical area of lymph
nodes. The B cell area comprises the follicles which after
antigenic stimulation enlarge to secondary follicles with a
germinal centre, and the so-called marginal zone (MZ) that is

separated from PALS and follicles by a marginal sinus. The MZ is a broad band of medium-sized lymphocytes that borders the red pulp. Plasma cells in the spleen are mainly found in the red pulp cords.

Mucosa associated lymphoid tissue The digestive, respiratory and genito-urinary tracts contain lymphoid tissue which is organized into non-encapsulated accumulations of lymphocytes or occurs diffusively in the subepithelial lamina propria. The former includes tonsils, small intestinal Peyer's patches and caecal appendix which show separation of lymphocytes into B cell (follicles) and T cell areas, whereas the latter includes isolated solitary follicles as well as lymphocytes, macrophages and plasma cells (mainly producing immunoglobulin A class antibodies) scattered in the loose connective tissue under the mucossaal surfaces.

HISTOLOGICAL METHODS

Conventional histopathology In many studies it has been shown that routine histopathology of lymphoid organs, as based on hematoxylin and eosin staining of formalin fixed and paraffin embedded tissue, is quite useful in assessing the immunotoxicity of a chemical; in particular when these results are combined with the effects observed on the weight of thymus, spleen and lymph nodes (Vos, 1977; Dean et al, 1982; Luster et al, 1982 & Dean et al, 1984). Depending on the route of exposure it may also be necessary to examine the mucosa associated lymphoid tissue, e.g. the Peyer's patches in the small intestine in orally exposed animals. A proper evaluation of intestinal lymphoid tissue can be facilitated by preparing so-called Swiss rolls of the intestinal tract (Moolenbeek & Ruitenberg, 1980). Since the bone marrow is an integrated part of the immune system, containing stem cell populations that are precursor cells for B and T lymphocytes and macrophages, morphologic examination of bone marrow is an essential in any immunotoxicity assessment . Morphological analysis can be done on tissue sections (preferably 1μm sections of plastic embedded materials) on marrow smears or on cytospin preparations e.g. of cells collected by flushing the femoral cavity. the latter technique has the advantage that cell viability (e.g. by a dye exclusion test) and cell number may be determined as well. Similarly, enumeration and characterization of free alveolar cells obtained by lung lavage appears to be a good quantitative method to detect the effect of inhalation exposure to a compound. Evaluation of bronchoalveolar lavage has yielded important information on immune and inflammatory processes in the human lung (Hunninghake et al, 1979).

In the morphological assessment of lymphoid tissues, changes in the number of lymphoid cells may be indicative of immunotoxicity. Thus, atrophy and lymphocyte depletion of the thymic cortex appears to be a sensitive parameter of many immunosuppressive compounds. Because of the structural division of secondary lymphoid organs into thymus-dependent and thymus-independent areas, an indication can be obtained regarding the relative effect of the chemical for T or B cell compartments. Suppression or stimulation of cell-mediated immunity may be reflected microscopically in hypoplasia or hypercellularity of the paracortical area in lymph nodes and of PALS in the spleen. The number of lymphoid follicles, germinal centers and plasma cells in lymph nodes and spleen, and size and cellularity of the marginal zone in the spleen can provide indications whether the B cell system is affected. Microscopical evaluation may indicate a cytotoxic action of the chemical, reflected by cellular degeneration. Confirmation of cytotoxicity can be obtained by a dye exclusion test using cell suspensions.

In the evaluation of changes in lymphoid tissues of chemically exposed animals, it is necessary to correlate these findings with other toxicological parameters (Vos, 1977; Dean et al, 1982; Luster et al, 1982 & Dean et alm 1984). For example, thymic atrophy is not necessarily a specific indicator of immunotoxicity, since stress, severe weight loss or general toxicity can also induce a similar lesion.

Although routine histopathology may be useful for the identification of an immunotoxic compound, special techniques may be required for a better understanding of the nature of the chemically-induced lesion in the lymphoid system. These techniques, such as enzyme histochemistry, immunocytochemistry and electron microscopy, mostly rely on the use of special fixation or embedding procedures.

Enzyme histochemistry This histological method depends on the production of an intensely stained precipitate at the site of enzymatic activity, by the action of the enzyme on a specific substrate. Enzyme histochemistry has been shown to be valuable for the identification and enumeration of macrophages by staining for nonspecific esterase activity (Koski et al, 1976), e.g. in lung lavage fluid.This technique is normally performed on unfixed cryostat sections of tissue frozen in liquid nitrogen. Recent advances in fixation and embedding techniques have enabled the characterization of macrophages by enzyme histochemical markers, even in $1-2\mu$m plastic sections, which greatly improved the cytological detail (Souflevis et al, 1982).

Immunohistochemistry This is a technique for detection and localization of antigen in tissue sections by the use of specific antibodies, which are coupled to a marker such as the fluorescent dye fluorescein isothiocyanate. Currently, enzyme markers (e.g. peroxidase) are widely used , as they enable the visualization of the reaction product by ordinary light microscopy.For the localization of antigen at the ultrastructural level, electron dense markers (e.g. ferritin) are used.

In the immunoperoxidase technique, there are different ways in which the test is carried out, i.e. the peroxidase labelled antibody method that can be divided in a direct and an indirect method, the unlabelled antibody method of peroxidaseantiperoxidase (PAP) and the avidinbiotin-peroxidase complex (ABC) method (reviewed in Falini & Taylor, 1983). In all techniques, peroxidase is localized through an antigenantibody reaction in areas where specific antigen is present. The sites of peroxidase localization are visualized by addition of a substrate solution which is transformed by the peroxidase label to an insoluble colored product.

Most cytoplasmic antigens e.g. immunoglobulins, are readily demonstrated in formalin-fixed paraffin sections. In particular, fixation with formalin containing mercuric chloride (sublimate) offers good preservation of antigens. Cell surface antigens, which are only present in small amounts, are better preserved in frozen sections (e.g. surface markers of macrophages, T helper and T suppressor cells that can be identified with monocolonal antibodies). However, with a proper fixative, paraffin and even plastic embedding can now also be employed (Gendelman et al, 1983; Ward et al, 1983 & Franklin, 1984) which enables the cutting of thinner (1-2 m) tissue sections in which enhanced cytological detail of lymphoid tissues can be observed.

Quantification of tissue lesions A difficulty for the pathologist in the evaluation of often minor chemically-induced lesions is making objective classifications. By randomizing and coding the slides, bias in reading can be avoided and qualitative analysis is possible. Classification is being improved by morphometric analysis since quantitative measurements on cells and tissues can be made by this method. In this context, it is of interest to mention that recent developments in monoclonal antibodies, computer processing and cytometric instrumentation has led to the new field of clinical flow cytometry. this field has already found specific applications in diagnostic immunopathology, including the study of congenital and acquired immune deficiency diseases (reviewed in Lovett et al, 1984). The application of this technique to immunotoxicology may be of great value e.g. in the enumeration of bone marrow stem cell populations, which can currently only be identified by complex culture methods, and of lymphocyte subpopulations.

CHEMICALLY INDUCED ALTERATIONS

The value of histopathology in the identification and elucidation of the immunotoxic property of a compound can be illustrated by results of toxicity experiments with chemicals causing different lesions.

Halogenated aromatic compounds The group of halogenated chemicals includes biphenyls, dibenzodioxins and dibenzofurans which have been shown to be capable of altering immunocompetence, in particular thymus-dependent immune responses (reviewed in Dean et al, 1982; Dean et al, 1984; Vos et al, 1980 & Vos, 1985 , see also Vecchi , this volume.) The prototype for these compounds is 2,3,7,8-tetrachlorodibenzo-p-dioxin (TCDD). Experimental studies indicate that TCDD and isosteric analogs act through a common receptor protein to produce characteristic toxic responsesm including thymus atrophy in all species investigated. Histopathologically, the thymus atrophy is characterized by lymphocyte depletion of the cortex, without evidence of thymocyte destruction. Recent data indicates that TCDD can act directly on thymic epithelial cells which thereby lose the ability to promote thymocyte maturation (see paper by Greenlee, Dold and Osborne in this volume).

Although major attention has been given to the effects of halogenated aromatic hydrocarbons on thymus and thymus-dependent cellular immunity, humoral responses are affected as well. In this regard it is of interest to note that the first indication for immunotoxicity of brominated biphenyls came from a study in chickens showing lymphocyte depletion in the bursa of Fabricius, the central lymphoid organ of the B cell system in birds ; and subsequently it was shown that the humoral immune response to tetanus toxoid was suppressed in guinea pigs following exposure to this fire retardant, has been demonstrated by an indirect immunofluorescent antibody technique and by serum antibody titrations (Vos & Genderen, 1973).

Organotin compounds It is now well established that certain organotin compounds e.g. di-n-butyltin dichloride and di-n-octyltin dichloride are potent immunotoxic chemicals (Seinen & Penninks, 1979). In short-term feeding studies in rats, these dialkyltins produced lymphocyte depletion of the thymic cortex and of the thymus-dependent areas in spleen and lymph nodes, due to a selective lymphocytoxicity. No myelotoxicity or involvement of non-lymphoid organs was noted. As a consequence thymus-dependent cellular and humoral immune responses appeared suppressed (Seinen & Penninks, 1979). Bis(tri-n-butyltin)oxide (TBTO) has been recently shown to cause similar effects on thymus and on thymus-dependent immunity (Krajne et al, 1984; Vos et al, 1984). Evidence for a direct toxic action of TBTO for thymocytes was obtained by light microscopic evaluation of plastic embedded thymic tissue .Lymphocyte depletion of T cell areas in spleen was confirmed by immunohistochemistry and by flow cytometric analysis of T and B lymphocytes using monoclonal antibodies. TBTO appeared not only to suppress specific immunity, but also nonspecific resistance as evidenced by a reduced activity of natural killer cells and macrophages. In addition, a pronounced feature in TBTO-exposed rats, which was not observed in the studies with dialkyltins, was the occurrence of rosettes of erythrocytes around macrophages in the medullary sinuses of mesenteric lymph nodes .Although the mechanism of rosette formation is as yet unclear, it might be a morphological expression of deficient phagocytosis of dying erythrocytes. This is supported by the finding of decreased bacterial clearance.

Hexachlorobenzene The immune effects of hexachlorobenzene (HCB) are exceptional as HCB exposure leads to lymphoid tissue hyperplasia in rats, both in young-adult animals and after pre- and postnatal treatment (Vos et al, 1979 & Vos et al, 1983), and in dogs (Gralla et al, 1977), whereas corresponding histological effects do not occur in HCB-exposed mice (reviewed in Loose et al, 1978). The splenomegaly in rats is characterized by enlarged marginal zones, prominent follicles and extramedullary haemopoiesis . Enlarged mesenteric and popliteal lymph nodes revealed an increase in the number of high endothelial venules in the paracortical area with many lynphocytes migrating through the endothelium , a phenomenon that normally occurs in antigen-stimulated lymph nodes. A similar effect was observed in the high-endothelial venules in the interfollicular area of Peyer's patches. Upon functional testing, these morphological changes indeed reflect immune stimulation, as evidenced by increased humoral and cellular immune responses (Vos et al, 1979 & Vos et al, 1983). On the other hand, suppression of various functional immune parameters has been observed in the mouse (Louse et al, 1978). The effect of HCB on endothelial cells of the rat was not limited to lymphoid organs, as proliferation of the lining endothelial cells was observed in lung capillaries and venules accompanied by perivascular infiltrates of lymphocytes and mast cells, and focal accumulation of macrophages in the alveoli (Vos et al, 1983). This latter findingt indicates that HCB in some way affects the mononuclear phagocyte system of the rat, although in function tests no clear effects were found. On the other hand, there are experimental data showing that HCB decreases the Fc receptor activity of rat alveolar macrophages (Ziprin & Fowler, 1977).

Nitrogen dioxide The lung is a primary target organ for air pollutants such as the oxidant gases nitrogen dioxide (NO$_2$) and ozone. In several studies it has been shown that these agents alter host resistance of mice as evidenced by increased mortality following aerosol challenge with bacteria. Decreased resistance is thought to be due to impaired phagocytic and bactericidal activity of pulmonary macrophages (re- viewed in Gardner, 1984; vide Gardner & Graham , this volume). In experiments in which the influence of concentration, exposure pattern and length of NO$_2$ exposure on degree and extent of morphological alterations in rat lung was studied, it appeared that influx of macrophages occurred early after continuous exposure , the accumulation of macrophages in the lung alveoli being a sensitive parameter (Rombout et al, 1985).

Mercury Immunological alterations caused by exposure to heavy metals, industrial chemicals or drugs, and resulting in autoimmune or hypersensitivity reactions, have received increasing attention in the last decade (reviewed in Dean et al, 1984 & Greally & Silano, 1983). Mercury is one of the heavy metals which has been shown to cause autoimmune processes. Depending on the rat strain used, immune complex glomerulonephritis with the appearance of antinuclear antibodies, or anti-glomerular basement membrane nephritis may be induced (Druet et al, 1982). Regarding the mechanism of this autoimmune phenomenon, recent studies in the PVG/c rat strain indicate that mercury inhibits the generation of T suppressor lymphocytes. This interference with the regulatory T cell system seems to be of pathogenetic significance in the observed anti-self response (Weening et al, 1981; see also Lawrence , this volume).

REFERENCES

Dean, J.H., Luster, M.I. & Boorman, G.A. 1982. Immunotoxicology. In Sirois, P. & Pola-Pleszczynski, M.(Eds). Immunopharmacology, Elsevier Biomedical Press, New York. pp. 349-397.

Dean, J.H., Murray, M.J. & Ward, E.C. 1984. Toxic modifications of the immune system. In Doul, J., Klaassen, C.D. & Amdur, M.O.(Eds). Cesarett and Doull's Toxicology: The Basic Science of Poisons, 3rd edition. In press.

Druet, P., Bernard, A., Hirsch, F., Weening, J.J., Gengoux, P., Mahieu, P. & Birkeland, S. 1982. Immunologically mediated glomerulonephritis by heavy metals, Arch. Toxicol., 50, 187-194.

Falini, B & Taylor, C.R , 1983. New developments in immuno-peroxidase techniques and their application, Arch.Pathol.Lab.Med., 107, 105-117.

Franklin, R.M. 1984. Immunohistochemistry on semi-thin sections of hydroxypropyl methacrylate embedded tissues, J.Immunol.Methods, 61-72.

Gardner, D.E. 1984. Alterations in macrophage functions by environmental chemicals, Environm.Health Perspect., 55, 343-358.

Gendelman, H.E., Moench, T.R., Narayan, O. & Griffin, D.E. 1983. Selection of a fixative for identifying T-cell subsets, B-cells, and macrophages in paraffin-embedded mouse spleen, J. Immunol.Methods, 65, 137-145.

Gralla, E.J., Fleischmann, R.W., Luthra, Y.K., Hagopian, M., Baker, J.R., Esber, H. & Marcus W. 1977. Toxic effects of hexachlorobenzene after daily administration to beagle dogs for one year. Toxicol.Appl.Pharmacol., 40, 227-239.

Greally, J.F. & Silano, V. (Eds.) 1983. Allergic Responses and Hypersensitivities Induced by Chemicals. Health Aspects of Chemical Safety, Interim document 12. World Health Organization, Copenhagen and Commission of the European Communities, Luxembourg.

Heymer, B., Niethammer, D., Spanel, R., Galle, J., Kleihauer, E. & Haferkamp, O. 1977. Pathomorphology of humoral, cellular and combined primary immunodeficiencies, Virchows Arch.A.Path. Anat. and Histol., 374, 87-103.

Hunninghake, G.W., Gadek, J.E., Kawanami, O., Ferrants, V.J. & Crystal, R.G. 1979. Inflammatory and immune processes in the human lung in health and disease: evaluation by bronchoalveolar lavage, Am.J.Pathol., 97, 149-206.

Koski, I.R., Poplack, D.G. & Blaese, R.M. 1976. A nonspecific esterase stain for the identification of monocytes and macrophages. In. Blood, B. & David, J.R.(Eds.): In Vitro Methods in Cell-Mediated and Tumor Immunity, Academic Press, New York, pp. 359-362.

Krajnc, E.I., Wester, P.W., Loeber, J.G., van Leeuwen F.X.R., Vos, J.G., Vaessen, H.A.G. & Van der Heijden, C.A. 1984. Toxicity of bis(tri-n-butyltin)oxide in the rat. I. Short-term effects on general parameters and on the endocrine and lymphoid system. Toxicol.Appl.Pharmacol., 75, 363-386.

Loose, L.D., Pittman, K.A., Benitz, K.F., Silkworth, J.B., Mueller, W. & Coulston, F. 1978. Environmental chemical-induced immune dysfunction, Ecotoxicol.Environ.Safety, 2, 173-198.

Lovett, E.J., Schnitzer, B., Keren, D.F., Flint, A., Hudson, J.L. & McClatchey, K.D. 1984. Application of flow cytometry to diagnostic pathology, Lab.Invest., 50,115-140.

Luster, M.I., Dean, J.H. & Moore, J.A. 1982. Evaluation of immune functions in toxicology. In. Hayes, A.W.(Eds). Principles and Methods of Toxicology, Raven Press, New York, pp. 561-586.

Moolenbeek, C. & Ruitenberg, E.J. 1980. The Swiss Roll: a simple technique for histological studies of rodent intestine, Lab. Anim., 15, 57-59.

Rombout, P.J.A., Dormans, J.A.M.A., Marra, M. & van Esch, G.J. 1985. Influence of exposure regimen on nitrogen dioxide induced morphological changes in the rat lung. Submitted for publication

Seinen, W. & Penninks, A. 1979. Immune suppression as a consequence of a selective cytotoxic activity of certain organometallic compounds on thymus-dependent lymphocytes, Ann.N.Y.Acad.Sci. 320, 499-517.

Soufleris, A.J., Pretlow, T.P., Bartolucci, A.A., Pitts, A.M., Macfadyen, A.J., Boohaker, E.A. & Pretlow, T.G. 1982. II, Cytologic characterization of pulmonary alveolar macrophages by enzyme histochemistry in plastic, J,Histochem.Cytochem., 13, 1412-1418.

Vos, J.G. & van Genderen, H. 1973. Toxicological aspects of immunosuppression. In. Deichmann, W.B.(Eds). Pesticides and the Environment: A Continuing Controversy. Intercontinental Medical Book Corp., New York, pp. 527-545.

Vos, J.G. 1977. Immune suppression as related to toxicology, CRC Crit.Rev.Toxicol., 5, 67-101.

134

Vos, J.G., van Logten, M.J., Kreeftenberg, J.G. & Kruitzinga, W. 1979. Hexachlorobenzene-induced stimulation of the humoral immune response in rats, Ann.N.Y.Acad.Sci., 320, 535-550.

Vos, J.G., Faith, R.E. & Luster, M.I. 1980. Immune Alterations. In. Kimbrough, R.D.(Eds).Halogenated biphenyls, Terphenyls, Naphthalenes, Dibenzodixins and Related Products, Elsevier/North- Holland Biomedical Press, Amsterdam, pp. 241-266.

Vos, J.G., Brouwer, G.M.J., van Leeuwen F.X.R. & Wagenaar, Sj. 1983. Toxicity of hexachorobenzene in the rat following combined pre- and postnatal exposure: comparison of effects on immune system, liver and lung. In.Parke, D.V., Gibson, G.G. and Hubbard, R.(Eds). Immunotoxicology, Academic Press, London, pp.219- 235.

Vos, J.G., de Klerk, A., Krajnc, E.I., Kruitzinga, W., van Ommen, B. & Rozing, J. 1984. Toxicity of bis(tri-n-butyltin)oxide in the rat. II. Suppression of thymus-dependent immune responses and of parameters of nonspecific resistance after short-term exposure. Toxicol.Appl.Pharmacol., 75, 387-408.

Vos, J.G. 1985. Dioxin-induced thymic atrophy and suppression of thymus-dependent immunity. In. Poland, A. & Kimbrough, R.D. (Eds). Biological Mechanisms of Dioxin Action. Banbury Report no 18, Cold Spring Harbor Laboratory, New York, In press.

Ward, J.M., Argilan, F. & Reynolds, C.W. 1983. Immunoperoxidase localization of large granular lymphocytes in normal tissues and lesions of athymic nude rats, J.Immunol., 131, 132-139.

Weening, J.J., Hoedemaeker, Ph.J. & Bakker, W.W. 1981. Immunoregulation and anti-nuclear antibodies in mercury-induced glomerulopathy in the rat, Clin.Exp.Immunol., 45, 64-71.

Ziprin, R.L. & Fowler, Z.F. 1977. Rosette-forming ability of alveolar macrophages from rat lung: Inhibition by hexachlorobenzene, Toxicol.Appl.Pharmacol., 39, 105-109.

EXPERIENCE WITH VALIDATION OF METHODOLOGY FOR IMMUNOTOXICITY ASSESSMENT IN RODENTS

Jack H. Dean, Lloyd D. Lauer, Robert V. House,
Edward C. Ward & Michael J. Murray

Department of Cell Biology Chemical Industry
Institute of Toxicology Research Triangle Park,
NC, U.S.A.

INTRODUCTION

This report summarizes our experience over the past two years in selecting and validating methodology for the immunotoxicity assessment of chemicals. Methods to assess lesions of humoral or cell-mediated immunity, natural resistance and host suscep- tibility to tumor cell or bacterial challenge are described. A major focus of this report will be the limitations and utility of methods proposed, selection of appropriate controls; assay variation and indications for data trans- formation, a quality control program; correlations between altered immune function and susceptibility to bacterial or tumor cell challenge; the concept of a functional immune reserve and its estimation; and, the need for an interna- tional interlaboratory validation of methods.

The sensitivity and utility of the immune system for detecting subclinical toxic injury has been recognized since Vos (1977) focused attention on the immune system as an important target organ of toxic insult. The susceptibility of the immune system to toxic injury may stem from several factors: funct- ionally immunocompetent cells are required for host resistance to opportunistic infectious agents or spontaneous neoplasia; immunocompetent cells require continued proliferation and differentiation for self-renewal and are, thus, sensitive to agents which affect cell proliferation or differentiation; and finally, the immune system is a tightly regulated organi- zation of lymphoid cells which are interdependent in function. Immunocompetent cells communicate through soluble mediators and cell-cell interactions. Any agent altering this delicate regulatory balance, affecting a particular cell type or altering intercellular communiciations can lead to immune alteration. An imbalance of the immune system resulting from cellular injury might be expressed as either immune enhance- ment (e.g., leading to autoimmunity or hypersensitivity) or immune suppression (e.g., or altered host resistance). Some believe that any immune alteration observed in rodents follo- wing xenobiotic exposure is of potential consequence for man. Others are more conservative and believe that only immune alteration associated with hypersensitivity or altered host resistance to infectious agents or neoplastic cells in rodents are of potential concern.

Experience by various workers over the past 8 years has shown that toxicological manifestations in the immune system follo- wing xenobiotic exposure in experimental animals may appear as

changes in lymphoid organ weights and/or histology; quantitative or qualitative changes in cellularity of lymphoid tissue,
bone marrow or peripheral leukocytes; impairment of immune
cell function; and, altered host resistance. A major cause
of previous failures in identifying immunotoxic compoounds
during routine toxicity assessment was the failure to include
even simple indicators of immunotoxicity such as thymus weight
or spleen and bone marrow cellularity measurements.

IMMUNOTOXICITY ASSESSMENT

Practical Consideration

In designing protocols for immunotoxicity assessment, special
attention should be given to the choice of species and age of
animals as well as duration, dosage and route of exposure.

The rationale for selecting the B6C3F1 mouse for immunotoxicity studies at the National Toxicology Program (NTP) was
based on the fact that the immune system of the mouse is best
characterized of all rodents, functional assays are better
defined, challenge models have been developed and monoclonal
antibodies are available to analyze lymphoid subpopulations.
Although the rat is more frequently used for toxicity
assessment, there is adequate precedent for selecting a
species other than the rat for special studies (e.g., dog for
drug evaluation, rabbit for teratology). Tumor resistance
models are more difficult in the rat because of the number of
animals required and the lack of well-defined transplantable
tumor models. Additionally, many of the immunological methods
used in the mouse are available or can be easily adapted for
subsequent work in the rat and human.

The exposure interval required for a chemical to produce
immune dysfunction depends on the type of immunological
injury, chemical threshold, toxicokinetics of the compound,
and the functional reserve of the immune parameteer affected.
In general, a subacute repeat exposure regimen of 14-30 days
is employed in young adult animals (6-8 weeks) for assessment
of chemically-induced alterations in immune competence. Few
systematic studies have examined the effects of chronic
exposure on immune function and such studies are desperately
needed, since low level chronic exposure may produce no effect
or more severe or persistent effects than subacute exposure.
Additionally exposure regimens and dosages should be selected
commensurate with the intended use of the compound.

Dose selection is critical in immunotoxicity assessment. High
doses producing overt toxicity should be avoided, since severe
stress and malnutrition are known to impair immune responses.
For proper dose selection, information on the effect of the
chemical on general toxicological parameters (e.g., LD_{50},
LD_{10}, type of acute or subchronic toxicity associated with
exposure) is important. To establish dose-effect relationships, three exposure levels are recommended. Ideally, the
highest dose should be less than the LD_{10} (e.g., 0.1 LD_{10}),
and have no associated mortality. The lowest dose ideally
should cause no alteration in immune function.

The route of exposure should, if possible, be the same as the natural route of exposure in man. for the majority of environmental chemicals, oral exposure (i.e., feeding or gavage) is preferred. When an accurate delivered dose is desirable, parenteral exposure is used. In the case of airborne agents, inhalation exposure is recommended.

A Tier Approach

Procedures currently used to detect immunotoxicity in rats include: weight and histology of thymus, spleen and mesenteric or popliteal lymph nodes; peripheral lymphocyte and monocyte counts; and, serum immunoglobulin levels (Vos, 1977). Functional measurements include induction of delayed hypersensitivity, proliferative responsivenesss to mitogens or allogeneic leukocytes, NK cell activity, macrophage phagocytosis, and splenic clearance of Listeria. However, results of early immune assessment in rats exposed to 17 different pesticides (Vos et al., 1983a; 1984a,b), which induced alterations in lymphoid organ weights, histology, or cellularity of lymphoid organs, did not always equate with functional immune alterations. Likewise, House et al. (1985) reported thymus atrophy in mice following exposure to ethylene glycol monomethyl ether and its principal metabolite, methoxy-acetic acid, which did not result in a functional immune defect in short term follow-up. Collectively, these, and other examples, demonstrate the need for functional assessment in addition to quantitation of lymphoid cells and examination of lymphoid tissue histology to assure that the significance of descriptive findings are understood in functional terms.

A flexible tiered approach for immunotoxicity assessment was proposed for the mouse which encompassed functional assays as well as host challenge models (Dean et al., 1979). The screening portion of this tier was adapted by the National Toxicology Program as part of their Special Studies Panel for Immunotoxicity Assessment (Deanb et al., 1982; Moore et al., 1982) and has since undergone validation. The screening panel currently used at the Chemical Industry Institute of Toxicology (CIIT) and in the National Toxicology Program for immunotoxicity evaluation in the mouse is shown in Table 1 and encompasses both in vivo and in vitro measures of quantitative and functional changes in immune statuts.

Methodology

Routine histophathology of lymphoid organs is useful in assessing the immunotoxicity of a chemical, particularly when these data are combined with effects observed on the weight and cellularity of thymus, spleen and peripheral lymph nodes. Because of the structural division of the spleen and lymph nodes into thymus-dependent and thymus-independent areas, careful microscopic examination may indicate preferential effects of the chemical for T or B cells.

Morphological examination of the spleen and bone marrow is essential in immunotoxicity assessment and can be performed on tissue sections, marrow smears or on cytocentrifuge preparations of single cell suspensions from these tissues. The latter technique allows the determination of cell numbers and viability. The paper by Vos in these proceedings , describes these approaches to immunopathology assessment.

Recent developments in monoclonal antibodies, computer proces- sing and cytometric instrumentation have found application in immunotoxicology and may be of potential value through the enumeration of bone marrow stem cell populations, quantitation of T and B lymphocytes and subpopulation of each in the spleen, lymph nodes or peripheral blood, or the identification of cells in various stages of activation using newly emerging reagents (Irons et al., 1983). Recently, observations of altered T and B cell distribution have been made in mice exposed to tumor promoting phorbol diesters (Murray et al., 1984). These techniques will not quickly replace functional analysis since Dean et al. (1984b) reported functional defects in mice exposed to dimethylbenzanthracene even though the percentages of T and B subpopuluations were unaltered.

Immune Function Tests

During the past 10 years, a number of assays have been deve- loped and refined to examine cell-mediated immunity, humoral immunity and natural resistance. The assembly of these assays into a tier is slightly different among the various groups working in immunotoxicology, partly because of the use of different animal species. This is particularly true for bacterial, viral and tumor challenge models. Selection of functional assays also depends on whether inbred or random-bred animals are employed. For example, at the Natio- nal Institute of Public Health, The Netherlands, random-bred Wistar rats are utilized in toxicity testing , and immunotoxi- city screening is based on assessment of immunopathology parameters included as part of a subacute toxicity study protocols. When the results of screening studies indicate that a chemical may be immunotoxic, function tests are perfor- med as part of a confirmatory tier in the same random-bred strain. Technical details of these methods are provided elsewhere (Vos, 1977). In contrast, initial screening (Tier I) for immunotoxicity at CIIT and in the NTP's Special Studies Panel for Immunotoxicity (Dean et al., 1982b; Moore et al., 1982) includes functional as well as host resistance assays (Table 1). It should be noted that the in vitro assays described in this Tier are performed following in vivo expo- sure of the animal to the test compound (ex vivo). Detailed information on these assays (Luster et al., 1982) and the effects of environmental chemicals on immune function in rodents should be obtained from several reviews (Vos, 1977; Dean et al., 1982a, 1984a) Assays to examine CMI at CIIT or in the NTP protocol include the in vitro techniques of lymphocyte proliferation and generation of one-way mixed lymphocyte responses. Lymphoproliferative responses are widely used correlates of CMI and can be defective in the absence of lymphocytopenia (Oppenheim and Rosenstreich, 1976). In the microculture assay, T or B cell mitogens (e.g. plant lectins, bacterial products), or allogeneic leukocytes (e.g., tissue transplantation antigens) are used to stimulate lymphocyte proliferation as measured by (3H)TdR incorporation into DNA. Depressed responses in humans or animals with normal numbers of lymphocytes are usually interpreted as a defect in cell activation.

Tumoricidal effector function assays have been evaluated at CIIT and recently incoporated in the NTP protocol. These assays quantitate both natural and acquired tumor resistance mechanisms (Figure 1). Spontaneous natural cytotoxicity is an important cytolytic effector mechanism in tumor resistance (Warner and Dennert 1982), limiting viral infections (Bukowski et al., 1983) and in resistance to intracellular parasites (Hatcher and Kuhn, 1982). NK tumoricidal activity is assessed in a four-hour microcytotoxicity assay by culturing splenocytes or peripheral blood lymphocytes with a 51Cr-labeled cell line sensitive to NK lysis (e.g., YAC-1 lymphoma cells).

The generation of cytotoxic T lymphocytes (CTL) is another manifestation of CMI which represents an important acquired effector mechanism in resistance to viral infections and surveillance against neoplastically transformed cells (Figure 1). Induction of CTL can be accomplished in vivo by immunization with allogeneic lymphocytes or tumor cells, or in vitro in a one-way mixed lymphocyte culture (MLC) or mixed lymphocyte-tumor cell interaction (MLTI). At CIIT, CTL-mediated-tumor cytolysis is assessed in a four hour 51Cr-release assay following a 5 day in vitro sensitization to allogeneic tumor cells (Murray et al., 1984b). In contrast to the ease with which mouse lymphocytes can be sensitized, it is rather difficult to generate CTL in rats (Weiss and Fitch, 1977).

Measurement of CTL activity has proven to be a valuable tool in immunotoxicity testing and has been reported to be suppressed by exposure to polycyclic aromatic hydrocarbon carcinogens (Dean et al., 1984b; Wojdani, 1983) and extremely low doses of TCDD (Nagarkatti, et al., 1984; Clark et al., 1981). The CTL assay is still used primarily for mechanistic studies, but will probably become an important component of Tier I following additional validation. Before this assay becomes routinely used, further correlation of its in vivo relevance and reserve capacity must be established.

Functional assessment of humoral immunity is most commonly accomplished by quantitating the number of antibody plaque-forming cells (PFC), or specific serum antibody titers. The Cunningham (1965) antibody plaque assay is extensively used for quantitating the number of antibody PFC. In this assay, lymphoid cells from an animal immunized 4 days previously with the T-dependent antigen, sheep red blood cells (SRBC), are incubated in a slide chamber with the target SRBC plus lytic complement. Plaques (hemolysis) in the SRBC lawn will be seen around each antibody-producing cell due to complement fixation and subsequent lysis of SRBCs that become coated with specific antibody produced by sensitized B cells (IgM). The PFC assay can also be applied to the measurement of IgG plaques. The PFC response to T-independent antigens (e.g., endotoxin or TNP-Ficoll) can also be measured by coating the surface of SRBCs with the sensitizing antigens. The PFC assay has proven to be a sensitive method for detecting chemical-induced alterations in humoral immunity.

It is now well established that cells of the mononuclear phagocyte system (MPS) not only provide nonspecific phagocytic and cytotoxic functions but are also directed and regulated by T-cell products (e.g., lymphokines). They also produce factors having regulatory roles in immune responses (e.g., prostaglandins and monokines). Dysfunction of the MPS can lead to indirect tissue damage through altered host resistance to infectious agents or neoplastically transformed cells, or through direct tissue injury by the mononuclear phagocytes themselves or their products (e.g., reactive oxygen intermediates). Xenobiotics, especially fibers, particulates and gases (see review Loose et al., 1981; Dean and Adams, 1985). The effects on macrophage function have been difficult to characterize precisely. This difficulty may be attributable, in part, to the fact that macrophage functions are closely related to their stage of maturation and that their development follows a complex and dynamic cascade of differentiation starting with bone marrow precursors (Adams and Dean, 1982; Adams and Marino, 1984). The effects of xenobiotic exposure are also often pleiotropic, so that a rational basis for studying and characterizing dysfunction of the MPS has been difficult to establish. A knowledge of macrophage function is pivotal to our understanding of immune responses and assessment of chemically-induced immunotoxicity.

Assessment of MPS function in vivo involves the measurement of RES clearance using the uptake of 125I-triolein (DiLuzio and Riggi, 1964) or the clearance of colloidal carbon (Stuart, et al., 1973). In vitro assessment includes phagocytosis of radiolabelled SRBC, macrophage bactericidal capacity (e.g., infection with Listeria monocytogenes). Besides their capacity of intracellular digestion, macrophages can destroy cells by a process of exocytosis, which is thought to play a role in the surveillance against malignancies (Higgs, 1977; Adams and Synderman, 1979). Tumor cytolysis activity of macrophages is commonly assessed in a microcytotoxicity assay by measuring the release of radioisotope from tumor target cells added to cultures of adherent peritoneal effector cells. More recently, the measurement of macrophage ecto- or lysosomal enzymes appears to offer another promising approach (Morahan et al., 1981).

For assessment of macrophage function it is recommended that peritoneal cells from mice treated with phylogistic agent or lymphokine should be given to a subset of control and exposed animals to determine activation potential following chemical exposure as well as basal function. Agents frequently used for in vivo activation include pyran copolymer (MVE-2), Cornybacterium parvum or the bacillus of Calmett and Gueirn (BCG) while macrophage activation factor and lipopolysaccharide are more frequently used as in vitro activating agents. The activational status of the macrophage appears to provide a more sensitive indicator than does basal level of macrophage injury following chemical exposure. Some have proposed using discrete markers for activation to assess the mechanism of chemical induced lesions of the mononuclear phagocyte system (Adams and Dean, 1982).

The application of one or more host resistance assays following exposure to chemicals has indicated that certain chemicals can alter host resistance to bacteria, viruses and parasites in rodents (see reviews of Vos, 1977; Faith et al., 1980; Bradley and Morahan, 1982; Dean et al., 1982b). Workers have utilized such infectious agents as Klebsiella pneumoniae, Listeria monocytogenes, Streptococcus pyogenes, Salmonella bern, Salmonella typhimurium, pseudorabies virus, duck heptitis virus, encephalomyocarditis virus, Trichinella spiralis and Plasmodium berghei. Resistance in most models appears to require T-cell immunity and functional mononuclear phagocytes. Resistance to Streptococcus pyogenes and Plasmodium berghei are exceptions, and require phagocytic cells whose function is facilitated by opsonizing antibodies.

Resistance to Listeria monocytogenes involves a combination of nonspecific phagocytosis by macrophages, which limits the growth or kills the organism during the first few days (1-3 days) after infection, and CMI which develops from day 2 postinfection (Tripathy and Mackaness, 1969; Cheers, et al., 1978). Nonspecific phagocytosis and killing can be measured on days 1 and 2 after an intravenous inoculation of Listeria, at a time when acquired CMI is not yet developed. Challenge of mice and rats with L. monocytogenes and the subsequent determination of mortality over 14 days has proven to be a reproducible model for detecting altered macrophage or T-cell function after chemical exposure (Dean, et al., 1980, 1982; Vos, et al., 1984a).

The ability of an animal to reject a challenge inoculation (TD 10-30%) of tumor cells can be a sensitive in vivo measure of general immunocompetence following chemical exposure (Dean et al., 1980, 1982b; see review Murray et al., 1984). Tumor challenge models using MKSA sarcoma (BALB/c background) and PYB6 sarcoma (C57BL/6 background) cells have been validated for detecting immune alterations following in vivo administration of the immuno-suppressive chemotherapeutic agent, cyclophosphamide (Dean et al., 1979b). Likewise, exposure to a variety of immunotoxic chemicals has been found to alter host susceptibility to tumor cells which can be correlated with deficits in T-lymphocyte function (Dean et al., 1982b). Chemically-induced immune suppression is expressed in these models as an increased incidence of tumors, a decreased latency to tumor appearance, an increased tumor growth rate, and/or decreased mean host survival time. Conversely, agents which stimulate immune function may facilitate resistance to tumor development through enhancement of transplantation rejection and/or immunosurveillance mechanisms. Immune enhancement can be detected in these models by using a higher challenge level of tumor cells (e.g., TD 70-90%).

Several metastatic models adaptable for host tumor resistance evaluation are available. The B16F10 melanoma model provides a convenient and reproducible means for detecting modulation

of host resistance parameters involved in solid, transplantable tumor growth , and the establishment of spontaneous or
experimental metastases as well as in vivo assessment of NK
activity. Intravenous challenge with the B16F10 subline
results in hematogenous dissemination of tumor cells, and
their subsequent growth in the lungs (i.e. experimental
metastasis). Since the B16 melanoma forms pigmented metastatic foci, visual quantitation of organ-associated metastases
is relatively simple. Alternatively, radioisotopic labelling
of tumor cells in vivo provides a reliable means of determining relative organ tumor burden between control and treated
mice. In this method (Murray et al., 1984a), after an initial
tumor growth period (21 days) animals receive an intraperitoneal injection of 1 Ci of $125I$-iododeoxyuridine, a radiolabelled DNA precursor which is incorporated into the nuclei of
proliferating cells. The mice are killed 18 hours after the
isotope injection and organs are removed and counted for
radioactivity.

ASSAY VALIDATION

Appropriate Controls

The selection of appropriate control groups is critical in
interpreting the data. For most studies, naive and vehicle
control animals must be included. These are animals of the
same strain and birth date as the exposed groups which receive
either nothing (naive) or vehicle using the same dosing
schedule as is used for the exposed animals. Since corn oil
or phosphate buffered saline are frequently used as vehicles
in toxicology studies and these have not been shown to produce
alterations in the function assays assessed in Tier I, a
separate naive group is not always included when either of
these two vehicles are employed.

A positive control group should also be considered, especially
during the development of a new assay, or when dealing with a
chemical of unknown immune status. Animals exposed to
cyclophosphamide, dexamethasone or cyclosporin A have frequently been used to verify the detection limits of the in
vitro assays, for a relative comparison between the test
chemical and a known immunosuppressant, or determining the
sensitivity of the challenge models. The inclusion of cyclophosphamide (180 mg/kg) in all challenge assays of infectious
agents or tumor cells is recommended, especially when one is
using an LD20 challenge dose, as this dose is subject to some
variation. By including a cyclophosphamide control group in
experiments employing low challenge inoculation we have been
able to utilize certain data although no mortality was noted
in the vehicle control group. Positive controls such as
cyclophosphamide have also frequently been used to determine
if the challenge model was sensitive to immunosuppression. We
periodically titrate our tumor models in cyclophosphamide
treated animals to determine if the tumor has drifted antigenically and is no longer sensitive to immunosuppression.

Assay Variation and Quality Control Procedures

Assay variation is an enigma of most in vitro biological methods. Immune function measurements are no exception. Some assays have more inherent variation than others, and the ultimate goal during assay refinement is to develop procedures that minimize variation. A minimization of variation can be accomplished by preliminary screening of serum, media and reagent lots; through the use of electronic cell counters to obtain accurate and reproducible cell counts; and, by careful pipetting of all reagents using repeating pipettes. Care should be taken not to use virally infected rodents, as certain rodent viruses will contribute to variation or failure of immune function assays. For example, mouse hepatitis virus induces suppressor macrophages (Boorman et al., 1982) and Sendai virus results in depressed lymphoproliferative and PFC responses (Kay, 1978). Although assay variation can be minimized, in vitro immune function assays will always include some inherent variation.

When the routine evaluation of chemicals is necessary it may be important to set up a quality control (QC) program to track assay variation and drift. To accomplish this, the responses of normal animals can be plotted over time as the mean $+$ 2 standard deviations (SD) (e.g., 95% confidence interval) as is shown in Figure 2. This figure presents data from natural killer cytolysis in control mice from the previous 2 1/2 years. Note that only 1 out 39 assays was outside the acceptable limits (+ 2SD(during this period, and this outlier was from animals that exhibited elevated NK activity for which no biological explanation was found. in other assays, (e.g., lymphoproliferative responses) the data were distributed over a range of several logs and frequently lacked normal distribution. Since these data are bounded by zero and skewed away from zero (i.e., not normally distributed), they should be transformed (e.g., normalized) to $\log_{10}$ or square root before standard comparisons are performed or quality control plots are developed. Figure 3 present histograms of lymphoproliferation data from control animals obtained over the preceding two years before (3A) and after log transformation (3B). Note the skewed distribution (i.e., non-normal) of the data prior to log transformation (Figure 3A). When transformed these data become normally distributed and can be statistically analyzed. Alternatively, for combining repeated experiments it may be possible to also use data expressed as a percentage of control response or percentage of suppression.

By developing the same type of quality control program frequently used in clinical hematology and chemistry, it should be possible to analyze the performance of each of the assays utilized in Tier I and determine if an assay has failed during the course of the immunological assessment of a chemical. On this basis, an objective decision as to the success or failure of an assay could be arrived at. This would allow one to rationally discard a particular test. Figure 4 demonstrates our experience for the past two years with the other measurement included in our Tier I panel. Note that some assays such as the plaque-forming cell response

(Panel B), can be used after a several month lay-off with results similar to values obtained previously. This probably indicates a small inherent variation in this assay. Other assays in which transformation of the data is required are also illustrated in this figure. Data presented in this figure which have not been transformed and were normally distributed by the Wilk-Shapiro test. The frequency of assays outside the acceptable limits was quite low in all cases.

Reporting Parameter

It is frequently desirable to express some immune function data for publication as both absolute counts and as a percentage of the response of the control animals. this allows the reader to assess the performance of the assay and also allows a comparison of these data with similar studies using the same assays. When describing the response of a cell population (e.g., the number of plaque-forming cells per 10_6 lymphocytes), these values should also be expressed on an organ basis (e.g., the number per spleen or the absolute values). Absolute values may have more meaning than the simple expression of a percentage or response per unit of cells. When reporting cytolysis assays, it is necessary to report the counts spontaneously released if the reader is to accurately judge the conditions of the assay. It may also be desirable to report the data from some assays as a percentage of suppression relative to a positive control chemical (e.g., cyclophosphamide).

Limitations and Utility of the proposed Methods

Frequently in biology the selection of what are believed to be appropriate methods is based upon standardized, readily available procedures without fully appreciating the biological interpretation of the results. For example, the biological consequence of marginally depressed lymphoproliferation in response to the mitogen PHA is beyond our current realm of interpretation. It is not known if a 30% decrease in PHA responsiveness, although statistically significant, has any biological significance. Thus, it is intuitively appealing to discard assays whose ultimate biological meaning is beyong our present understanding and adopt methodology involving more tangible aspects of biological relevance. Effector cell assays tend to require intercellular cooperation which ultimately results in the expression of a measurable function. Thus, assays requiring cellular interactions are often intuitively more appealing (e.g., PFC or CTL assays). During the past two years our laboratory has adopted assays measuring cell-mediated effector function by incorporating NK-, macrophage- and T cell-mediated cytolysis assays into our assessment repertoire. These methods have proven helpful in identifying lesions induced by chemical exposure, and seem related to changes in tumor susceptibility. It is hoped that once the pattern of associations between the in vitro and in vivo assays is established, some of the in vivo assays may be discontinued. For example, if correlation is consistently observed between host susceptibility in a particular tumor model and suppression of NK or CTL activity, and the threshold for this effect is known, then the NK or CTL assay might be used in place of the in vivo tumor model. One could envision in vitro assays of macrophage or lymphocyte function replacing bacterial and viral challenge models as well.

MECHANISMS

Correlations between Immune Function Measurements and Altered Host Resistance

Determining how loss of immune function, as measured in vitro, produces a significant biological effect in vivo is a goal of an applied discipline such as immunotoxicology. Furthermore, it is now recognized that the immune system possesses a resilience and reserve functional capacity which must first be lost before any in vivo alterations are seen. To address the question of correlations between in vitro immune function measurements and altered host susceptibility to challenge with infectious agents or tumor cells, we have assembled data obtained over the last two years with a variety of chemicals tested at three different doses in host resistance models and which have produced varying degrees of functional modulation. The lack of independence of these two parameters was evaluated with Spearman's rank correlation coefficient. Figure 5 shows a significant correlation (Spearman's Rho = -0.758) between depressed NK cytolysis and increased susceptibility to in vivo challenge with B16F10 melanoma cells (p < 0.01). Similarly, Figure 6 demonstrates a correlation between loss of CTL activity and increased susceptibility to challenge with PYB6 sarcoma cells (p < 0.05). Conversely, loss of CTL activity was not correlated with increased susceptibility to B16F10, and NK suppression was only weakly associated with increased susceptibility to PYB6. From these figures it is also possible to estimate the functional reserve in these two effector functions which must be lost before altered suscepti- bility to tumor challenge is seen, assuming host resistance to the particular tumor is predominantly by a single effector mechanism. In the CTL assay, the functional reserve appears to be approximately 40-50 percent since this much activity must be lost before a significant increase in tumor frequency is seen following PYB6 tumor challenge. NK activity seems to have a higher functional reserve. Sixty to 70 percent of this activity must be lost before increased susceptibility to B16F10 tumor challenge is noted. The level of functional reserve may be different for each host parasite model depen- ding on the pleiotropic nature of immune responses that govern the model. These types of correlations, albeit preliminary, provide insight into the biological significance of the various in vitro measures of immune function (Table 2). Information in this area should be expanded if we are to accurately assess chemical safety and risk. A detailed understanding of effector mechanisms involved in host resis- tance is required to establish the relationships between immune function alterations and altered susceptibility in challenge models.

Interlaboratory Validation

During the past three years, under the auspices of the
National Toxicology Program/NIEHS/NIH, an interlaboratory
methods development and validation effort was initiated in two
contract laboratories (i.e., Medical College of Virginia and
Illinois Institute of Technology Research Institute), one
government (NIEHS) and one private laboratory (CIIT). In this
interlaboratory validation effort, the Tier I panel was used
to study immunotoxic effects in B6C3F1 mice exposed to several
chemicals. The data in Table 3 represent a preliminary
analysis of this effort. The first two years of the study
were directed at methods development and standardization. In
several of the assays there is good agreement between the
different laboratories on the frequency and amount of immunosuppression observed with a particular chemical. These data
suggest that immune alterations induced by chemicals can be
accurately assessed by different groups employing
well-controlled and stadardized methodologies. The contributors of these data should be commended for the high quality
achieved in the standardization and performance of the assays
included in this analysis.

This interlaboratory validation effort is quite preliminary
and should be expanded on an international scale to assess and
improve the reproducibility of methodology throughout the
world. This will facilitate the interpretation of data and
accurate assessment of the immunotoxic potential of chemicals.
One goal of such a comparison might be to determine if both
mice and rats are equally appropriate species and interchant-
geable for the safety assessment of chemicals for
immunotoxicity. Additionally, this approach would expedite
progress in expanding our limited data base regarding the
potential of chemicals of various classes to alter the immune
response. An international program of interlaboratory validation would have to be organized within the framework of an
international organization such as the World Health Organization (WHO) or the Commission of European communities (CEC)
in order to provide the infrastructure needed for the successful completion of such an ambitious project. One goal of
such a comparison might be to determine if both mice and rats
are equally appropriate species and interchangeable for the
safety assessment of chemicals for immunotoxicity. In
addition, an expanded effort in methods selection might also
be accomplished by such an international comparison. The
ultimate goal of such an international interlaboratory validation would be to provide the scientific community with a
validated and reproducible panel of well-selected methods to
obtain data for assessment of chemical safety relative to the
immune system and to allow better human risk extrapolation.

SUMMARY

The application of immunologic methods for toxicity assessment
has developed rapidly and been widely accepted. Programs to
determine the immunotoxic potential of chemicals and drugs are
being developed in many governmental, university and industrial laboratories throughout the world. Since a single

immune function assay cannot be used to comprehensively evaluate immunomodulation following exposure to chemicals or drugs, a flexible tier of sensitive in vivo and in vitro assays was developed to assess immunotoxicity in rodents and is currently being refined and validated in several laboratories. The tier approach to immunotixicity assessment consists of a screening panel (TIER I) which enables the quick identification of compounds which may produce immune alterations. Agents positive in TIER I assays can be further evaluated with assays selected from a more comprehensive panel (TIER II). Tier II assays allow confirmation and an indepth evaluation of the underlying mechanism(s) of immunotoxicity.

The interpretation of immune alterations observed in rodent toxicity studies in terms of risk for man deserves continued consideration and discussion. A larger data base in rodents correlating immune function measurements and altered suscepti- bility to challenge with infectious agents or tumor cells, spontaneous tumor development and development of hypersensiti- vity or autoimmunity is needed. Only through the incorpora- tion of reliable methods for assessing immune function into toxicity testing will the information necessary for the rational safety assessment of chemicals be made available for risk estimation.

Further development in this area should include an internati- onal interlaboratory validation of test methods using com- pounds with known immunotoxic effects. This would ultimately provide a more standardized protocol for immunotoxicity and immunopharmacological testing. Such a tier of validated methods should not rely solely on state-of-the-art function tests, but incorporate immunopathology, immunohistochemistry or flow cytometry methods, as well as host challenge models.

The next few years present a new challenge to the field of immunotoxicology because of the required efficacy and safety assessment of new recombinant biologicals (e.g., growth hormones, interferons, interleukins, and new vaccines); biorational pesticides; biological response modifiers (i.e., drugs such as muramyl dipeptide designed to enhance immunores- ponsiveness against tumors and infections); and, monoclonal antibodies designed as drug delivery vehicles or for detoxification. Many of these agents will present new and varied immunotoxicology problems and will require the develop- ment of new and better models. Careful study of these agents should provide insight into mechanisms of immunotoxicty and immunopharmacological effects which should lead to the design of safer chemicals and more efficacious drugs.

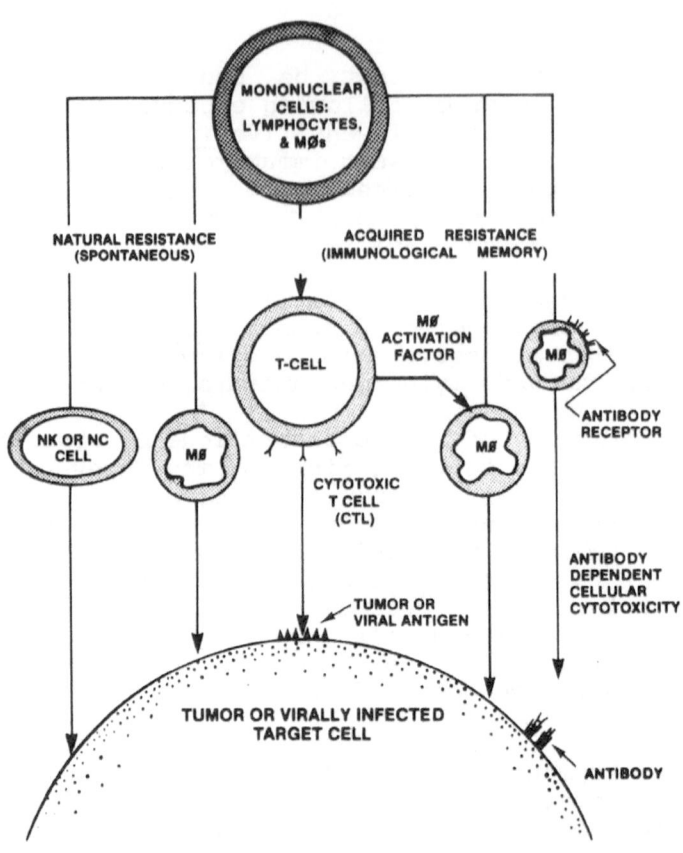

Figure 1. Schematic of effector cells active in resistance to tumor and virus showing both natural and acquired mechanisms. Macrophages (MØ), natural killer cells (NK) and thymus-dependent lymphocytes (T-cells) are illustrated.

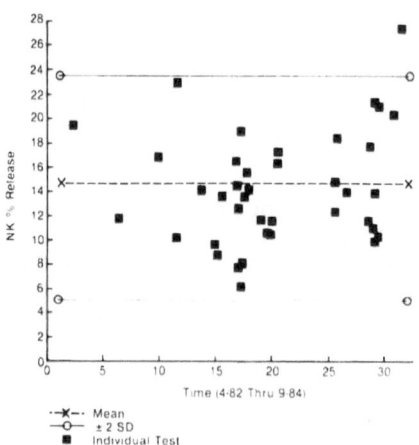

Figure 2. Plot of the percentage of NK cytolysis over past 2 1/2 years observed in lymphocytes from normal (control groups) B6C3F1 mice against YAC-1 target cells showing mean (x) SD (0) (e.g., 95% confidence limits).

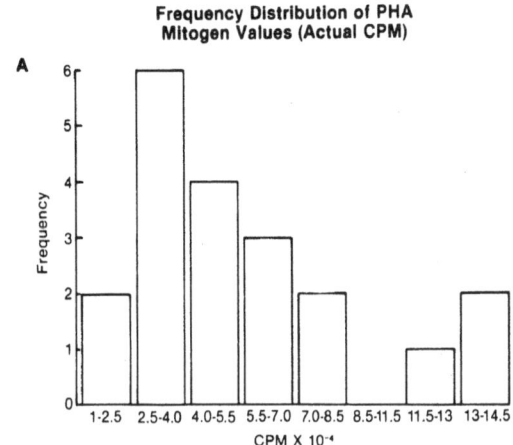

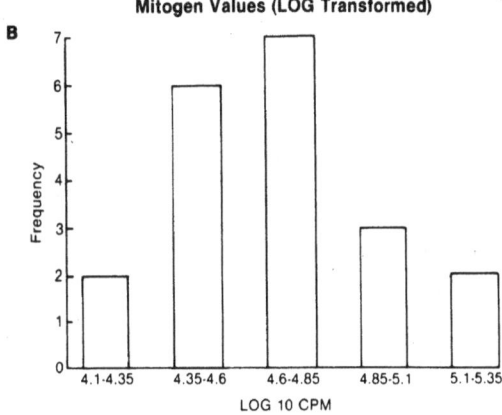

Figure 3. Frequency distribution of lymphoproliferative response to phytohemagglutinin (PHA) in splenocytes from normal B6C3F1 mice (control groups)
over the past 2 years showing actual CPM (3A) and $\log_{10}$ transformed CPM
(3B). Note the skewed distribution (i.e., non-normal) of the data prior
to log10 transformation.

150

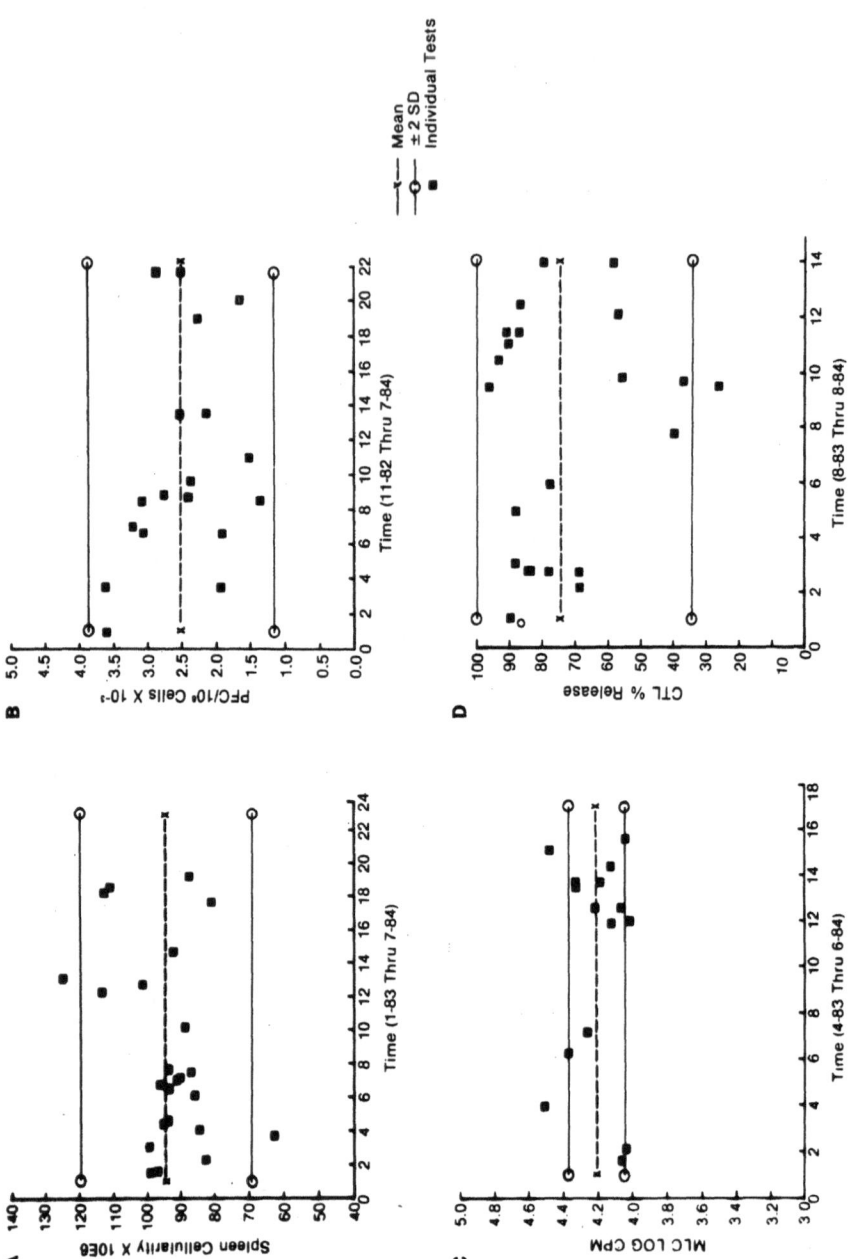

Figure 4. Historical plots of data from Tier I assays (i.e., spleen cellularity (A), antibody PFC (B), mixed leukocyte (C) and cytotoxic T-cell response (D) performed on control mice during the previous 2 years. Individual values and mean (X) ± SD (0) (e.g., 95% confidence limits) are represented.

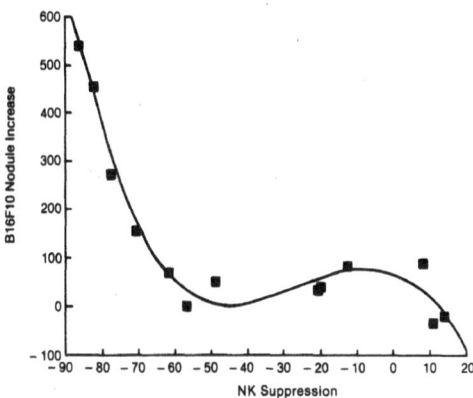

Correlation of NK Suppression With Susceptibility To B16F10 Lung Nodule Formation

Spearman's Rho = − 0.758242   p<0.01

Figure   5.   Plot showing correlation of chemical-induced depression of NK cytolysis and increased susceptibility to nodule formation following in vivo
challenge with B16F10 melanoma cells. Note Spearman's rho and probability
values at bottom of panel. Values are given as percentage increase to
nodule formation and percentage suppression of NK cytolysis from all
chemicals studied during previous 2 years.

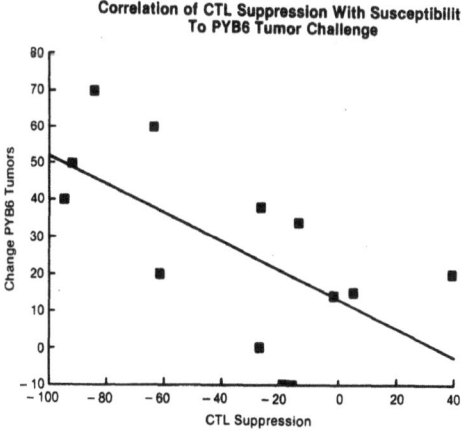

Correlation of CTL Suppression With Susceptibility To PYB6 Tumor Challenge

Spearman's Rho = − 0.626207   p<0.05

Figure   6.   Plot showing correlation of chemical-induced depression of CTL cytolysis and increased susceptibility to PYB6 tumor formation following in
vivo challenge. Note Spearman's rho and probability values at bottom of
panel.   Values are given as percentage increase in PYB6 tumor takes and
percentage suppression of NK cytolysis from all chemicals studied during
the previous 2 years.

Table 1

Methods for Detecting Immunotoxic Alterations Currently Being Evaluated at CIIT

Parameters	Procedures
Immunopathology	Routine hematology.
	Lymphoid organ weights (spleen, thymus) and histology.* Spleen and bone marrow cellularity
Cell-mediated immunity	
Proliferation	Mitogen responses and one-way mixed leukocyte cultures*.
Tumoricidal	Natural killer cell cytolysis* and cytotoxic T cell induction
Surface markers	Quantification of lymphocyte sub-populations using monoclonal antibodies.
Antibody-mediated immunity	Antibody plaque-forming cells (PFC) response.*
Macrophage function	Resident peritoneal macrophage number,* phagocytosis, cytostasis and enzyme levels* in activated and non-activated cells.
Host resistance	Tumor challenge model: PYB6 sarcoma* B16F10 melanoma Bacterial challenge model: Listeria monocytogenes*

*Currently included in the National Toxicology Program's Special Studies Panel for Immunotoxicity Assessment.

Table 2. Correlations Between Altered Susceptibility In Challenge Models and Antibody Plaque Forming Cell Response With Loss of In Vitro Immune Function

Parameter	Correlation Values:				
	NK	CTL	MLC	LPS	PHA
Listeria monocytogenes susceptibility	.31[a]	.66	.54*	.06	.44
PYB6 susceptibility	.56*	.63*	.51*	-	.32
B16F10 susceptibility	.76**	.36	.51	-	.56
Loss of PFC response	-	-	-	.62*	.08

[a]Correlation coefficient as determined by Spearman's rank correlation test.

*Significantly different from control at $P< 0.05$.

**Significantly different from control at $P< 0.01$.

-Not Tested

Table 3. Interlaboratory Variability of Methods Used in Tier I Immunotoxicity Testing Following DES Administration in B6C3F1 Mice[a]

Parameter	Laboratory	DES Exposure (mg/kg)[b]			
		0	2	10	40
Listeria challenge					
No. Dead/No. Tested	I	21/61(34)	25/27(93)*	ND	34/39(87)*
(% Mortality)	II	4/20(20)	19/20(95)*	18/20(90)*	16/20(80)*
	III	4/15(27)	9/14(64)*	11/15(73)*	14/15(93)*
MLC [CPM±SEM of	I	29 ± 2	18 ± 2(-38)*	9 ± 1(-69)*	11 ± 2(-62)*
^{3}H-TdR Incorp.	II	19 ± 3	18 ± 3(-5)	12 ± 2(-37)*	9 ± 1(-53)*
× 10^3 (% change)]	III	24 ± 2	26 ± 2(+8)	10 ± 1(-58)*	9 ± 1(-63)*
Antibody PFC	I	1.67 ± .34	1.04 ± .06(-38)	1.65 ± .34(-1)[a]	.76 ± .46(-54)*
to SRBC: 10^{-3}	II	ND	ND	ND	ND
PFC/10^6 Spleen	III	3.87 ± .50	3.62 ± .52(-6)	3.34 ± .56(-14)	1.87 ± .06(-52)*
Cells ± SEM					
(% change)					
PFC/Spleen ± SEM	I	16.2	13.0(-20)	8.7(-54)*	9.1(-44)*
× 10^4	II	39.0	ND	24(-38)*	12.3(-68)*
(% change)	III	22.0	20.7(-6)	11.9(-46)*	5.5(-75)*

[a]Summarized from Dean, Luster and Munson, 1985.

[b]Female B6C3F1 mice, 6-8 weeks of age were exposed to a total dose of DES at 2, 10 or 40 mg/kg over either a 1 week (Lab I) or 2 week (Labs II and III) period. DES was dissolved in corn oil] and diluted such that each mouse received a volume of 0.1 ml injection subcutaneously in the dorsal cervical region. Controls received an equal volume of corn oil. Animals were challenged with Listeria or tested for immunological function 3 to 5 days following the last exposure. Each value in the mixed leukocyte culture (MLC) or antibody PFC response represents a minimum of 6 mice/group.

*Significantly different from control values at P< 0.05.

REFERENCES

Adams, D.O. & Dean, J.H., 1982, Analysis of macrophage objective markers to characterize the stages of activation. Natural cell-mediated immunity. II. Ed. Herberman, R., Academic Press, pp. 511-518.

Adams, D.O. & Marino, P., 1984, Activation of mononuclear phagocytes for destruction of tumor cells as a model for study of macrophage development. In: Contemporary Hematology - Oncology. (Eds Gordon, A.S., Silber, R. & LoBue, J.), Vol. III, pp. 69-136.

Boorman, G.A., Luster, M.I., Dean, J.H., Campbell, M.L., Lauer, L.D., Talley, F.A., Wilson, R.E. & Collins, M.J., 1982, Peritoneal macrophage alterations caused by naturally occurring mouse hepatitis virus. Amer. J. Path., 106, 110-117.

Bradley, S.G. & Morahan, P.S., 1982, Approaches to assessing host resistance. Environ. Health Perspect., 43, 61-69

Bukowski, J.F., Woda, B.A., Habu, S., Okumura, K. & Welsh, R.M., 1983, Natural killer cell depletion enhances virus synthesis and virus-induced hepatitis in vivo, J. Immuno., 131, 1531-1538.

Cheeers, C., McKenzie, I.F.C., Pavlov, H., Waid, C. & York, J., 1978, Resistance and susceptibility of mice to bacterial infection: course of listeriosis in resistant or susceptible mice. Infect. Immun., 19, 763-770.

Clark, D.A., Gauldie, J., Szewczuk, M.R. & Sweeney, G., 1981, Enhanced suppressor cell activity as a mechamism of immunosuppression by 2,3,7,8-tetrachlorodibenzo(p)dioxin. Proc. Soc. Expt. Biol. Med., 168, 290-299.

Cunningham, A.J., 1965, A method of increased sensitivity for detecting single antibody-forming cells. Nature, 207, 1106-1107.

Dean, J.H., Padarathsingh, M.L. & Jerrels, T.R., 1979a, Assessment of immunobiological effects induced by chemicals, drugs, or food additives. I. Tier testing and screening approach. Drug Chem. toxicol. 2, 5-17.

Dean, J.H., Padarathsingh, M.L., Jerrells, T.R., Keys, L. & Northing, J.W., 1979b, Assessment of immunological effects induced by chemicals, drugs or food additives. II. Studies with cyclophosphamide. Drug Chem. Toxicol. 2, 133-153.

Dean, J.H., Luster, M.I., Boorman, G.A., Luebke, R.W. & Lauer, L.D., 1980. The effect of adult exposure to diethylstilbestrol in the mouse: alterations in tumor susceptibility and host resistance parameters. J. Reticuloendoth. Soc., 28, 571-583.

156

Dean, J.H., Luster, M.I. & Boorman, G.A., 1982a, Immunotoxicology. In (Eds. Sirois, P. & Rola-Pleszczynski, M.) Immunopharmacology, pp. 349-397. elsevier Biomedical Press, Amsterdam.

Dean, J.H., Luster, M.I., Boorman, G.A. & Lauer, L.D., 1982b, Procedures available to examine the immunotoxicity of chemicals and drugs. Pharmacol. Rev. 34, 137-148.

Dean, J.H., Murray, M.J. & Ward, E.C., 1984a, Toxic modifications of the immune system. In: Casarett & Doull's Toxicology: The basic science of poisons (Eds. Doull, J., Klaassen, C.D. & Amdur, M.O.), 3rd edition, in press.

Dean, J.H., Ward, E.C., Murray, M.J., Lauer, L.D., House, R.V., Stillman, W. & Adams, D.O., 1984b, Immunosuppression following 7,12-dimethylbenz(a)anthracene exposure in B6C3F1 mice. II. Altered cell-mediated immunity and tumor resistance. Cellular Immunol., in press.

Dean, J.H., Luster, M.I. & Munson, A.E. (1985). Approaches and methodology for immunotoxicity assessment. In Eds. Dean, J.H., Munson, A.E., Luster, M.I. & Amos, H. Toxicology of the Immune System (in press), Raven Press, New York.

Faith, R.E., Luster, M.I. & Vos, J.G. (1980). Effects on immunocompetence by chemicals of environmental concern. In Eds. Hodgson, E., Bend, J.R. & Philpot, R.M.. Reviews in Biochemical Toxicology 2, pp. 173-211. Elsevier/North Holland, New York.

Gardner, P.E. (1984). Alterations in macrophage function by environmental chemicals. Environ. Health Perspect., in press.

House, R.V., Lauer, L.D., Murray, M.J., Ward, E.C. & Dean, J.H. (1985). Immunological studies in B6C3F1 mice following exposure to ethylene glycol monomethyl ether and its principal metabolite methoxyacetic acid. Toxicol. Appl. Pharmacol., in press.

Irons, R.D., Stillman, W.S. & Dean, J.H. (1983). Application of flow cytometric methods in immunotoxicology. U.S.A.F. Conference Proceedings, 13th Conference on Environmental Toxicology. Publication no. AFAMRL-TR-82-101, United States Air Force, pp. 24-32.

Kay, M.M. (1978); Long term subclinical effects of parainfluence (Sendai) infection on immune cells on aging mice. Proc. Soc. Explt. Biol. Med. 158, 326-331.

Loose, L.D., Silkworth, J.B., Charbonneau, T. & Blumenstock, F. (1981). Environmental chemical-induced macrophage dysfunction. Environ. Health Perspect. 39, 79-81.

Luster, M.I., Dean, J.H., Moore, J.A., (1982). Evaluation of immune functions in toxicology. In: Methods in Toxicology, Ed. Hayes, A.W. (Raven Press, New York) pp. 561-586.

Moore, J.A., Huff, J.E. & Dean, J.H. (1982). The National Toxicology Program and Immunological Toxicology. Pharmacol. Rev. 43, 13-16.

Morahan, P.S., Edelson, P.J. & Gass, K. (1980). Changes in macrophage ectoenzymes associated with anti-tumor activity. J. Immunol. 125, 1312-1317.

Murray, M.J., Lauer, L.D., Luster, M.I., Luebke, R.W., Adams, D.O. & Dean, J.H. (1984a). Correlation of murine susceptibility to tumor parasite and bacterial challenge with altered cell-mediated immunity following systemic exposure to the tumor promoter phorbol myristate acetate. Int. J. Immunopharmacol., in press.

Murray, M.J., Kerkvliet, N.I., Ward, E.C. & Dean, J.H. (1984b). Models for the evaluation of tumor resistance following chemical or drug exposure. In: Toxicology of the Immune System, Target Organ Toxicity Series (Eds. Dean, J.H., Munson, A.E., Luster, M.I. & Amos, H.E.), Raven Press, New York.

Nagarkatti, P.S., Sweeney, G.D., Gauldie, J. & Clark, D.A. (1984). Sensitivity to suppression of cytotoxic T-cell generation by 2,3,7,8-tetrachlorodibenzo-p-dioxin (TCDD) is dependent on the Ah genotype of the murine host. Toxicol. Appl. Pharmacol., 72, 169-176.

Oppenheim, J.J. & Rosenstreich, D.L. (1976). Mitogens in Immunobiology. Academic Press, New York.

Tripathy, S.P. & Makaness, G.B. (1969). The effect of cytotoxic agents on the primary immune response to Listeria monocytogenes. J. Exp. Med., 130, 1-16.

Vos, J.G. (1977). Immune suppression as related to toxicology. CRC Crit. Rev. Toxicol., 5, 67-101.

Vos, J.G., Krajnc, E.I., Beekhoff, P.K. & van Logten, M.J. (1983a). Methods for testing immune effects of toxic chemicals: evaluation of the immunotoxicity of various pesticides in the rat. In Eds. Miyamoto, J. et al., IUPAC Pesticide Chemistry. Human Welfare and the Environment, pp. 497-504. Pergamon Press, Oxford.

Vos, J.G., de Klerk, A., Krajnc, E.I., Kruizinga, W. (1984b). Effect of triphenyltin hydroxide on the immune system of the rat. Toxicology, 29, 325-336.

158

Ward, E.C., Murray, M.J., Lauer, L.D., House, R.V. & Dean, J.H. (1984). Immunosuppression following 7,12=dimethylbenz°a§anthracene exposure in B6C3F1 mice. I. Effects on humoral mediated immunity and host resistance. Toxicol. Appl. Pharmacol. 75, 299-305.

Warner, J.F. & Dennert, G. (1982). Effects of a cloned cell line with NK activity on bone marrow transplants, tumour development and metastasis in vivo. Nature, 300, 31-34.

Weiss, A. & Fitch, F.W. (1977). Macrophages suppress CTL generation in rat mixed leukocyte cultures. J. Immunol., 199, 510-516.

Wojdani, A., Nieto, M., Alfred, L.J. (1983). Carcinogenic PAH compound suppressed cell-mediated immune functions, and alter T-cell subsets in splenic lymphocyte populations. Proc. Amer. Assoc. Cancer Res. 24, 242.

AN IN VITRO MODEL FOR STUDYING CELLULAR AND MOLECULAR MECHANISMS OF THYMIC ATROPHY INDUCED BY CHLORINATED AROMATIC COMPOUNDS

William F. Greenlee, Karen M. Dold & Rosemarie Osborn
CIIT Postdoctoral Fellow

Department of Cell Biology Chemical Industry,
Institute of Toxicology Research Triangle Park,
NC, U.S.A.

INTRODUCTION

2,3,7,8-Tetrachlorodibenzo-p-dioxin (TCDD) is the prototype for certain isomers from several classes of halogenated aromatic compounds, including the polychlorinated biphenyls (Goldstein, 1980; Poland et al., 1979). Studies carried out in inbred murine strains have shown that the induction of cytochrome P_1-450 and other xenobiotic metalbolizing enzymes by TCDD is regulated by a genetic locus (designated the Ah locus) (reviewed in Poland and Knutson, 1982; Nebert and Jensen, 1979). It has been postulated (Nebert et al., 1984; Poland et al., 1979), that the Ah locus codes for a receptor Protein (to be designated in this report as the Ah receptor). The Ah receptor originally was identified in murine liver (Poland et al., 1976) and subsequently has been detected in several epithelial tissues (Glasiewicz, 1983) and animal (Guenthner and Nebert, 1977) and human (Hudson et al., 1983) cells in culture. In mice this receptor has been shown to be involved in two toxic responses to TCDD: epidermal hyperplasia (Knutson and Poland, 1982) and thymic atrophy (Poland and Glover, 1980; see below). The actions of TCDD on targets such as the skin and thymus appear to result in altered patterns of growth and differentiation (reviewed in Greenlee and Neal, 1985).

ACTIONS OF TCDD ON THE IMMUNE SYSTEM

Evidence obtained in various animal and cell culture models indicate that TCDD exerts diverse actions on the immune system, suggesting the involvement of several cellular target sites. Luster et al. (1984) have shown that TCDD can act directly on bone marrow stem cells and splenocytes in culture to suppress the formation of granulocyte-macrophage colonies and plaque forming cells, respectively. In adult mice TCDD has been reported to suppress antibody production at doses which do not alter cell mediated (T-lymmphocyte) immunity (CMI) (Mantovani et al., 1980; Vecchi et al., 1980). In young animals, the adverse actions of TCDD on the immune system appear to be selective for cells participating in the differentiation and expression of CMI and T-lymphocyte-dependent antibody responses (Dean et al., 1982; Vecchi et al., 1983; Vos, 1977). Comparison of the responsiveness of the immune system to TCDD in adult and perinatally exposed animals indicate that the developing immune system is a particularly sensitive target, with thymic atrophy being the most common pathologic finding (Gupta et al., 1973; Luster et al., 1982). The histopathology of the thymic lesions induced by TCDD is characterized by a depletion of cortical thymocytes (Vos and Moore, 1974; McConnell et al., 1978) and is similar to that reported for cortisone-treated animals (Bach, 1975).

TCDD-INDUCED THYMIC ATROPHY: INVOLVEMENT OF THE AH RECEPTOR AND PROPOSED CELL TARGET SITES

Studies carried out in inbred murine strains differing in sensitivity to TCDD indicate that TCDD-induced thymic atrophy is mediated by the Ah receptor:(1) thymic atrophy segregates with the Ah locus; and (2) this response is stereospecific (i.e., chlorinated aromatic compounds isosteric with TCDD produce thymic atrophy) (Poland and Glover, 1980). The Ah receptor is detected in thymic cytosol and nuclear fractions from rats (Lund et al., 1982) and in the thymus from strains of mice with greatest sensitivity to TCDD (Poland and Glover, 1980). In these studies, receptor binding was measured in subcellular fractions prepared from whole thymus. The relative distribution of the receptor in the various thymus cell populations (e.g., thymocytes versus thymic epithelial cells) was not determined. Although the involvement of the Ah receptor in TCDD-induced thymic atrophy appears to be well-established, cellular targets and specific responses regulated by the Ah receptor relevant to thymic pathogenesis have not been established by the available animal data.

Immunosuppressive agents with the potential to compromise CMI can act at one or more target sites: prethymic stem cells in the bone marrow, intrathymic precursor cells, thymic macrophages and epithelial cells, or peripheral T-lymphocytes. Toxicity to T-lymphocytes also can result from modulation of pituitary or adrenal gland function (e.g., glucocorticoid-induced thymic atrophy and suppressed CMI). TCDD is not cytotoxic to murine lymphoma or virus-transformed lymphocyte cells lines (Knutson and Poland, 1980) and does not adversely affect peripheral lymphocytes in vitro at concentrations which suppress CMI in vitro (Luster et al., 1979). Further, TCDD does not appear to act through modulation of serum corticosteroid levels (Van Logten et al., 1980) and does not appreciably alter macrophage function (Luster et al., 1982). These observations have led to the hypothesis that lymphocyte precursors, thymic epithelium, or both may be possible target sites (Vos, 1977; Poland and Knutson, 1982).

IN VITRO MODEL FOR THYMIC ATROPHY

In order to study the cellular and molecular mechanisms for TCDD-induced thymic atrophy, an in vitro system was established for co-culturing thymocytes on thymic epithelial (TE) monolayers (Greenlee et al., 1985a). Several methods have been reported for cultivation of TE monolayers including the use of conditions selecting against thymic fibroblasts and macrophages (Boniver et al., 1981), and co-culture with lethally irradiated murine 3T3 fibroblasts (Sun et al., 1984). TE cells obtained by these methods have been shown to be of epithelial origin as judged by the expression of prekeratin filaments (Fig 1).

Thymocytes from C57BL/6 (Ah-positive) mice were co-cultivated on TCDD treated syngeneic TE monolayers, or cultured in TE-conditioned medium from TCDD treated cultures and then assayed for responsiveness to the mitogens concanavalin A (Con A and phytohemagglutinin (PHA), according to the experimental protocol shown in Fig. 2 (Greenlee et al., 1985a). Cocultivation of thymocytes on control monolayers (Fig. 3) or in conditioned medium from control cultures (Table 1) resulted in an enhanced response to both mitogens. Treatment of the TE monolayers with TCDD (at noncytotoxic concentrations) resulted in a concentration-dependent (Fig. 3) and stereospecific (Greenlee et al, 1985a) suppression of the enhanced response of co-cultivated thymocytes to both Con A and PHA, whereas the enhanced mitogen response mediated by TE supernatant was not suppressed in thymocytes incubated in conditioned medium from TCDD treated cultures (Table 1). These findings indicate that TCDD can act directly on TE cells to suppress thymocyte maturation. This response is not mediated by soluble factors produced by TE cells (Table 1). It has been proposed (Greenlee et al., 1985a) that TCDD may alter early stages in the complex process of thymus-dependent T-lymphocyte maturation requiring direct contact between precursor cells and the thymic microenvironment (Bach and Papiernik, 1981).

The concentration-dependence and stereospecificity for the suppression of TE-dependent maturation of thymocytes by TCDD in vitro (Greenlee et al., 1985a) correspond with the values for these same parameters for TCDD-induced thymic atrophy in vivo (Poland and Glover, 1980), indicating that modulation of TE cell function by TCDD is mediated by the Ah receptor. The concentration of the Ah receptor in cytosol fractions from cultured TE cells was measured directly by adsorption onto hydroxylapatite and was found to be 3 and 3.5 times greater than that measured in cytosol fractions prepared from whole thymus and thymocytes, respectively (Greenlee et al., 1985a). The value obtained for the cultured TE cells (86 fmol/mg protein) (Greenlee et al., 1985a) was nearly identical to the value reported for the number of hepatic receptor sites (84 fmol/mg protein) (Poland et al., 1976) in the same strain of mice.

COMMON ACTIONS OF TCDD ON EPIDERMAL AND TE CELLS

TCDD-induced epidermal hyperkeratinization has been studied in cultured human epidermal cells derived from neonatal foreskin (Greenlee et al., 1985c; Osborne and Greenlee, 1985) and in human squamous cell carcinoma lines of epidermal origin (Hudson et al., 1985). These cells can be serially cultivated in the presence of lethally-irradiated murine 3T3 fibroblasts (Rheinwald and Green, 1975; Rheinwald and Beckett, 1980; 1981) and from colonies which essentially maintain the structural and functional dynamics of the epidermis in vivo (Green, 1979). The differentiation of epidermal cells can be monitored with monoclonal antibodies directed against human thymus (Haynes, 1984). Both epidermal and TE cells appear to undergo an analogous pattern of terminal differentiation as judged by the expression of similar surface antigens (Table 2) (Haynes, 1984).

Treatment of confluent cultures of normal human epidermal cells with TCDD results in enhanced differentiation analogous to hyperkeratinization observed in vivo (Greenlee et al., 1985c; Osborne and Greenlee, 1985). The enhanced differentiation response in the TCDD treated cultures can be quantitated and is characterized by a decrease in the number of proliferating (basal) cells and DNA synthesis, and an increase in the number of differentiating (envelope competent) and terminally differentiated (with spontaneous envelopes) cells (Table 3). This response to TCDD appears to be mediated by the Ah receptor (Osborne and Greenlee, 1985).

The observations on the actions of TCDD on human epidermal (Osborne and Greenlee, 1985) and TE (Greenlee et al., 1985a) cells suggest that TCDD may be altering similar regulatory events in both cell targets. Hyperkeratinization, one of the toxic responses of the epidermis to TCDD, is characterized in vitro to result from enhanced differentiation mediated by the Ah receptor (Osborne and Greenlee, 1985). It has been proposed that thymic atrophy also can result from TCDD-induced terminal differentiation of TE cells (Greenlee et al., 1985b). It is assumed that the terminally differentiating TE cell loses the ability to support thymocyte maturation. Impaired thymocyte maturation may lead to increased thymocyte death contributing to the depletion of cortical thymocytes characteristic of TCDD-induced thymic atrophy.

CONCLUDING COMMENTS

The available data do not support a definitive association between TCDD exposure in humans and immune dysfunction. The inability to detect adverse effects may indicate that the human immune system is not a major target for TCDD. However, it is possible that subtle changes in the differentiation or function of the cellular components of the immune system may not be detected by the immunotoxicity screening assays routinely used. Several strains of human TE cells have been successfully cultivated in our laboratory (Fig. 1B). Comparison of the responses of murine and human TE cells to TCDD should provide insight into the mechanisms of potential interspecies differences in the susceptibility of this thymus target cell population. Should a response to TCDD be observed in the human TE cells, detailed study of the mechanisms involved may lead to a predictive model for potential immunotoxic actions of TCDD in humans.

Footnote

Abbreviations used include: CMI, cell-mediated immunity; Con A, concanavalin A; CTL, cytotoxic T-lymphocyte; PCB, polychlorinated biphenyls; PHA, phytohemagglutinin; TCDD, 2,3,7,8-tetrachlorodi ben zo-p-dioxin; TE, thymic epithelial.

Table 1 Lymphoproliferative responses of thymocytes from C57BL/6J
mice cultured in TE-conditioned medium[a]

TE Treatment (nM TCDD)	TE-conditioned Medium	[^{3}H]-Thymidine Incorporation (cpm)	
		Con A	PHA
0	-	11,416 ± 1870	2,945 ± 619
0	+	33,273 ± 2993	12,321 ± 1835
0.1	+	36,307 ± 1827	11,677 ± 1707
1	+	29,143 ± 3135	12,476 ± 1386
10	+	33,826 ± 2050	17,620 ± 3046
30	+	35,447 ± 5306	16,117 ± 2007

[a]Confluent monolayers of TE cells from C57BL/6J mice were treated with
either solvent vehicle (DMSO, 0.1%), or the indicated concentrations of TCDD
for 48 hrs and then were washed two times with DMEM containing 5% fetal calf
serum. Conditioned medium was prepared by culturing washed monolayers in the
presence of RPMI 1640 medium supplemented with 5% heat-inactivated human AB
serum, 2 mM glutamine and 50 µg/ml gentamycin for 24 hrs. Thymocytes were
prepared and incubated in either control or conditioned RPMI 1640 medium for
48 hrs. Lymphoproliferative responses to Con A and PHA were measured as
described previously (Greenlee et al., 1985a). Each value represents the
mean ± S.D. of 4 determinations. Taken from Greenlee et al. (1985a).

Table 2. Actions of TCDD on selected parameters of cell growth and differentiation in normal human epidermal cells[a,b]

	DMSO	TCDD
Total cell number ($\times 10^{-6}$)	1.9 ± 0.2	2.0 ± 0.1
Small (basal) cell number ($\times 10^{-6}$)	0.80 ± 0.60	0.37 ± 0.02[c]
Cell protein (mg)	0.69 ± 0.03	0.74 ± 0.01
^{3}H-Thymidine incorporation (DPM/mg protein $\times 10^{-3}$)	7.82 ± 1.20	3.85 ± 0.70[c]
Spontaneous envelopes ($\times 10^{-4}$)	1.5 ± 0.02	3.5 ± 0.2[c]
Envelope competence ($\times 10^{-6}$)	0.92 ± 0.06	1.9 ± 0.05[c]
EGF bound (DPM/mg protein $\times 10^{-3}$)	5.57 ± 0.09	3.34 ± 0.14[c]

[a]Confluent cultures of normal human epidermal cells in 6-well dishes were treated 4 days with 0.01% DMSO or 10 nM TCDD. At the end of the treatment period, the parameters indicated were measured in replicate dishes. The mean and SEM of values from triplicate wells are given. Taken from Osborne and Greenlee (1985).

[b]A cytochrome P_1-450 mediated monooxygenase activity, 7-ethoxycoumarin O-deethylase (measured as described by Hudson et al., 1983), was increased 12-fold by TCDD in this experiment, from 0.44 ± 0.01 pmol/mg protein/min in controls, to 5.3 ± 0.46 pmol/mg protein/min in TCDD treated cells.

[c]$p < 0.05$ versus DMSO control values (Student's t test).

Table 3. Co-expression of thymus antigens by epidermal keratinocytes and thyic epithelium[a]

Organ	Antigens
Skin	
Basal layer	TE-4[+], TE-8[-], TE-15[-]
Stratum granulosum	TE-4[-], TE-8[+], TE-15[-]
Stratum corneum	TE-4[-], TE-8[-], TE-15[+]
Thymus	
Medullary epithelium	TE-4[+], TE-8[-], TE-15[-]
Hassall's bodies	TE-4[-], TE-8[+], TE-15[+]

[a]Data from B. N. Haynes (1984)

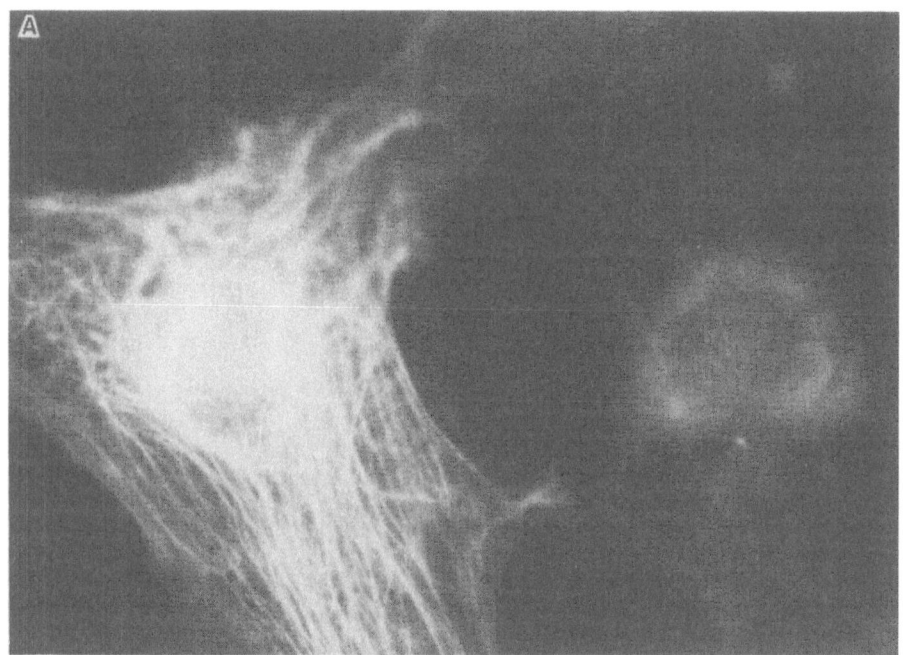

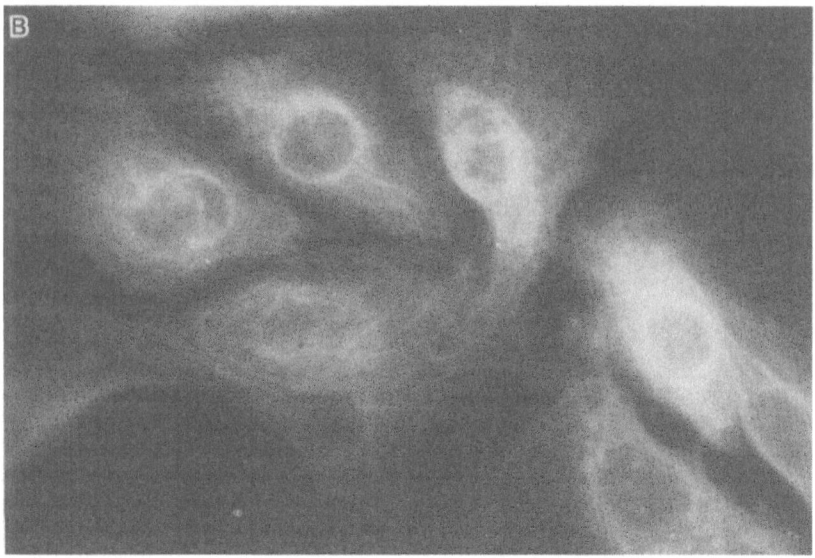

Figure 1. Visualization of prekeratin filaments in cultured
TE cells from A murine B human thymus. TE cells were
plated at a density of 2 x lo 4/ml on Lab-Tek chamber
slides and prokeratin filaments were visualized as
described previously (Greenlee et al., 1985a).

166

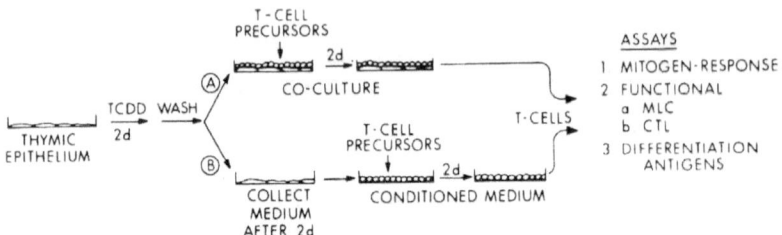

Figure 2. Protocol for co-culture and conditioned medium maturation of T-lymphocyte precursors.

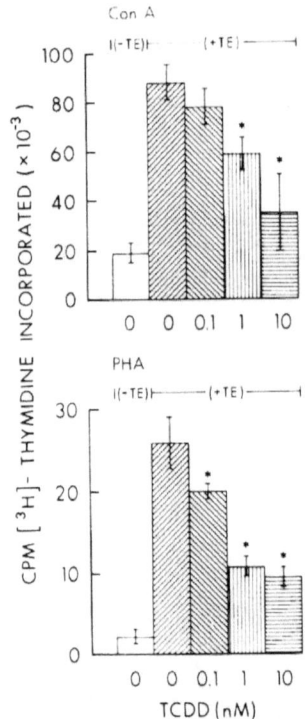

Figure 3. Lymphoproliferative responses of thymocytes from C57BL/6J mice co-cultivated on TCDD-treated syngeneic TE monolayers. Confluent cultures of TE cells were treated with either solvent vehicle (DMSO, 0.1 %), or the indicated concentrations of TCDD for 48 hrs. Thymocytes were isolated (Boniver et al., 1981) from thymuses of 6 week old mice, co-cultivated on the treated TE monolayers, and assayed for mitogenic responses to Con A and PHA as described previously (Greenlee et al., 1985a). Each bar represents the mean SD of 4 determinations. Asterisks indicate values significantly different ($p < 0.05$) from the DMSO-treated co-culture controls. Taken from Greenlee et al., 1985a.

REFERENCES

BACH, J.F. (1975) Cortisteroids. In The Mode of Action of Immunosuppressive Agents (eds., A. Neuberger & E.L. Tatum) pp. 21-91. North-Holland Publishing Co., Amsterdam.

BACH, J.F. & PAPIERNIK, M. (1981). Cellular and molecular signals in T cell differentiation. In Microenvironments in Hematopoietic and Lymphoid Differentiation. pp. 215-235. Ciba Foundation Symposium 4, Pitman, London.

BONIVER, J., DECLERE, A., DAILEY, M.O., HONSI, C., LIBERMAN,M. & KAPLAN, H.S. (1981). Macrophage and lymphocyte-depleted thymus reticulo-epithelial cell cultures: establishment and functional influence on T-lymphocyte maturation, C-type virus expression and lymphomatous transformation in vitro. Thymus, 2: 193-213.

DEAN, J.H., LUSTER, M. I. & BOORMAN, G.A. (1982). Immunotoxicology. In Immunopharmacology (eds., P. Sirois and M. Rola-Pleszczynski) pp. 349-397. Elsevier Biomedical Press, New York.

GASIEWICZ, T. A. (1983) Receptors for 2,3,7,8-tetrachlorodi-benzo-p- dioxin: their interand intra-species distribution and relationship to the toxicity of this compound. In Proceedings of the 13th Annual Conference on Environmental Toxicology, pp. 250-269. University of California, Dayton, OH.

GOLDSTEIN, J.A. (1980). Structure-activity relationships for the biochemical effects and the relationship to toxicity. In Halogenated Biphenyls, Terphenyls, Naphthalenes, Dibenzodioxins and Related Products, (ed., Kimbrough, R.D.) pp. 151-190. Elsevier/North-Holland Biomedical Press, New York.

GREEN, H. (1979). The keratinocyte as differentiated cell type. The Harvey Lectures, 74:101-139.

GREENLEE, W.F., DOLD,K.M., IRONS, R.D., & OSBORNE, R. (1985a). Evidence for direct action of 2,3,7,8-tetrachlo- rodibenzo-p-dioxin (TCDD) on thymic epithelium. Toxicol. Appl. Pharmacol., in press.

GREENLEE, W. F., DOLD, K. M. & OSBORNE, R. (1985). A proposed model for the actions of TCDD on epidermal and thymic epithelial target cells. In Biologic Mechanisms of Dioxin Action. (eds. Poland, A. and Kimbrough, R. D.), pp. 435-44o. Banbury Report No. 18, Cold Spring Harbor Laboratory, New York.

168

GREENLEE, W.F. & NEAL, R. A. (1984). Ah receptor: a biochemical and biologic perspective. In The Receptors (Vol.2) (ed. J.M. Conn) Academic Press, New York, in press.

GREENLEE, W. F., OSBORNE, R., DOLD, K.M., HUDSON, L. G. & TOSCANO, W.A., Jr. (1985c). Toxicity of chlorinated aromatic compounds in animals and humans: in vitro approaches to toxic mechanisms and risk assessment. Environ. Health Perspect., in press.

GUPTA, B.N., VOS, J.G., MOORE, J. A., ZINKL, J. G. & BULLOCK, B.C. (1973). Pathologic effects of 2,3,7,8-tetrachlorodibenzo-p-dioxin in laboratory animals. Environ. Health Perspect., 5:125-140.

GUENTHNER, T.M. & NEBERT, D.W. (1977). Cytosolic receptor for aryl hydrocarbon hydroxylase induction by polycyclic aromatic compounds. Evidence for structural and regulatory variants among established cell culture lines. J. Biol. Chem., 252:8981-8989.

HAYNES, B. F. (1984). The human thymic microenvironment. Adv. in Immunol., 36:87-142.

HUDSON, L.G. SHAIKH, R. TOSCANO, W.A., JR., & GREENLEE, W. F. (1983). Induction of 7-ethoxycoumarin O-deethylase activity in cultured human epithelial cells by 2,3,7,8-tetrachlorodibenzo-p-dioxin (TCDD: Evidence for TCDD receptor. Biochem. Biophys. Res. Commun., 115:611-617.

HUDSON, L.G., TOSKANO, W.A., JR., & GREENLEE, W. F. (1985). Regulation of epidermal growth factor binding in a human keratinocyte cell line by 2,3,7,8-tetrachlorodibenzo-p-dioxin. Toxicol. Appl. Pharmacol., in press.

KNUTSON, J.C. & POLAND, A. (1980). 2,3,7,8-Tetrachlorodibenzo-p-dioxin: failure to demonstrate toxicity in twenty-three cultured cell types. Toxicol. Appl/ Pharmacol., 54:377-383.

KNUTSON, J.C. & POLAND, A. (1982). Response of murine epidermis to 2,3,7,8-tetrachlorodibenzo-p-dioxin: Interaction of the Ah and hr loci. Cell, 30:225-234.

LUND, J., KURL, R.N., POELLINGER, L. & GUSTAFFSON, J.A. (1982). Cytosolic and nuclear binding proteins for 2,3,7,8-tetrachlorodibenzo-p-dioxin in the rat thymus. Biochem. Biophys. Acta, 716:16-23.

LUSTER, M.I., CLARK, G. , LAWSON, L.D. & FAITH, R,E, (1979). Effect of brief in vitro exposure to 2,3,7,8-tetrachlorodibenzo-p-dioxin (TCDD) on mouse lymphocytes. J.Environ. Pathol. Toxicol., 2:965-977.

LUSTER, M.I., TUCKER, A.N., HONG, L., BOORMAN, G. and PATTERSON, R. (1984). In vivo and in vitro effects of TCDD on stem cell and B cell differentiation. In Biologic Mechanisms of Dioxin Action (Eds Poland, A. & Kimbrough, R.), pp. . Banbury Report, Vol.18, Cold Spring Harbor Laboratory, New York.

MANTOVANI, A., VECCHI, A., LUINI, W., SIRONI, M., CANAIANI, G.P., SPREAFICO, F. & GARATTINI, S. (1980). Effect of 2,3,7,7-tetrachlorodibenzo-p-dioxin on macrophage and natural killer cell-mediated cytotoxicity in mice. Biomedicine, 32:200-204.

McCONNELL, E.E., MOORE, J.A., HASEMAN, J.K. and HARRIS, M.W. (1978). The comparative toxicity of chlorinated dibenzo-p-dioxins in mice and guinea pigs. Toxicol. Appl. Pharmacol., 44:335-356.

NEBERT, D.W., EISEN, H.J. & HANKINSON, O. (1984). The Ah receptor: binding specificity only for foreign chemicals? Biochem. Pharmacol., 33:917-924.

NEBERT, D.W. and JENSEN, N.M. (1979). The Ah locus: genetic regulation of the metabolism of carcinogens, drugs, and other environmental chemicals by cytochrome P-450-mediated monooxygenases. CRC Crit, Rev, Biol., 6:401-437.

OSBORNE, R. & GREENLEE, W.F. (1985). 2,3,7,8-Tetrachlorodibenzo-p-dioxin (TCDD) enhances termical differentiation of cultured human epidermal cells. Toxicol. Appl. Pharmacol., in press.

POLAND, A. & GLOVER, E. (1980). 2,3,7,8-Tetrachlorodibenzo-p-dixin: segregation of toxicity with the Ah locus. Mol. Pharmacol., 17:86-94.

POLAND, A., GLOVER, E. & KENDE, A.S. (1976). Stereospecific, high affinity binding of 2,3,7,8-tetrachlorodibenzo-p-dioxin by hepatic cytosol. Evidence that the binding species is receptor for induction of aryl hydrocarbon hydroxylase. J. Biol. Chem., 251:4936-4946.

POLAND, A., GREENLEE, W.F. & KENDE, A.S. (1979). Studies on the mechanism of action of the chlorinated dibenzo-p-dioxins and related compounds. Ann. N.Y. Acad. Sci., 320:214-230.

POLAND, A. & KNUTSON, J.C. (1982). 2,3,7,8-Tetrachlorodibenzo-p-dioxin and related halogenated aromatic hydrocarbons: examination of the mechanism of toxicity. Ann. Rev. Pharmacol. Toxicol., 22:517-554.

RHEINWALD, J.G. & BECKETT, M.A. (1980). Deffective terminal differentiation in culture as a consistent and selectable character of malignant human keratinocytes. Cell, 22:629-632.

170

RHEINWALD, J.G. & BECKETT, M.A. (1981). Tumorigenic keratinocyte lines requiring anchorage and fibroblast support cultured from human squamous cell carcinomas. Cancer Res., 41:1657-1663.

RHEINWALD, J.G. & GREEN, H. (1975). Serial cultivation of strains of human epidermal keratinocytes: the formation of keratinizing colonies from single cells. Cell, 6:331-344.

SUN, T.-T., BONITW, P. & BURNS, W.H. (1984). Cell culture of mammalian thymic epithelial cells: growth, structural, and antigenic properties. Cellular Immunol., 83:1-13.

VAN LOGTEN, M.J., GUPTA, B.N., McCONNELL, E.E. & ;OORE, J.A. (1980). role of the endocrine system in the action of 2,3,7,8-tetrachlorodibenzo-p-dioxin (TCDD) on the thymus. Toxicology, 15:135-144.

VECCHI, A., MANTOVANI, A,, SIRONI, M., LUINI, W., CAIRO, M. & GARATTINI, S. (1980). Effect of acute exposure to 2,3,7,8-tetrachlorodibenzo-p-dioxin on humoral antibody production in mice. Chem.-Biol. Interact., 30:337-342.

VECCHI, A., SIRONI, M., CANEGRATI, M.A., RECCHIA, M. & GARATTINI, S. (1983). Immunosuppressive effects of 2,3,7,8-tetrachlorodibenzo-p-dioxin in strains of mice with different susceptibility to induction of aryl hydrocarbon hydroxylase. Toxicol. Appl. Pharmacol., 68:434-441.

VOS, J.G. & MOORE, J.A. (1974). Suppression of cellular immunity in rats and mice by maternal treatment with 2,3,7,8-tetrachlorodibenzo-p-dioxin. Int. Arch. Allergy Appl. Immunol, 47:777-794.

VOS, J.G. (1977). Immune suppression as related to toxicology. CRC Crit. Rev. in Toxicol., 5:67-101.

THE GUT ASSOCIATED LYMPHOID TISSUE AS A MODEL OF A SPECIALIZED IMMUNE SUBSYSTEM

J. G. Hall

Department of Tumour Immunology,
Institute of Cancer Research, Sutton,
Surrey, United Kingdom

INTRODUCTION

It has been recognised for centuries that the gut of many animals is richly endowed with what we now describe as lympho/reticular tissue. It is agreed generally now that the primary function of such lympho/reticular tissue is to generate immune effector mechanisms which protect the body against the onslaughts of pathogenic bacteria, viruses and toxins. Because the gut is designed to absorb nutriment and has a vast surface area that is in contact with the outside world , it is more than usually at risk and requires special protection. The protection afforded to the gut by the gut associated lymphoid tissue (GALT) is by no means absolute; even in developed communities, which have sophisticated sanitary arrangements and medical supervision, occasional illness caused by enteric infections is by no means rare. In undeveloped communities, especially where population density is high such infections cause continual morbidity and mortality. The young of both man and animals are particularly at risk; the adaptation (in an immunological sense) to pathogenic and commensal bacterial flora necessarily takes time, and, in many species, the GALT is poorly developed at birth. During this process of adaptation the GALT very occasionally over reacts and produces antibodies and immunocytes directed at normal dietary constituents so that states of clinical hypersensitivity, or allergy, may develop.

In considering these complicated interactions between the GALT and the miriad antigenic macromolecules present in the lumen of the gut, it is often very difficult to draw the line between the processes of normal, physiological development and genuinely pathological processes. Of necessity the experimental approach to the investigation of these problems often involves the use of experimental animals. Unfortunately, even among mammals, there are important species differences and these must be borne in mind continually. Much confusion and some bad feeling has been caused because individual investigators or clinicians have attempted to draw general conclusions from the small amount of evidence with which they are personally familiar. The truth is that even where the most familiar species are concerned, our knowledge of how the GALT functions is fragmentary and superficial.

BASIC ANATOMY

From an anatomical standpoint the GALT is comprised of three components; the diffuse lymphoid tissue in the lamina propria of the intestine, the Peyer's patches (aggregates of lymphoid follicles that are distributed along the length of the intestine) and the mesenteric lymph nodes. (A physiologist might add a fourth component , i.e. the pool of circulating lymphocytes , the components of which continually migrate from the blood, into the wall of the gut and the mesenteric nodes, enter the local lymph and so find their way back to the blood).

The lamina propria. The lympho-reticular tissue is distributed along the whole length of the gut, in between the basement membrane of the epithelium and the muscular coats. It extends into the villi and surrounds the crypts. It is most abundant in the small gut, and immunologists tend to concentrate on this part of the alimentary tract as being typical and, quantitatively, the most important. However, the large bowel, too, is a significant lymphoid organ but the traffic of lymphoid cells through its walls, and the population of resident lymphoid cells, are usually an order of magnitude less than those of the small gut. In monogastric mammals the traffic of lymphoid cells through the laminae of the oesophagus and stomach is usually small, though in ruminants the abomasum (which corresponds to the glandular stomach of monogastric mammals) has a lamina that contains a substantial population of immunologically active cells.

Cytologically, the cells of the lamina are of three main types; macrophages (often dendritic), lymphoid cells (small lymphocytes, large lymphoid immunoblasts and particularly, mature, antibody-secreting plasma cells) and granulocytes (in health, these are relatively sparse and consist mainly of eosinolphils and mast cells). Unless special means of investigation are the used the macrophages are often rather inconspicuous but modern techniques (1,2,3) have shown the tissue spaces of the gut to be abundantly supplied with dendritic macrophages which are especially important in the presentation of antigens to immunologically competent B and T lymphocytes. A feature of the lymphoid cells in the laminae of adults is the large number of plasma cells; these are characterised ultrastructurally by their content of concentric lamellae of endoplasmic reticulum, which indicates a vigorous synthesis of antibody protein. In man and laboratory rodents most of these plasma cells secrete immunoglobulin A (IgA), the principal antibody of the external secretions.

The Peyer's patches. This term is properly applied to the macroscopic aggregates of lymphoid tissue which Joseph Conrad Peyer described in 1677. These aggregates are situated in the anti/mesenteric wall of the intestines. In rodents they are easily visible without opening the gut but in large animals they are best seen after the gut is opened. In the rat they are a few mm. in diameter but in man and large animals they may be several cm. long. A rat may have 5-10 substantial patches; larger animals, a score or more. The detailed structure of these patches cannot be gone into here but a few salient features require comment. The overlying epithelium loses its villous pattern and becomes a flat membrane composed of columnar epithelial cells. Some of the epithelial cells are specialized and have a "phagocytic" function (4,5). Although they are genuine epithelial cells and not true macrophages these 'M' (the 'M' stands for membranous) cells seem able to take "samples" of the contents of the gut and pass small amounts of material to the dense masses of lymphoid tissue which underly them. Much of this lymphoid tissue is arranged in follicles, not unlike the germinal centres found in lymph nodes, and these follicles are comprised principally of small B lymphocytes, while the interfollicular areas between them are the areas where small T lymphocytes recirculate from blood to lymph. In spite of the fact that the follicles are B cell areas, the Peyer's patches contain very few mature, antibody forming plasma cells.

The mesenteric lymph nodes. These nodes receive and filter the lymph that is formed in the wall of the intestine and conveyed to them by the afferent lymphatics. These afferent lymphatics are referred to sometimes as 'lacteals' because they necessarily contain the macromolecular products of digestion, principally the chylomicra, or fat globules, which give the lymph the milky appearance, from which the lacteals take their name. It cannot be stressed too often that macromolecular material, be it derived from the diet or intestinal microorganisms, that has succeeded in penetrating the epithelium, depends absolutely for its transport on the lymphatic system. Except in the case of gross injury or pathology, macromolecules cannot enter the blood capillaries or venules directly, and so the portal blood cannot, in health, contain antigenic material of this sort. Those antigenic macromolecules that do penetrate the gut wall must impinge first on the local lymphoid tissue in the lamina and, second, on the mesenteric nodes to which the lymph will carry them. It is probably for this reason that, even in healthy animals, the mesenteric nodes usually display the histological stigmata of antigenic stimulation.

The general structure of the mesenteric nodes is similar to that of nodes elsewhere in the body. They have the usual cortex, containing the germinal centres (A B cell area), and a deeper 'para-cortex' which is the principal area through which T cells recirculate from blood to lymph. Deeper still, is the medulla which is replete with plasma cells. Most of these synthesise conventional IgG and IgM antibodies but a certain amount of IgA synthesis goes on as well. This observation highlights a peculiar feature of the mesenteric nodes. They are unusual in being downstream of the diffuse lymphoid tissue in the wall of the gut and of the Peyer's patches. Thus small lymphocytes, immunoblasts and macrophages from these tissue are conveyed in significant numbers (1) to the mesenteric nodes. Many of these itinerant immunoblasts are, in fact, IgA plasma blasts and they become trapped in the lymph sinuses of the mesenteric nodes, where they mature into IgA plasma cells. It is likely, then, that much of the IgA synthesis that occurs in the mesenteric nodes, was induced and initiated in the wall of the gut.

Intra epithelial lymphocytes (IEL). Mention must be made of the lymphocytes which are present actually inside the epithelium, i.e. between epithelial cells and above the basement membrane. Compared with the cells of the lamina such IEL are sparse and may represent nothing more than a random selection of wandering lymphocytes which have fortuitously penetrated the basement membrane. They show considerable heterogeneity; a minority is of 'B' origin and may be precursors of basophilic granulocytes or mast cells (6,7), others have T cell markers (8), and appear to belong to the suppressor/cytotoxic series rather than the helper/inducer category (9). The biological functions and significance of these cells are uncertain at present but some believe that they play a part in the epxression of cell mediated immunity (CMI) in the gut (q.v.).

Developmental considerations. One of the most intriguing findings of modern immunobiology was the observation that, at any rate in fowls, the GALT plays a crucial part in the development of the whole system of B lymphocytes. Avian species have a substantial lymphoid organ, the Bursa of Fabricius, situated near the cloacal end of the gut. When the bursa was surgcally excised, or hormonally suppressed, before hatching took place, the chick failed to develop a system of B lymphocytes and could not make antibody globulin. The implications of this finding for the understanding of the congenital hypogammaglobulinaemias of man were obvious but no structure analogous to the avian bursa was found in man or laboratory rodents. It was believed that some part of the GALT of these species might function as did the bursa but it was apparent that this function was not associated with a discrete anatomical compartment of the mammalian GALT.

Recently it has been observed in sheep that some of the Peyer's patches may have this function. Foetal sheep have, in addition to the conventional Peyer's patches, a vey substantial and continuous patch that extends up the ileum for many cm. from the ileo/caecal junction. In post/natal life this patch involutes, as does the thymus, as sexual maturity approaches and may be scarcely discernible in the adult. When the gut containing this patch was removed surgically from the foetus the lamb suffered no later nutritional consequences, but the number of circulating B lymphocytes were severely reduced, and this impairment appeared to be life long (10,11). One may anticipate that this finding will be common to all ruminants, and data is accumulating that suggest a similar situation may exist in the pig (12).

LYMPHOCYTE MIGRATION AND RECIRCULATION

Gowans's demonstration that small lymphocytes recirculate continually from blood to lymph by traversing the walls of the post capillary venules in the lymph nodes and Peyer's patches (and also, probably in the spleen and the wall of the intestine generally) is now a quarter of a century old. This work has been amply confirmed and seems common to all mammalian species, though the pig shows some peculiar differences (13).

For some time after the phenomenon of lymphocyte recirculation was established and generally accepted it was believed that small lymphocytes recirculated more or less randomly through any part of the fixed lymphoid tissue to which the blood stream happened to carry them. In 1976 it was shown that this was not so in the sheep; small lymphocytes collected from the intestinal lymph recirculated preferentially through the GALT, while those from peripheral somatic nodes (PSLN) recirculated through oter PSLN but tended to avoid the GALT (14). The original experiments were carried out using unfractionated small lymphocytes but later experiments showed that purified populations of T lymphocytes behaved in the same way (15). For technical reasons these experiments cannot be repeated on rats and mice and there is some doubt, therefore, as to whether this is a general phenomenon. Also, it seems to be an acquired characteristic, in that it cannot be demonstrated in foetal sheep in utero (16). In any event, it must be empha- sized that the preferential recirculation of small lymphocytes from GALT through their tissue of origin is by no means an "all or nothing" phenomenon, it is only a bias. Thus, some GALt lymphocytes are capable of recirculating through the PSLN, and vice versa. The most striking and generally agreed feature of the migratory behaviour of lymphoid cells from the GALT relates not to small lymphocytes but to large ones. The capacity of lymph-borne immunoblasts from the gut to "home"back to the lamina propria almost as soon as they reach the blood is a major feature of the cellular economy of the GALT.

Migration of lymph-borne immunoblasts from the GALT. Mention has been made already of the fact that the lymphoid tissue of the GALT is subject, even in health, to continual antigenic stimulation. One consequence of this is that the lymphocytes in the intestinal lymph of all mammalian species that have been investigated include a few percent of immunoblasts (small lymphocytes that have transformed into large lymphoid blast cells as a result of appropriate stimuli). Again, it was Gowans (17) who first noticed that these cells had a striking ability to extravasate in the lamina propria of the small gut after they had been injected intravenously into syngeneic recipients. This work has been confirmed amply (18,19) and the process occurs in ruminants (1) as well as in monogastric mammals. The mechanism is unknown; antigen does not seem to be involved for the mechanism can be made to operate in antigen-free foetuses (1, 20). Similarly, the isotype of the immunoglobulin that the immunoblasts make seems not to be a factor in guiding them to their destination; cells making IgM and IgG as well as those making IgA can extravasate in the small gut (1), while T immunoblasts (which make no Ig at all) can also be shown to 'home' to the gut (21). Even though very large numbers of cells are involved the reason for this circulatory odyssey is unknown. It does mean that immuno- blasts generated in a restricted part of GALT, in response to a local stimulus, have the opportunity to become disseminated throughout the whole length of the gut, and this may have survival value. What is certain is that the B immunoblasts which extravasate in the small gut soon turn into mature

plasma cells (19) which populate the lamina and which, during
a life span of only a few days (22), secrete the immunoglobulins which protect the gut (see Fig. 1).

IMMUNOGLOBULIN TRANSPORT BY THE GUT AND THE LIVER

The plasma cells in the lamina propria of the gut of rodents
and man secrete immunoglobulins mainly of the IgA isotype but
significant numbers of cells produce IgG, IgM and IgE as well.
Any type of antibody can only become really effective in
preventing the attachment or ingress of pathogens if it is
present on the surface of the mucosa. However, any major
non-specific "leakage" of protein from the tissue spaces of
the gut into the lumen would soon lead to circulatory
collapse, and death, so a special active transport mechanism
has evolved to ferry the specialized IgA antibodies across the
epithelium, while the other antibodies and protein constituents of the tissue fluid are retained beneath the epithelium.
The mechanims is an example of receptor mediated endocytosis,
and works as follows.

The IgA molecule is secreted from the plasma cells in the form
of a dimer, the two immunoglobulin units being linked by a
joining or 'J' chain. In this form (or in the form of higher
polymers) it is spoken of as pIgA. The pIgA molecule has an
affinity for a receptor known as the 'secretory piece' (SC)
or, in more modern terminology, a "poly Ig receptor", a glycoprotein which is displayed on the baso/lateral aspects of the
enterocytes. After pIgA has united with SC the whole complex
is internalized into an endocytic vesicle, conveyed across the
cytoplasm and discharged en bloc onto the luminal surface of
the enterocyte. The pIgA-SC complex is now termed secretory
IgA (sIgA) and the glycoprotein moiety of the SC may help to
"anchor" the molecule in the boundary layer of mucus which
covers and protects the luminal surface of the gut (Fig. 2).

Not all the IgA produced by the submucosal plasma cells is
transported directly into the lumen. There is no active
transport mechanism to convey newly synthesised IgA from the
plasma cells to the enterocytes, this process depends on
simple diffusion. Because of this, and particularly during
the post absorptive state when the net fluid flow across the
gut wall is directed inwards, much of the IgA produced in the
submucosa is swept up into the regional lymph. It is for this
reason that the intestinal lymph of experimental animals (and
man) is relatively rich in IgA. Surprisingly, the concentration of IgA is much higher in the intestinal lymph than in the
blood. Although substantial amounts IgA-rich lymph are
discharged continually into the blood, the concentration of
IgA in the blood remains low. How does this come about? The
short answer is that the IgA is extracted from the blood and
secreted into the bile. The portal sinusoids of the liver are
lined with a discontinuous, or fenestrated, endothelium so
that the proteins in the blood plasma can make rapid and
intimate contact with the sinusoidal facets of the
hepatocytes. In many rodent species the hepatocytes function
like enterocytes (embryologically their origin is the same);

they display SC on their cytoplasmic membranes and transport the pIgA into the bile by exactly the same means as the enterocytes transport it into the lumen. in this way the bile is endowed with high concentrations of sIgA and so freshly ingested food (and microorganisms) can be douched with specific antibody as soon as it enters the duodenum. The experimental work which elucidated this situation is extensive and has been reviewed (23).

Special features of the IgA system in man. Unlike many animals man is unusual in having relatively large numbers of plasma cells that secrete monomeric IgA (mIgA). Some of these cells are to be found in the gut but many are remote from the GALT, e.g. in the bone marrow. Because monomeric IgA contains no J chain it does not qualify for active transport by the gut or the liver, and thus it tends to accumulate in the blood so that, in man, at least 75% of the total IgA in the blood is of monomeric form. This can lead to a good deal of confusion. Assessments of the amount of IgA in the blood measured by methods which cannot distinguish between molecules of differing sizes, yield results that are difficult to interpret from the point of view of secretory immunity.

Another distinguishing feature of human IgA is that it can belong to one of two subclasses, and although similar subclasses may exist in experimental animals they remain to be discovered. The subclasses are distinguished on the basis of serological (i.e. antigenic) differences which reflect differences in strucutre and are referred to as IgA1 and IgA2. In blood serum the amounts of each subclass are similar but, in secretions IgA2 predominates. The reason for this is not entirely clear; in the gut the IgA1, which is said to be more susceptible to proteolytic enzymes, may be broken down rather more rapidly than IgA2.

Although the hepato/biliary excretion of pIga undoubtedly occurs in man (24) it is likely that the rapidity and scale of the transport are relatively less than in the rat, and are said to be similar to those which occur in the dog (25). Reports of the occurrence of SC on human hepatocytes are conflicting, and now the consensus view is that human hepatocytes do not display SC. The hepato/biliary transport of human IgA probably takes place through specialized "biliary epithelial" cells which display SC (26). Because these are not as numerous as hepatocytes the transport of IgA from blood to bile in man is less striking than it is in the rat.

BIOLOGICAL FUNCTIONS OF ANTIBODIES IN THE GUT

IgA. Many enteropathogenic microorganisms can only succeed in infecting their potential victim by first attaching themselves to specific receptors on the surfaces of the enterocytes or other mucosal epithelia. If these receptors are, for genetic reasons, absent the organism cannot gain a foothold and, as far as that particular individual is concerned, may be considered non-pathogenic. Similarly, if the complementary group on the bacterium or virus is masked by the attachment to it of a specific IgA antibody, it is likewise unable to gain a foothold and is swept away to excretory oblivion by the motion of the gut contents. This simple "steric hindrance" by IgA antibodies is probably their most important function but they have others. Suppose an antigenic entity, be it a pathogenic microorganism or a dietary immunogen, does succeed in penetrating the epithelium, it is still liable to the attachment of pIgA antibodies. These pIgA antibodies have not yet acquired SC and so the pIgA-antigen complex is able to unite with the SC and be secreted back immediately in the lumen. Indeed, even if the complex enters the lymph stream and gains the systemic blood circulation it may still be excreted by the bile. This scenario is not just idle fancy; it has been shown to occur by direct experiment (27), and because IgA does not activate complement this mechanism represents a way of eliminating dietary antigen that has no damaging, allergic sequelae.

Monomeric IgA has no function in the gut because it is not secreted. Its function in the blood and tissue spaces is unknown. It has been suggested that, because it does not activate complement or promote opsonisation, it may moderate immune reactions that might become dangerously damaging if IgG and IgM antibodies were allowed to operate without competition.

IgE. Although in absolute terms the amounts of IgE synthesised in the wall of the gut are vey low, the ability of even small amounts to sensitize mast cells has extremely important consequences. Small amounts of antigen which succeed in penetrating the mucosa will, if they confront a specifically sensitised mast cell, cause such cells to degranulate immediately. The histamine released from the granules act on the local blood vessels to increase their permeability and thus the transudation of conventional IgG andf IgM antibodies from the blood. At the same time, protease released by the degranulating mast cells are believed to destabilize the intercellular functions between the enterocytes so that the antibodies that have escaped from the blood can gain direct and rapid entry into the lumen of the gut. this type of IgE "triggering" can produce an almost expolosive effect which probably underlies the hyper acute, "self-cure" reactions with which animals purge themselves of a burden of intestinal, helminthic parasites (Fig. 3). Similar reactions, on a smaller, sub-clinical scale may occur in response to dietary antigens where, paradoxically, the general "leakyness" induced in the gut may favour the absorption of successively larger amounts of dietary antigens. In this way, hypersensitivity to a particular dietary constituent may lead to the ingress of unrelated antigens and the establishment of allergy to a progressively expanding repertoire of antigenic epitopes from the environment.

IgG and IgM. Although IgM (a pentamer) can to some extent substitute for IgA in cases of congenital or acquired deficiency of IgA, the amounts of IgM, and IgG in the secretions is usually quite small. As has been detailed above their massive entry, into the gut is a special circumstance. However, antibodies of any isotype are capable of playing an important role in modulating the biology of the bacterial flora of the gut. Recently, evidence has become available which indicates that antibodies of appropriate specificity may be able to inhibit the transfer of plasmids between bacteria (28). Since many of the virulence determinants on the surface of bacteria are coded for by plasmids, the presence of appropriate antibodies may be important in preventing the acquisition of dangerous characteristics by bacteria (such as E. coli) which are otherwise usually harmless.

CELL MEDIATED IMMUNITY (CMI) IN THE GUT

Cell mediated immunity is difficult to define; its classical manifestations are the allograft reaction, and the cutaneous delayed type hypersensitivity reaction and, as with the tuberculin (Mantoux) reaction, the reactions are characterized by the infiltration of mononuclear cells which, in the most florid examples, are able to destroy the tissue in which they find themselves. This killing of cells or "cytotoxicity" is carried out by a subset of T lymphocytes and is quite independent of specific immunoglobulin antibodies (even though these may well be present too). Such cytotoxic reactions are also a crucial feature of the defense against viruses, for they allow the immune system to destroy any cell which is harbouring viruses and expressing viral antigens on its surface.

The hallmark of CMI is a mononuclear cell infiltrate but it is very difficult to see by straightforward methods whether it is taking place in the gut, because this organ is always well provided with mononuclear cells. One cannot see the wood because of the trees. However, it is unlikely that such an important component of the immunological defense would be absent from the gut and there are now some cogent ideas about how the system may operate (29,30).

A feature of several hypersensitivity states (e.g. like gluten hypersensitivity) is the shortening of the villi which occurs after exposure to the alleged antigen. This is known as "villous atrophy"; part of the shortening appears to be due to the shedding of mature enterocytes from the tips of the villi, though how exactly this comes about is not known (perhaps the IEL may be involved). At the same time, T lymphocytes in the lamina, activated presumably by contact with antigen, begin to secrete lymphokines. These in turn act upon the stem cells of the crypt epithelium and increase the mitotic rate by a factor of 5 or so. The net result of all this activity is to produce a shortened villus (and/or deeper crypts) covered with relatively less mature enterocytes. It is known that immature enterocytes express more SC (i.e. they can secrete more IgA) than mature ones but, on the other hand, they seem to be less efficient at absorbing materials from the gut. This chain of events, it is argued, leads to a situation in which the intestine is able to secrete more antibody, and at the same time absorb less antigen. It is certainly possible to show that when experimental animals are challenged, by feeding, with an antigen to which their gut has been sensitized, they undergo a period of relative malabsorption (as evidenced by e.g. xylose excretion tests). This period of malabsorption appears to correlate with the villus atrophy, though it may have causes other than the ones outlined above.

THE ENTRY OF ANTIGEN INTO THE GALT

Readers may think that I have been perverse in delaying the consideration of this topic until now. Logic would surely dictate that, because antigen is the principal initiator of the events under discussion, it should be considered first. This may be true, but there is some method in my madness. One cannot discuss the entry of antigen in realistic terms without knowing something of the structure and function of the GALT, its relationship to the gut epithelium on the one hand, and the systemic circulation on the other.

The study of the absorption by the gut of intact macromolecules from the gut presents problems. Most "physiological" macromolecules presented to the gut are dietary proteins and carbohydrates and, in health, most of these are almost entirely cleaved into small fragments by the digestive enzymes. In spite of this, some molecules that are big enough to be antigenic do get through the gut and enter the systemic circulation. Fifty years ago (31) it was shown quite unequivocally that after dogs were fed ovalbumin in sufficient quantity, ovalbumin (which could be precipitated with a specific antiserum) appeared transiently in the dog's intestinal lymph. Long before this it was, of course, known that certain dietary proteins (e.g. boiled fish, in the Prausnitz-Kustner reaction) could provoke cutaneous urticaria etc. in sensitized individuals, and this was strong circumstantial evidence that intact, antigenic moieties from the diet could get into the blood. The questions that have not been satisfactorily answered is exactly how and where such antigens cross the gut.

It has been noted already (vide supra) that degranulating mast cells may destabilize the intercellular junctions between enterocytes so that in individuals who are already sensitzed, antigens may pass between the enterocytes. Presumably, it is for this reason that some patients suffering from diet-iddnduced urticaria can be treated prophylactically with disodium cromoglycate, which inhibits mast cell degranulation. Similarly, non-specific damage to the gut by agents like alcohol can also destabilize the intercellular junctions and permit the ingress of antigen (32). However, the entry of macromolecules into undamaged gut is less easy to demonstrate under physiological conditions (32). The entry of antigen into the 'M' cells of the Peyer's patches has been described already, and while this undoubtedly happens, its quantitative significance has not been assessed.

In some species, the placenta is unable to transmit maternal antibody to the foetus and the offspring are born in an

essentially agammaglobulinaemic state. In these cases the
maternal antibody can only get to the newborn animal via the
colostrum that it ingests, and thus in these species the
neonatal enterocytes have the ability to absorb maternal IgG
which passes, intact, into the blood. Although this faculty
soon atrophies, vestiges of it remain, and it may be that this
is the basis of much antigen absorption by the gut. Again,
the mechanism is one of receptor mediated endocytosis. Thus,
on the enterocytes of neonatal rats there is a receptor for
homologous IgG, and, as soon as it has bound the
immunoglobulin, it becomes internalized in an endocytic
vesicle and transported across the cell. Not only does this
patway diminsh with age but such protein as is absorbed
becomes increasingly susceptible to degradation by lysosomal
enzymes, so that little intact protein survives its journey
across the cell. Of course, there may not be receptors for
all antigens but materials like cholera toxin, E coli endotoxin and many plant lectins can bind to enterocytes and may be
transported in this way. Although, in the adult the process
may be very inefficient it could, because of the large number
of enterocytes, be sufficient to ferry immunologically significant amounts of protein aross the gut. It is believed that
this sort of process is particularly susceptible to steric
hindrance by secreted antibody, and there is certainly experimental evidence that secretory antibody specific for a given
antigen will inhibit significantly its uptake by the gut (33).
This phenomenon is spoken of as "immune exclusion", and those
individuals with a congenital or acquired deficit of secretory
IgA are said to be more vulnerable to the onslaughts of
dietary antigen (33).

In spite of these uncertainties it is clear that some antigen
does penetrate the epithelium of the gut and when it does so
it will be confronted immediately by the macrophages and
lymphocytes that lie in wait in the lamina propria, the
Peyer's patches, and the mesenteric nodes.

ORAL TOLERANCE

Perhaps the most significant thing about allergic reactions to
dietary constituents is that they are so rare. We all eat
about 30 grams of protein a day, to say nothing of polysacca-
ride and bacterial antigens and, although most of us have
measurable antibodies to such materials, we can live for
25,000 days without sufferinge overt allergic reactions. How
can this paradoxical situation be reconciled? One group of
theories (which has some experimental justification) is based
on the concept of "oral tolerance". In general terms these
ideas envisage that dietary antigens may stimulate a local,
protective immunity in the gut (e.g. IgA mediated immune
exclusion) while, at the same time, they induce an immunologically specific, systemic unresponsiveness (tolerance). Even
supposing that this occurs, the mechanisms are to some extent
conjectural, and rely on the presumptive presence in the body
of appropriate subsets of T cells which have suppressor and
contra suppressor functions. This subject is complicated and
has been reviewed (34). It is believed that antigen, when

presented by the oral route, stimulates effector cells in the GALT as well as generating a cohort of suppressor T cells that are distributed round the body. The suppressor cells abrogate the activities of T and B effector cells and so prevent systemic allergic reactions. The T and B effector cells in the gut are shielded from the effects of suppression by a resident population of specific contra suppressor cells which inhibit the suppressors. When the effector T and B cells migrate out of the gut (as we know they do) they are no longer shielded from suppression and so their activities are abrogated and they are unable to mediate allergic reactions. This, then, is the theory; there are some facts which support it, and there are some which don't.

Anecdotal reports emanating from American medical men in the first half of the 19th century claimed that aboriginal Indians were able to protect themselves from the effects of cutaneous hypersensitivity to poison ivy by deliverately eating the small amounts of the leaves of the plant. Much later, in 1946 Chase (35) showed experimentely that prior feeding of skin-sensitizing agents could inhibit the development of cutaneous contact sensitivity. Since then, there have been many experiments in which the feeding of chemical haptens appears to suppress responses to later, parenteral challenges with the same material. However, before rushing to embrace the suppressor T cell explanation one should consider other findings. In the first place, haptens are small molecules and will thus, if eaten, be aborbed directly into the portal blood and conveyed, initially, to the liver. Antigens presented in this way are known to be especially liable to suppress sensitization ()36,37), and evidently the liver plays some special role in the process. Probably, the immunogenic moiety of the test material is captured by the hepatic Kuppfer cells (macrophages), while that part of the material that cannot react with such macrophages is free to continue circulating and induce systemic tolerance or 'immune paralysis'.

Whatever the explanation of oral tolerance may be, it is by no means a universal phenomenon; otherwise the oral polio vaccine could hardly have been as successful as it has been. Many antigens, like cholera toxin, that bind firmly to enterocytes can be made to induce antibodies after oral administration (38), and even simple protein antigens like egg albumin can often be immunogenic when given by the oral route (39). It is an unfortunate fact that orally administered antigens may induce allergy, or they may induce tolerance, or they may have no detectable effect. For this reason it is impossible to predict the outcome of any given confrontation between the GALT and a dietary antigen.

Whatever view one takes of the importance, or otherwise, of allergic reactions to dietary antigens, there are two groups of people which seem to be particularly at risk. The groups in question are children, and adults who move to a region that is alien to them in terms of climate, culture and dietary habit. It is in the nature of things that prospective clinical trials are difficult to carry out on such groups, particularly when the actual incidence of unequivocal overt clinical diasease is low.

At first, infants depend upon maternal immunoglobulin for much of their immunity, and it is agreed generally that the presence of maternal antibody actually suppresses the infant's potential ability to make their own. When weaning occurs the infant (or young animal) is deprived suddenly of antibodies in the gut and it will be some time before the independent intrinsic activity of the GALT can take over. This period of sub-optimal defense coincides often with drastic changes in the composition of the diet, as the available food tends toward the "adult" pattern. It is believed that it is during this period of adaptation that dietary allergies are likely to arise. In man, the picture may be complicated by the fact that sucking infants receive feeds that may be formulated from cows' milk which contains heterologous and potentially antigenic proteins. Some believe that the ingestion of such material is an important factor in the aetiology of infantile eczema (40). The exact cause of chronic, dietary-induced skin lesions remote from the gut are matters for speculation but the formation of immune complexes (i.e. complexes of food antigens with antibody) may be important (41).

The basis of apparent allergic reactions to foods in, e.g. Asian migrants to the U.K. is even less easy to pinpoint; the fact that it occurs suggests that the gut of individuals adapts in a complex way to the antigenic spectrum engendered by a particular environment, and that if this environment is suddenly and permanently altered a minority of adult individuals may not be able to readapt without developing symptoms.

These problems do not apply to man alone; they are not unobtrusive in animal husbandry, and economically significant disorders of the bowel in weaning lambs, calves and pigs are familiar problems in animal husbandry. Some of the problems may be caused by bacteria and viruses, and some by inert dietary antigens. What has been written above can do little more than indicate the infinite complexity of the interactions of antibodies, CMI effectors and environmental antigens in which the GALT is continually involved, and warn against the adoption of facile explanations1.

THE GALT AND SYSTEMIC RESPONSES: TECHNICAL PROBLEMS

In spite of claims to the contrary I know of no really well documented case in which immune responses initiated in the GALT remain truly local. Always, activated lymphoid cells are released into the systemic circulation and, in my experience, some IgM and IgG antibodies are formed as well as IgA. Immune responses in the gut and mucosa may often <u>seem</u> to be local. For example, an immune response in the lymphoid tissue associated with the eye may endow the tears (a relatively small volume) with high titres of antibody. The same amount of antibody diluted in the whole pool of circulating proteins may become almost undetectable. However, this does not mean that it is not there, and by the same token some immunologically activated cells will have become systematized.

This systematization of immunologically activated cells from (e.g.) the GALT has lead to the concept of the MALT - mucous associated lymphoid tissue (42). This concept is based on the proposition that lymphoid cells activated in the GALT (or other mucous-associated lymphoid tissue) migrate to other mucosae and so endow them with specific responsiveness. My own experience is that while this undoubtedly occurs, and is easily demonstrable at the experimental level, the number of cells involved is often quite insufficient to provide the cellular wherewithal to produce enough IgA to endow the local secretions with the amount of antibody that actually exists. Again, species differences are particularly obtrusive. In animals like rats, where the hepato-biliary excretion of pIgA keeps the concentration of such immunoglobulin in the blood very low, the peripheral exocrine glands (e.g. salivary, lachrymal etc.) cannot rely on the blood for a supply of IgA and must rely on their intrinsic lymphoid cells to make it. No doubt some of these cells, are, indeed, migrants from the GALT. On the other hand, larger animals like sheep (and probably man) have less efficient "IgA pumps" in their livers, and so the blood levels of IgA tend to be higher. In such species, the satellite exocrine glands can extract from the blood sufficient IgA to populate their secretions with anti-body and rely less on local synthesis. In health, the number of lymphoid cells in these glands is often low. Of course, when the picture is complicated by local infection, inflamma-tion and gross pathology the cell traffic is likely to be enormously expanded, and such situations must be considered separately.

A further difficulty in quantitative studies of the activity of the GALT is that of measuring accurately amounts of immuno-globulins and antibody activity in secretions contaminated with mucus, proteolytic enzymes and detritus. Even when these difficulties have been solved there is still the problem of measuring the rate of flow of the secretions. Some, like bile or ruminant saliva, have rates of flow that can be relatively high but which fluctuate widely. Unless the flow rates, throughout the period of an immune response (several days, if not weeks) are known precisely no accurate quantitation of the secretory immune response can be made. It must always be born in mind that the secretory immune system is, as far as its immunoglobulin goes, an "open" system in which fluid and antibodies are lost continually. Antibody activity cannot therefore accumulate, to give the impressively high titres that are encountered in traditional serology, which is is concerned with "closed" system of the circulating protein pool of the blood and lymphatic systems. Thus, quite modest titres of antibody in fast flowing secretions can reflect a level of antibody production that is much greater than the actual titration result would suggest.

In man it is, of course, difficult often to measure or even obtain, normal secretions from patients or healthy subjects and, in my view the dynamic aspects of the secretory immune system are lost sight of too often. Much reliance is placed on the immuno-histological examination of small mucosal biopsies, while these can provide qualitative demonstrations with compelling aesthetic appeal, the enormous sampling error involved makes accurate quantitation difficult, and at best they show what happened in a minuscule measure of time and space in a vast and often protracted process.

ACKNOWLEDGEMENTS

The author's research is supported by a programme grant from the joint committee of the Medical Research Council and the Cancer Research Campaign. Figure 1 is reproduced from "Blood Cells": (5, 470-492, 1979), Figure 2 from "The Africal Journal of Clinical and Experimental Immunology" (45, 169-176, 1981), and Figure 3 from "Immunotoxicology" (pp 315-327, Academic Press, 1983).

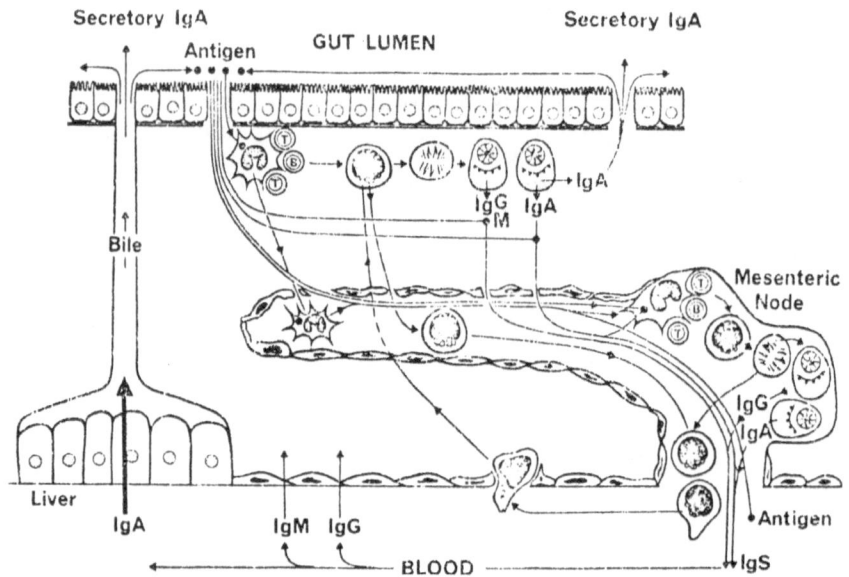

Figure 1: *Diagram to show the principal cellular events in the delivery of immunoglobulin to the lumen of the gut. Antigen that penetrates the epithelium is liable to react with dendritic macrophages which present it to T and B lymphocytes, which undergo transformation into immunoblasts. The B immuno-blasts either develop into plasma cells in situ or migrate (together with macrophages and antigen) to the mesenteric node, where a similar sequence of events going on. Immuno-blasts and immunoglobulins are discharged into the intestinal lymph and reach the blood. Many of the immunoblasts extra-vasate in the wall of the gut and turn into plasma cells which, together with their fellows that arose in situ, secrete IgA antibodies which are transported to the lumen of the gut by the overlying enterocytes.*

IgA antibodies also reach the gut by active transport from blood to bile.

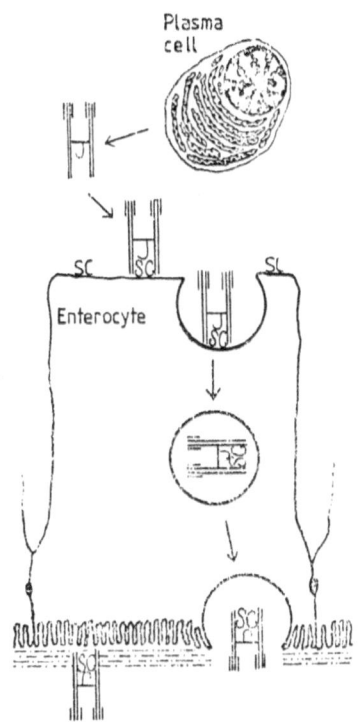

Figure 2: Diagram to show the mechanism of IgA transport by enterocytes:- The plasma cell secretes dimeric IgA - two immunoglobulin units linked by J chain - which binds to secretory component (SC) which is displayed on the baso-lateral aspect of the enterocyte's cytoplasmic membrane. The IgA-SC complex is internalized in endocytic vesicles, transported across the cell, and discharged enbloc into the lumen, where the SC anchors it in the boundary layer of mucus.

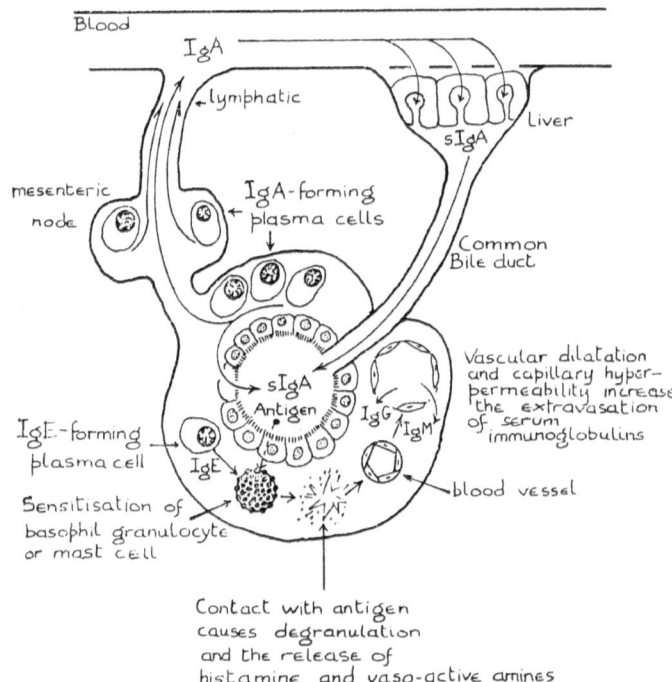

Figure 3: Summary diagram to show how IgE can facilitate the transudation of IgG and IgM antibodies into the gut.

REFERENCES

1) Hall, J.G., Hopkins, J. & Orlans, E. (1977). Eur. J. Immunol. 7, 30.

2) Hall, J.G. (1979)_. Blood Cells 5, 479.

3) Mayrhofer, G., Pugh, C.W. & Barclay, A.N. (1983).

4) Owen, R.L. (1977). Gastroenterology 72, 440

5) Cottier, H., Hess, M.W. & Keller, H.V. (1980). Monogr. Allergy 16, 50.

6) Mayrhofer, G. (1980). Blood 55, 532.

7) Guy/Grand, D. & Vassalli, P. (1982). p. 301 Recent Advances in Mucosal Immunity, Raven Press, New York.

8) Arnaud-Battandier (1982).289. Recent Advances in mucosal Immunity. Raven Press, New York.

9) Lamm, M.E. (1982). p. 313 Recent Advances in Mucosal Immunity. Raven Press New York.

10) Reynolds, J. & Morris, B. (1983). Eur. J. Immunol. 13, 627.

11) Morris, B. (1983). Personal communication

12) Binns, R.M. (1984). Personal communication.

13) Binns, R.M. & Hall, J.G. (1966). Br. J. Exp. Path. 47, 275.

14) Scollay, R.G., Hopkins, J. & Hall, J.G. (1976). Nature 260, 528.

15) Cahill, R.N.P., Poskitt, D.C., Frost, H. & Trnka, Z. (1977). J., exp. Med. 145, 420.

16) Cahill, R.N.P. & Trnka, Z. (1980). Monogr. Allergy. 16, 38.

17) Gowans, J.C. & Knight, E.J. (1964). Proc. Roy. Soc. B. 159, 257.

18) Griscelli, C., Varsalli, P. & McCluskey, R.T. (1969). J. exp. Med. 124, 1017.

19) Hall, J.G., Parry, D.M. & Smith, M.e. (1972), cell, tissue Kinet. 5, 269. 20) Halstead, T. and Hall, J.G. (1972). Transplantation 14, 339.

21) Sprent, J. (1976). Cell. Immunol. 21, 278.

190

22) *Mattioli, C.A. & Tomasi, T.VB. (1973). J. exp. Med.* 138, 452.

23) *Hall, J.G. & Andrew, E.M. (1980). Immunology Today* 1, 100.

24) *Orlans, E., Peppard, J.V., Payne, A.W.R. Fitzharris, B.M., Mullock, B.M., Hinton, R.H. & Hall, J.G. (1983). Ann. N.Y. Acad. Sci.* 409, 411.

25) *Delacroix, D.L., Furtado-Barreira, G., De Hemptinne, B., Goudswaard, J., Dive, C. & Vaermann, J.P. (1983). Hepatology* 3, 980.

26) *Nagura, H., Smith, P.D., Nakane, P.K. & Brown, W.R. (1981). J. Immunol.* 126, 587.

27) *Peppard, J.V., Orlans, E., Payne, A.W.R. & Andrew, E. (1981). Immunology* 42, 83.

28) *Porter, P., Linggood, M.A. & Chidlow, J. (1978). Adv. Exp. Med. Biol.* 107, 133.

29) *Fergusson, A. (1978). p. 145 in Antigen Absorption by the Gut. (Ed. W.a. Hemmings) M.T.P. Press, Lancaster.*

30) *Fergusson, A. & Mowat, A.M. (1981). p. 107 in The Mucosal Immune System. Current Topics in Veterinary Medicine and Animal Science. Vol. 12. Martinus Nijhoff, The Hague & London.*

31) *Alexander, H.L., Shirley, K. & Allen, D. (1936). J. Clin. Invest.* 15, 163.

32) *Draper, L.R., Gyure, L.A., J.G. Hall & Robertson, D. (1983). Gut* 24, 399.

33) *Walker, W.A. (1981). Immunol. Today* 2, 30

34) *Tomasi, T.B. (1980). Transplantation* 29, 353.

35) *Chase, M.W. (1946). Proc. Soc. Exp. Biol. Med.* 21, 257.

36) *Cantor, H.M. & Dumont, A.E. (1967). Nature* 215, 744.

37) *Battisto, J.R. & Miller, J. (1962). Proc. Soc. Exp. Biol. Med.* 111, 111.

38) *Lycke, N, Lindholm, L. & Holmgren, J. (1983). Int. Archs. Allergy appl. Immun.* 72. 119.

39) *Strannegard, O. & Yurchision (1969). Int. Archs. Allergy appl. Immun.* 35, 579.

40) Atherton, D.J., Soothill, J.F., Sewell, M., Wells, R.S. & Chilvers, C.E.D. (1978). Lancet, 1, 401.

41) Levinsky, R.J., Paganelli, R., Robertson, D.M. & Atherton, D.J. (1981). p. 154 in The Mucosal Immune System. Current topics in Veterinary Medicine and Animal Science. Vol. 12. Martinus Nijhoff, The Hague & London.

42) Bienenstock, J. & Befus, A.D. (1980). Immunolgoy 41, 249.

IMMUNODEPRESSIVE DRUGS AS PROTOTYPE IMMUNOTOXICANTS

F. Spreafico, A. Merendino, L. Braceschi & S. Sozzani

Istituto di Ricerche Farmacologiche "Mario Negri", Milano, Italy

INTRODUCTION

In spite of the fact that indisputable advancements have been made in recent years in various areas of immunotoxicology, it can easily be argued that several problems of both conceptual and practical importance are still outstanding in this young discipline (1,2), as is readly apparent from various chapters in this volume. Since agents that are therapeutically employed with the objective of obtaining a state of modified immune responsiveness can be regarded as being in many respects prototype immunotoxicants, experience acquired in the characterization and use in animals and humans of immunomodulatory drugs can be of direct relevance for a number of current problems in immunotoxicology, and especially for that domain of this composite, three-pronged speciality (2) concerned with the effects of xenobiotics on immune cells and their function. These levels of relevance include a better understanding of the mechanism(s) of action of immunoactive xenobiotics, sounder approaches to the prospective identification of actual and/or potential immunotoxicants, a clearer appraisal of the spectrum of immune effects inducible by exogenous substances, and finally guidance in evaluating the possible human health implications of immunological disturbances effected by exposure to foreign compounds. In a single chapter it is not possible to present an extensive review of the immunological phenomenology of so-called non-specific immunodepressive drugs . The interested reader is referred for detailed descriptions of these and other groups to references 3-9. Rather, this discussion will concentrate on a number of more recent findings regarding the mode of action of chemical immunodepressive drugs focussing on those aspects that we believe possess a more direct and general significance for Immunotoxicology.

ON THE MODE OF ACTION OF IMMUNOMODULATORY DRUGS

Immunologically active compounds used therapeutically are commonly divided into immunodepressants and immunostimulants, and these categories are often regarded as being strictly separate and opposing ones. For the purpose of this discussion it is however important to emphasize that such a strict categorization represents a simplification and that the more appropriate term for both types of agents is that of immunomodulator, a term that more aptly conveys the complexity of the effects that can be exerted by these compounds. In fact both immunodepressants and immunostimulants can produce apparently paradoxical immune effects with moreover the possibility of inducing a condition of split-immunomodulation, i.e. the coexistence of immune effects of contrasting sign.

Table 1 presents in very schematic form the general mechanisms through which drugs can be expected to influence the expression of immunity. In view of their general relevance, a number of points related to this listing of possible mechanisms deserve comment. In the first place, it can be readily deduced that the same general immunological result may be obtained via mechanisms of opposite sign. A condition of depressed expression of immunity can in fact be achieved not only through destruction or inhibition of cells sustaining the inductive and/or effector phases of the immune response, but also through prevalent stimulation of the immunocytes participating in the various down-regulatory circuits that consitute a very important physiological component of the immune system. This eventuality is not only theoretical but can indeed be observed both experimentally and clinically with many if not all "true" immunostimulants when administered according to selected treatment conditions. In parallel, prevalent inhibition of suppressor cells by an immunodepressant can lead to a state of partial or complete enhanced immunity, and thus both types of agents can have bell-shaped rather than straight line dose-response curves, although depending not only on the category of the agent but also on its individual mode of action, the characteristics of the curve will obviously differ among compounds.

In connections with Table 1, a second point is that the division among mechanisms presented is per force an artificial categorization, and that within each general mechanism further subdivisions can be made. The multiplicity of possible mechanisms, and the fact that an essential feature of the immune apparatus is its richnesss in interactions among cells in a complex web of amplifying and regulatory networks, render it often problematic to identify with confidence primary from secondary targets affected by an agent. Classification of these agents, that ideally should be based not only on the immune target(s) (cellular or subcellular) primarily affected but also on the biochemical mechanism through which the effect is exerted (8), is also hindered by our large ignorance of many aspects of the molecular mode of action not only for newer immunodepressants but also for agents that have been in use for decades. On the other hand, this multiplicity of mechanisms and the fact that agents can differ quantitatively if not qualitatively in the influence exerted primarily and/or secondarily at the various levels, implies that treatment with exogenous immunomodulators can be expected to be associated with non-stereotyped but more or less individualized effects. Thirdly, Table 1 also alludes to the possibility that a state of modified down-expression of immunity may be sustained not only through a gross mechanism such as cellular destruction, but also via more "functional" effects on the immune cells and/or their products. Although this aspect has so far been explored to only a limited extent with most immunodepressants, an expanding body of evidence (9) indicates that also for compounds inhibiting cell proliferation, that is the majority of available therapeutic imuunodepressants, a major component of their mode of action may actually be represented by more discrete, and not necessarily lethal effects, on immunocytes'

functional capabilities, such as effects on mediator production and/or responsiveness, or membrane expression of immunologically relevant receptor or constituents. By way of
example, Table 2 summarizes the effects of a number of classical cytotoxic agents on various functions of cells of
monocyte-macrophage lineage.

THE HETEROGENOUS SENSITIVITY OF IMMUNOCYTES TO DRUGS

Although the majority of classical, first generation immunodepressants have been in clinical use for nearly three decades
either for the treatment of autoimmunity and graft rejection
or, and on a larger scale, in cancer chemotherapy, a sufficiently detailed picture of the immunopharmacological activity
of such compounds has been obtained only recently. In this
effort, evidence has been obtained that such cytotoxic agents
differ among themselves in their immunological effects both
quantitatively and qualitatively, in the sense that they
exhibit individualized immunopharmacological profiles as a
reflection of at least partial selectivity in their influence
on the various types and subsets of immune cells.

An example of this heterogeneity among drugs and among cells
in their sensitivity to a given drug, is given in Table 3.
This setsout schematically a summary of data from this group
(7) on the effects of a number of drugs, representative of
widely employed classes of cytotoxic chemicals, on murine NK
cell and macrophage-mediated cytotoxic activity. NK-cells
have recently been credited with a crucial role in host
natural resistance mechanisms towards various types of infectious agents, as well as in the control of cancerous
dissemination; whereas it is well established that macrophages have an essential role in the initiation, regulation
and expression of immunity. In addition to showing that cells
participating in front-line host resistance can be differentially affected by a given drug, these results also indicate
that a given type of immunocyte can display a different
susceptibility to agents that are chemical analogues and are
believed to affect cellular biochemical processes through
similar if not identical mechanisms. This was the case for
instance for the close chemical analogs Doxorubicin (DXR) and
Daunorubicin (DNR), anthracyclines that are in wide use in the
treatment of neoplasia and are believed to act essentially as
DNA intercalators. Treatments with doses up to the LD_{10} of
the former compound did not affect the number of murine
macrophages nor the capacity of these cells to expresse
antibody-mediated and non-specific direct cytotoxicity as well
as phagocytic activity. In contrast with the analog DNR was
clearly inhibitory to this cell type both in terms of total
population size and functional ability per unit cell number.
A parallel differential has been observed with these drugs in
vitro on both murine and human cells of this lineage (10).
Evident differences in immunopharmacological profiles among
chemical analogs have also been described for other classes of
cytotoxic drugs, such as the nitrosoureas and the vinca
alkaloids (11).

NK cells and macrophages are known to derive from different cellular lineages and can therefore be expected to differ vis-a-vis several characteristics (e.g. proliferative kinetics, capacity to repair cellular damage, biochemical processes involved in mediating effector functions) that may be of relevance in determining their differential sensitivity to a given drug in vivo or in vitro. However, it is also important to emphasize that in experimental conditions it is now well established that even within the same general popu-lation of immunocytes, elements belonging to different sub-populations can exhibit a different sensitivity to a given immunodepressive agent, so that certain cells (and the func-tion they subserve) can be more easily affected than others. An example of this is shown in Table 4 where treatment of mice with Cyclosporin A (CS-A).(An immunodepressive drug of fungal origin that can be regarded as a truly second-generation agent in view of its substantially improved immunological and pharmatoxicological properties (12)), did not significant affect the response to the mitogen ConA while markedly inhi-biting that to PHA (13). The same table also shows that CS-A did not significantly affect macrophage mediated effector function, evaluated in terms of cytotoxic activity, whereas it inhibited, although transiently, NK-mediated cytotoxicity (14). In parallel it is known that committed T effector lymphocytes are unaffected by this agent, which conversely severely impairs the generation of cytotoxic T lymphocytes (CTL) (12). This drug blocks in fact the expression on T cells of the receptors for IL1 and IL2, a mechanism that coupled to a block in the production by T-helper-inducers elements (Th) of the signal for IL1 production by macrophages, ultimately leads to inhibition of T cell proliferation and clonal expansion (see 9).

Although sufficiently complete data are available for only a minority of the agents known to depress immunity, enough data exist for the most widely employed drugs for drawing an operational hierarchy of the relative susceptibility among lymphocyte subsets. Thus for instance, this hierarchy (listed in order of decreasing sensitivity) for Corticosteroids can be delineated as follows : Th > precursors of CTL (CTL p) and precursors of T suppressors (Tsp) > CTL and Ts "effectors" (Tse) > B cells; whereas that for Cyclophosphamide is : Tsp > Th, CTLp > B > CTL, Tse (see 9). Because of its possible immunotoxicological relevance, it should additionally be noted, that even within a given subset of immune cells of the same lineage and subserving the same general function, certain agents may display at least a degree of preference in their inhibitory effect.

This possibility is illustrated in Table 5. This summarizes the data obtained for this group in mice by examining the effect of a number of immunodepressants on the generation and expression of T-lymphocyte-mediated specific suppressive activity for cell mediated (delayed type hypersensitivity, DTH) and antibody production to the same antigen, sheep erythrocytes (7,15). It can be seen, for example, that whereas single low doses of DNR were capable of markedly inhibiting supressive capacity for DTH, the same doses were incapable of affecting suppressive activity for antibody production that was inhibited only after a repeated subtoxic treatment. In contrast, DXR was inhibitory of both types of suppressive activity in single well tolerated doses. For these studies, T suppressors were induced by injection of a supraoptimal antigen load, drugs being administered either before or after this stimulation. Suppressive activity was subsequently assessed in secondary recipients that at the time of optimal antigen immunization were also injected with cells from the primary hyperstimulated and drug-treated host. Since multiple cells are involved in these regulatory network (16) and no formal dissection of drug' effects on each cellular component was made, the terms Tsp and Tse are used in this table only operationally. In addition to showing that, in the conditions of this model, the ability of certain compounds to affect T-mediated suppression varied, depending on whether the treatment was before immunization (the drug thus presumably acting only on the precursors of Tse), or after it (presumably influencing more committed elements including the actual Tse). Table 5 also shows the effect of the same compounds in vivo on the subsequent capacity of purified preparations of macrophages to develop, upon in vitro incubation, non-specific "spontaneous" suppression, evaluated in terms of inhibition of mitogen responsiveness of syngeneic untreated splenocytes.

In connection with the complexity of the effects of drugs (and, by implication of xenobiotics) on the various cells of the immune apparatus, two further aspects may be mentioned. The first aspect is related to the possibility that at least certain chemicals while being strongly depressive of the functional capacities of given immunocytes, can at the same time not only spare other immune elements (in terms of number and/or function), but actually produce directly or indirectly a stimulation of given immune reactivities. Although the possibility of observing, after treatment with several bona fide immunodepressants, not only a "rebound" immunostimulation (i.e. a phase of augmented reactivity following a previously reduced immunity), but also an increase in given reactivities (e.g. DTH) concomitant to a depression of others e.g. antibody production has been recognized since many years (8), the mechanisms sustaining such split-immunomodulation have for long remained essentially speculative. Following more in-depth investigations on the cellular effects of such drugs, it is now well established that a number of cytotoxic agents produce such apparently paradoxical increases in the expression of immunity by virtue of their greater inhibition of the cells physiologically involved in the down-regulation of the immune response vis-a-vis elements involved in the afferent and/or effector phases. An example of such a mechanism will be discussed below. More recent on the other hand is the demonstration that a number of immunodepressants, through biochemical mechanisms still unresolved in most cases, can directly stimulate given immune cells to express an enhanced function. For instance, Vincristine has been reported to stimulate NK cell activity and Cis platinum and 1-phenylalanine mustard to augment macrophage mediated functions after _in vivo_ or _in vitro_ treatments (see 11). Table 6 shows that MCI and PAP-S, protein synthesis inhibitors of plant origin having close structural and biochemical resemblance to the A chain of Ricin, thus being the focus of current interest for the preparation of antibody-toxin conjugates, were capable of inducing _in vivo_ and _in vitro_ a very marked increase in macrophage-mediated cytotoxicity at doses that drastically reduced a number of other immune functions (17). A second aspect of possible practical importance for a sounder evaluation of immunological data, as well as for the best choice of testing conditions, is related to the fact that at least certain immunodepressants may differentially affect a given type of immune cell, depending on the coexistence or not of other immune stimuli that may change its functional level and/or its maturational stage. At variance with the finding that resting and previously-activated macrophages were qualitatively similar in their sensitivity to various cytotoxic chemicals, as assessed in terms of capacity to inhibit the _in vitro_ growth of transformed cells (18), we have also observed that certain immonodepressants (e.g. CS-A, Cyclophosphamide) that were clearly capable of inhibiting baseline NK activity did not significantly affect Interferon-induced stimulation of this reactivity, a differential whose mechanistic basis is still speculative.

In view of the fact that data do far available on the way that different immunocytes vary in their susceptibility to immuno-modulatory drugs have mostly been obtained in rodents, the question can be raised as to their relevance for man. Although such analyses are difficult to perform in humans due to the prevalent use in the clinic of drugs in combinations and moreover at the largest tolerated doses, the available evidence though admittedly limited, suggests that by and large the same general conclusion also apply to man. As recently discussed (9), _in vitro_ and _in vivo_ studies of several groups have revealed that human immune cells of different populations and subpopulations can vary in their modulability by a given agent, and that, for at least a number of drugs, similar hierarchies of sensitivity among immunocytes as delineated for animals can also be recognized for human cells.

ORGAN-RELATED HETEROGENEITY IN IMMUNOCYTES SENSITIVITY TO DRUGS

Data discussed in the preceding section have provided evidence to support the conclusion that:(a) immune cells of different lineages and even from different subsets of the same population, can vary markedly in their modulability by a given immunodepressive agent and:(b) this inter-cells hierarchy can differ substantially in sensitivity among closely related chemical analogs. It should be noted however that the evidence examplified above on the existence of an heterogeneity in sensitivity to drugs among immunocytes has been obtained by comparing cells obtained, especially in the case of experimental animals, from lymphoid organs such as the spleen or lymph nodes, i.e. organs that are not the common sites for the first encounter between xenobiotics and the host. On the

other hand, studies from other groups have shown that immune
cells of a given lineage, but obtained from different organs,
can display marked differences in at least some functional
capabilities. For instance, Table 7 shows that, in mice,
after in vitro incubation, alveolar macrophages are markedly
more efficient than peritoneal or spleen phagocytes in mediating non-specific suppression, as evaluated by their capacity
to inhibit mitogen-induced proliferation of syngeneic lymph
node cells.Such a differential activity is presumably linked,
according to preliminary data, to differences in the relative
quantities of the various prostaglandins produced by cells of
the three regions (19). Conversely, no differences between
the phagocytic activity of macrophages from the three organs
were seen. It is also well known that physiologically a
number of nonlymphoid peripheral organs are richly endowed
with types of fixed immune cells (e.g. marophages in the
lung) or are the site of specialized immune subsystems, as is
the case of the intestinal lymphoid apparatus (Vide Hall,this
volume). Although certain types of immune cells are known to
recirculate between the periphery and the more "internal"
lymphoid organs, keeping also in mind that chemicals can vary
markedly in their initial distribution and/or persistence in
different regions, the possibility that a drug may differently
affect immune cells present in lymphoid and non-lymphoid
organs should be considered. In order to approach such a
question, a series of studies were initiated to test the
effect of a series of immunodepressants on immune reactivities
assessed simultaneously in "central" lymphoid sites, such as
the spleen, and in "peripheral" organs. In these preliminary
studies, we have concentrated on organs, i.e. lung and
intestine, that in addition to being the initial sites of
exposure for most xenobiotics, are also important barriers in
the interaction between host and environment (e.g. infectious
agents), and on those immune cells that are primarily involved
in natural host resistance. Data so far obtained support the
concept that immunomodulatory agents may indeed exhibit
organ-related differences in their effects on immune elements.
As presented schematically in Table 8, while certain drugs
exhibited concordant effects at each of the sites for one
(e.g. Cy) or both (e.g. DXR) immune activities-tested, other
compounds revealed at least a degree of organ related
preference. Thus subcutaneous Azathioprine (Aza) reduced NK
activity, on a unit cell number basis, in spleen but not in
lung and intestine. Doses of Hydrocortisone (OHCort) capable
of clearly depressing this reactivity in spleen and lung were
not inhibitory for the intestine. In parallel, 5-Fluorouracil
depressed macrophage, cytotoxicity in lung and peritoneal
cavity but not in the spleen. Aza spared this activity in
alveolar macrophages while inhibiting that of peritoneal and
spleen phagocytic adherent cells. Table 8 also shows that
oral or intraperitoneal 5FU treatment markedly impaired NK
activity in lung and spleen cells, whereas it was associated
with a marked and long-lasting (up to 8 days after a single
200 mg/kg oral dose) increase in this reactivity in intraepithelial lymphocytes that were (IEL) obtained from the small
intestine of similarly treated mice. This immunomodulatory
effect of 5FU is not sustained by a stimulation of intestinal

NK effectors by the drug, but rather by an inhibition of cells down-regulating thse effectors. In fact, the addition of a small proportion of normal IEL to 5FU IEL was capable of bringing the latter's NK activity to control values, whereas normal spleen cells were incapable of modifying the reduced NK activity of splenocytes from 5FU-treated animals.

The mechanism(s) responsible for this organ-related differential susceptibility of immune reactivities to drugs remains to be explored. Whereas initial data suggest the existence for some agents (e.g. OHcort) of a correlation between drug biovailability in the various organs and effect herein exerted, such correlation was not apparent in preliminary investigations for other compounds, such as 5FU. Therefore, the relative role played by drug biovailability and other possible mechanisms (e.g. differences among organs in the cytokinetics of the immunocytes assayed and/or their regulatory cells, intrinsic differences in susceptibility among cells depending on their maturational stage or level of "spontaneous" activation, local richness in other cells capable of modulating immunocytes function) is still a matter of speculation for the majority of compounds. Also essentially unresolved are the bases for the differential sensitivity to a given compound clearly recognizable among the various immune cells present in a given lymphoid organ, as discussed above.This heterogeneity is incidentally detectable for the so-called immunostimulatory drugs (20). The difficulty in advancing a satisfactory mechanistic pictures for these inter-cell and inter-drug heterogeneities derives, on one hand from present ignorance of many critical aspects of the physiology of the various immune cells,particularly as regards for instance their turnover rates in resting conditions and after stimulation, and on the other on the presence or not of critical individualized biochemical pathways and thus capacity to withstand or repair cytotoxic damage. This ignorance is compounded by our current very limited understanding of many aspects of the molecular pharmacology of cytotoxic compounds that have been in use for many years. For istance, it has been reported that Cy, a prototype alkylating agent, could inhibit immunocyte function at doses below those capable of inducing nucleic acid alkylation (21). Although the major mechanism of cytotoxic damage of DXR and DNR is believed to be trough DNA intercalation, the latter compound was markedly more inhibitory for non-replicating macrophages in vitro and of affecting T suppressor cell in vivo.

CONCLUDING REMARKS

From the above discussion of selected aspects of the cellular mode of action of chemical immunodepressants, a number of points that appear to have general relevance to immunotoxicology emerge. The first of these points is related to the conclusion that chemical immunodepressants, even when chemically analogous and /or thought to exploit similar modes of subcellular action, at least in interfering with cell replication, can in fact be markedly heterogenous in their effects on the various populations and subpopulations of immune elements present in a given lymphoid region or organ. This obviously implies the possibility that within a chemical class different molecules, though structurally closely related, may nevertheless display immunotoxicological profiles individualized, not only in quantitative, but also in qualitative terms. In view of the fact that hierachies in susceptibility to modulation by drugs can be recognized among immunocytes, and that some cells can be relatively or absolutely spared, even at doses having clear general toxicity, it can be expected that many xenobiotics will not affect equally each and every expression of immune reactivity. Indeed, it can be expected that the final profile of immunological activity, of at least a proportion of foreign substances, may represent the algebraical sum of a series of individual effects that may also be of opposing sign. Quite apart from the consideration that excessive deviation in either direction from the normal immune level should be considered as potentially harmful, and thus bona fide immunoenhancers should be included among immunotoxicants, the fact that, for at least certain drugs, down-regulatory cells may be more sensitive than helper-inducer or effector immunocytes, suggests additionally that in a least some conditions, exposure to a true immunodepressive xenobiotic may actually be first revealed by an augmented expression of some form of immune reactivity.

The possibility that with drugs possessing antiproliferative capacity, immunodepression could be sustained not only by lymphoid cell destruction, but also by "functional" inhibition of immune elements, is a further point of practical importance. This possibility in fact implies that the absence of pathological changes in lymphoid organs after exposure to a foreign compound, does not necessarily exclude that it may be an immunotoxicant. Considering the very marked variations that can exist among chemicals in their bioavailability in different body organs because of their route of entry and/or physicochemical properties, the possibility that immune reactivities may be differentially affected in lymphoid and non-lymphoid peripheral organs appears also of significance in immunotoxicology. This organ-related heterogeneity has in fact obvious implications with regard to the use of realistic routes of exposure in the testing of xenobiotics and to the potential non-representativeness of assays conducted exclusively on immune cells taken from "central" lymphoid districts.

ACKNOWLEDGEMENT

Supported in part by Progetto Finalizzato CNR (Rome) "Medicina Preventiva e Riabilitativa", Contract No. 82.02058.56.

Table 1 - Possible Mechanisms for Drug-Induced Immunodepression

---

- Affect antigen distribution and/or persistence

- Influence production-differentiation of precursors immunocytes

- Affect traffic and/or number of inducer, effector and/or regulatory
  immune cells

- Influence activation threshold of immunocytes to antigen and/or growth
  and differentiation factors (e.g. responsiveness to lymphomonokines,
  expression of receptors)

- Affect production, release and/or metabolism of Lymphomonokines and/or
  other substances (e.g. λ-fetoprotein) modulating immune cell function

- Influence quantity, quality, persistence of effector products of immune
  cells (e.g. antibody)

- Affect number, traffic, functional capacity of other cells (e.g. platelets,
  neutrophils) and dependent mediators

- Affect indirect regulatory circuits (e.g. CNS-endocrinological homeostasis).

Table 2 - Modulatory Effects of Immunodepressants on Macrophage-Monocyte
Functions

Direct cytotoxicity: $\downarrow$ DNR, Azathioprine, Steroids, Dacarbazine, Actinomycin D,
Vinblastine, 5FU; = DXR, Cy; $\nearrow$ Cisplatin, 1-PAM

Responsiveness-Production of LK: $\downarrow$ Steroids, Azathioprine, Cyclosporin, MTX,
Vinblastine

Suppressive activity: $\downarrow$ DNR, Azathioprine; = Cy, DXR

Ag.processing-phagocytosis: $\downarrow$ Steroids, Vinca alk, Actinomycin D; = Azathioprine

Chemotaxis-migration: $\downarrow$ Steroids, MTX, Azathioprine, Vinca alk.

$\downarrow$: inhibitory agent; = inactive agent; $\nearrow$: augmenting agent

Table 3 - Effect of Chemical Immunodepressants on Murine NK Cells Activity and Spontaneous and Activated Macrophage-Mediated Cytotoxic Capacity

Drug	NK activity	Macroph. Cytotox. Activity	
		Spont.	BCG-activ.
Cy	- 58*	- 2	- 6
DTIC	- 6	-58*	-67*
OHCort	- 53*	-41*	-64*
Aza	- 48*	-49*	-58*
DXR	- 4	+ 2	- 3
DNR	- 32*	-53*	-61*

* : p < 0.01

Results are expressed as % decrease in specific cytotoxicity. Cytolytic capacity of spleen macrophages was assessed on mKSA TU5 target with 48 h incubation; data shown are for 20 : 1 A : T. YAC 1 targets were used to test spleen NK activity; data are for 20 : 1 A : T after 4 h incubation. Drugs were given 48 h before test. Cy : cyclophosphamide; DTIC : dacarbazine; OHCort : hydrocortisone; Aza : azathioprine; DXR : doxorubicin; DNR : daunorubicin.

Table 4 - Spleen cells responsiveness to mitogens, NK activity and macrophagic cytotoxic capacity after Cyclosporin A treatment in mice

Exp. Group	NK[a]	Macroph.[b]	ConA[c]		PHA[c]	
			1	10	5	10
Control	32.8 ± 2.0	21.2 ± 1.8	6.5 ± 0.7	57.0 ± 3.8	76.0 ± 3.1	25.2 ± 2.5
CS-A	16.7 ± 1.7*	23.3 ± 2.0	4.3 ± 1.0	49.6 ± 4.3	34.2 ± 10.2*	13.7 ± 1.2*

*: p<0.01

a: data are% specif. cytotox. values at 50:1 A:T on YAC-1 targets after 4 h incubation;

b: % specif. cytotox. at 20:1 A:T on mKSATU5 targets after 72 h incubation;

c: data are values of stimulation index at mitogen concentrations (in $\mu g/ml^{-1}$).

Tests performed 48 h after 70 mg/kg os x 4 CS-A.

204

Table 5 - Schematic Summary of the Effect of Chemical Immunodepressants
on the Expression of Murine Non-Specific Macrophage-Mediated
and T-dependent Antigen Specific Suppression for Humoral (abs)
and Cell-Mediated (dth) Reactivity to SRBC

D r u g	Macroph. suppress.	Ts — abs		Ts — dth	
		precursors	effectors	precursors	effectors
DNR	++	=	=	++	++
DXR	=	+++	+++	+++	+++
Aza	++	++	+	=	=
Cy	=	+++	+	++	+̲

= : no significant inhibition;

+ : significant inhibition

Table 6 - Non-Specific Suppressive Activity of Macrophages from Different
.Murine Sites

% macroph. added	lung macroph.	perit. macroph.	spleen macroph.
0	123,150	96,780	116,445
6	31,210*	52,805*	109,680
12	1,885*	23,460*	126,175
25	1,340*	12,575*	138,040

* = p < 0.01

Data are cpm of ConA-stimulated splenocytes in the presence of
different % of syngeneic macrophages from different sources.

Table 7 - Immunomodulatory Effects of the Protein Synthesis Inhibitors
MCI and PAP-S

Exp. group	Dose (mg/kg)	NK^a	$Macroph.^b$	$SRBC^c$	$ConA^d$
Control	—	49.8	18.7	39,650	66,345
MCI	0.4	36.3*	37.6*	1,350*	21,115*
PAP-S	0.2	32.4*	39.7*	410*	19,710*

*p < 0.01

a : % specif. activity splenocytes at 100: 1 A:T; b : % specific activ. of spleen macrophages at 25:1 A:T; c : nos. spleen PFC; d : cpm of splenocytes at 2 μg/ml ConA.

Table 8 - Schematic summary of effects of chemical immunodepressants
on NK activity and macrophage-mediated cytotoxic capacity
in different murine organs.

Drug	Route of admin.	NK activity in			macroph. cytotox. in		
		spleen	lung	gut	spleen	lung	perit.
DXR	i.v.	=	=	=	=	=	=
Aza	s.c.	↙	=	=	↙	=	↙
OHCort	s.c.	↙	↙	=	↙	/	↙
5FU	os	↙	↙	↗	=	/	↙
Cy	i.v.	↙	↙	↙	=	=	↙

= : no significant effect; ↙ or ↗ : at least 25% reduction or increase in specific. cytotox. values at 3 A:T ratios. Gut refers to intestinal intraepithelial lymphocytes, and perit. to peritoneal macrophages

REFERENCES

1. Spreafico, F., A. Vecchi, M. Sironi & S. Filippeschi, 1983. Problems in immunotoxicological assessment : Examples with different classes of xenobiotics, in Immunotoxicology, C.G. Gibson, R. Hubbard and D.V. Parke (Eds.) Academic Press, London pp.343-357.

2. Spreafico, F., 1984. Immunomodulation by xenobiotics. The open field of immunotoxicology, in Immunomodulation. New Frontiers and Advances, H.H. Fudenberg, H.D. Whitten and F. Ambrogi (Eds.) Plenum Press, New York pp. 311-330.

3. Bach, J.F., 1975. The Mode of action of Immunosuppressive Agents. Elsevier/North Holland, Amsterdam.

4. Spreafico, F. & A. Anaclerio, 1977. Immunosuppressive agents. in Immunopharmacology, J.W. Hadden, R.G. Coffey, and F. Spreafico (Eds.) Plenum Press, New York, pp.245-278.

5. Webb, D.R. & A. Winkelstein, 1980. Immunosuppression and immunopotentiation, in Basic and Clinical Immunology, H.H. Fudenberg, D.P. Stites, J.L. Caldwell and J.V. Wells (Eds.). Lange Medical Publ., Los Altos, CA., pp.313-326.

6. Moller, G. (Ed.), 1982. Immunosuppressive agents. Immunol Rev., 65 1-178.

7. Spreafico F. , S. Alberti, M. Allegrucci, A. Canegrati, F. Colotta, W. Luini, A. Merendino, E. Pasqualetto, M. Romano, M. Sironi & A. Vecchi, 1983. On the mode of action of immunodepressive agents, in Advances in Immunopharmacology 2, J.W. Hadden, L. Chedid, P. Dukor, F. Spreafico and D. Willoughby (Eds.). Pergamon Press, New York, pp. 745-752.

8. Spreafico, F., A. Tagliabue & A. Vecchi, 1982. Chemical immunodepressants in Immunopharmocology, P. Sirois (Ed.) Elsevier Biomedical Press, New York, pp.315-347.

9. Spreafico, F,M. Allegrucci, A. Merendino & W. Luini, 1984. Chemical immunodepressants. Their action on the cells of the immune system and lymphokines. In Toxicology of the Immune System, J. Dean (Ed.) Raven Press, New York, in press.

10. Mantovani, A., 1982. The interaction of cancer chemotherapy agents with monoclear phagocytes. Ad. Pharmacol. Chemother., 19. 35-66.

11. Spreafico, F., & A. Vecchi, 1984. The immunomodulatory activity of other cancer chemotherapeutic agents. in Biological Responses in Cancer. Progress Towards Potential Application, E. Mihich (Ed.) Plenum Press, New York, in press.

12. Ritton, S., & R. Palacios, 1982. Cyclosporin A. Usefulness, risks and mechanism of action. Immunol. Rev., 65. 5-22.

13. Alberti, S., D. Boraschi, W. Luini & A. Tagliabue, 1981. Effects of in vivo treatment with cyclosporin A on mouse cell-mediated immune responses. Int. J. Immunopharmacol., 3. 357-364.

14. Introna, M., P. Allavena, F. Spreafico & A. Mantovani, 1981. Inhibition of human natural killer activity by cyclosporin A. Transplantation, 31. 113-116.

15. Anaclerio, A., G. Conti,, G. Goggi, M.C. Honorati, A. Ruggeri, M.L.Moras & F. Spreafico, 1980. Effect of cytotoxic agents on suppressor cells in mice. Eur. J. Cancer, 16. 53-58.

16. Cantor, H., R.K. Gershon, 1979. Immunological circuits: Cellular compositon. Fed. Proc., 38. 2058-2064.

17. Spreafico, F., C. Malfiore, M.L. Moras, L. Marmonti, S. Filippeschi, L. Barbieri, P. Perocco & F. Stirpe, 1983. The immunomodulatory activity of the plant proteins Momordica Charantia inhibitor and Pokeweed Antiviral Protein. Int. J. Immunopharmacol., 5. 335-343.

18. Mantovani, A.,W. Luini, G.P. Candiani & F. Spreafico, Effect of chemotherapeutic agents on natural and BCG-stimulated macrophage cytotoxicity in mice. Int. J. Immunopharmacol, 2. 333-339.

19. Vicenzi A., A. Biondi, C. Bordignon, A. Rambaldi, M.B.Donati & A. Mantovani, 1984. Human mononuclear phagocytes from different anatomical sites differ in their capacity to metabolize arachidonic acid, Clin. Exp. Immunol., 57. 385-392.

20. Spreafico, F., 1984 . The complex galaxy of immunomodulatory drugs. Int. Arch. Allergy Appl. Immunol. in press.

21. Ozer, H., J.W. Cowens, M. Calvin, A. Nussbaum-Blumenson & D. Sheedy, 1982. In vitro effects of 4-hydroperoxycyclophosphamide on human immunoregulatory T subset function I.J.Exp.Med., 155. 276-290.

THE TOXICOLOGY OF BIOLOGICAL RESPONSE MODIFIERS

E. Mihich, P.M. Kanter

Grace Cancer Drug Center, Roswell Park Memorial Institute, Departement of Health Buffalo NY. U.S.A.

INTRODUCTION

Major advances have been achieved in cancer therapeutics during the past 30 years. At this time patients with many different types of neoplasms can be brought into complete remission by therapeutic means and are free of detectable disease 5 years or longer after diagnosis. Despite these advances substantial obstacles still remain to be overcome before medical treatments can be generally useful in the management of cancer, particularly of the more common solid tumors.

While new and more effective drugs and treatments are continuously sought through the identification of new sites of pharmacological intervention and an increased knowledge of the mode of action of available agents, new modalities of treatment are also being actively investigated. Among these, the possibility is being considered that new therapies may be developed through a favorable modification of the interactions between tumor and host defense mechanisms directed against the tumor.

The programmatic concept of Biological Response Modifiers (BRMs) has been formulated based on the hypothesis that these agents or approaches may modify in an efficacious way the antitumor responses of the host through augmentation or restoration of existing effector mechanisms or inhibition of suppressing components of the host response; the administration of natural or synthetic mediators or effectors, including cells, is a part of this programmatic approach. Changes in tumor cells may also be induced that might lead to an increased stimulation of the host response or sensitivity of the tumor cells to a host response. The induction of differentiation of tumor cells by natural or synthetic regulators or drugs is also being considered as having potential for therapeutic applications. The possibility that certain BRMs may reduce the development of opportunistic infections related to disease state and/or chemotherapy has also been visualized.

The development of a BRM towards clinical trial, like that of a cytotoxic antitumor agent, requires a thorough evaluation of its toxicological features for the purpose of identifying potential toxicity that may be encountered in humans. Major toxicological differences are expected to exist between a BRM and an antiproliferative agent in the sense that, as a group, cytotoxic agents are likely to be generally more toxic than BRMs. Indeed, BRMs are expected to stimulate, magnify and/or mimic physiological responses of the host to tumor. Moreover, in the case of cytotoxic agents, their toxicity to normal tissues is often directly related to the very antiproliferative action which is the basis of their antitumor activity. Although generalization would be unwarranted and imprudent at this time, in the case of BRMs it is conceivable that their untoward toxicity may not be directly related to their mode of antitumor action.

As it may be perceived from the above comments, the toxicological studies of BRMs may require the evaluation of endpoints which may be somewhat different from those required in the evaluation of cytotoxic antitumor agents; nevertheless equally rigorous studies are needed. It is the purpose of this presentation to bring into focus some of the salient features of BRM toxicology, in terms of both preclinical studies and initial experiences in humans. The few examples selected for discussion concern the interferons (IFNs), monoclonal antibodies (Moabs), and some immunomodulating agents. By necessity the discussion is reduced in scope with reference made, whenever possible, to recently published review articles.

GENERAL CONSIDERATIONS

In the case of most antiproliferative cytotoxic agents, effective antitumor and toxic dose-response curves are in parallel and consequently maximum tolerated doses (MTD) must be determined in animals and in Phase I trials so that appropriate doses may be identified for Phase II and III clinical trials. For many BRMs, the "BRM effective" dose-response curve is not in parallel with the toxicity dose-response curve and in fact may be bell-shaped. Because of these features, and because the optimal dose for BRM action may be much lower than the MTD, it is necessary to determine also the optimal BRM dose (OBRMD) in animals and during Phase I clinical trials by measuring the biological responses which are expected to be modified by the agent. The essential differences between OBRMD and MTD must be recognized and indeed the need for a modified Phase I trial that would include the necesssary idendification of the OBRMD has been proposed since the inception of the BRM program (Mihich and Fefer, 1983) and is now broadly accepted. The MTD should be determined also in animals unless the BRM is species-specific or strictly antigen-specific or non-toxic up to reasonably high doses.

The assumption that BRMs offer a selective means to affect the tumor is reasonable as it is based on the specificity of antigen-dependent immune responses; in addition, selectivity may be expected even in the case of antigen-independent mechanisms as one is essentially dealing with augmentation of physiological responses of the host. Toxicity is nevertheless seen with most BRMs in preclinical test systems and has been shown in some cases to limit the degree of achievable antitumor selectivity. In certain of these cases the question of whether or not a BRM's antitumor and toxic action may be directly related is still moot.

PRECLINICAL APPROACHES TO TOXICITY EVALUATION

Any new compound expected to undergo a clinical trial as an antineoplastic agent must undergo rigorous toxicology testing. Such studies are normally carried out in two or more species, with single and multiple adminstrations of varying amounts of agent. Preclinical toxicology studies stress evaluations at or near lethal dose levels to demonstrate the fullest possible spectra of toxicities. The potential of the agent to produce lethality, the formation and regression of specific organ toxicities, sex and species differences, are studied and documented to serve as a guide for a human clinical trial (Mihich, 1966). Such studies have to be carried out also in the case of BRMs and may have to be altered and expanded in scope in order to increase the probability that possible unique toxicities evoked by BRMs may be identified. The extreme toxicities of these agents have to be evaluated at their maximally tolerated levels, provided that these are not totally unreasonable with respect to dosing practicalities, lower doses, which may induce important functional and mor-phologic alterations of the immune system, should also be studied. Indeed changes may be missed if the animal is overwhelmed by the toxicities induced by high dosage.

Numerous <u>in vitro</u> and <u>in vivo</u> assays have been developed to evaluate drug effects on the various functional aspects of the immune system. i.e., cell mediated immunity, macrophage function, humoral immunity, lymphocyte proliferation, host resistance, etc. While information from such assays is useful in elucidating the mechanism of action of an agent, and of practical use in monitoring a clinical trial if human testing correlates exist, they are difficult to superimpose on toxi-cology protocols that are designed chiefly to evaluate the safety of an agent. Most immune function tests rely on administration of foreign substances (e.g., tuberculin, sheep red blood cells, etc.) which would complicate the evaluation of toxicities induced by the drug itself. Furthermore, these tests frequently require serial sampling of organs such as thyms, spleen or lymph nodes wihich may require sacrifice of the test animal. This form of testing is impractical in large animals (i.e., dogs and primates) and would add greatly to the already costly process of preclinical toxicology testing, and delay the timely completion of such testing.

The emphasis on the evaluation of the immunotoxicity of BRMs and related noncytotoxic agents is on procedures that by themselves do not alter the normal physiology of test animals. The primary goal of these test procedures is to adequately evaluate the potential for untoward effects on the immune system that could lead to concerns for the health of the recipient. Disturbances in immune function could result in, (a) immune suppression, which might lead to opportunistic infections, or enhanced tumor growth;(b) immune enhancement, which may result in development of autoimmune disease or allergic syndromes; and (c) immune complex formation which might lead to drug inactivation, glomerulonephritis, etc.

The specific tests one may employ to evaluate effects on the immune system are as follows:

Morphology. Gross and histopathologic observations are made of the lymph nodes, spleen Peyers patches and bone marrow of test animals. Organ weights are taken as a measure of atrophy or hypertrophy, a procedure which is generally more sensitive and reliable than microscopic evaluations. Immune complex deposition in the kidneys is evaluated by standard fluorescence techniques.

Hematology. Serial blood samples are evaluated for total leukocyte count, and films are made for differential counts. Platelet numbers are determined serially, as a potential measure of autoimmune processes.

Serum Chemistry. Acute phase reactants such as cortisol, C-reactive protein and fibrinogen are evaluated serially as a sensitive measure of inflammation. Serum cortisol assay also aids in the evaluation of immune suppression that may be induced directly by drugs, or indirectly through adrenal steroid release. The potential for autoimmune disease is evaluated by Coombs test, SLE (latex slide agglutination), titer of anti-DNA antibodies, and the bentonite flocculation test for rheumotoid factor. Total serum globulins, as well as quantitation by immunodiffusion of IgG, IgM, and IgA are carried out on all serums samples. Immunodiffusion is also used to screen serum for the presence of antibodies directed against the drug being evaluated. Serum agarose gel electrophoresis is conducted on all serum samples, a method far more sensitive than routine electrophoresis on cellulose acetate plates.

Urinalysis. Standard urinalysis procedures are used to evaluate onset and duration of nephrotic syndromes, a possible consequence of immune complex formation and deposition.

Body Temperature. Rectal temperatures are checked daily to monitor inflammatory syndromes and opportunistic infections.

Bacterial Cultures. Heart blood samples are taken at the time of necropsy to aid in the diagnosis of opportunistic infections.

In conclusion, while customary toxicology, well seasoned by many years of experience in the development of anticancer drugs and their use in therapy must be mandatory in the development of BRMs, flexibility in approaches, and a continuous evaluation of new assays and tests appropriate for the particular requirement of a BRMs, is an equally important consideration.

THE TOXICOLOGY OF INTERFERONS

This group of agents comprises glycoproteins which are made by mammalian cells in response to viral infection or to stimulation with several types of inducers (Borden et al., 1982). Proteins with antiviral activity comparable to that of natural IFNs have been recently obtained from E. coli or other microorganisms through recombinant DNA technology. The biological actions of the natural IFNs, namely and include antiviral, antitumor and immunomodulation effects, actions which are shared by the natural interferons and, to the extent that they have been so tested, by the recombinant DNA IFNs. Heterogeneity occurs within and among IFN types (Stewart, 1984), but species specificity is prevalent, if not unequivocally absolute (Borden et al., 1982).

In the case of agents like the IFNs, which are essentially species specific, toxicological data in animals are limited in value. In such cases MTD and OBRMD usually cannot be obtained for preclinical studies and testing is limited to verification of biological activity in vitro and assessment of pyretic activity in animals, plus exclusion of obvious toxicities, possibly related to impurities derived from the preparative procedures.

In humans, the toxicities of the IFNs have been identified primarily with IFN , the clinically most extensively studied member of the group, but it has been essentially verified, albeit to a more limited extent, with the other IFNs. These toxicities can be divided into acute and subacute (Kirkwood and Ernstoff, 1984).

The acute toxicity is essentially an influenza-like syndrome with fever, chills, myalgia, arthralgia, malaise, anorexia, fatigue, headache and, in some patients, nausea and vomiting. As treatments continue, these symptoms decrease in intensity suggestive of the onset of a type of tachyphylaxis.

The subacute or chronic toxicities are often dose-limiting and somewhat dependent on schedule and route of administration; tolerance is less rapidly achieved after i.m. or s.c. than after i.v. administration. These toxicities include:

> (a) hematological effects, particularly neutropenia and dose-limiting thrombocytopenia (it appears that this toxicity is due to a reversible inhibition of myeloid maturation, possibly with some sequestration);

> (b) reversible hepatotoxicity which is dose-related, is seen primarily at high doses and is reflected in increases of serum glutamic oxaloacetic transaminase and serum pyruvic transaminase;

(c) neurological toxicity has been seen in some cases and consists of somnolence, lethargy, malaise and progressively more severe debilitation with occasional stupor and psychosis, a toxicity which appears to have ECG counterparts; peripheral neuropathy has also been observed in some patients;

(d) mild gastrointestinal toxicity, commonly with anorexia and less frequently nausea, vomiting and diarrhea; at high doses stomatitis not dissimilar from that observed with anticancer agents is also noted;

(e) cardiotoxicity is infrequent with sinus tachyarrhythmias as the prominent sign; this toxicity was seen primarily in patients with prior history of cariopathy or cardiotoxic drugs;

(f) hypocalcemia, hyperkalemia, transient elevations of creatinine and urea nitrogen levels have been observed occasionally. Despite the evidence that antibodies are formed against exogenous IFNs and that relatively broad specificities pertain, possible physiopathological consequences of these antibodies or related complexes have not been reported except for abolition of biological effects.

MONOCLONAL ANTIBODIES

To date Moabs have been primarily obtained from mouse hybridomas and are by definition antigen-specific; in this sense their preclinical toxicological study would seem at first glance to be unnecessary. Such a statement, although not unreasonable in principle, is however not valid. In fact, the exquisite specificty of Moabs for single epitopes makes it likely that cross-reactivities with tissues other than tumor, bearing the same epitope, will occur. Moreover, when Moabs are used as carriers of toxic moieties, the additional potential toxicities may be related to inappropirate release of toxins or uptake into the RES with consequent toxicity (Vitetta and Uhr, 1984). Therefore appropriate in vitro and/or in vivo tests are required, as discussed below.

The use of Moabs in cancer therapeutics is dependent on the existence of larger amounts of tumor asssociated antigens (TAA) on tumor cells than on normal cells; notwithstanding the fact that most TAA are differentiation antigens, it is likely that this quantitative difference occurs in many cases. Two major uses of Moabs have been visualized in therapeutics, namely Moabs by themselves as presumed effectors and MOabs as vectors for cytotoxic moieties or isotopes. To date the clinical studies of Moabs per se have been only preliminary in nature (Mastrangelo et al, 1984; Oldham, 1984; Miller et al, 1982; Mihich, 1984). Studies with Moabs as vectors are only now beginning to appear (Mihich, 1984; Oldham, 1983; Bernstein et al., 1982). In discussing the prerequisites for preclinical toxicology of Moabs, one should distinguish between these two major applications.

The preclinical toxicological study of Moabs to be used as effectors need not involve extensive animal experimentation, provided that in vitro tests of specificity against a battery of human cells and cell lines of human origin does not show cross-reactivities with cells of normal origin. If cross-reactivites are seen, toxicology studies in baboons may be indicated under the assumption that they would reveal potentially toxic cross-reactivities of relevance to humans. Possible cross-reactivities may also be assessed in early clinical trials through biodistribution studies with a labeled Moab; such studies may provide useful verification of previously in vitro identified cross-reactivities. Regardless of proof of specificity, Moabs must be rigorously tested for the possible presence of viruses of mouse or human origin which may be pathogenic; lymphocytic choriomeningitis, Reo virus type 3, polyoma, mouse adenovirus, mouse hepatitis and LDH viruses are just a few examples of possible sources of concern. With the possible advent of human Moabs, the presence of human pathogenic viruses would also have to be excluded. Essentially all the other required toxicological studies would be those aimed at excluding the presence in the final preparation of potentially toxic materials derived from the various preparative steps; this is indeed a general prerequisite in the development of most biological products. Allergic or anaphylactoid reactions may occur with Moabs but as no good animal model is available to identify human allergies, these possible toxicological effects should be excluded in cautious clinical trials.

The preclinical toxicological study of Moabs to be used as vectors would require essentially the same evaluation but, in addition, would require thorough studies in animals aimed at identifying potential toxicity due to inappropriate release of the conjugated toxin and/or toxicity related to non-specific concentration of the complex in the RES (Vitetta and Uhr, 1984).

Moabs have not yet been extensively and systematically studied in humans (Oldham, 1983). Based on the results obtained to date, some of the toxicities that may be expected to occur can be identified. Above certain doses, pulmonary toxicity may be expressed in acute dyspnea and wheezing. Hypotension, anaphylactoid reactions, serum sickness, increased creatinine, fever, chills, urticaria, rash and nausea with vomiting have been seen in some patients (Oldham, 1983). In the future, attention will also have to be given to toxicities possibly due to immune complex formation such as the alterations in renal function already noted in some cases (Bernstein et al., 1982). Toxicities due to cross-reactions with epitopes present on normal cells or to non-specific uptake by macrophages may be particularly worrisome with Moabs conjugated with cytotoxic moieties (Vitetta and Uhr, 1984).

IMMUNOMODULATING AGENTS

Within the context of this discussion, agents affecting both antigen-dependent and antigen-independent mechanisms are considered together. Indeed most of these agents affect a multiplicity of mechanisms, some involving specific T or B effector or regulatory cells, some involving presumed antigen-independent effectors such as macrophages or NK cells. In most cases it is relatively difficult to ascertain which effect at the cellular level is primarily related to the ultimate antitumor effect observed.

Immunomodulation may be elicited by natural products, chemical agents, cytokines or antibodies directed against specificities present on subsets of cells of the immune system. Several anticancer cytotoxic agents have also been shown to cause immunomodulation through effects on specific cell subsets within the immune szstem. The toxicology of immunomodulators will vary, depending on the specific agent studied; it is often related to such phenomena as autoimmune-like reactions, modification of RES function and anaphylactoid reactions. Consequently, for some of these effects appropriate animal models are lacking. For the purpose of this discussion, the toxic effects of BCG, C. Parvum and levamisol will be briefly considered as examples.

In humans, BCG has been studied extensively in the treatment of various types of neoplastic disease. Excluding the thera-peutic advantages achieved by the intralesional injection of BCG in patients with metastatic melanoma (Mihich, 1981; Mastrangelo an Bird, 1982), significant effects reflected primarily in a prolongation of survival time were noted only in a few disease types (Mastrangelo and Bird, 1982; Torti and LUm, 1984). The systemic toxicity of BCG consists of fever, chills, anorexia, nausea and, in some patients, vomiting and myalgias; all of these effects occur shortly after treatment and subside within 48 hours. C. Parvum has similar toxic effects except that cardiorespiratory toxicity is also seen in this case (Mastrangelo and Bird, 1982). Levamisol toxicity may be divided into non-hematoligical and hematological. The former includes sensorial reactions such as alteratrions in taste and smell, allergic reactions such as rash and influenza-like syndrome, and gastrointestinal symptoms which are relatively mild. Hematotogical toxicity consists primari-ly of agranulocytosis, which was fatal in a few cases and appeared with greater frequency in patients with rheumatoid arthritis and, less so, in patients with cancer. Leukopenia and thrombocytopenia were also seen. A significant genetic predisposition to agranulocytosis seemed related to HLA-B27; in most cases this toxic effect was readily reversible (Mihich and Fefer, 1983).

As is apparent from these brief comments, immunoaugmenting agents may cause unique toxicological effects even when the common basic background of relatively mild syndromes is elicited by them; thus each agent should be carefully studied in animals for possible unique toxicities which may not be necessarily shared by known agents with similar BRM actions.

CONCLUDING CONSIDERATIONS

The development of BRMs as cancer therapeutic agents is still in its infancy. Clinical studies with lymphokines are starting only now, essentially due to the recent availability of sufficient quantities of material obtained by recombinant DNA technology. Adoptive transfer of immune cells sensitized against TAA, with or without anti-suppressor cell treatment or IL2 administration, is likely to be studied in the future. It is likely that allogeneic T cell grafts may cause graft versus host disease; autoimmune toxicities may be the consequence of selective inhibition of T-suppressor cells or may be caused by the administration of cultured autologous lymphocytes sensitized against cross-reacting TAA (Mihich, 1984). Chemically induced immunological hypersensitivities have been known to occur widely in humans and should also be mentioned. Toxicity to the immune system derived from inappropriate immunomodulation may result in the onset of opportunistic infections which may be lethal. Selective tissue toxicities such as the arteritis caused by certain muraminic acid derivatives have also been observed in animal models. Thus future opportunities for the therapeutic development of BRMs will no doubt increase the spectrum of specific toxicities encountered beyond the autoimmune, allergic or influenza-like syndromes elicited by most immunomodulating agents tested to date.

In conclusion, the toxicity of BRM as a functional group of agents has been relatively modest and somewhat uniform in its features. Nevertheless unique toxicities related to the BRM function of the specific agents tested or seemingly to different pharmacological actions may also be encountered. While different approaches are needed in studying this complex group of relatively non-toxic agents, absence of severe toxicity cannot be taken for granted especially in the case of chemical structures and in each case the spectrum of toxicological effects should be rigorously evaluated following with judicious flexibility the well established procedures which have been developed in studies of cytotoxic agents.

REFERENCES

BERNSTEIN, I.D., NOWINSKI, R.C., & RIGHT, P.W. (1982) Monoclonal antibodies: Prospects for cancer treatment. In: Immunological Approaches to Cancer Therapeutics (ed. Mihich, E.) pp 277-297. John Wiley & Wand Sons, New York.

BORDEN, E.C., EDWARDS, B.S. HAWKINS, M.J., & MERRITT, J.A. (1982) Interferons: Biological response modification and pharmacology. In:Biological Responses in Cancer: Progress Toward Potential Applications, (ed. Mihich, E.) Vol 1, pp 169-218. Plenum Publishing Corp., New York.

KIRKWOOD, J.M. & ERNSTOFF, M.S. (1984). Interferons in the treatment of human cancer. J. Clin. Oncol 2:336-352.

MASTRANGELO, M.F. & BERD, D. (1982) Immunotherapy with microbial products. In: Immunological Approaches to Cancer Therapeutics (ed. Mihich, E.) pp. 75-105. John Wiley and Sons, New York.

MASTRANGELO, M.J., BERD, D., & MAGUIRE, H.C. (1984) Current conditon and prognosis of tumor immunotherapy: A second opinion. Cancer Treatment Reports 68:207-219.

MIHICH, E. (1966) Prediction of the Potential Toxicity of Anticancer Agents from Studies in Animals. In: Methods in Drug Evaluation (eds. P. Mantegazza and Piccinini, F.) pp 393-41o. North-Holland Publishing Co., Amsterdam.

MIHICH, E., (1981) Biological response modifiers in cancer therapeutics. In: Cancer Achievements, Challenges and Prospects for the 1980's (eds. Burchenal, J.H. & Oettgen, H.F.) pp. 135-146, Grune and Stratton, New York.

MIHICH, E. (1984) Biological response modifiers: Potentialities and limitations in cancer therapeutics. Clinical Investigation, in press.

MIHICH, E. & FEFER, A. eds. (1983). Report on the biological response modifiers by the subcommittee of the DCT Board of Scientific Advisors. J. Natl. Cancer Inst. Monograph 63.

MILLER, R.A. MAlONEY, D.G., WARNICKE, R., & LEVY, R. (1982) Treatment of B cell lymphoma with monoclonal anti-idiotype antibody. New Engl. J. Med. 306:517-522.

OLDHAM, R.K. (1983) Monoclonal antibodies in cancer therapy. J. Clin Oncology 1:582-590.

OLDHAM, R.K. (1984) Biologicals and biological response modifiers: Fourth modality of cancer treatment. Cancer Treatment Reports 68:207-219.

218

STEWART, W.E. (1984). Heterogeneities of human interferons In: Biological Responses in Cancer: Progress Toward Potential Applications,(ed. Mihich, E.) Vol 2, pp 19-44, Plenum Publishin Corp., New York.

TORTI, F.M. & LUM, B.L. (1984) The biology and treatment of superficial bladder cancer. J. Clin. Oncology 2:505-531.

VITETTA, E.S. & UHR, J.W. (1984) The potential use of immunotoxins in transplantation, cancer therapy, and immunoregulation. Transplantation 37:535-538.

MTP-PE, A SYNTHETIC LIPOPHILIC MURAMYLTRIPEPTIDE: BIOLOGICAL AND TOXCOLOGICAL PROPERTIES

D.G. Braun, P. Dukor, B. Lukas, G. Schumann,
L. Tarcsay, M. Court, J.C. Schaffner, T. Skripsky,
M. Fischer & P. Graepel
IBA- Geigy Limited, Basel,
Switzerland

BRIEF ACCOUNT OF THE BIOLOGICAL PROPERTIES OF MTP-PE

Muramyl peptides are biological response modifiers (BRM), and by virtue of this property they exert immune stimulating and immune modulating properties in model systems of antigenic stimulation and also increase prophylactically the resistance to some bacterial and fungal infections (1-4).

Among the currently known BRMs MTP-PE (an N-acetyl-muramyl-L-alanyl-D-isoglutaminyl-L-alanyl-2-(1',2'-di palmitoyl -sn-gly-cero-3'-phosphoryl)-ethylamide-mono-sodium salt, CGP 19 835A) deserves special attention because it stimulates both in vitro and in vivo mouse and rat macrophages to become tumoricidal (5-8). Entrapping of this compound in multilamellar liposomes appears to be particularly effective in this regard, for repeated intravenous injections of liposome encapsulated MTP-PE into B16 BL6 melanoma bearing mice is mandatory to eradicate spontaneous lung metastanses typical for this model, and survival correlates with the activation of tumoricidal macrophages (9-12). Tumor cells derived from metastases of unsuccessfully treated mice were not resistant to macrophage-mediated lysis and the degree of alveolar macro-phage mediated lysis was indistinguishable from that of the parent B16 BL6 tumor (11). Furthermore, surviving tumor-free animals were not immune to a second tumor challenge suggesting that resistance to the B16 BL6 melanoma is short lived. In this model system no activation of tumoricidal macrophages and, therefore, also no eradication of lung metastases was achieved with free agent given intravenously in doses effec-tive when injected entrapped in liposomes.

Recently is was reported that MTP-PE also activates human blood monocytes to attain tumoricidal properties (13,14). This finding is considered an important step towards the development for its applicability as a putative "anti-cancer agent".

The hitherto observed and described anti-tumor effects achie-ved with MTP-PE are summarized in Table 1. For putative human use it is relevant to note that the in vitro and the in situ or ex vivo modes of activation are good parameters for judging the expected tumoricidal state of alveolar macrophages, blood monocytes, Kupffer cells of the liver or peritoneal exudate cell. So far correlation has always been observed. MTP-PE induced macrophages have proven tumoricidal to a variety of different tumors as listed in Table 1. The decisive experiment, however, has to aim at the human situation once the toxicological requirements both for MTP-PE and its liposome encapsulated form as well as for free liposomes have been fulfilled.

In the past tumoricidal alveolar macrophages have always been induced with MTP-PE entrapped in multilamellar liposomes. Recent evidence suggests that multiple intranasal application of the free agent is similarly effective both in the induction of tumoricidal alveolar macrophages and in achieving survival of B16 BL6 melanoma bearing mice (A.F. Brownbill et al. 1984, submitted for publication). This finding clearly contrasts with the low efficacy of intravenously administered free drug, and it may entail significant considerations for therapeutic schemes.

MTP-PE has another exciting biological property. When solubilized in buffers as free agent it exerts prophylactic and therapeutic antiviral effects after single intranasal, peroral, intravaginal and intravenous administration depending on the virus model used (15), a feature quite distinct from its weak protective properties against bacterial and fungal infections (4). MTP-PE proved to be highly active in a variety of experimental RNS virus infections in the mousse (e.g. influenza A & B, strains). It was also active both therapeutically and prohylactically in DNS virus infection models, (e.G. herpes simplex and herpes simplex virus 2) in mice and guinea-pigs. (Dietrich and Lukas, 1985; Lukas and Dietrich, 1985, in preparation)

Furthermore, the experimentally proven antiviral efficacy of free MTP-PE in animal models finds its correlate - as in the tumor models described above - in the fact that MTP-PE inserted into the phospholipid bylayer of multilamellar liposomes can activate human peripheral blood monocytes to lyse herpes simplex virus 2- infected human cells but not uninfected cells (16).

Finally, M. Kende from the USAMRIID at Frederick, Maryland, reported that liposomally entrapped MTP-PE also exerted prohylactic and therapeutic efficacy in experimental murine rift valley fever virus infections (17).

Taken together these findings suggest that in model systems MTP-PE shows highly interesting anti-tumoral and anti-viral effects. In order to become an investigational drug for human use this agent must next pass the hurdles of toxicological scrutiny. The description of the initial available data constitutes the major part of this contribution.

Toxicological Findings with MTP-PE

Immunotoxicology must be tentatively understood in two ways. Firstly, it comprises the toxic effects of any drug on all cellular compartments required for unimpaired immune responsiveness, and, secondly, it encompasses adverse properties of drugs specifically designed to influence cells of the immune system. General and specific immunotoxicological aspects must be taken into account when one deals with MTP-PE, a situation which makes a safety assessment even more difficult.

The terms "toxic" and "adverse" in drug development are usually associated with high, non-physiological, in most cases excessive doses, which lie orders of magnitude above those used or intended for use in therapeutic schemes in man. The "mission" of toxicological testing, is to produce undesired reactions, and the study of the underlying mechanisms is one of the important end-points in the study objectives. The toxicological testing programm for MTP-PE is based on criteria similar to the usual drug development plan. However, by only following the standard registration checklist approach this compound would probably be abandonned very early in the process. The ordinary 90-day-toxicity routine as a prerequisite to clinical testing must be very carefully adapted in this case. In this paper the initial toxicological testing program primarily designed for the intranasal formulation of MTP-PE developed at CIBA-GEIGY in Basel will be highlighted and our first results will be discussed.

Following intranasal application both systemic effects and local reactions at the application site were studied. At this stage of development no pharmacokinetic data are available that would have allowed any quantitation of the absorption of MTP-PE through the nasal mucosa. Therefore, in order to derive a standard for comparison of systemic effects between different modes of administration the intravenous route was chosen first as this is the most direct way to establish the response to systemic exposure to MTP-PE.

The choice of animal species was based on own experiments with MDP-derivatives and on experience in other laboratories from which we learned that rats and mice were almost unsusceptible to MTP-PE as far as toxic reactions are concerned. The guinea-pig, probably the most susceptible animal (Fidler, I.J., personal communication, 1983) is only suited for short-term toxicity experiments. In pilot studies we were able to identify the dog and the rabbit as satisfactory responders and so these two species were chosen for intravenous administration of MTP-PE at daily doses of 0.001, 0.01,0.1 and 1.0 mg/kg of body weight for a total of 14 consecutive days. Three of five animals per groupe were killed 24 hours after the last administration and the remaining two animals per group 6 weeks later. The results indicated that clinical, laboratory and microscopical lesions were confined to the two top dose groups (1.0 and 0.1 mg/kg) while the two lower dose groups were free of effects that could be associated with the experimental treatment. Clinical symptomatology and laboratory data are summarized in Tables 2 and 3. Although no clearly identifiable pattern of events was observed it can be stated that pronounced acute inflammatory responses prevailed. A considerable inter-individual variation of the response was also noticeable.

After standard histological processing of the tissues harvested at autopsy, the microscopical examination of one hematoxylin and eosin stained slide per organ yielded the distribution pattern of vascular lesions summarized in Table 4. The microscopical organ examination identified the vascular bed as the primary target system of MTP-PE for toxic effects. The main lesion comprised an accumulation of cells in the intimal/medial regions of small arteries and arterioles, sometimes markedly obstructing the vessel lumina and partially destroying the elastica membrane (Fig. 1-3). While the most common lesions were detected in small arteries and arterioles, a few animals had additional findings which were considered to be most probably secondary to the vascular lesions: extensive non-fatal brain necrosis in one dog at 1.0 mg/kg, necrotic foci with granulation tissue and fibrosis in the myocardium (same dog as above), and complete necrosis of the gall-bladder (one rabbit at 1.0 mg/kg) with aneurysms of blood vessels in the liver. Additional findings observed with non-systematic distribution and frequency are listed in Tables 5 and 6. Of these the epi-/peri-cardial and the synovial changes appear to be typical for the pathology of this group of compounds.

When the data of the above described experiments were available, the discussion of the subsequent steps in the development of MTP-PE focused on two issues. Firstly, the toxicological profile established so far for the drug by the intravenous route characterized MTP-PE as a very toxic compound with high-dose systemic effects with seriously implicationsas far as risk assessment for man is concerned. Secondly, it was felt that this systemic profile could nevertheless now serve as an acceptable basis for further comparatie studies. We decided to therefore conduct an experiment with intranasal application of the highest dose (1.0 mg/kg) used in the i.v. studies. Of our two animal species only the dog was suitable for the minimum volume requirements which could not be met with rabbits due to their lower bodey weight. In order to give approx. 1 mg MTP-PE per kg body-weight, a total of 1 ml of fluid had to be administered. To avoid excessive washing-down, the solution was instilled in 10 fractionated amounts over a period of 2 hours daily for 14 consecutive days. Three male and 3 female dogs were used.

Laboratory investigations this time included measurement of C-reactive protein, fibrinogen and erythrocyte sedimentation rate as possible indicators of an acute inflammatory process. Blood pressure measurements were carried out. For this procedure the dogs were trained before the experiment. The outcome of this study, in contrast to the i.v. study with the same high dose gave no indication of adverse effects, particularly with regard to the vascular bed. Only one dog developed a large hematoma around the site where the catheter for blood pressure determinations had been inserted. No other relevant finding were noted. In order to study onset and sequence of events leading to the vascular changes, further short-term studies with free MTP-PE are currently in progress.

Discussion of the Toxicological Findings

This paper contains a status report of the toxicological evaluation of MTP-PE, a promising candidate for a potent drug with established tumoricidal and antiviral properties in experimental animal modesl (5-17). The search for a relevant animal species resulted in the choice of the dog and the rabbit for reasons of susceptibility, ease of handling and also known pathological background data.

The study of systemic toxic effects by the most direct (intravenous) exposure of the animal was the first objective of toxicity testing. The dosing scheme was chosen on the presumption that after 2-week-toxicity studies in two species it would be possible to conduct first tolerability and drug disposition studies in man.

The systemic toxicological response of both animal species confirmed the expectation of a marked toxicity which is known and typical of practically all biologically active substances. In spite of marked clinical and morphological alterations all animals survived the two weeks of treatment. The target system identified for the main toxic effects was the vascular bed, especially the small arteries and arterioles. The origin of the cells obstructing these vessels and the mechanisms of their accumulation are under study by additional specialized techniques such as autoradiography, electron microscopy, cytochemistry and immunopathology. Irrespective of how these highly relevant questions are resolved, it must be emphasized that the vascular bed is, with the exception of the retinal arteries, practically inaccessible to preventive diagnostic assessment in man e.g. during clinical trials. Any risk of producing such changes as seen in the animal models is con-sidered unacceptable for the conduct of human trials. It is tho aim of further toxicity testing to make sure that no such unwanted effects will occur in situations which model human therapeutic use.

A study with a protocol similar to the i.v. study and with the highest dose (1 mg/kg) was conducted with the intranasal MTP-PE formulation. As no toxic effects attributable to MTP-PE were seen in this experimental set-up we consider a single intranasal application in man possible.

As a prerequisite, the no-toxic-effect level, i.e. the maximum dose tolerated without toxic effects, which is usually inferred from relevant toxicological tests, which was taken from the i.v. study data was regarded as the absolute baseline. There it was shown that doses up to 0.01 mg/kg produced no toxic reactions. This precautionary measure was necessary in view of the fact that no pharmacokinetic and resorption data existed. Therefore the possibility could not be totally excluded that MTP-PE is simply not adequately resorbed through the nasal mucosa in the dog. When it reaches the circulation, however, as evidenced in the i.v. tests, 0.01 mg/kg would not have caused any effects in rabbits and dogs that could be detected by standard toxicity testing procedures.

CONCLUSION / SUMMARY

MTP-PE (an N-acetyl-muramyl-L-alanyl-D-isogluta minyl-L-alanyl
-2- (1',2'- dipalmitoyl-sn-glycero-3'-phosphoryl) -ethylamide
-mono-sodium salt, CGP 19 835A) is a synthetic muramylpeptide
with significant anti-tumor metastatic and anti-viral properties mediated by macrophages in rodents when given
intravenously, encapsulated into multilamellar liposomes, or
intranasally as free substance. Additionally, as is typical
for this class of compounds, MTP-PE increases prophylactically
the resistance to bacterial and fungal infections.

The statuts of the safety evaluation program of MTP-PE is as
follows:

1) 2-week intravenous toxicty studies (free MTP-PE) in rabbits
and dogs with 6-week recovery periods have yielded a
no-toxic-effect level of 0.01 mg/kg body weight in both animal
species. Accumulations of cells orginating from or proliferating in the intimal/medial regions of small arteries and
arterioles, sometimes markedly obstructing the vessel lumina,
constituted the most characteristic morphological change,
accompanied by clinical and laboratory findings suggesting
acute inflammatory events.

2) A 2-week intranasal toxicity study in dogs (1 mg/kg of free
MTP-PE) has not yielded any toxic effects that could be
associated with MTP-PE. Most importantly no vascular changes
were seen. The biochemical parameters tested did not indicate
inflammatory processes.

Acknowledgement. We are very grateful to Mrs. Dorette
Moeschli for her expertise secretarial help in compiling this
manuscript.

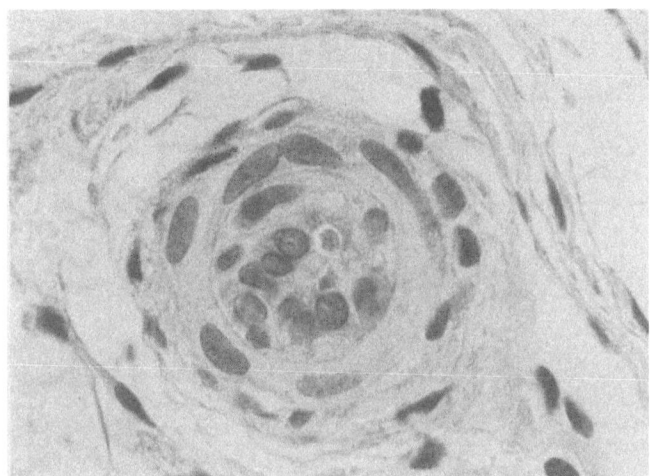

Figure   **1**   Dog adrenal arteriole (hematoxylin-eosin, 1250 x; MTP-PE 1 mg/kg i.v. 2 weeks). Subtotal obliteration of lumen caused by cellular accumulation.

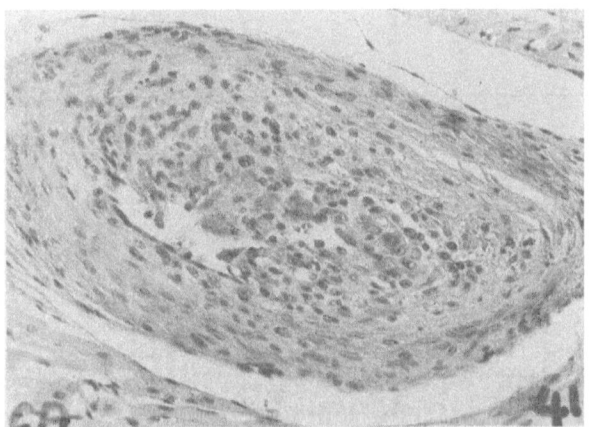

Figure   **2**   Rabbit heart (hematoxylin-eosin, 312 x; MTP-PE 1 mg/kg i.v. 2 weeks). Small artery with subtotal occlusion and intima/media destruction by cell aggregation of unidentified origin.

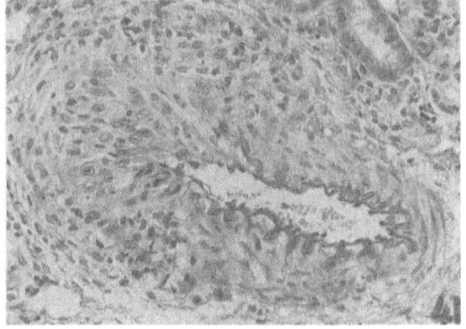

Figure   **3**   Rabbit kidney (hematoxylin-eosin, 312 x; MTP-PE 1 mg/kg i.v. 2 weeks). Arteria arcuata showing focal cellular accumulations involving intima and media cinfined to the left part of the artery with destruction of the elastic membrane.

Table 1

MTP-PE (CGP 19 835); ANTI-TUMOR REACTIVITY BY MACROPHAGE ACTIVATION

Form of Agent	Source of Cells	Mode of Activation	Target Tumor Cells	References
MTP-PE/MLV	AM rat	in vitro	MADB-200	Fidler, I.J. et al. J.Biol.Resp.Modifiers 1982, 1: 43-55.
MTP-PE/MLV	AM mouse	in vitro	P16 BL6	
MTP-PE/MLV	AM mouse	in situ (i.v.)	B16 BL6	
MTP-PE/MLV	AM mouse	in vivo (i.v.)	B16 BL6 metastases lung	Fidler, I.J. et al. Adv.Immunopharmacology 1983, 2: 235-241.
MTP-PE/MLV	AM mouse	in vivo (i.v.)	B16 BL6	Key, M.E. et al. JNCI 1982, 69: 1189-1198.
MTP-PE/MLV	B Mo man	in vitro	A375	Kleinerman, E.S. Cancer Res. 1983, 43: 2010-2014.
MTP-PE/MLV	B Mo man	in vitro	HT-29	
MTP-PE/MLV	B Mo man	in vitro	Natusch	
MTP-PE/MLV	B Mo man	in vitro	A375	Bucana, C.D. et al. Amer.J.Pathol. 1983, 112: 101-111.
MTP-PE/MLV	PEC mouse	in vitro	T241	Barna, B.P. et al Cancer Res. 1984, 44: 305-310.
MTP-PE/MLV	macrophages	in vivo (i.v.)	UV induced	Talmadge, E. et al. Behring Inst. Mitt. 1984, 74: 219-229.
MTP-PE/MLV	B Mo man	in vitro	A375	Sone, S. et al. J.Immunol. 1984, 132: 2105-2109.
MTP-PE	Kupffer cells, mouse	in situ (i.v.)	B16 BL6 UV 2237	Zuliang, Xu & Fidler, I.J. Cancer Immunol. Immunother. 1984 in press

MADB-200, mammary adeno-carcinoma of F344 rats; B16 BL6 melanoma of the C57 BL6 mouse; A375, human melanoma line; HT-29, human colon carcinoma line; Natusch, human glioblastoma line; T241, fibrosarcoma mouse. UV 2237, UV-induced autochthonous fibrosarcoma; AM, alveolar macrophages; B Mo, peripheral blood monocytes; PEC, peritoneal exudate cells.

PUB1/mö.

TABLE 2   CGP 19 835A, TWO WEEK INTRAVENOUS TOXICITY STUDY IN BEAGLE DOGS

Parameter	Dose in mg/kg daily i.v.			
	0.001	0.01	0.1	1.0
Mortality	-	-	-	-
Symptomatology				
spastic gait, diffi- culties in walking	-	-	-	10/10
swelling of the ankle and/or radiocarpal joint	-	-	-	4/10
limping, occasionally	-	-	2/10	some dogs
Body weight	-	-	1/10 $\downarrow$10-16 %	5/10 $\downarrow$10-16 %
Food consumption	-	-	reduced in dogs with body weight loss	
Total proteins	-	-	($\downarrow$)	($\downarrow$)
– albumins	-	-	2/10 $\downarrow$	10/10 $\downarrow$
– α3-globulins	-	-	$\uparrow\uparrow$	$\uparrow\uparrow\uparrow$
– ß1-globulins	-	-	$\uparrow$	$\uparrow$
			all changes reversible	
RBC-parameters	-	-	-	($\downarrow$)
monocytes	-	-	1/10 $\uparrow$	5/10 $\uparrow$
fibrinogen, ESR	-	-	$\uparrow\uparrow$	$\uparrow\uparrow\uparrow$
Bone marrow	-	-	-	1 dog: marked decrease in erythr.series
			all changes reversible	
Cardiography				
ST-segment	-	-	-	2/10
marked enlargement of T-wave	-	-	-	5/10
			all changes reversible	
Neurol. Examin.				
Depressed placing and hopping reactions	-	-	-	mostly all dogs
depressed flexor reflex	-	-	-	3 males
			all changes reversible	

- = no change; $\uparrow$ = increase; $\downarrow$ = decrease; ( ) = minimal

PUB1/mö.

TABLE 3   CGP 19 835A, TWO WEEK INTRAVENOUS TOXICITY STUDY IN RABBITS

Parameter	Dose in mg/kg daily i.v.			
	0.001	0.01	0.1	1.0
<u>Mortality</u>	−	−	−	−
<u>Symptoms</u>				
peripheral hyperaemia	−	(+)	(+)	+
dacryorrhoea	−	−	−	+
swollen eye lids, dry eyes	−	−	−	+
hair loss	−	−	−	+
cloudy cornea	−	−	(+)	+
<u>Body weight</u>	−	−	−	↓
<u>Blood chemistry</u>				
Potassium	−	−	−	↓
Alk. Phosphatase	−	−	↓	↓↓
BUN	−	−	−	↑
Albumins	−	−	(↓)	↓↓
Globulins	−	−	(↑)	↑
<u>Haematology</u>				
RBC-Parameters	−	−	(↓)	↓
Reticulocytes	−	−	−	(↑)
Aniso- / Anulocytes	−	−	−	+
Thrombocytes	−	−	−	↑
Fibrinogen	−	−	(↑)	↑
Segm.Neutr.Granulocytes	−	−	−	(↑)
Monocytes	−	−	(↑)	(↑)

+   = present   − = no change

↑   = increase   ↓ = decrease

( ) = minimal

TABLE 4   2 WEEK INTRAVENOUS TOXICITY STUDIES WITH MTP-PE - INCIDENCE OF VASCULAR LESIONS

| | Number of RABBITS with vascular lesions | | | | Number of DOGS with vascular lesions | | | |
| | End of treatment N = 6 | | 6 week Follow-up N = 4 | | End of treatment N = 6 | | 6 week Follow-up N = 4 | |
	1.0 mg/kg	0.1 mg/kg	1.0 mg/kg	0.1 mg/kg	1.0 mg/kg	0.1 mg/kg	1.0 mg/kg	0.1 mg/kg
Kidneys	6		3		3	1	2	
Heart	6	3	4		5	1	2	1
Lung	6	6	4		1			
Stomach	6	1	2					
Peritoneum	4	2	4					
Liver/Gall bladder	2		4					
Pancreas	2	1	1					
Mesent.lymph node	1							
Poplit.lymph node	6		2					
Axill. lymph node	1				6	5	4	1
Cervic.lymph node	4							
Thymus	2		2					
Thyroid	3		4		2			
Mediastinum	1		2					
Pericardium	3							
Prostate/Vesicular)			1					
Gl./Semin.vesicles)								
Uterus					2			
Ovaries					2			
Urinary bladder	3	1	1		1	1		
Adrenals	1				3			
Skin	1		2				3	1
Injection site			1		1	1		
Skeletal muscle	3		1		6	5		
Knee-joint	2	1	4					
Eyes	4		3					
Orbital glands	3		1					

N = Number of animals per dose group

TABLE 5   2 WEEK INTRAVENOUS ͜XICITY STUDY WITH MTP-PE - NATURE ͡D INCIDENCE OF OTHER FINDINGS IN RABBITS

Organs	Lesions	Number of RABBITS with lesions			
		End of treatment N = 6		6 week Follow-up N = 4	
		1.0 mg/kg	0.1 mg/kg	1.0 mg/kg	0.1 mg/kg
Liver	Bridging hepatic necrosis	2			
	Periportal subacute inflammation	3	4	2	
	Iron-positive pigment	5			
Gall bladder	Total necrosis	1			
Spleen	Neutrophilic infiltration	6	4	1	
	Acute congestion	3			
	Increased RHS-cells	3			
Lung	Neutrophilic infiltration	6	6	4	
Thymus	Atrophy	6			
Knee-joint	Synovitis	5			
Bone marrow	Hypercellularity	6		2	
Kidneys	Multifocal cortical fibrosis			3	
Testes	Disturbance of spermatogenesis			1	

N = number of animals per dose group

TABLE 6.   2 WEEK INTRAVENOUS TOXICITY STUDY WITH MTP-PE – NATURE AND INCIDENCE OF OTHER FINDINGS IN DOGS

Organs/tissues	Lesions	Number of DOGS with lesions			
		End of treatment N = 6		6 week Follow-up N = 4	
		1.0 mg/kg	0.1 mg/kg	1.0 mg/kg	0.1 mg/kg
Brain	Necrosis	1			
Heart	Necrotic foci with granulation tissue and fibrosis in the myocardium	1			
	Single cell necrosis in the myocardium	3	4		
	Epi-/Pericarditis	4	2	2	
	Fibrosis of epi-/pericardium			4	
Kidneys	Endothelial cell proliferation in the glomeruli	1		1	
Liver	Foci of single cell necrosis and mononuclear cell infiltrates	3			
Knee-joint	Synovitis		5		
Thymus	Atrophy	2			

N = number of animals per dose group

REFERENCES

1. LEDERER, E. (1980) J. Med. Chem. 23, 819-825.

2. DUKOR, P., L. TARCSAY, G. BASCHANG (1979) Ann. Reports Med. Chem. 14, 146-167.

3. CHEDID, L., L. CARELLI, F. AUDIBERT (1979) J. Reticulo-endothel. Soc. 26, 631-641.

4. DIETRICH, F.M., W. SACKMANN, O. ZAK, P. DUKOR 1980) In: Current Chemotherapy and Infectious Disease (eds. J.D. NELSON, C. GRASSI). Proc. 11th Int. Congr. Chemotherapy 2, 1730-1732.

5. FIDLER, I.J., S. SONE, W.E. FOGLER. Z.L. BARNES (1981) Proc. Nat. Acad. Sci. USA 78, 1680-1684.

6. FIDLER, I.J., G. POSTE (1981) In: The Prostatic Cell: Structure and Function, Part B. A.R. Liss, New York, 257-267.

7. SONE, S., E. TSUBURA. (1982) J. Immunology 129, 1313-1317.

8. GISLER, R.H., G. SCHUMANN, W. SACKMANN C. PERICIN, L. TARCSAY, F.M. DIETRICH (1982) In: Immunomodulation by microbial products and related synthetic compounds (eds. Y. YAMAMURA, S. KOTANI, Excerpta Medica, 167-170.

9. FIDLER, I.J., S. SONE, W.E. FOGLER, D. SMITH, D.G. BRAUN, L. TARCSAY, R.H. GISLER, A.J. SCHROIT (1982) J. Biol. Resp. Med. 1, 43-55.

10. SCHROIT, A.J., I.J. FIDLER (1982), Cancer Research, 42, 161-167.

11. FIDLER, I.J., W.E. FOGLER, L. TARCSAY, G. SCHUMANN, D.G. BRAUN, A.J. SCHROIT (1983) In: Advances in Immuno-pharmacology 2 (eds. J.W. HADDEN et al., Pergamon Press) 235-241.

12. KEY, M.E., J.E. TALMADGE, W.E. FOGLER, C. BUCANA, I.J. FIDLER (1982) J. Natl. Cancer Inst. 69, 1189-1198.

13. KLEINERMAN, E., K.L. ERICKSON, A.J. SCHROIT, W.E. FOGLER, I.J. FIDLER (1983) Cander Research, 43, 2010-2014.

14. SONE, S., S. MUTRSUURA, M. OGOWARA, E. TSUBURA (1984) J. Immunology 132, 2105-2110.

15. DIETRICH, F.M., B. LUKAS, K.H. SCHMIDTRUPPIN, (1983) Proc. 13th Int. Congress Chemotherapy, Vienna, 91, 50-53.

16. KOFF, W.C. I.J. FIDLER, S.D. SHOWALTER, M.K.
     CHAKRABARTY, B. HAMPAR, L. M. CECCORULLI, E.S.
     KLEINERMAN (1984) Science 224, 1007-1009.

17. KENDE, M. (1983) Abstract No. 153, 23rd ICAAC, Las
     Vegas, October 24th-26th.

ALTERED IMMUNE FUNCTION AND HOST RESISTANCE FOLLOWING EXPOSURE TO COMMON AIRBORNE POLLUTANTS

Donald E. Gardner,*, *** & Judith A. Graham **.

*Northrop Services, Inc. Environmental Sciences Research Triangle Park,
North Carolina U.S.A.

**Toxicology Branch (MD-82) Health Effects Research Laboratory Environmental Protection Agency Research Triangle Park,
North Carolina U.S.A.

***Person to whom correspondance should be addressed.

INTRODUCTION

The ambient air consists of a multitude of air pollutants that differ geographically and temporarily by concentration and chemical identity. They can be classed as either gases or particles. Only a limited number of these pollutants has been studied for immunotoxic effects. Those chemicals that have been studied are relatively common, such as ozone (O_3), nitrogen dioxide (NO_2), sulfur dioxide, sulfates (including sulfuric acid), and fly ashes. Other chemicals which are common, but less widely distributed, such as metals, have also been investigated.

The purpose of this paper is to describe the immunotoxic potential of common air pollutants. To accomplish this with brevity, while illustrating concepts and needed areas of research on this topic, we have chosen to focus on O_3, NO_2, and complex, real-world particles. The photochemical oxidants, O_3 and NO_2, are the most intensely studied common air pollutants. Even so, the following discussion will show the limitations in knowledge of their toxicity. Complex particles were chosen since they represent a more difficult research endeavor than pure chemicals, like metals. Reviews on the immunotoxicity of inhaled metals, sulfates, and sulfur dioxide are available elsewhere (Graham and Gardner, 1984; Gardner 1979, 1982; EPA, 1978, 1982a,b). The lung, which is the first target organ of air pollutants, is an active immunologic organ which can have specific local responses without a generalized systemic response. The role of the macrophage in pulmonary immunological responses has been reviewed recently (Bice, 1984; Bitterman et al., 1981; Schwartz and Bellanti, 1977; Brody and Davis, 1982; Green et al., 1977). Major classes of immunoglobulins are found in the respiratory tract with secretory IgA being the principal immunoglobulin in the upper respiratory tract and IgG being predominant in the lower respiratory tract. Cells lavaged from the lung include functional B, T, and null lymphocytes, as well as plasma cells. The interactions between these immunoglobulins, lymphoid cells, and alveolar macrophages is complex and incompletely understood (Bice, 1984, Green et al., 1977).

The vast majority of the air pollutant immunotoxicology literature is on non-specific anti-bacterial host defense mechanisms, such as mucociliary clearance and alveolar macrophage defenses. Little research has focused on anti-viral defenses or humoral and cell-mediated immunity. In the following text, this literature will be discussed generally and key details will be provided in tables.

EFFECTS OF PHOTOCHEMICAL OXIDANTS

Introduction

Photochemical oxidants arise from a complex series of atmospheric reactions of hydrocarbons and nitrogen oxides in the sunlight, producing O_3 , NO_2 , and other complex chemical compounds. Both gases generally produce similar types of effects, but O_3 is more potent (EPA, 1978, 1982b).

Ozone:

The cells most vulnerable to O_3 -induced injury in the conducting airways are the ciliated cells, resulting in loss of the effectiveness of mucociliary clearance as measured by reduced rate of transport of deposited particles (Kenoyer et al., 1981; Friberg et al., 1972; Abraham et al., 1980; Phalen et al., 1980; Fragern et al., 1979), increased mucus secretions (Last et al., 1977, 1980); and altered size, number and distribution of various mucous secreting cells (EPA, 1978). However, low levels of O_3 alone failed to produce any loss in ciliary beating activity (Grose et al., 1980). Altering these defense mechanisms can result in an accumulation of viable and non-viable inhaled substances that could significantly increase the incidence of upper respiratory tract disease. Few studies have systematically explored the clinical implications resulting from the effects of long-term exposure or long-term recovery from such insults on this host defense system.

A number of studies (Table 1) have shown that acute exposure to O_3 can significantly decrease the ability of alveolar macrophages to phagocytize foreign particles, reduce ability to migrate, disrupt macrophage membrane integrity, reduce lysosomal enzymatic activity, decrease the ability to produce superoxide anion radicals, impair interferon production, and reduce the number of free macrophages available for pulmonary defense. With longer exposure (Table 1), there is a significant influx of new macrophages within the airways. Such accumulation of macrophages may play a role in the development of future chronic pulmonary disease due to the numerous cytolytic and proteolytic enzymes released by the damaged macrophage in its attempt to phagocytize, digest, and transport material out of the lung. Impairment of macrophage functions would alter the lungs' capability for maintaining sterility within the gaseous exchange regions of the lung. Such adverse effects would reduce the host's ability to resist infection and may be involved in the pathogenesis of chronic diseases. An increased incidence of pulmonary infections due to exposure to oxidizing pollutants has been reported by numerous investigators (Table 2), as well as reviewed by Coffin and Gardner (1972), Gardner and Graham (1976), Gardner, (1982). In most cases, these data indicate that O3 acts by prolonging the residence time of the viable infectious organisms and thus enhances the establishment of the opportunistic microorganisms. A wide range of infectious agents have been used including Streptococcus sp. (Group C), Pasturella haemolytica, and Mycobacterium tuberculosis.

The effects of subchronic exposure to O3 on the systemic immune system was studied using the blastogenic response of splenic lymphocytes to mitogens and alloantigens and plaque forming cells' response to sheep red blood cells (Aranyi et al., 1983). A significant suppression in blastogenesis to the T cell mitogen PHA and Con A was detected. There was no effect using the B cell mitogen, LPS, or alloantigen. The immunosuppressive effect of O3 has also been suggested to explain why mice which were immune to tetanus toxoid had an increase in mortality rate, as compared to clean air controls after challenged by the toxin (Campbell et al., 1976). In guinea pigs infected with M. tuberculosis, the cutaneous sensitivity to purified protein derivative (PPD) was significantly reduced in the O3-exposed animals indicating a depressed cell-mediated response (Thomas et al., 1981).

The possibility that O3 may be responsible for enhancement of allergic sensitization has important implications for human health effets. Gershwin et al. (1981) reported that O3 exposure of mice caused a 34-fold increase in the number of IgE containing cells in the lungs that correlated positively with levels of anaphylactic sensitivity. Oxidant damage also caused an increase in IgA containing cells in the lungs and a rise in IgA content in respiratory secretions (Osebold et al., 1979). These authors showed a significant increase in anaphylactic sensitivity when antigen-stimulated and O3 exposed animals were compared to controls (Osebold et al., 1980).

Since there is little doubt that O3 can alter various host defense mechanisms in the laboratory animal, human defense systems have also been examined to determine if these are also impaired by O3 . Although the biological endpoints measured are different, any relationship between the animal data and human subject would be of significant interest. The data indicate that polymorphonuclear neutrophils isolated from the blood of persons exposed to O3 did have a reduced ability to phagocytize and a depressed bactericidal function (Peterson et al., 1978a). The authors proposed that O3 either produced indirect effects on neutrophils through toxicity to the granulocytic stem cell or by altering humoral factors that facilitate phagocytosis. In other studies, peripheral blood T lymphocyte rosette formation was not altered by acute exposure to O3,but B-lymphocyte rosette formation was depressed (Savino et al., 1978) Mitogen-induced transformation of circulating T lymphocytes was also decreased in these studies (Peterson et al., 1978b).

Nitrogen Dioxide

With NO_2 , the individual host defenses are affected in a manner similar to those described for O_3 . The major difference appears to be that the concentration required to elicit a significant response has to be much greater than with O_3 . This difference in toxicity is easily recognizable when one compares a single response such as increases in susceptibility to pulmonary infections. With O_3 , a 3-hr exposure to levels as low as 0.1 ppm O_3 (Miller et al., 1978) produces the same significant response as a 3-hr exposure to 3.5 ppm of NO_2 (Gardner et al., 1977a,b). Other investigations of the effects of NO_2 on susceptibility to laboratory-induced infections are described on Table 3. A series of studies (EPA, 1982b) in Britain and the U.S. suggest that children exposed to NO_2 have a higher incidence of respiratory infection. These epidemiological studies compared subjects in homes with gas cooking stoves vs. homes with electric stoves. The causative pollutant in these studies has not been proven, but it has been interpreted to be NO_2 based on animal studies.

The distribution of cellular injury from NO_2 extends throuh out the conducting airways to the alveoli. In the conducting airways, NO_2 reacts with the ciliated epithelium, causing a decrease in ciliary beating rates and as a consequence, a significant reduction in mucus transport (Kita and Omichi, 1974; Giordano and Morrow, 1972). Such impairment could render this physiological line of defense less effective in the process of lung clearance.

At the alveolar level, the host defense system that receives direct exposure to the inhaled pollutant is the alveolar macrophage. Measuring the functional integrity of macrophages isolated from the lungs of NO_2 -exposed animals indicates that macrophages can be depressed to such a degree that the host can no longer effectively maintain pulmonary sterility (Brody and Davis, 1982). The importance of these defenses in maintaining pulmonary sterility against invading microorganisms becomes clearly evident when these "impaired" animals have to cope with a labatrrory-induced pulmonary infection (Table 3). Animals exposed to NO_2 succumb to the bacterial or viral infection quickly and in a concentration-response manner (Acton and Myrvik, 1972; Ehrlich 1975; Gardner and Graham, 1976; Gardner et al., 1977a,b; Gardner et al., 1979; Ito, 1971; Sherwood et al., 1981). Evidence clearly indicates that these cells are no longer capable of isolating, transporting, or detoxifying these desposited microbes due to their reduced level of phagocytosis, lytic potential, ability to produce interferon (Table 4), and other responses. Morphological indicators of NO_2 damage to this cell are also recognizable after either in vivo or in vitro exposure.

Since NO_2 has been shown to cause an increase in susceptibility to both bacterial and viral infections, a few investigators have examined the immune system to explain this change in susceptibility. However, this research has focused on the systemic immune system which would be less directly involved in pulmonary infections. Nitrogen dioxide decreases the production of serum neutralizing antibody to viruses (Fenters et al., 1971, 1973; Ehrlich 1975) and humoral primary antibody responses to red blood cells (Nakamura et al., 1971; Hidekazu et al., 1981). Other significant immunological effects attributed to NO_2 exposure include an increase in IgM, IgG, and IgG and a decrease in IgA serum levels (Ehrlich et al., 1975). Hemagglutination inhibition titers were unchanged with NO_2 exposure (Fenters et al., 1971, 1973).

Acute exposure to high concentrations of NO_2 significantly decreased the number of spleen and thymus cells, however, at a lower concentration, the number of spleen cells actually increased (Hidekazu and Fujio, 1981). The same authors reported that NO_2 is capable of depressing primary humoral antibody response and that the degree of suppression deferred with respect to time. Fujimaki (1981) showed that the reduction in primary antibody response against sheep red blood cells was more influenced by a suppression of B cell function; for the secondary antibody response, T cells were more affected. Holt et al. (1979) showed that chronic intermittent NO_2 exposure results in a biphasic response.

Antibody titers to sheep red blood cells were increased after 10 weeks of exposure, unchanged at 20 weeks, and decreased at 30 weeks. There were no effects when a T-independent antigen (PVP) was used. A similar biphasis response was observed for a graft vs. host reaction. Response of lymphocytes to PHA was depressed at all exposure times tested. An earlier study (Maigetter et al., 1978) had also reported that the splenic T and B cell response to mitogens was suppressed by NO_2.

In a study of the pulmonary immune system, Joel et al. (1982) observed a temporary decrease in response after a short-term exposure of sheep to NO_2. Pulmonary lymphocytes (from a cannulated mediastinal lymph node) exhibited a reduction in plaque forming cell numbers and response to PHA in animals immunized 2 days, but not 4 days, after exposure to NO_2 ceased.

Complex Particles

Industrial and energy-related processes emit complex particles containing many chemical elements. With few exceptions, these particles have not been investigated for effects on pulmonary defenses. Fly ash is the most notable exception. However, the chemical composition of fly ashes differ, depending based on energy source and combustion techniques (Abbott and Prehnel, 1979; Davidson, et al., 1974), thus a study of one fly ash cannot be taken as necessarily representative of other fly ashes. Since carbon is a major constituent of fly ashes, it too has been investigated. In a few cases carbon or fly ash have been studied in combination with SO_2 and H_2SO_4. The results of this work are only mentioned briefly here. The key studies are summarized in Tables 5 and 6.

Subchronic exposures to high levels of carbon black (Rylander, 1969) decrease pulmonary bactericidal activity, but lower concentrations increased bactericidal activity (Fenters et al., 1979). Alveolar macrophage numbers and viability were unchanged (Fenters et al., 1979). Acute (Gardner, 1981) or subchronic (Fenters et al., 1979) exposures to carbon did not alter bacterial or viral infectivity as measured by excess mortality.

Studies of the effects of carbon on humoral and cell-mediated immunity are complex, being affected differently in relation to time of exposure and route of antigen challenge. Zarkower and Morges (1972) exposed mice to air or carbon for 3-4 or 14-16 days prior to antigen (Ag) challlenge (E. coli, erythrocytes), after which time all the mice received exposure until sacrifice. The most significant alterations were when the Ag challenge was via inhalation as opposed to IV or IP injection. In the spleen, the number of plaque-forming cells was decreased with either a 4 or 15 day pre-exposure. In the mediastinal lymph nodes (MLN), plaque forming cells increased only in the 4 day group. Serum hemagglutination titers were decreased at both exposure times. The increased response in the mediastinal lymph nodes might have been due to the hyperplasia of the nodes; however, the response was observed when the data were expressed per 10 cells or per node. Cell-mediated immunity was also affected in that splenic cells had a transiently decreased Con A-induced transformation (Miller and YZarkower, 1974). LPS-induced transformation was unaffected. In the mediastinal lymph nodes., this decrease with Con A was present at all examination times (7-28 days) and after 14-28 days of exposure, the incorporation of H-thymidine into LPS-treated lymphocytes was increased. Other mice were sensitized to M. tuberculosis via inhalation or subcutaneous injection. When splenic lymphocytes were stimulated with PPD, there was an increased response which was of greater magnitude when the sensitization was via subcutaneous injection.

Zarkower (1972) also conducted similar studies after longer exposure periods (up to 192 days). In the spleen, the number of plaque forming cells/10 cells had a trend towards a decrease at 135 days of exposure which became significant at 192 days. No such effects were observed on the mediastinal lymph nodes, but a similar response was observed when serum hemagglutination titers were measured. Fensters et al. (1979) found a biphasic response when determining effects of carbon on splenic plaque forming cells (Ag. sheep red blood cells). Immunoenhancement was observed after 4 wk of exposure, and suppression occurred by 2o wk.

As mentioned earlier, fly ashes can have quite different chemical compositions. Even more complex is the question of bioavailability. For example, an elemental analysis of fly ash may not increase our understanding of toxicity since some of the elements may not be on the surface, and even then, may not be bioavailable. Garrett et al. (1981) compared the cytotoxicity of fly ashes from 3 energy processes (conventional coal combustion, fluidized bed combustion, and coal gasification) to alveolar macrophages after in vitro exposure. Under equivalent conditions, conventional coal combustion ash was the most toxic whereas coal gasification particles caused little effects. Effects noticed were a decrease in viability, the viability index (a relation between cell lysis and viability), and ATP, with the latter being the most sensitive indicator. When lactate dehydrogenase enzyme release from alveolar macrolphages was measured after in vitro exposure to fly ashes from pulverized coal, stoker-fed, and fluidized bed processes were studied, no effects were observed (Hill and Hobbs, 1982). Fly ash from a fluidized bed process also caused no effects on surface morphology (Hill et al., 1982)

Alveolar macrophages from mice which were exposed acutely to a high concentration of a fine (1.6 m mass median aerodynamic diameter) fraction of ash of conventional coal (low sulfur) combustion process showed a decrease in phagocytosis several days post exposure. It appeared that there was a hematogenous recruitment of alveolar macrophages. The delayed effects are not unexpected since particulate burdens within alveolar macrophages incrased with time post exposure. Clearance of fly ash from the lungs was slow, with only about 6% of the burden being removed in 30 days (Wehner, 1979).

Zarkower and colleagues performed a series of subchronic and chronic exposures to fly ash on alveolar macrophages (Zarkower et al., 1982) and the immune system (Eskew et al., 1982). Exposure for 21, 56, and 148 days to conventional coal fly ash decreased the ability of alveolar macrophages to phagocytocize bacteria. Higher concentrations decrased the ability of alveolar macrophages to enhance mitogenesis of T cells from normal spleens. Longer exposures to higher levels, caused no effect on pulmonary delayed-types hypersentitivity reaction. Little change was observed in the response of splenic lymphocytes to mitogens or target lymphoma cells. The number of antibody-producing cells against an inhaled Ag (E. coli) were not altered in the mediastinal lymph nodes, but a decrease in the spleen was observed at 5 wks. When the length and concentration of fly ash exposure were increased, splenic plaque-forming responses were decreased when Ag was administered by inhalation.

Aranyi et al. (1981, 1982) studied fly ashes and industrial particulate samples after in vitro and in vivo exposure. Using the in vitro rabbit alveolar macrophage assay, potency ranking for effects of viability, cell lysis, and ATP were equivalent with the ranking from high to low toxicity being: copper smelter dust >> aluminum smelter dust >> 2 samples of conventional coal fly ash = fluidized bed fly ash = steel-foundry sample. Inhalation exposure correlates were sought for copper smelter dust and 2 of the coal fly ashes and were found.

The eruption of Mt. St. Helens in 1980 resulted in extremely high levels of human exposure, causing several animal studies of the effects of volcanic ash to be initiated. This research has been reviewed (Martin et al., 1983). Generally, no significant effects were observed on alveolar macrophages following in vitro or intratracheal instillation exposure. When positive controls were used, quartz was substantially more toxic. More recent acute inhalation studies (Grose et al., 1984) showed no or minimal effects on the host defense parameters examined. Thus, it appears that short-term exposures to volcanic ash are without major influence on immunotoxicity.

SUMMARY

The most common ubiquitous air pollutants decrease the function of pulmonary host defense mechanisms against infection. Most of this knowledge is based on animal studies and involves cellular antibacterial defenses such as alveolar macrophage and mucociliary function. Information on viral infectivity is more sparse. Since there is no routine treatment for viral infections, this gap in knowledge is of concern.

In the cases in which lung humoral and cell-mediated immunity have been investigated, effects have been observed. These findings illustrate the complexity of pulmonary immunotoxicity since the direction of the effect (i.e. increase or decrease) was dependent upon concentration, the time of exposure, furthermore systemic and pulmonary immune responses sometimes differed. Thus, future research needs to take into account the kinetics of the immune response vis-a-vis toxicokinetics and dose-rate influences on toxicity. Such considerations raise the level of difficulty of pulmonary immunotoxicity considerably, and without an increase in our basic understanding of these responses, a plethora of studies are required. Hence, it is unreasonable to expect significant improvements of knowledge unless mechanisms of both lung immunolgy and lung immunotoxicity are better understood. An important factor for this future research would be the development of more sensitive and descriptive animal models of lung immunotoxicity and the broader, but selective, utilization of those advanced models that are now available. The establishment of the relevance of the animal model system to the human situation is crucial if extrapolation of the animal results to man under conditions for which human research is impossible/impracticalis to be achieved. The attainment of realistic correlations will require the development of techniques which could ethically be performed in human clinical or epidemiology studies. With such techniques it would be possible to make proper measurements of pulmonary immunotoxicity in the species of greatest interest-man.

When one considers the state-of-the-art of immunotoxicity in general, pulmonary immunotoxicity falls below the norm. Because the lung is one of the major portals of entry of pollutants into the body and there is a degree of compartmentalization between the pulmonary and systemic immune systems, the low level of the state-of-the-art of pulmonary immunotoxicity must be a matter of considerable concern.

There are at present such major gaps in knowledge, that a reasonably accurate assessment of the immunotoxicity of air pollutants is not possible. When the limited data base is reviewed relative to ambient levels of the common pollutants, it appears that acute exposures to O3 and chronic exposures to NO2 are the major exposures of concern for immunotoxic effects. It should be emphasized that until information is available for chronic exposures to low levels of metals and sulfates and for exposures to common organic vapors, the immunotoxicity of air pollutants cannot be assessed.

TABLE 1
EFFECTS OF OZONE ON ALVEOLAR MACROPHAGES (AM)

ppm[a]	Length of Exposure	Effects	Species	Reference
0.1 1.0	2.5 hr in vivo or 30 min in vitro	Lung protective factor partially inactivated, increasing fragility of AM (concentration-related).	Rabbit	Gardner, et al., 1971
0.2	8 hr/day for 7 days	Increased number of AM in lungs (morphological).	Monkey	Castleman et al., 1977 Stephens et al., 1976
0.25 0.50	3 hr (in vivo and in vitro)	Decreased activity of the lysosomal enzymes lysozyme, acid phosphatase, and β-glucuronidase.	Rabbit	Hurst et al., 1970, 1971
0.5	8 hr/day for 7 days	Increased osmotic fragility.	Rabbit	Dowell et al., 1970
0.5	3 hr	Decreased enzyme activity and increased influx of polymorphonuclear leukocytes.	Rabbit	Alpert et al., 1971
0.5	3 hr	Decreased red blood cell rosette binding to AM.	Rabbit	Hadley et al., 1977
0.5 0.67	3 hr	Decreased ability to ingest bacteria.	Rabbit	Coffin et al., 1968b Coffin and Gardner, 1972b
0.5, 1	2 hr (in vitro)	Decreased agglutination in the presence of concanavalin A.	Rat	Goldstein et al., 1977
0.54	23 hr/day for 34 days	Increased number of AM (morphological).	Mouse	Zitnik et al., 1978

ppm[a]	Length of Exposure	Effects	Species	Reference
0.8	11 and 24 days (in vivo)	No effect on in vitro interferon production.	Mouse	Ibrahim et al., 1976
0.8	90 days	Eightfold increase in number of AM at 7 days, reducing to fourfold after days.	Rat	Boorman et al., 1977
0.8	7 days	Decreased number of migrating AM and total distance migrated.	Monkey	Schwartz and Christman, 1979
0.8	3, 7, 20 days	Increased phagocytosis.	Rat	Christman and Schwartz, 1982
1,5	3 hr	Decreased ability to produce interferon in vitro.	Rabbit	Shingu et al., 1980
1	4 hr	Decreased in vitro migrational ability, as evidenced by decreased number of AM able to migrate.	Rat	McAllen et al., 1981
1.6 to 3.5	2 hr to 3 hr	Decreased superoxide anion radical production.	Rat	Amoruso et al., 1981 Witz et al., 1982
2.5	5 hr	Loss of β-glucuronidase and acid phosphatase in AM with ingested bacteria; decreased rate of bacterial ingestion and killing; increased numbers of intracellular staphylococcal clumps; lack of lysozyme in AM with staphylococcal clumps.	Rat	Goldstein et al., 1978b Kimura and Goldstein, 1981

[a] ppm = parts per million

TABLE 2

EFFECTS OF OZONE ON SUSCEPTIBILITY TO INFECTIOUS AGENTS

ppm[a]	Length of Exposure	Effects	Species	Reference
0.08, 0.1	3 hr	Increase in mortality during and after O_3 exposure (Streptococcus pyogenes). Exercise enhances mortality.	Mouse	Coffin et al., 1968 Miller et al., 1978 Ehrlich et al., 1977 Illing et al., 1980
0.1	5 hr/day, 5 days/wk for 103 days	Increased mortality to bacterial infection (S. pyogenes).	Mouse	Aranyi et al., 1983
0.2-0.7	3-4 hr	Increase in mortality ($<$ 0.4 ppm) to Klebsiella pneumoniae.	Mouse	Bergers et al., 1982
0.3	3 hr/day for 2 days	Enhancement of severity of bacterial pneumonia (Pasturella haemolytica).	Sheep	Abraham et al., 1982
1.0	3 hr/day, 5 days/wk for 8 weeks	Increase in Mycobacterium tuberculosis lung titers.	Mouse	Thomas et al., 1981
1.5	4 hr/day, 5 days/wk for 2 months	No effect on resistance to M. tuberculosis.	Mouse	Thienes et al., 1965

[a] ppm = parts per million

TABLE 3

EFFECTS OF NITROGEN DIOXIDE ON SUSCEPTIBILITY TO INFECTIOUS AGENTS

ppm[a]	Length of Exposure	Exposure / Effects	Species	Reference
0.3-0.5	6 mo	No enhancement of effect of NO_2 on influenza infection.	Mouse	Motomiya et al., 1973
0.5	(6 or 18 hr/day Intermittent, 12 mo.	Increased mortality to K. pneumoniae after 6 mo intermittent exposure or after 3, 6, 9, or 12 mo continuous exposure.	Mouse	Ehrlich and Henry, 1968
0.5-1	39 days, continuous	Increased susceptibility to influenza.	Mouse	Ito, 1971
0.5 5	3-8 mo, continuous 7 days, continuous	Increased mortality to K. pneumoniae at 5 ppm	Mouse	McGrath and Oyervides
1-6.6	17 hr	Decreased bactericidal activity $\geq$ 2.3 ppm.	Mouse	Goldstein et al., 1973b
1.5-28		Increased mortality to streptococcus sp. with increased time and concentration.	Mouse	Gardner et al., 1979
1,3	3 hr	Exercise increased mortality to streptococcus sp. (3 ppm).	Mouse	Illing et al., 1980
1.5	Continuous or intermittent (7 hr/day)	After 1 wk, mortality to streptococcus sp. with continuous exposure greater than that for intermittent. After 2 wk, no difference between exposure regimens.	Mouse	Gardner et al., 1979
3.5	Continuous or intermittent (7 hr/day) to 15 days.	Increased mortality with increased duration of exposure. No difference between continuous and intermittent exposure.		

TABLE 3 Cont'd

ppm[a]	Length of Exposure	Effects	Species	Reference
1.9-14.8	4 hr	Decrease in bactericidal activity $\geq$ 7 ppm.	Mouse	Goldstein et al., 1973b
2	3 hr	Increased mortality to Streptococcus sp.	Mouse	Ehrlich et al., 1977
3.5 35 50	2 hr 2 hr 2 hr	Increased mortality to K. pneumoniae.	Mouse Hamster	Ehrlich, 1975 Henry et al., 1969, 1970

[a] ppm = parts per million

TABLE 4

EFFECTS OF NITROGEN DIOXIDE ON ALVEOLAR MACROPHAGES (AM)

ppm[a]	Length of Exposure	Effects	Species	Reference
0.5	33 wks, cont. (5 days/wk, 1 hr peaks to 2 ppm)	AM surface morphological alterations after 21 wk. Surface morphological changes.	Mouse	Aranyi et al., 1976
2	6 mo	Decreased response to migration inhibition factor.	Baboon	Green and Schneider, 1978
3.6, 12.1	1 hr, 2 hr	Increase in Con-A agglutination of AM.	Rat	Goldstein et al., 1977
7	24 hr	Increased rosette formation in AM treated with wheat germ lipase.	Rabbit	Hadley et al., 1977
8-60	3 hr	Increased number of polymorphonuclear leukocytes in lavage.	Rabbit	Gardner et al., 1969
10, 25	24 hr	Phagocytic activity unchanged. Depressed phagocytosis on 3rd day of culture.	Rat	Katz and Laskin, 1975
10	7 wk continuous	Increased number of AM.	Guinea Pig	Sherwin et al., 1968
10	3 hr	Inhibition of phagocytosis.	Rabbit	Gardner et al., 1969
25	3 hr	No development of resistance with NO_2 exposure immediately after infection with parainfluenza-3 virus or up to 24 hr before viral inoculation. Increased lung absorption of virus. No effect on viral potency.	Rabbit	Valand et al., 1970 Williams et al., 1972
25	3 hr	Uptake of parainfluenza-3 virus not affected. Twice as many virus attached and penetrated AM.		

[a] ppm = parts per million

Pollutant	Concentration (gas, ppm) (particles, mg/m³)	Length of Exposure	Effects	Species	Reference
Carbon black	15 mg/m³	6 hr/day 4 days/wk 4 wk	No effect on tracheobronchial clearance of bacteria.	Guinea pigs	Rylander 1969
Carbon black + SO$_2$	15 mg/m³ and 10 ppm	6 hr/day 5 days/wk 4 wk	Slowed tracheobronchial clearance of dead bacteria. Synergistic effect.	Guinea pigs	Rylander 1969
Carbon black	1.5 mg/m³	3 hr/day 5 days/wk 4, 12, 20 wk	No effect on cell numbers or viability.	Mouse	Fenters et al., 1979
Fly ash (conventional coal)	0.2 mg/l	2 hr	6 and 15, but not 2, days post-exposure, ↓ phagocytosis. No effect on viability. 2 days post-exposure ↓ adherence to glass. No effect on AM precursors in bone marrow. Initial (2 day) ↓ in AM, followed by (day 6, 15) AM ↑.	Mouse	Fisher & Wilson, 1980
Fly ash (conventional coal)	0.5 0.8 mg/m³	24 hr/day 7-148 days	↓ Phagocytosis (0.5 mg/m³; ↓ ability to enhance PHA-induced mitogenesis of splenic lymphocytes (0.8 mg/m³).	Mouse	Zarkower et al., 1982

TABLE 5 Cont'd

Pollutant	Concentration (gas, ppm) (particles, mg/m³)	Length of Exposure	Effects	Species	Reference
Volcanic ash	9.4 mg/m³	2 hr	Mice: No effect on mortality due to Streptococcus sp. aerosol. Rats: Inflammatory response; no effect on alveolar macrophage phagocytosis; decrease in ciliary beating frequency.	Mouse Rat	Grose et al., 1984
Carbon black	1.5 mg/m³	3 hr/day 5 days/wk 4, 12, 20 wk	Carbon only: Increased bactericidal activity at 4 and 12 wk of exp; No effect on influenza virus-induced mortality. Carbon + H$_2$SO$_4$: Same as above, except increase in mort.	Mouse	Fenters et al., 1979
Carbon black SO$_2$	15 mg/m³ 10 ppm	6 hr/day 5 days/wk, 4 wk	Greater number of viable bacteria in lungs (carbon only). When SO$_2$ added, no effect.	Guinea pig	Rylander, 1969
Carbon	5 mg/m³	2 hr	No effect on streptococcal-induced mortality.	Mouse.	Gardner, 1981

TABLE 6

EFFECT OF COMPLEX PARTICLES ON IMMUNE SYSTEM

Pollutant	Concentration (gas, ppm) (particles, mg/m³)	Length of Exposure	Effects	Species	Reference
Carbon black	0.8-1.9 1.9	24 hr/day 3/4 or 14/18 days before antigen (Ag) 4-5 days after Ag.	Ag by inhalation: ↓ PFC/spleen, ↑ PFC/mediastinal lymph nodes, ↓ hemagglutination inhibition titer	Mouse	Zarkower and Morges, 1972
Carbon black	1.5 mg/m³	24 hr/day 7, 14, 21, or 28 days	Spleen: ↓ response to Con A at 7 days; ↑ at later times; no change in LPS response; after sensitization to M. tuberculosis; ↑ response to PPD. Mediastinal lymph nodes: ↓ Con A response; no change in LPS response at 7 days, but ↑ thereafter.	Mouse	Miller and Zarkower, 1974
Carbon black SO_2 SO_2 + Carbon	0.56 mg/m³	100 hr/wk 102, 135, 192 days	Spleen: ↓ PFC (192 days), all 3 exposure groups Mediastinal lymph node: no effect on PFC, carbon or SO_2; ↑ PFC (192 days), SO_2 + Carbon. Hemagglutination inhibition titers ↓ 192 days, all 3 exposure groups, ↑ 135 days in SO_2 group.	Mouse	Zarkower 1972
Carbon black H_2SO_4	1.5 mg/m³ 1.4 mg/m³	3 hr/day 5 days/wk 4, 12, 20 wk	Carbon only: ↑ PFC (4 wk), no effect (12 wk), ↓ PFC 20 wk. Serum Ig altered (most ↓) at 1 wk, not later times. Carbon + H_2SO_4: Similar effect, except Ig altered at all exposure times.	Mouse	Fenters et al., 1979
Fly ash (conventional coal)	2.2 mg/m³	24 hr/day 160 days	No effect on ability of BCG-sensitized mice to respond to intratracheal instillation of PPD.	Mouse	Zarkower et al., 1982

TABLE 6 Cont'd

Pollutant	Concentration (gas, ppm) (particles, mg/m³)	Length of Exposure	Effects	Species	Reference
Fly ash conventional coal	0.7-2.2 mg/m³	24 hr/day 9 mo	Increase in response of splenic lymphocytes to Con A only after 1 wk exposure; no effect with LPS or PPD (in BCG-sensitized mice. No effect on cytolytic activity. Decrease in splenic plaque response at 5 wk and 9 mo of exposure.	Mouse	Eskew et al., 1982
Volcanic ash	9.4 mg/m³	2 hr/day 5 days	Slight increase in response of splenic lymphocytes to LPS. No change in PHA response.	Mouse	Grose et al., 1984

REFERENCES

Abbott, J.H. & Drehnel, D.C. (1979). Control of particulates from combustion. In Proceedings, Symposium on the Transfer and Utilization of Particulate Control Technology. EPA-600/7-79-044b, pp. 383-405. U.S.E.P.A., Research Triangle Park, NC.

Abraham. W.M. Januszkiewicz, A.J., Mingle, M., Welker, M., Wanner, A. & Sackner, M.A. (1980). Sensitivity of bronchoprovocation and tracheal mucous velocity in detecting airway responses to O3 . J. Appl. Physiol. Respirat Environ. Exercise Physiol., 48 : 789-793.

Abraham. W.M., Lauredo, I., Sielczak, M., Yerger, L., King, M.M. & Ratzan, K. (Supplement 1982). Enhancement of bacterial pneumonia in sheep by ozone exposure. (Abstract Am. Rev. Resp. Dis. p. 148.

Acton, J.D. & Myrvik, Q.N. (1972). Nitrogen dioxide effects on alveolar macrophages. Arch. Environ Health, 24: 48-52.

Alpert, S.M. Gardner, D.E., Hurst, D.J., Lewis, T.R. & Coffin, D.L. (1971). Effects of exposure to ozone on defensive mechanisms of the lung. J. Appl. Physiol., 31: 247-252.

Amoruso, M.A. Witz, G. & Goldstein, B.D. (1981). Decreased superoxide anion radical production by rat alveolar macrophages following inhalation of ozone or nitrogen dioxide. Life Sci., 28: 2215-2221.

Aranyi, C., Fenters, J., Ehrlich, R. & Gardner, D. (1976). Scanning electron microscopy of alveolar macrophages after exposure to O3 , NO2 and O3 . Environ. Health Persp., 16: 180.

Aranyi, C. Gardner, D.E. & Huisingh, J.L. (1981). Evaluation of potential inhalation hazard of particulate silicious compounds by in vitro rabbit alveolar macrophage tests - application to industrial particulates containing hazardous impurities. In Health effects of Synthetic Silia Particulates, (eds. Dunnon, D.D.) ASTM STP732, pp. 48-57. American Society for Testing and Materials.

Aranyi, C., Bradof, J., Gardner, D.E. & Huisingh, J.C. (1981). In vitro and in vivo evaluation of potential toxicity of industrial particulates. In Short Term Bioassays in the Analysis of Complex Environmental Mixtures, (eds. Waters, M.D., Sandhu, S.S., Huisingh, J.L., Claxton, L. and Nesnow, J.) pp. 431-444. Environmental Science Research, Plenum Press, Vol. 22.

Aranyi, C., Vana, S.C., Thomas, P.T., Bradof, J.N., Fenters, J.D., Graham, J.A. & Miller, F.J. (1983). Effects of subchronic exposure to a mixture of O3 , SO2 and (NH4) SO4 on host defenses in mice. Environ Res., 12: 55-71.

Bergers, W.W.A., Gerbrandy, J.L.F., Stap, J.G. & Dura, E.A. (1982). Influence of air polluting components vis. ozone and the open air factor on host-resistance towards respiratory infections. In International Symposium on the Biomedical Effects of Ozone and Related Photochemical Oxidants, March 1982; Pinehurst, N.C., (eds. Lee, S.D., Mustafa, M.G.and Mehlman, M.A.) pp. 459-467. Princeton Scientific Publishers, Inc., Princeton, N.J.

Bice, D.E. (1984). Methods and approaches for assessing immunotoxicity of the lower respiratory tract. In Toxicology of the Immune System, (eds. Dean, J.A., Munson, A. and Luster M.) (in press). Raven Press, New York.

Boorman, G.A., Schwartz, L.W., McQuillen, N.K. & Brummer, M.E. (1977). Pulmonary response following long-term intermittent exposure to ozone: structural and morphological changes. Am. Rev. Resp. Dis., 115: 201-210.

Brody, A.R. & Davis, G.A. (1982). Alveolar macrophage toxicology. In Mechanisms in Respiratory Toxicology Vol. II, (eds, Witschi H. and Nettersheim, P.) pp. 4-24. CRC Press, Inc., Florida.

Brummer, M.E.G., Schwartz, L.W. & McQuillen, N.K. (1977). A quantitative study of lung damage by scanning electon microscopy. Inflammatory cell response to high-ambient levels of ozone. Scan. Elec. Micros., 2: 513-518.

Campbell, K.I. & Hilsenroth, R.H. (1976). Impaired resistance to toxin in toxoid-immunized mice exposed to ozone on nitrogen dioxide. Clin. Toxicol., 9: 943-954.

Castleman, W.L., Tyler, W.S. & Dungworth, D.L. (1977). Lesions respiratory bronchioles and conducting airways of monkeys exposed to ambient levels of ozone. Exp. Mol. Pathol., 26: 384-400.

Coffin, D.L., Blommer, E.J. Gardner, D.E. & Holzman, R. (1968). Effect of air pollution on alteration of susceptibility to pulmonary infections. In Proceedings of the 3rd Annual Conference on Atmospheric Contaminants in Confined Spaces, pp. 71-80. AMRL-TR-67-200, Aerospace Medical Research Laboratories, Wright-Patterson Air Force Base, Dayton, Ohio.

Coffin, D.L. & Gardner, D.E. (1972). Interaction of biological agents and chemical air pollutants. Ann. Occup. Hyg., 15: 219-235.

Davidson, R.L., Natusch, D.F.S., Wallace, J.R. & Evans, C.A., Jr. (1974). Trace elements in fly ash. Dependence of concentration on particle size. Environ. Sci. Technol., 8: 1107-1113.

Dowell, A.R., Lohrbauer, L.A. Hurst, D. & Lee, S.D. (1970). Rabbit alveolar macrophage damage caused by in vivo ozone inhalation. Arch. Environ. Health, 21: 121-127.

Ehrlich, R. (1975). Interaction between NO₂ exposure and respiratory infections. In Scientific Seminar on Automotive Pollutants, EPA-600/9-75-003. U.S. Environmental Protection Agency, Washington, D.C.

Ehrlich, R. & Fenters, J.D. (1973). Influence of nitrogen dioxide on experimental influenza in squirrel monkeys. In Proceedings Third International Clean Air Congress A11-A13. Dusseldorf, W. Germany.

Ehrlich, R., Silverstein, E., Maigetter, R., Fenters, J.D. & Gardner D.E. (1975). Immunologic response in vaccinated mice during long-term exposure to nitrogen dioxide. Environ. Res., 10: 217-223.

Ehrlich, R., Findlay, J.C. & Gardner, D.E. (1977). Effects of repeated exposures to peak concentrations of nitrogen dioxide and ozone on resistance to streptococcal pneumonia. J. Toxicol. Environ. Health, 5: 631-642.

Environmental Protection Agency (1978). Air Quality Criteria for Ozone and Other Photochemical Oxidants EPA-600/8-78-004, Ch. 8-10, U.S. Environmental Protection Agency, ECAO, Research Triangle Park, North Carolina.

Environmental Protection Agency (1982a). Air Quality Criteria for Particulate Matter and Sulfur Oxides, Vol. III, EPA-600/ 8-82-0298, Ch. 11-14, U.S. Environmental Protection Agency, ECAO, Research Triangle Park, NC.

Environmental Protection Agency (1982b). Air Quality Criteria for Nitrogen Oxides, EPA-600/8-82-026, Ch. 14-15. U.S. Environmental Protection Agency, ECAO, Research Triangle Park, NC.

Eskew, M.L., Zarkower, A., Scheuchenzuber, W.J. & Graham, J.A. (1982). Effects of fly ash on murine immune functions: Effects on systemic response. Environ. Res., 28: 375-385

Fenters, J.D. Bradof, J.N., Aranyi, C., Ketels, K., Ehrlich, R. & Gardner, D.E. (1979). Health effects of long-term inhalation of sulfuric acid mist-carbon particle mixtures. Environ. Res., 19: 244-257.

Fenters, J.D., Ehrlich, P., Spangler, J. & Tolkacz, V. (1971). Serologic response in squirrel monkeys exposed to nitrogen dioxide and influenza virus. Am. Rev. Resp. Dis., 104: 448-451.

Fenters, J.D., Findlay, J.P., Port, C.D., Ehrlich, R. & Coffin, D.L. (1973). Chronic exposure to nitrogen dioxide: immunologic, physiologic and pathologi effect in virus-challenged squirrel monkeys. Arch. Environ. Health, 27: 85-89.

Fisher, G.L. & Wilson, F.D. (1980). *The effects of coal fly ash and silica inhalation of macrophage function and progenitors.* J. Reticuloendothel. Soc., 27: 513-524.

Frager, N.B., Phalen, R.F. & Kenoyer, J.L. (1979). *Adaptations to ozone in reference to mucociliary clearance.* Arch. Environ. Health, 34: 51-57.

Friberg, L., Holman, B. & Rylander, R. (1972). *Animal lung reactions after inhalation of lead and ozone.* Environ. Physiol. Biochem., 2: 170-178.

Fujimaki, H., Shimizu, F. & Kubota, K. (1981). *Suppression of antibody response in mice by acute exposure to nitrogen dioxide: In vitro study.* Environ. Res. , 26: 490-496.

Gardner, D.E. (1979). *Impairment of pulmonary defense following inhalation exposure to cadmium, nickel and manganese.* In Aerosols in Science , Medicine and Technology, (eds. Stober, W. and Jaenicke, R.) pp. 120-132. *Max Planck Institute for Chemie, Mainz, Germany.*

Gardner, D.E. (1982). *Effects of gases and airborne particles on lung infections.* In Air Pollution - Physiological Effects, (eds. McGrath, J.J. and Barnes C.D.) pp. 47-79. *Academic Press.*

Gardner, D.E. & Graham, J.A. (1976). *Increased pulmonary disease mediated through altered bacterial defenses.* In Pulmonary Macrophage and Epithelial Cells, (eds. Schneider, R.P., Doyle, G.E. and Ragan, H.A.) pp. 1-21. *Proceedings Sixteenth Annual Hanford Biology Symposium, Richland, Washington.*

Gardner, D.E., Holzman, R.S. & Coffin, D.L. (1969). *Effects of nitrogen dioxide on pulmonary cell population.* J. Bacteriol., 98: 1041-1043.

Gardner. D.E., Coffin, D.L., Pinigin, M.A. & Sidorenko, G.I. (1977a). *Role of time as a factor in the toxicity of chemical compounds in intermittent and continuous exposures. Part I. Effects of continuous exposure.* J. Toxicol. Environ. Health, 3: 811-820.

Gardner, D.E., Miller, F.J., Blommer, E.J. & Coffin, D.L. (1977b). *Relationship between nitrogen dioxide concentration, time and level of effect using an animal infectivity model.* In Proceedings International Conference on Photochemical Oxidant Pollution and ist Control, Vol.I pp.513-525. *EPA-600/3-77-001a. U.S.Environmental Protection Agency.*

Gardner, D.E., Miller, F.J., Blommer, E.J. & Coffin, D.L. (1979). *Influence of exposure mode on the toxicity of NO_2 .* Environ Health Persp., 30: 23-29.

Gershwin, L.J., Osebold, J.W. & Zee, Y.C. (1981). Immuno-globulin E containing cells in mouse lung following allergen inhalation and ozone exposure. Int. Arch. Allergy Appl. Immun., 65: 266-277.

Giordano, A.M. & Morrow, P.E. (1972). Chronic low-level nitrogen dioxide exposure and mucociliary clearance. Arch. Environ. Health, 25:443-449.

Goldstein, B.D., Hamburger, S.J., Falk, G.W. & Amoruso, M.A. (1977). Effect of ozone and nitrogen dioxide on the agglutination of rat alveolar macrophages of concanavalin A. Life Sci., 21: 1637-1644.

Goldstein, E., Eagle, M.C. & Hoeprich, P.D. (1973). Effect of nitrogen dioxide on pulmonary bacterial defense mechanisms.Arch. Environ Health, 26: 202-204.

Goldstein. E., Warshauer, D., Lippert, W. & Tarkington, B (1974). Ozone and nitrogen dioxide exposure. Arch. Environ. Health, 28:85-90.

Graham, J.A. & Gardner, D.E. (1984). Immunotoxicity of air pollutants. In Toxicology of the Immune System, (eds. Dean, J.A., Munson, A. And Luster, M.) (in press). Raven Press, New York.

Greene, N.D. & Schneider, S.L. (1978). Effects of NO2 on the response of baboon alveolar macrophages to migration inhibitory factor. J. Toxicol. Environ Health, 4: 869-880.

Grose, E.C., Gardner, D.E. & Miller, F.J. (1980) Response of ciliated epithelium to ozone and sulfuric acid. Environ. Res., 22: 377-385

Grose, E.C., Grady, M.A., Illing, J.W., Daniels, M.J., Selgrade, M.J.K. & Hatch, G.E. (1984). Inhalation studies of Mt. St. Helens volcanic ash in animals: Host defense mechanisms. Environ Res., accepted for publication.

Hadley, J.G. Gardner, D.E., Coffin, D.L. & Menzel, D.B. (1977). Effects of ozone and nitrogen dioxide exposure of rabbits on the binding of autologous red cells to alveolar macrophages. In Proceedings International Conference Photochemical Oxidant Pollution and its Control, Vol. I, pp. 505-511. EPA-600/3-77-001a. U.S. Environmental Protection Agency.

Hidekazu, F. & Fujio, S. (1981). Effects of acute exposure to nitrogen dioxide on primary antibody response. Arch. Environ. Health, 36: 114-119.

Hill, J.O., Gray, R.H., DeNee, P.B. & Newton, G.J. (1982). Comparative damage to alveolar macrophages after phagocytosis of respirable particles. Environ. Res., 27: 95-109.

Hill, J.O. & Hobbs, C.H. (1982). Comparative cytotoxicity of DQ12-quart and fly ash particles from coal combustion. Toxicol. Lett., 10: 399-403.

Holt, P.G., Finlay-Jones,L.M., Keast, D. & Papadimitrou, J.M. (1979). Immunological function in mice chronically exposed to nitrogen oxides. Environ. Res., 19: 154-162.

Hurst, D.J. & Coffin, D.L. (1971). Ozone effect on lysosomal hydrolases of alveolar macrophages in vitro. Arch. Intern. Med., 127: 1059-1063.

Hurst, D.J., Gardner, D.E. & Coffin, D.L. (1970). Effect of ozone on acid hydrolases of the pulmonary alveolar macrophage. Res. J. Reticuloendothel. Soc., 8: 288-300.

Ito, K. (1971). Effect of nitrogen dioxide inhalation on influenza virus infection in mice. Jap. J. Hygiene, 26: 304-314 (in Japanese).

Joel, D.D., Chandra, P. & Chanana, A.D. (1982). Effects of NO2 on immune responses in pulmonary lymph of sheep. J. Toxicol. Environ. Health, 10: 341-348.

Katz, G.V. & Laskin, S. (1977). Effect of irritant atmospheres on macrophage behavior. In Pulmonary Macrophage and Epithelial Cells , (eds. Sanders, C.C., Schneider, R.P., Dagle, G.E. and Ragan, J.)pp. 358-373. Tech. Inf. Center,Oak Ridge, Tenn.

Kenoyer, J.L., Phalen, R.F. & Davis, J.R. (1981). Particle clearance from the respiratory tract as a test of toxicity: Effect of ozone on short and long term clearance. Exp. Lung. Res., 2: 111-120.

Kimura, A. & Goldstein, E. (1981). Effect of ozone on concentrations of lysozyme in phagocytizing alveolar macrophages. J. Infect. Dis., 143: 247-251.

Kita, H. & Omichi, S. (1974). Effects of air pollutants on cilia movement in airways. Jap. J. Hyg., 28: 100 (in Japanese).

Last, J.A. & Kaizu, T. (1980). Mucus glycoprotein secretion by tracheal explants: effects of pollutants. Environ. Health Perspect., 35: 131-138.

Last, J.A., Jennings, M. & Cross, C.E. (1977). Mucus glycoprotein secretion by tracheal explants from rats exposed to ozone. Fed. Proc., 36: 413.

Maigetter, R.Z., Fenters, J.D., Findlay, J.C., Ehrlich, R. & Gardner, D.E. (1978). Effect of exposure to nitrogen dioxide on T and B cells in mouse spleen. Toxicol. Letters, 2: 157-161.

Martin, T.R., Wehner, A.P. & Butler, J. (1983). *Pulmonary toxicity of Mt. St. Helens volcanic ash.* Amer. Rev. Resp. Dis., 128: 138-143.

McAllen, S.J., Chiu, S.P., Phalen, R.F. & Rasmussen, R.E. (1981). *Effect of in vitro pulmonary alveolar macrophage mobility.* J. Toxicol. Environ. Health, 7: 373-381.

McGrath, J.J. & Oyervides, J. (1983). *Response of NO2-exposed mice to Klebsiella challenge.* In The Biome-dical Effects of Ozone and Related Photochemical Oxidants, (eds. Lee, S.D. Mustafa, M.G. and Mehlman, M.A.) pp. 486-495. Princeton Scientific Publishers, Inc., Princeton, N.J.

Miller, F.J., Illing, J.W. & Gardner, D.E. (1978). *Effects of urban ozone levels on laboratory induced respiratory infections.* Toxicol. Letters, 2: 163-169.

Miller, F.J., Gardner, D.E., Graham, J.A., Lee, R.E., Wilson, W.E. & Bachman, J.D. (1979). *Size considerations for establishing a standard for inhalable particles.* J. A. P. C. A., 26: 610-615.

Miller, S.D. & Zarkower, A. (1974). *Effects of carbon dust inhalation on the cell-mediated immune response in mice.* Infect. Immunity, 9: 534-539.

Miller, S.D. & Zarkower, A. (1974). *Alterations of murine immunologic responses after silica dust inhalation.* J. Immunol, 113: 1533-1543.

Motomiya, T., Ito, K., Yoshida, R., Ide, G. & Nakishima, Y. (1973). *The effects of exposure to NO2 gas in the infection of influenza virus of mouse.* Resp. Environ. Res. Organ. Chiba Univ.

Nakajima, T., Kusumoto, S., Oda, H., Nogami, H. & Shingu, H. (1980). *Biological effects of exposure to photochemical reaction mixture.* In Proceedings of V, pp. 785-789. Clean Air Congress, Buenos Aires, S.A.

Nakamura, S., Nakayama, Y., Miura, T. & Mori, K.J. (1971). *Effects of NO2 gas exposure on antibody formation.* Osaka Prefect. Inst. Public Health, 9: 20-22.

Osebold, L.W., Gershwin, L.J. & Zee, Y.C. (1980). *Studies on the enhancement of allergic lung sensitization by inhalation of ozone and sulfuric acid aerosols.* J. Environ. Pathol. Toxicol., 3: 221-234.

Osebold, J.W., Owens, S.L., Zee, Y.C., Dotson, W.M. & La Barre, D.D. (1979). *Immunological alterations in the lungs of mice following ozone exposure: Changes in immunoglobulin levels and antibody-containing cells.* Arch. Environ. Health, 34: 258-265.

Peterson, M.L., Harder, S., Rummo, N. & House, D.   (1978a).
Effect of ozone on leukocyte function in exposed human
subjets. Environ. Res., 15: 485-493.

Peterson, M.L., Rummo, N., House, D. & Harder, S.   (1978b).
Effect of ozone on human immunity: In vitro responsi-
veness of lymphocytes to phytohemmagglutinin. Arch.
Environ. Health, 33: 59-63.

Phalen, R.F., Kenoyer, J.L., Crocker, T.T. & McClure, T.R.
(1980). Effects of sulfate aerosols in combination with
ozone on elimination of tracer particles inhalated by
rats. J. Toxicol. Environ. Health, 6: 797-810.

Rylander, R. (1969). Alterations of lung defense mechanisms
against airborne bacteria. Arch. Environ. Health, 18:
551-555.

Savino, A., Peterson, M.C., House, D., Turner, A.G., Jeffries,
H. & Baker, R. (1978): The effect of ozone on human
cellular and humoral immunity. Environ. Res., 15:
65-69.

Schwartz, L.K. & Christman, C.A. (1979). Alveolar macrophage migration. Influence of lung lining material and
acute lung insult. Am. Rev. Respir. Dis., 120:
429-439.

Sherwin, R.P., Richters, V., Brooks, M. & Buckley, R.D.
(1968). The phenomenon of macrophage congregation in
vitro and its relationship to in vivo NO2 exposure of
guinea pigs. Lab. Invest., 18: 169-277.

Sherwood, R.L., Lippert, W.E., Goldstein & Tarkington, B.
(1981). Effect of ferrous sulfate aerosols and nitrogen
dioxide on murine pulmonary defense. Arch. Environ.
Health, 36: 130-135.

Shingu, H., Sugiyama, M., Watanabe, M. & Nakajima, T.
(1980). Effects of ozone and photochemical oxidants on
interferon production by rabbit alveolar macrophages.
Bull. Environ. Contam. Toxicol., 24: 433-438.

Thomas, G.B., Fenters, J.D., Ehrlich, R. & Gardner, D.E.
(1981). Effects of exposure to ozone on susceptibility
to experimental tuberculosis. Toxicol. Lett., 9:
11-17.

Valand, S.B., Acton, J.D. & Myrvik, Q.N. (1970). Nitrogen
dioxide inhibition of viral-induced resistance in alveolar monocytes. Arch. Environ. Health, 20: 303-309.

Wehner, A.P., Moss, O.R., Milliman, E.M., Dagle,G.E. &
Schirmer, R.E. (1979). Acute and subchronic inhalation
exposures of hamsters to nickel-enriched fly ash.
Environ. Resp., 19: 355-370.

Witz, G., Amoruso, M.A. & Goldstein, B.D. (1982). Effect of ozone on on alveolar macrophage function: membrane dynamic properties. In International Symposium on Biomedical Effects of Ozone and Related Photochemical Oxidants, Pinehurst, N.C. (eds. Lee. S.D. and Mustafa, M.G.) pp. 263-272. Princeton Scientific Publishers, Inc. Princeton, N.J.

Zarkower, A. (1972). Alterations in antibody response induced by chronic inhalation of SO_2 and carbon. Arch.Environ. Health 25: 45-50.

IMMUNOTOXICITY OF ORGANOTIN COMPOUNDS.
A CELL BIOLOGICAL APPROACH
TO DIALKYLTIN INDUCED THYMUS ATROPHY

A.H. Penninks & W. Seinen.

Working Group Pathology-Toxicology,
Pathology-Toxicology Department,
Faculty of Veterinary Sciences, State University of Utrecht,
The Netherlands

INTRODUCTION

In the last decade immunotoxicity has developed into a new area of drug and chemical toxicity as result of a growing number of compounds that are known to alter immunological responsiveness, either by an immunosuppression or an immunostimulation. The most conspicuous need is for much more information about the underlying molecular mechanisms. Only then will it be possible to explain why in some cases components of the immune system are so extremely sensitive. From reported data it is apparent that various compounds i.e. 2,3,7,8-tetrachlorodibenzo-p-dioxin (TCDD), 2,3,7,8-tetra chlorodi benzofuran (TCDF), polychlorinated biphenyls (PCBs), polybrominated biphenyls (PBBs), diethylstilbestrol (DES) and some di- and tri-alkyl substituted organotins act more or less preferentially on the thymus and therefore probably on thymus dependent functions (1-4). Although these compounds all produce thymic injury, they probably act at several different levels. To get more insight in the diand trialkyltin induced immune suppression studies our group has focussed on their ability to produce selective thymus atrophy. After a short overview of organotin applications, toxicity and immunosuppressive effects, the mechanisms that might be involved in the dialkyltin induced thymolytic effects are discussed in more detail.

ORGANOTINS AND THEIR APPLICATION

Organotins is the common name assigned to the group of compounds with at least one bond between carbon and tin. commercially, major subgroups are referred to as di- and tri-substituted organotin compounds, R2SnX2 and R3SnX respectively. Usually R stands for an alkylchain of different length or an aryl group and X for chloride, fluoride, oxide, hydroxide, carboxylate or thiolate. Recently a new class of organotin compounds was introduced into the market, the estertins in which an ester group is incorporated in aliphatic alkylchain (5).

The organotin compounds of industrial importance are used in three major types of application: (1) as heat stabilizers in polymers, (2) as biocides and (3) as catalysts (6-8). Dialkyltins, in particular di-n-butyltin and di-n-octyltin derivatives are used as stabilizers for PVC plastics to protect against degradation by heat and light during the production phase and use as well. Recently dimethyltin and diestertin compounds have also been found to be suitable for this purpose. Dialkytin derivatives are also used as catalysts in the production of polyurethane foam products and as vulcanizing agent for silicone rubbers. Trialkyltins are widely used as industrial and agricultural biocides. Triphenyltin and tricyclohexyltin derivatives have important use as agricultural fungicides and acaricides and tributyltin compounds have many applications as industrial biocide. In particular bis (tri-n-butyltin) oxide (TBTO) is used as preservative for wood, paper, textiles, leather and glass, and as an antifoulant and disinfectant. Tributyltin derivatives have also been proposed as a molluscicide for the control of the aquatic snails, that are the intermediate hosts for the parasite that causes Schistosomiasis in man (9-10).

This multiplicity of applications has resulted in an enormous growth in the worldwide production of organotin compounds. In 1976 the synthesis of organometallics was approximately 27000 tons and is expected to grow to about 63000 tons in 1986 (11) of which 70 percent will be used to heat-stabilize PVC plastic products. This enormous growth may have profound implications for environmental and occupational exposure to organotins. However, no serious environmental effects of organotins have been observed so far, although a number of occupational hazards have been described (12). The use of an organotin compounds (diethyltin, diiodide stalinon), for the treatment of staphylococcal skin infections resulted in a mass poisoning in 1954. Due to a contamination of a badge with triethyliodide, a powerful neurotoxin, 110 patients died of the 217 known to have been poisoned (13).

TOXICITY OF ORGANOTIN COMPOUNDS

The toxicity of organotin compounds is mainly determined by the number and nature of the organic groups. In general the toxicity decreases with increasing chain length of the alkyl group linked to the tin. In mammals the toxicity of di-and trialkyltins differ considerably; dialkyltins are found stringly hepatotoxic, whereas trialkyltins are potent neurotoxins (8,10,14,15). The dialkyltin compounds with methyl to hexyl substitutions induce bile duct lesions in rat and mice, but not in the guinea pig or cat (16). The higher homologs-octyl or above- were found to be much less toxic by oral administration, and even considered to be biologically inactive (14). In the dialkyltin series the lower homologs cause skin irritation (17). Although little is known about the toxicity of estertins diestertin compounds appear to be much less toxic than dialkyltins (5,18). From the trialkyltins the lower homologues are extremely neurotoxic (17). Trimethyltin compounds (TMT) induce degradation and necrosis in various areas of the central nervous system, particularly in the hippocampus but also in the brain stem and spinal cord (19). Triethyltin compounds (TET) induce severe oedema and destruction of the myelin sheaths (20). Trialkyltins substituted with alkyl groups of increasing chain length or arylgroups (phenyl) are not neurotoxic and are considered to be less toxic in general (10,21).

Effects of organotin compounds on the immune system

Recent studies have revealed that some di- and trialkyltin as well as triaryltin compounds, share immunotoxic properties, which were also found to be a sensitive criteria of their toxicity. The dialkyltin homologs, in particular di-n-butyltin (DBTC) and di-n-octyltin (DOTC) dichlorides, induced a dose and time-related decrease of thymus, spleen and lymph node weight (22). The lower dialkyltin homologs did not (dimethyl-substituted) or only slightly (diethyl substituted) reduce thymus weights, whereas no thymus atrophy was observed with the higher homologs (23,24). Diestertin compounds did not induce lymphoid atrophy (18), possibly because there is a rapid hydrolysis of the ester bond (25). To evaluate the functional significance of the dialkyltin induced reduction of lymphoid organ weights, various immune function studies were performed. From these studies is was apparent that immune reactions in which T lymphocytes participate were suppressed by DBTYC and DOTC treatment, without significant compromise of the humoral immunity or the mononuclear phagocyte system. Suppression of cell mediated immunity was shown by a delayed type of hypersensitivity to tuberculine (26), by skin graft rejection (26), and graft versus host reactivity (27), by the mitogenic responsiveness of thymocytes, spleen cells and peripheral lymph node cells to T cell mitogens (27) and by a reduced resistance to bacterial infections (28).

From the trialkyltin substituted compounds tri-n-butyltin chloride (24) and bis (tri-n-butyltin) oxide (29,30) were found to induce a marked thymus atrophy which was associated with a less severe reduction in spleen and lymph node weights. Immune function studies in rats revealed that low-dose feeding of TBTO suppressed various parameters of the thymus dependent immunity as well as the mononuclear phagocyte system (31). The triaryltin compounds triphenyltin chloride (TPTC) (24), triphenyltin acetate (TPTA) (31) and triphenyltin hydroxide (TPTH) (33) were also active against the lymphoid system. Depending on the laboratory species used, a reduced number of circulating lymphocytes, a reduction of spleen weights and a moderate degree of thymus atrophy were observed. It was concluded from immune function studies in the rat that TPTA exposdure suppresses cell mediated immunity without compromising humoral immunity. This finding is at variance with the results of Verschuuren (32) who reported a suppression of the primary and secondary antibody response to tetanus toxoid in guinea pigs exposed to the related compound TPTA.

The induction of selective thymus atrophy by dialkyltin compounds

Thymus atrophy is the most remarkable feature of dialkyltin toxicity in vivo (22). Histologically, lympochyte depletion is observed particularly in the thymic cortex, without signs of cell destruction (karyorhexis and "starry sky" formation), as is seen after treatment with corticosteroids (34, 35), antimetabolites or alkylating agents (36). Electron microscopic examination revealed no distinct signs of lymphocyte destruction, and no activation of macrophages in the thymic cortex was observed (37,38). Since cell divisions are part of the maturation process of bone marrow derived stem cells into immune comptent T cells in the thymic cortex, the absence of clear signs of cell destruction indicates that dialkyltins probably induce an inhibition of thymocyte proliferation. This might result in a decreased migration of mature T-cells into the peripheral lymphoid organs, as was demonstrated by the observed depletion of lymphocytes in the T cell dependent areas of spleen and lymph nodes, and consequently to a reduced T cell dependent immunity.

Disturbances of thymocyte proliferation within the thymus could be mediated by an interference of dialkyltin compounds with various mechanisms implicated in thymocyte population dynamics. Either indirectly, through changes in endocrine control or the reticular epithelial cells, or directly effect on precursor T cells or on the intrathymic rapidly dividing cells.

Interference with precursor T cells seems unlikely since neither the number, viability or the mitotic activity of bone marrow cells were affected after treatment with DOTC and DBTC, in contrast to the number and viability of isolated thymocytes (24). In addition, the number of colony forming stem cells from bone marrow cells of DBTC treated mice were not affected (24,38), as measured by the spleen colony assay. However a selective interference of DBTC with the input of precursor T cells cannot be excluded definitively, since in the spleen colony assay the pre T cell is not separated from the other bone marrow stem cells. However, a selective effect of organotins on precursor T cells without an affect on the other stem cells seems unlikely.

Distribution studies with ^{14}C-labeled DBTC and DOTC have revealed that after oral, as well as i.v. application, the dialkyltins did not accumulate in the thymus (39). The highest amounts were recovered from liver and kidney. Therefore the specificity was not simply due to an accumulation of dialkyltins within the thymus. Glucocorticosteroids, growth hormone as well as thymic factors (hormones) are considered to be involved in the differentiation and proliferation of precursor T cells into mature classes of T lymphocytes (34, 40-42). There is substantial evidence that a stress related increase of corticoteroids can be excluded. After dialkyltin treatment neither the adrenal weight nor the histology of the adrenal cortex was affected (22). Moreover, thymus-weights of adrenalectomized as well as sham operated DOTC fed rats were equally decreased (22). Growth hormone (STH) deficiency is also associated with thymus atrophy and a depressed cell mediated immunity, which can be reversed by STH supplement-ation (43,44). However, daily injections of STH did not modify the DOTC induced thymus atrophy, whereas this treatment was sufficient to restore hypophysectomy induced thymus involution in control rats (38,39). Therefore it seems unlikely that a diminished STH production mediates the immuno-toxic effects of dialkyltins. A decreased production and/or excretion of thymic factors ("hormones") from thymic epithe-lial cells (REC's) could also result in a reduced cellularity of the thymus. Miller et al (37) suggested that DOTC acts selectively on the thymus in such a way that the humoral function of the organ may be affected. After 2 weeks feeding they observed besides normal appearing REC's adjacent to a number of vacuolated REC's. In short time studies after a single i.p. injection of DOTC we only observed an increased vacuolisation of REC's when the thymus was already markedly involuted (38). However, extensive vacuolisation of REC's is a common finding when the reticular meshwork of the thymus collapses after depletion of cortical lymphocytes (45). Probably this type of vacuolisation is rather a consequence than a cause of thymus atrophy. Since it seems unlikely that indirect mechanisms are involved it seems justified to consider a direct effect on thymocytes. The absence of any clear signs of cell destruction suggests a cytostatic rather than a cytotoxic effect. However, since under physiological conditions most of the cortical thymocytes die in situ without histological evidence of cell destruction a cytotoxic activity cannot be excluded (46-48).

EFFECTS OF DIALKYLTINS ON CELLULAR BIOLOGY

Dialkyltin effects on mitochondrial respiration.

The biological activitry of dialkyltin compounds was first studied by Aldridge and Cremer (49). They observed that in isolated rat liver mitochondria diethyltindichloride (DETC) inhibited oxygen and substrate consumption. Moreover substrate oxidation resulted in an accumulation of ketoacids expecially 1-glutamate. Further studies showed that other dialkyltin homologs (methyl to hexyl substituted) inhibited the alpha-ketoacid oxidation like DETC (50-53). The reduction of α-ketoacids oxidation is believed to be the result of an inhibition of the α-ketoacid dehydrogenase system. The mechanism of this inhibition is almost certainly a binding of dialkyltins with dithiols in either the coenzyme lipoic acid or the catalytic centre of the lypoyldehydrogenase.

Cain et al (51) suggested that besides an the inhibition of the α-ketoacid dehydrogenase systems, at higher concentrations DBTC also affected oxidative phosphorylation in mitochondria, similar to inhibitors like oligomycine and trialkyltins. An interaction was suggested with the lipoic acid cofactor pool found in the membrane bound, oligomycine sensitive ATP-ase complex (54). More recently an uncoupling of the mitochondrial respiration by DBTC was observed (53). This uncoupling effect may also be the result of sulfhydryl interactions, since a direct involvement of thiolgroups is implied in the uncoupling action of the known uncoupler and sulfhydryl reagent carbonyl-cyanide-p-trifluoromethoxy-phenylhydrazine (FCCP). The uncoupling activity of FCCP could be prevented and fully reversed by sulfhydryl compounds like dithioerythritol (55,56). Moreover the thiol oxidizing agent diamide exhibits an analogy to the FCCP uncoupling effect, that was completely restored by the addition of dithioerythritol 56.

Dialkyltin effects on thymocyte metabolism.

To evaluate the significance of the dialkyltin effects in mitochondrial suspensions at the cellular level, thymocytes were exposed to various dialkyltin compounds in order to investigate their interference with cell energy metabolism. Exposure of thymocytes to dialkyltins (methyl- to octyl-substituted) resulted in an impairment of their glucose metabolism, characterized by an increased glycolytic activity (51). For DBTC a dose and time dependent increase in glucose consumption as well as an accumulation of lactate and pyruvate was observed up to levels of 5 M DTBC (Fig. 1). Maximal stimulation of the glycolytic activity of thymocytes was observed at this level, since glucose consumption was equally increased as under anaerobiosis (52). A further increase of the DBTC concentration resulted in a rapid decline of glucose metabolism associated with only a slight decrease in cell viability. The increased glycolytic activity was also reflected by the stimulation of the pyruvate kinase activity, that was almost doubled after incubation of thymocytes with 5 M DBTC for 2 hr (39). From the accumulation of lactate and pyruvate, it is obvious that the increased amount of glucose consumed is hardly metabolized oxidatively. These results suggest an inhibition of the entrance of the glycolytic end products into the tricarboxylic acid cycle, possibly due to an interference of DBTC with the pyruvate dehydrogenase system. This was confirmed by the disturbed metabolism when lactate or pyruvate was used as oxidizable substrates in dialkyltin exposed thymocytes (52).

In spite of the inhibition of the oxidative respiration of thymocytes by DBTC, the increased glucose consumption was able to support nearly optimal ATP concentrations up to levels of $5 \mu M$ DBTC (Table 1). However, at levels of $10 \mu M$ DBTC the ATP levels declined. This is possibly due to a lesser degree of glycolytic activation at this concentration (52), which is supported by the lower accumulation of lactate compared with the $5 \mu M$ DBTC level (Table 1). Upon exposure of thymocytes to DBTC in the absence of glucose or the presence of β-OH-butyrate it is shown that an increased glycolytic activity is essential to maintain the ATP levels. In the absence of glucose the metabolism in the control incubations of endogenous substrates was nearly sufficient to maintien the ATP levels as high as those seen with glucose (Table 1). However in the presence of 5 and $10 \mu M$ DBTC the ATP level decreased in a dose and time dependent fashion.

Also with β-OH-butyrate the oxidative generation of ATP was not sufficient in thymocytes in the presence of $5 \mu M$ DBTC (Table 2. An inhibition of the alpha-keto-glutarate dehydrogenase complex by DBTC may be responsible for the observed decrease in β-OH-butyrate oxidation (Table 2) which will result in a diminished oxidative ATP production.

Dialkyltin effects on hepatocyte metabolism.

By __in vivo__ exposure of rats to dialkyltins it has been shown by Seinen et al (23) that the liver was not affected at concentrations that induced a remarkable lymphoid atrophy. In a paired feeding study at 100 ppm DBTC for 16 days the relative thymus weights were decreased to 47 per cent of the controls, whereas the relative liver weight was not changed (Table 3).

Moreover the endogenous levels of glucose, glycogen and lactate in liver homogenates of the DBTC exposed rats were not affected. Although in the distribution studies with radiolabeled dialkyltins the highest amount of activity was recovered from the liver (39), the hepatocyte metablolism was not disturbed seriously. Also in vitro, liver cells were less sensitive to dialkyltin exposure than thymocytes. In the presence of graded amounts of DBTC no stimulation was observed of the glycolytic activity of hepatocytes oxidizing their endogenous substrates. Neither an accumulation of lactate or pyruvate nor a stimulation of the pyruvate kinase activity could be detected up to levels of 40μM DBTC (Penninks, unpublished results). Moreover fatty acid oxidation, as well as gluconeogenesis, both studied as overall parameter of hepatocyte integrity, were only affected at relatively high levels of 20 to 40μM DBTC (39). Additional studies revealed that at 40 M DBTC the decreased oleate oxidation as shown by a diminished ketone body formation of approximately 25 per cent, was associated with an equal fall in ATP concentration (Table 4).

These results indicate that in hepatocytes the α-ketoacid dehydrogenase systems are probably not affected by DBTC, at least not at concentrations of 1μM DBTC that already clearly disturbed these enzyme systms in insolated thymocytes (52). Diethyltin dichloride (DETC) seems also to be less toxic for hepatocytes than for thymocytes. Wiebkin et al (57) observed that 10μM DETC did not affect the viability and lactate dehydrogenase release from liver cells after a 1 hr incubation period. At extremely high levels of 100μM DETC these parameters for cell integrity were decreased by 30 per cent only.

In contrast, levels as low as 10 M DETC induced a maximal increase of glycolytic activity in thymocytes (52), whereas at levels of 100μM DETC thymocyte viability was seriously affected. The different subcellular distribution patterns in liver and thymus cells, as observed after in vitro exposure to ^{14}C-DBTC, may account for the differential effects on these cells (39). In contrast to a mitochondrial accumulation in thymocytes, ^{14}C-DBTC accumulated in the cytoplasmic fraction of hepatocytes. This indicates the possibility of a cytoplasmic scavanger in hepatocytes, that might be less effective in thymocytes. Since dialkyltin compounds show a high affinity to vicinal thiols a possible role of metallothionines is postulated.

Dialkyltin effects on thymocyte proliferation

In previous studies of Seinen et al (27) is was shown that the blast transformation of rat thymocytes in response to the mitogens PHA and Con A was inhibited in a dose-related manner in the presence of graded amounts of DBTC. At a concentration of 0.1 μg DBTC/ml medium (0.33μM) the thymidine (3H-TdR) incorporation, measured after 72 hr of incubation, was already completely inhibited. In short term incubation experiments of 1 hr without mitogenic stimulation, it was found that the basal DNA synthesis of thymocytes, as measured by their incoporation of ^{3}H-TdR, was dose relatedly diminished from a level of 1 μM DBTC (39). The 3H-TdR incorporation was decreased to about 70 per cent of the control value at 2.5 μM DBTC, which further decreased to 25 per cent at 5μM DBTC (Fig. 2). At higher levels of 10μM DBTC the DNA replication was almost completely inhibited, although only a slight decrease in thymocyte viability was observed, as scored by trypan blue exclusion.

In contrast to the diminished incorporation of the DNA precursor thymidine, the incorporation of the RNA precursor 3H-uridine was dose relatedly increased (Fig. 2). It was already stimulated at a level of 0.5μM DBTC and increased to a maximum of approximately 270 per cent of the control value at a level of 5μM DBTC. At concentrations up to 10μM DBTC the incorporation declined but was still higher than those in the controls.

The incorporation of precursors for protein synthesis, as measured by the incorporation of ^{14}C-leucine, was similar to the incorporation of precursors for DNA replication dose relatedly decreased (Fig. 2). The ^{14}C-leucine incorporation was found to be a very sensitive in vitro parameter since a 50 per cent inhibition was observed at a level of 0.5μM DBTC. In the presence of 2.5μM DBTC it was almost completely inhibited.

Since up to levels of 5μM DBTC the viability of thymocytes was not affected, the functional inhibition of thymidine and leucine incorporation and the stimulation of the uridine incorporation cannot be accounted for by cell loss or reduced viability. Moreover, it seems unlikely that these effects are secondary to a limited energy supply, since up to 5μM DBTC the ATP levels in thymocytes were maintained as high as those in the controls during the 1 hr incubation period (Table 1).

Dialkyltin effects on Camp generation

When thymocytes were preincubated with graded amounts of DBTC for 5 min, the PGE1 induced cAMP response was found to be dose relatedly decreased both in the presence or absence of a phosphodiesterase inhibitor (39). In Fig. 3 it is shown that this inhibition of cAMP production can be prevented by the addition of increasing amounts of the dithiol compound 2,3-dimercaptopropanol (BAL), whereas BAL itself did not affect the PGE1 induced cAMP production. The disturbance of cAMP generation by DBTC is probably caused by an interference with the adenylate cyclase activity (Fig. 3). In lysates of thymocytes that were exposed to 5μM DBTC for 10 min, the adenylate cyclase activity decreased by 55 per cent as measured by the production of cAMP. BAL was also able to restore the reduced cAMP production in the adenylate cyclase assay (Fig. 3). Although in the initiation of thymocyte proliferation cAMP elevations are probably not involved (58,59), the maturation and differentiation of thymocytes are considered to be cAMP dependent. Kook and Trainin (57) have shown that the thymic humoral factor (THF) promoted maturation of T lymphocytes is associated with an obligatory early rise in cAMP. They also found that immature rather than differentiated T lymphocytes are the target cells influenced by the THF. These results are in agreement with those of Singh and Owen (60,61), who showed that thymic stem cell maturation can be stimulated by cAMP or compounds that elevate cAMP production. Therefore the DBTC induced disturbances in cAMP generation may result in a decreased maturation and differentiation of thymocytes.

VIVO-VITRO RELATION OF DIALKYLTIN EFFECTS ON THYMOCYTE PROLIFERATION

The in vivo exposure of rats to DBTC also resulted in a disturbance of the nucleoside and amino acid incorporation, as well as a diminished camp induction of thymocytes. The 3H-thymidine, 3H-uridine and 14C-leucine incorporation of thymocytes time dependently decreased up to 48 hr after a single intravenous injection of 2.5 mg DBTC/kg body weight. Twenty-four hours after DBTC application the ^{3}H-thymidine incorporation of thymocytes was already diminished to approximately 50 per cent, which further decreased to about 20 per cent of the control value after 48 hr (Fig. 4). In contrast to the in vitro observed stimulation of 3H-uridine incorporation, in vivo exposure to DBTC resulted in an inhibition. A maximal reduction of 50 per cent was reached at 36 hr after DBTC application, whereas after 48 hr it started to increase again, although the incorporation was still inhibited (Fig. 4).

At 72 hr after the single injection of DBTC the uridine incorporation reached control values again. Also the 14C-leucine incorporation of thymocytes was inhibited maximally 36 hr after DBTC injection. Like the uridine incorporation it was less inhibited at 48 hr and was stimulated to 120 per cent of the control value at 72 hr after DBTC dosage. At that time 3H-thymidine incorporation also started to increase although it was still inhibited by 60 per cent.

Thymus weight was initially diminished at 48 hr after DBTC injection, declined to 68 per cent of the control weights at 72 hr and recovered thereafter. Up to 36 hr after DBTC injection thymus weight as well as the number and viability of thymocytes were not affected. Therefore, the inhibition of DNA, RNA and protein synthesis already observed from 24 hr after DBTC exposure is not caused by a loss of thymocytes or a diminished cell viability. Moreover, it is unlikely that the decreased thymidine, uridine and leucine incorporation are caused by a limited energy supply. The ATP levels of in vivo exposed thymocytes did not differ from those of the controls. Also during an additional 2 hr incubation period of the thymocytes, in the presence of glucose as substrate, the ATP concentration remained at control levels (Penninks, unpublished results). Since lactate did not accumulate during this incubation period the maintenance of the ATP levels was not the result of an increased glycolytic activity, as was observed after in vitro exposure of thymocytes to DBTC.

The combined _in vivo-in vitro_ effects of dialkyltins on the DNA-, RNA- and protein-synthesis of thymocytes support the postulated anti-proliferative effect. The selectivity of this effect is further stressed by combined _in vivo-in vitro_ studies with rat bone marrow cells. Upon _in vitro_ exposure of bone marrow cells a comparable inhibition of blastransformation was noted, as with rat thymocytes, although some higher concentrations of DBTC were needed to obtain an equal inhibition of the ^{3}H-TdR incorporation (24,62). A 50 per cent decrease of the basal incorporation of 3H-Tdr of rat bone marrow cells were observed at 6.3 μM DBTC, whereas in thymocytes this was already reached at a level of 3.6 μM (62). After _in vivo_ exposure the differences in sensitivity between bone marrow and thymus cells are more remarkable. After a single i.v. injection with 2.5. mg DBTC/kg body weight, neither the blast transformation, nor the PGE1 induced cAMP response of bone marrow cells were affected at all (62).

Although the molecular mode of action of dialkyltins has not been elucidated yet, it seems justified to suppose that their selective immunotoxicity is related to an interference with lymphocyte proliferation.

CONCLUDING REMARKS ON THE MODE OF ACTION OF DIALKYLTINS

Inhibition of thymocyte proliferation is the most prominent feature of dialkyltin toxicity. Whether the inhibition is the result of an indirect effect on the input of precursor T cells, the humoral function of thymic epithelial cells or a direct effect on the proliferative activity of thymocytes still needs further research. However, the marked decrease of DNA synthesis by DBTC in isolated thymocyte suspensions, in which epithelial cells are absent, suggest a direct anti-proliferative effect on dividing thymocytes. At the cellular level an interference with the energy metabolism by interaction with the α-ketoaciddehydrogenase systems, as found in isolated mitochondria and thymocytes, seems not to be involved. Still, it cannot be excluded that the selectivity for the thymus is based on a selective effect on the energy metabolism of the pre-T-cells in the bone marrow or the proliferating thymocytes in the thymus, since they form only a minority of the total bone marrow and thymocyte populations, respectively. Moreover, it cannot be exlcuded that minor changes in energy metabolism could account for a reordering of metabolic priorities, for instance a decreased proliferation of thymocytes in favour of processes essential for cell survival.

Since the _in vivo_ (63) and _in vitro_ (49,50) observed disturbances of biological functions by dialkyltin compounds can be reversed or even prevented by dithiol compounds (i.e. BAL), and moreover their effects on the energy metabolism are believed to be caused by an interaction with dithiol lipoic acid, it is obvious that dialkyltins readily react with SH-groups. The particular affinity of dialkyltins for dithiols in a correct conformation is further confirmed by direct chemical interaction with sulfhydryl containing compounds (39,49,51). Therefore we suppose that the dialkyltin

effects may be mediated by an interference with intra- or
extracellular SH-groups. In biological systems SH groups play
important roles in enzymatic activity and properties of
proteins. In particular membrane associated functions, like
receptor functions, hormone binding, guanyl- and adenyl-
cyclase activity and transport of sugars, amino acids and
nucleosides are known to be disturbed by sulfhydryl reagents
(64). For lymphocyte proliferation SH-interactions at the
plasma membrane are considered to be of importance (65,66).
Lymphocyte blastogenesis may also be inhibited by membrane
penetrating sulfhydryl reagents by a disruption of cytoskeletal microtubulin assembly (67,68). The similarity in effects
of dialkyltins with known sulfhydryl reagents as NEM, further
support the hypothesis of dialkyltins interaction with membrane and/or cytoskeletal SH-groups. Like DBTC, NEM also
induced a disturbance of the DNA, RNA and protein synthesis of
thymocytes, although at slightly higher concentrations (Fig.
5). Preliminary experiments have also shown that at least
with DBTC the reduction of protein synthesis may be due to a
decreased transport of amino acids across the plasma membrane,
since the uptake of the unmetabolizable amino acid -amino
isobutyric acid was decreased by DBTC.

Further research is needed to evaluate the postulated interference of dialkyltins with membrane and/or cytoskeletal
associated sulfhydryl groups as a cause of the observed
anti-proliferative effects.

Table 1. Concentrations of ATP and lactate of isolated thymocytes incubated with or without glucose in the presence of various concentrations of DBTC.[a]

Concen-tration DBTC µM	Incuba-tion period min	ATP concentration + glucose	ATP concentration − glucose	Lactate concentration + glucose	Lactate concentration − glucose
		nmol/10[7] thymocytes			
0	60	5.2 ± 0.2	5.3 ± 0.1	4 ± 1	2 ± 1
	180	4.4 ± 0.2	4.2 ± 0.3	17 ± 2	3 ± 1
5	60	5.4 ± 0.5	4.6 ± 0.2*	37 ± 4**	4 ± 1
	180	4.4 ± 0.2	2.2 ± 0.2**	142 ± 4**	5 ± 1
10	60	4.3 ± 0.1*	3.3 ± 0.2**	33 ± 1**	4 ± 1
	180	3.8 ± 0.2*	1.6 ± 0.3**	121 ± 4**	7 ± 3

[a] Results are mean values ± SD of a typical experiment performed in triplicate.
* p < 0.05; ** p < 0.001, Student t-test.

Table 2. Concentrations of ATP and the consumption of β-OH-butyrate of isolated thymocytes utilizing glucose or β-OH-butyrate as substrate in the presence of 0 and 5 µM DBTC.[a]

Concen-tration DBTC µM	Incuba-tion period min	ATP concentration + glucose	ATP concentration + β-OH-butyrate	β-OH-butyrate consumption
		nmol/10[7] thymocytes		
0	60	5.9 ± 0.2	5.8 ± 0.1	26 ± 5
	180	5.1 ± 0.3	4.9 ± 0.2	56 ± 2
5	60	5.7 ± 0.3	5.1 ± 0.3*	13 ± 5*
	180	5.0 ± 0.2	3.5 ± 0.2**	26 ± 3**

[a] Results are mean values ± SD of a typical experiment performed in triplicate.
* p < 0.05; ** p < 0.001, Student t-test

Table 3. Body- and relative organ weights, and glucose, glycogen and lactate levels in liver homogenates after a paired feeding study at dietary levels of 0 and 100 ppm DBTC for 16 days.[a]

Time days	Dieta-ry level	Body weight g	Relative organ weight Thymus g/100 g b.w.	Relative organ weight Liver	Glucose µg glucose/mg ww	Glycogen	Lactate nmol/mg ww
8	0	189±4	0.222 ± 0.035	4.58 ± 0.29	40.6±5.6	343±66	62.2 ± 8.9
	100	187±6	0.104 ± 0.010*	4.61 ± 0.18	41.9±3.4	321±44	68.3 ± 6.1
16	0	217±2	0.232 ± 0.032	4.28 ± 0.26	54.7±8.4	387±63	49.7 ± 6.9
	100	220±10	0.113 ± 0.024*	4.32 ± 0.25	52.4±3.5	341±75	59.4 ± 14.6

[a] Mean values ± SD of 5 animals per group.
* p < 0.001, Student t-test.

Table 4. Ketone body production, ATP concentrations and viability of isolated hepatocytes incubated for 60 min with oleate as substrate in the presence of various concentrations of DBTC.[a]

Concentration DBTC µM	Ketone body production	ATP concentration	Viability in %
	nmol/mg ww		
0	79.0 ± 0.8	3.4 ± 0.1	90 ± 2
5	78.0 ± 1.1	3.3 ± 0.1	86 ± 2
20	73.0 ± 1.3*	3.2 ± 0.1	88 ± 2
40	58.0 ± 0.6**	2.9 ± 0.1*	80 ± 2

[a] Results are the means ± SE of a typical experiment performed in triplicate.
* p < 0.01; ** p < 0.001, Student t-test.

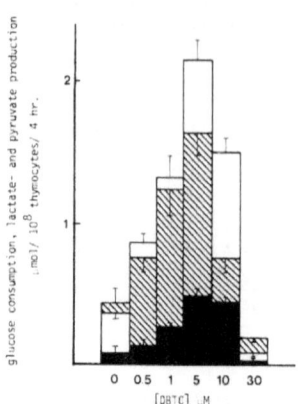

Fig. 1. Consumption of glucose (▨) and the production of lactate (□) and pyruvate (■) of isolated rat thymocytes incubated with various concentrations of DBTC for 4 hr.

Results are mean values ± SE of at least three incubations each performed in triplicate.

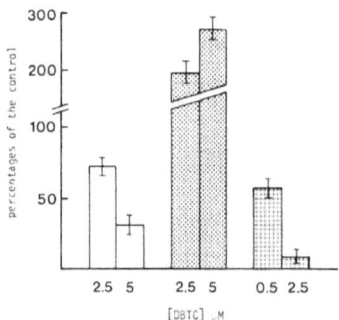

Fig. 2. The effects of various concentrations of DBTC on (^{3}H)-thymidine (□), (^{3}H)-uridine (▨) and (^{14}C)-leucine (▦) incorporation of isolated rat thymocytes.[a]

[a] DBTC was added 30 min prior to the addition of the radiolabeled recursors, and their incorporation was followed for 60 min.

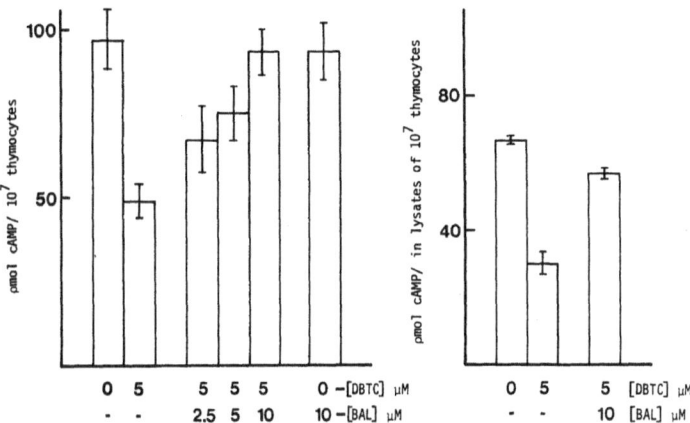

Fig. 3. Effect of DBTC on the PGE[1] induced cAMP response[a] and the adenylate cyclase activity[b] of rat thymocytes in the presence or absence of various concentrations of 2,3-dimercaptopropanol (BAL).

[a] After a 5 min preincubation period with 0 or 5 µM/DBTC with or without various concentrations of BAL, PGE[1] was added and the cAMP production of thymocytes measured after an additional incubation period of 10 min in the presence of the phosphodiesterase inhibitor 3-isobutyl-1-methylxanthine (10^{-3}M).

[b] After a 10 min preincubation period of thymocytes with 0 or 5 µM DBTC the cells were washed twice and lysed in a 50 mM Tris-HCl buffer pH 7.4 with 4 mM $MgCl_2$ for 10 min. The adenylate cyclase activity was measured by the production of cAMP in lysates after an additional incubation of 10 min with theophyline as phospho-diesterase inhibitor. After the 10 min incubation period 10 µM BAL was added to some incubation vials and the cAMP production measured after a successive 5 min incubation period.

Results are mean values ± SD of a typical experiment performed in triplicate

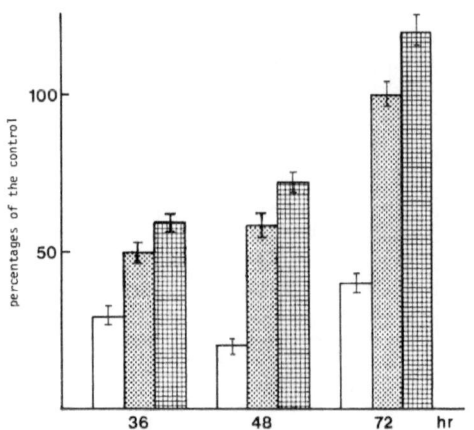

Fig. 4.   The (^{3}H)-thymidine (□), (^{3}H)-uridine (▨) and (^{14}C)-leucine

(▦) incorporation of thymocytes isolated at 36, 48 and 72 hr

after a single intravenous injection of 2.5 mg DBTC/kg.[a]

[a]   Results are mean values ± SD of 3 rats.

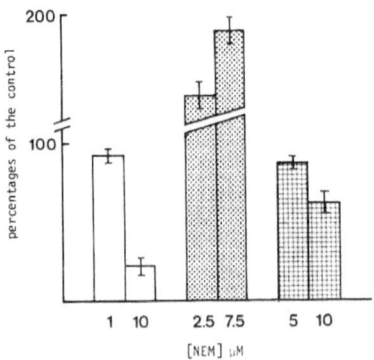

Fig. 5.   The effects of various concentrations of N-ethylmaleimide (NEM) on

the (^{3}H)-thymidine (□), (^{3}H)-uridine (▨) and (^{14}C)-leucine

(▦) incorporation of isolated rat thymocytes.[a]

[a]   NEM was added 30 min prior to the addition of the radiolabe-

led precursors and their incorporation was followed for 60 min.

REFERENCES

1.   Faith, R.E., M.I. Luster and J.G. Vos, 1980. Effects on immunocompetence by chemicals of environmental concern. In: Reviews in biochemical Toxicology (Eds. Hodgson, E., J..R. Bend and R.M. Philpot), Elsevier/North Holland, New York, Vol 2 173-212.

2.   Vos, J.G. 1977. Immune suppression as related to toxicology, CRC Crit.Rev. Toxicol., 5 67-101

3.   Vos, J.G., R.E. Faith and M.I. Luster 1980. Immune Alterations, Elsevier Holland Biomedical Press, Elsevier/North Holland, New York, 241-266.

4.   Dean, J.H., M.I. Luster and G.A. Boorman 1982. Immunotoxicology, In Immonopharmacology (Eds Sirois, P. and M.R. Pleszczynski) elsevier Biomedical Press, New York, 349-397.

5.   Lanigan, D. and E.L. Weinberg, 1976. The use of Estertin Stabilizers in PVC, In Organotin Compounds: New Chemistry and Applications. (Ed. Zuckermann, J.J.) American Chemical Society, Washington, D.C., 134-154.

6.   Ross, A., 1965. Industrial application of organotic compounds, Ann. N.Y. Acad. Sci., 107-123.

7.   Luyten, J.G.A. In Applications and Biological Effects of Organotin Compounds (Ed. Sawyer, A.K.) Dekker, New York, 3 931-974

8.   Environmental Health Criteria, 15 1980. Tin and Organotin Compounds: A preliminary review, WHO, Geneva.

9.   Cardarelli, N.F. 1974. Slow release molluscicides and related materials. In Molluscicides in schistosomiasis control (Ed. Cheng, T.C.) Academic Press, New York 177-240.

10. Duncan, J. 1980. The toxicology of Molluscicides. the Organotins, Pharmac. Ther., 10 407-429.

11. Midwest Research Institute 1977. Assessment of the need for the character of, and the impact resulting from limitations on selected organotins. Phase I Assessment of the need for limitations on organotins. Washington, D.C., U.S. Environmental Protection Agency, EPA, contract No 68-01-4313.

12. Occupational exposure to Organotin Compounds, 1976. U.S. Department of Health, Education, and Welfare. U.S. Government Printing Office, Washington, D.C.

13. Alajonanine, T., Derobert, L. and Thieffry, S., 1958, Etude clinique d'ensemble de 210 cas d'intoxication par les sels organiques d'etain, Rev. Neurol., 98, 85-96.

14. Barnes, J.M. & Stoner, H.B., 1959, The toxicology of tin compounds, Pharmac. Rev., 11, 211-231.

15. Piver, W.T., 1973, Organotin Compounds: Industrial applications and biological investigation. Environ. Health Perspect., 4, 61-80

16. Barnes, J.M. & Magee, P.N., 1958, The biliary and hepatic lesion produced experimentally by dibutyltin salts, J. Pathol. Bacteriol., 75, 267-279.

17. Barnes, J.M. & Stoner, H.B., 1958, toxic properties of some dialkyltin and trialkyltin salts, Br. J. ind. Med., 15, 15-22.

18. Penninks, A.H. & Seinen, W., 1982, Comparative toxicity of alkyltin and estertin stabilizers, Fd. Chem. Toxicol., 20, 909-916.

19. Chang, L.W., Tiemeyer, T.M., Wegner, G.R. & McMillan, D.E., 1983, Neuropathology of trimethyltin intoxication. III. Changes in the brain stem neurons, Environ. Res., 30, 399-411.

20. Watenabe, I., 1980, Organotins, In: Experimental and Clinical Neurotoxicity (Eds Spencer, P.S. & Schaumberg, H.H.) Williams & Wilkins, Baltimore, 545-557.

21. Stoner, H.B., 1966, Toxicity of triphenyltin, Br.J.ind.Med., 23, 222-229.

22. Seinen, W. & Willems, M.I., 1976, Toxicity of organotin compounds. I. Atrophy of thymus and thymus-dependent lymphoid tissue in rats fed di-n-octyltin dichloride, toxicol. Appl. Pharmacol.,35, 63-75.

23. Seinen, W., Vos, J.G., van Spanje, I., Snoek, M., Brands, R. & Hooykaas, H., 1977, Toxicity of organotin compounds. II. Comparative in vivo and in vitro studies with various organotin and organolead compounds in different animal with various organotin and organolead compounds in different animal species with special emphasis on lymphocytotoxicity, Toxicol. Appl. Pharmacol., 42, 197-212.

24. Seinen, W. & Penninks, A.H., 1979, Immune suppression as a consequence of a selective cytotoxic activity of certain organometalic compounds on thymus-dependent lymphocytes, Ann. N.Y. Acad. Sci., 320, 499-517.

25. Penninks, A.H. & Seinen, W., Detoxification of the estertin stabilizer Bis-(-carbobutoxyethyl0tin dichloride in rats by hydrolysis of the esterbond, Submitted.

26. Seinen, W., Vos, J.G., van Krieken, R., Penninks, A.H., Brands, R. & Hooykaas, H., 1977, Toxicity of organotin compounds. III. Suppression of thymus-dependent immunity in rats fed by di-n-butyltin dichloride and di-n-octyltin dichloride, Toxicol. Appl. Pharmacol., 42, 213-224.

27. *Seinen, W., Vos, J.>., Brands, R. & Hooykaas, H., 1979, Lymphocytotoxicity and immunosuppression by organotin compounds. Suppression of GVH activity, blast transformation and E-rosette formation by di-n-butyltin dichloride and di-n-octyltin dichloride, Immunopharmacol., 1, 343-355.*

28. *Seinen, W., 1981, Immunotoxicity of alkyltin compounds. In Immunologic considerations in Toxicology (Ed. Sharma, R.P.) Boca Raton: CRC Press, 1, 103-119.*

29. *Funahashi, N., Iwasahi, I. & Ide, G.I., 1980, Effects of bis(tri-n-butyltin) oxide on endocrine and lymphoid tissues of male rates, Acta Pathol. Jpn., 30, 955-966.*

30. *Krajnc, E.I., Wester, P.W., Loeber, J.G., van Leeuwen, F.X.R., Vos, J.G., Vaessen, H.A.M.G. & van der Heyden, C.A., 1984, Toxicity of Bis (tri-n-butyltin)oxide in the rat. I. Short-time effects on general parameters and on the endocrine and lymphoid systems. Toxicol. Appl. Pharmacol., 75, 363-386.*

31. *Vos., J.G., de Klerk, A., Krajnc, E.I., Kruizinga, W., van Ommen, B. & Rozing, J., 1984, Toxicity of Bis (tri-n-butyltin)oxide in the rat. II. Suppression of thymus-dependent immune responses and parameters of non specific resistance after short-time exposure. Toxicol. Appl. Pharmacol., 75, 387-408.*

32. *Verschuuren, H.G., Ruitenberg, E.J., Peetoom, F., Helleman, P.W. & van Esch, G.J., 1970, Influence of triphenyltin acetate on lymphatic tissue and immune response in guinea pigs, Toxicol. Appl. Pharmacol., 16, 400.*

33. *Vos, J.G., van Logten, M.J., Kreeftenberg, J.G. & Kruizinga, W., 1984, Effect of triphenyltin hydroxide on the immune system of the rat, Toxicology, 29, 325-336.*

34. *Dougherthy, T.F., Berliner, M.L., Schneebeli, G.L. & Berliner, D.L., 1964, Hormonal control of lymphatic structure and function, Ann. N.Y. Acad. Sci., 113, 825-843.*

35. *Claesson, M.G. & Ropke, C., 1969, Quantitative studies on cortisol induced decay of lymphoid cells in the thymolymphatic sustem, Acta Pathol. Microbiol. Scand., 76, 367-382.*

36. *Thompson, H.A. & Gale, G.R., 1971, Cis-dichlorodiamicne platinum. II. Hematopoietic effects in rats, Toxicol. Appl. Pharmacol., 19, 602-609.*

37. *Miller, K., Scott, M.P. & Foster, J.B., 1984, Thymic involution in rats given diets containing dioctyltin dicloride, Clini. Immunol. Immunopathol., 30, 62-70.*

38. Penninks, A.H., Kuper, F., Spit, B.J. & Seinen, W., On the mechanism of dialkyltin induced thymus involution, Submitted.

39. Penninks, A.H. & Seinen, W., 1983, The lymphocyte as target of toxicity: a biochemical approach to dialkyltin induced immunosuppression, In Advances in Immunopharmacology (Eds Hadden, J.E. et al), Pergamon Press, Oxford-New York, 2, 41-60.

40. Ernstroem, U., 1970, Hormonal influences on thymic release of lymphocytes into the blood. in Hormones and the immune response (Eds Wolstenholme, G.E.W. & Knight, J.), Churchill J. & A. Publishers, 53.

41. Greaves, M.F., Owen J.J.T. & Raff, M.C., 1973, In: T and B lymphocytes, Excerpta Medica, Amsterdam, 13.

42. Mosier, D. & Cohen, P.L., 1975, Ontogeny of mouse T-lymphocyte function, Fed. Proc. Fed, Am. Soc. Exp. Biol., 34, 137-140.

43. Pierpaoli, W. & Sorkin, E., 1968, I. Effects of heterologues anti-growth hormone (ASTH) antiserum on thymus and peripheral lymphatic tissue in mice. Induction of wasting syndrome. J. Immunol., 101, 1036-1047.

44. Pierpaoli, W., Baroni, C., Fabris, N. & Sorkin, E., 1969, Hormones and immunological capacity. II. Reconstitution of anti-body production in hormonally deficient mice by somatotropic hormone, thyrotropic hormone and thyroxine, Immunol., 16, 217-229.

45. Haelst, U. van, 1967, Light and electronmicroscopic study of normal and pathological thymus of lthe rat. II. The acute thymic involution, Zeitschr. fuer Zellforsch., 80, 153-182.

46. Claesson, M.G., Jorgenson, O. & Olsson, L., 1972, Comparative light and electron microscopical studies of decaying thymic lymphoid cells, Acta pathol. Microbiol. Scand., 80, 821-826.

47. Metcalf, D. & Brumby, M., 1966, the role of the thymus in the ontogeny of the immune system, J. Cell. Physiol., 76, 1, 149-168.

48. Weismann, I.L., 1976, Thymus cell migration, J. Exp. Med., 126, 291-294.

49. Aldridge, W.N. & Cremer, J.E., 1955, The biochemistry of organotin compounds. Diethyltin dichloride and triethyltin sulphate, Biochem. J., 61, 406-418.

50. Aldridge, W.N., 1976, The influence of organotin compounds on mitochondrial functions, In Organotin Compounds: New chemistry and application. (Ed. Zuchkermann, J.J._ American Chemical Society, Washington, D.C., 186-196.

51. Cain, K., Hyams, R.L. & Griffiths, D.E., 1977, Studies on the energy-linked reactions: Inhibition of oxidative phosphorylation and energy-linked reactions by dibutyltin dichloride, Feb Lett., 82, 23-28.

52. Penninks, A.H. & Seinen, W., 1980, Toxicity of organotin compounds. IV. Impairment of energy metabolism of rat thymocytes by various dialkyltin compounds, Toxicol. Appl. Pharmacol., 56, 221-231.

53. Penninks, A.H., Verschuren, P.M. & Seinen, W., 1983, Di-n-butyltin dichloride uncouples oxidative phosphorylation in rat liver mitochondria, Toxicol. Appl. Pharmacol., 70, 115-120.

54. Griffiths, D.E., 1976, Studies on energy-linked reactions. Net synthesis of adenosine triphosphate by isolated adenosine triphosphate synthese preparations: A role for lipoic acid and unsaturated fatty acids, Biochem. J., 160, 809-812.

55. Toninello, A. & Siliprandi, N., 1982, Restoration of membrane potential in mitochondria deenergized with carbonyl cyanide p-trifluoromethoxyphenylhydrazone (FCCP), Biochem. Biophys. Acta, 682, 289-292.

56. Kaback, H.R., Reeves, J.P., Short, S.A. & Lombardi, F.J., 1974, Mechanisms of active transport in isolated bacterial membrane vesicles. XVIII. The mechanism of action of Carbonylcyanide-m-Chlorophenylhydrazone, Arch. Biochem. Biophys., 160, 215-222.

57. Wiebkin, P., Prough, R.A. & Bridges, J.W., 1982, The metabolism and toxicity of some organotin compounds in isolatedrat hepatocytes, Toxicol. Appl. Pharmacol., 62, 409-42.

58. Kook, A.I. & Trainin, N., 1974, Hormone-like activity of a thymus humoral factor on the induction of immune competence in lymphoid cells, J. Exp. Med., 139, 193.

59. Goffey, R.G., Hadden, E.M. & Hadden, J.W., 1977, Evidence for cyclic GMP and Calcium mediation of lymphocyte activation by mitogens, J. Immunol., 119, 1387-1394.

60. Singh, U. & Owen, J.J.T., 1975, Studies on the effect of various agents in the maturation of thymus stem cells, Eur. J. Immunol., 5, 286-288.

61. Singh, U. & Owen, J.J.T., 1976, Studies on the maturation of thymus stem cells. The effect of catecholamines, histamine and peptide hormones on the expression of T cell alloantigens, Eur. J. Immunol., 6, 59-62.

62. Penninks, A.H. & Seinen, W., 1983, Immunotoxicity of organotin compounds, In Immunotoxicity (Eds Gibson, G.G., Hubbard, R. & Parke, D.V.) Academic Pres, London, 426-436.

278

63. *Stoner, H.B., Barnes, J.M. & Duff, J.I., 1955, Studies on lthe toxicity of alkyltin compounds, Br. J. Pharmacol., 10, 16-25.*

64. *Rothstein, A., 1970, Sulfhydrylgroups in membrane structure and function. In Current tropics in Membranes and Transport. Academic Press, Nez-York-London, 1, 135-176.*

65. *Chaplin, D.D. & Wedner, H.J., 1978, Inhibition of lectin-induced lymphocyte activation by diamide and other sulfhydril reagents, Cell. Immunol., 36, 303-311.*

66. *Noelle, R.J. & Lawrence, D.A., 1981, Modulation of T-cell function. II. Chemical basis for the involvement of cell surface thiol-reactive sites of T-cell proliferation, Cell. Immunol., 60, 453-469.*

67. *Pfeifer, R.W. & Irons, R.D., 1981, Inhibition of lectin stimulated lymphocyte agglutination and mitogenesis by hydroquinone: reactivity with intracellular sulhydril groups, Exp. Mol. Pathol., 35, 189-198.*

68. *Pfeifer, R.W. & Irons, R.D., 1983, Alteration of lymphocyte function by quinones through a sulfhydryl dependent disruption of microtubule assembly, Int. J. Immunopharmacol., 5, 463-470.*

Immunosuppressive Effects of Benzidine in BCF Mice

Michael I. Luster, Lily H. Hong, Anne N. Tucker,
Oscar Pung & Gary A. Boorman

National Toxicology Program,
National Institute of Environmental Health Sciences Research
Triangle Park, NC U.S.A.

INTRODUCTION

Benzidine (4,4'-diaminobiphenyl) is an acknowledged carcinogen, employed industrially in the synthesis of dyes as well as analytic reagents in various laboratory tests (rev. by Haley, 1975). Benzidine exposure is associated with urinary bladder tumors in humans and with hepatomas, mammary tumors, and, to a lesser extent lymphomas in rodents (IARC, 1982a, b; Baker, 1953; Grieswold, et al, ., 1968). Numerous studies have suggested that the immune response can modulate the growth of antigenic tumors (rev. by Stutman, 1975). Thus, it follows that an increased incidence or progression of neoplastic disease may occur by chemical carcinogens that are also immunosuppressive. In this respect, a strikingly high percentage of carcinogens are also immunosuppressive in experimental studies including diethylstilbestrol, certain polycyclic aromatic hydrocarbons, cyclophosphamide, benzene, nitrosamines, and phenytoin (rev. by Dean, et al., 1982). Furthermore, studies in laboratory animals have demonstrated an enhanced incidence of tumors induced by UV, methylcholanthrene or benzo(a)pyrene in mice treated with immunosuppressive agents (e.g. Kalland and Forsberg, 1981; Stjensward, 1966; Outzen, 1980). Of particular relevance to the present studies is a recent report which indicated a direct relationship between immunosuppression and neoplasia in workers engaged in the manufacture of benzidine (Gorodilova and Mandrik 1978). In this 4 year study, workers who were identified as having suppressed cell-mediated immunity, as assessed by skin tests, demonstrated pre-cancerous conditions and subsequent neoplasms. On the other hand, no cases of neoplastic diseases were registered in workers with normal immunological responses. The objectives of the present study were to characterize the immunotoxicity of benzidine at dose levels reported to induce tumors in mice using a comprehensive immune screening panel and to determine whether immunosuppression by benzidine was related to oxidative or nonoxidative metablolism of the parent compound. In vitro studies provided suggestive evidence that benzidine-induced suppression of lymphocyte proliferation is a consequence of changes in arachidonic acid/lipoxygenase conversion products and does not reflect a direct interaction of the lymphocyte with a reactive metabolite of benzidine.

MATERIALS AND METHODS

Chemicals: Benzidine (4,4'-diaminobiphenyl), 4-aminobiphenyl, indomethacin, 3,3',5,5'-tetramethylbenzidine (TMB) 8-bromoguanosine 3':5'-cyclic monophosphate(8 brc GMP)and arachidonic acid, were from Sigma Chemical Co. (St. Louis, MO). Other commercial compounds used were mono- and diacetyl-benzidine (ICN Pharmaceuticals, Inc.) and 4-aminophenol (Aldrich). ^{14}C-benzidine (S.A. 13.4 mCi/mM) was from Path-finders Lab., Inc. (St. Louis, MO) and nafazatrom (2,4-dihydro-5-methyl-2-(2-napthyloxy)ethyl-3H-pryazol-3-one was kindly supplied to Dr. Thomas Eling of this Institute from Bayer AG, West Germany. N-OH-Diacetyl benzidine was a gift from Dr. R.K. Lynn, Oregon Health Sciences University, Portland, OR.

Experimental Design: In vivo studies were conducted by exposing adult female BCF mice (C57BL/6N x C$_3$H; Charles River, Portage, MI) to benzidine (as the hydrochloride) for 5 consecutive days by gavage at a daily dose of 11,22 or 44 mg/kg body weight. The material was given in a volume of 0.2 ml of water per dose and controls received an equal volume of water. Mice were examined 3-5 days following the last exposure. Lymphocyte proliferation assays were used to examine direct cellular events associated with chemical exposure and were performed as described previously (Luster, et al., 1982), using lipopolysaccharide (LPS) and Con A to activate B cells and T cells, respectively. For in vitro studies, water insoluble chemicals were dissolved in ethanol and diluted in culture medium so as not to exceed a final concentration of 0.1% ethanol. This concentration of ethanol had no effect on cell viability. Water soluble compounds were dissolved in culture media and added directly to lymphocyte cultures at the indicated concentrations.

Histopathology: Mice were killed with CO$_2$ for necropsy. Body, liver, spleen, kidney, and thymus weights were recorded, and tissues were collected for histophathology. Tissues were fixed in 10% buffered formalin, stained with hematoxylin and eosin and examined histologically.

Hematology: Blood samples were obtained via cardiac puncture, and hematological parameters, including erythrocyte count (RBC), total white blood cell count (WBC), leukocyte diffe-rential and platelet counts, were examined. Cell numbers were determined with a Coulter counter.

Bone Marrow Cellularity and Function: Marrow cells were aseptically collected in RPMI 1640 culture media as described previously (Boorman, et al., 1984). Pluripotent bone marrow stem cells (CFU-S) were examined using the spleen colony method originally described by Till & McCulloch (1961). Bone marrow granulocyte-macrophage progenitor cells (CFU-GM) were determined in vitro using a modification (Boorman, et al., 1984) of the method previosly described by Bradley & Metcalf (1966).

Immune Function Tests: Antibody responses were measured to sheep red blood cells (SRBCs) by enumeration of direct splenic plaque forming cells (PFCs) (Luster, et al., 1982). The lymphoproliferative response of spleen cells to T- and B-cell polyclonal acitvators and allogeneic leukocytes (MLC) was performed as previously described in detail (Luster, et al., 1982; 1984). Delayed-type hypersensitivity reactions were measured to keyhole limpet hemocyanin (KLH, Pacific Biomarine, Venice, CA) by a radiometric ear assay (Luster, et al., 1982) as modified by Holsapple, et al. (1984). Natural killer (NK) cell activity was determined in spleen cells using YAC-1 tumour cells as described by Ortaldo, et al. (1977). Briefly, 5 x 10^3 ^{51}Cr-radiolabeled YAC-1 tumour cells were incubated with spleen cells for 4 hr at 37°C in wells of microtiter plates at effector target cell (E:T) ratios of 100:1 and 50:1. Supernatants were collected utilizing a rapid harvesting system and radioactivity released was quantified.

Host Resistance Assays: Mice were challenged intravenously with approximately 5 x 10^4 viable Listeria monocytogenes (Strain L242/73), originally obtained from a naturally infected mouse and maintained as a frozen stock. Mortality was monitored for 14 days. The nonlethal strain of malaria used in this study, Plasmodium yoelii 17XNL, was a gift from Mr. Charles Evans, Laboratory of Microbial Immunity, National Institute of Allergy and Infectious Diseases (NIH; Bethesda, MD). Five days following chemical exposure mice were injected intraveneously with 1 x 10^6 parasitized erythrocytes. Diff-Quik -stained thin films of tail blood were used to determine the percentage of parasitized cells on the day of peak parasitemia (day 12 after infection). Polyoma virus-induced tumor cells (PYB6), obtained from Dr. Jack Dean (Chemical Industry Institute of Toxicology, Research Triangle Park, NC) were inoculated (1 x 10^4 viable cells) s.c. into the right rear flank. Animals were palpated weekly for 60 days and tumor occurrence recorded.

Statistical Analysis The Mann-Whitney U-test was employed to assess the significance of treatment effects in all in vito tests except host resistance assays in which the Chi-square test was used. The significance of chemical treatment in the in vitro studies was determined by establishing confidence levels from replicate values of historical controls. LPS-stimulated lymphocyte cultures never varied more than 6% from the mean of replicate cultures which results in differences greater than 15% as being significant at the $P<0.01$ level.

RESULTS

None of the benzidine treated mice died or revealed overt signs of toxicity as a result of chemical exposure. As can be seen in Table 1, neither body, liver, kidney nor thymus weights were affected by chemical exposure. However, splenomegaly occurred at the two highest dose levels and histologically appeared to be due to an increase in extramedullary hematopoiesis, probably erythropoiesis. An increase in liver weight occurred in the 22 mg/kg dosed group but was not believed to be biologically significant because of a lack of dose response. There were no changes in hematological values including erythrocyte numbers, white blood cell numbers or differential counts (based upon percent or absolute values), associated with benzidine exposure.

In contrast to the absence of general toxicological changes, benzidine was myelotoxic. As shown in Table 2, although cellularity was not effected in mice exposed to benzidine, there was a marked inhibition of progenitor cell proliferation. The number of pluripotent stem cells (CFU-S) was suppressed at the two highest dose levels while CFU-GM progenitor cell formation was suppressed at all dose levels.

As summarized in Table 3, benzidine exposure suppressed a number of immune functions. At the highest dose level tested, benzidine suppressed natural killer cell activity, lymphoproliferative responses to polyclonal activators and delayed hypersensitivity responses. B cell activation (mitogen response to LPS) was suppressed in splenic lymphocytes from all chemically-treated animals although a dose response was not observed. In contrast, neither the IgM or IgG antibody PFC response to SRBC was significantly decreased at any dose level.

A marked increase in susceptibility to L. monocytogenes infection occurred in mice exposed to benzidine (Table 4). Increased mortality occurred in all chemically-treated groups ranging from 62% at the low dose level to 100% at the highest dose level compared to 23% in control animals. Increased susceptibility to infection with the parasite, P. yoelii,17X, as well as to growth of transplantable tumor cells also occurred following benzidine exposure; however, these increases were significant only in the highest dose groups. Benzidine suppressed lymphocyte proliferation in a concentration dependent manner when added directly to mitogen-stimulated lymphocyte cultures (Fig. 1). Suppression of B-cell proliferation in LPS-stimulated lymphocyte cultures occurred at concentrations of benzidine as low as 10^{-6} M while inhibition of Con A-activated T-cells occurred at 10-5 M benzidine.

Benzidine, in its parent form, is relatively innocuous; its carcinogenicity and toxicity are believed to result from reactive oxidative and/or hydroxylated metabolites (e.g., Eling, et al., 1983; Lynn, et al., 1984; Backer, 1953). Thus, the ability of the major hydroxylated metabolites of benzidine to inhibit LPS-induced lymphocyte activation was examined. As seen in Table 5, several of the metabolites that are found in the liver (hydroxylated series) were slightly antiproliferative, including monoacetylbenzidine and N-OH-diacetylbenzidine. However, the degree of inhibition of these metabolites did not exceed that which resulted from incubation with the parent compound. The oxidative products of benzidine metabolism, including the cation radical and nitrenium ion, are relatively unstable and have not been purified, thus these could not be directly evaluated. We instead examined a number of related compounds, which are not benzidine metabolites, but like benzidine serve as cooxidative substrates for hydroperoxidase in the arachidonate pathway. All of these compounds, particularly 4-aminophenol, inhibited LPS-induced lymphocyte activation at levels comparable to that required to suppress LPS responses by benzidine suggesting a common mode of action.

DISCUSSION

The relationship between the immune system and the development of cancer remains controversial. A correlation exists between the administration of selected chemical immunosuppressants and an increased incidence of certain types of neoplasia. This is supported by the enhanced incidence of UV-, methylcholanthrene-, or benzopyrene-induced tumors that occurs in mice treated with immunosuppressive agents (e.g. Kalland and Forsberg, 1981; Stjensward, 1966; Outzen, 1980) reported that the incidences of cancer in renal transplant recipients on prolonged immunosuppressive therapy was 25% at 1 year and 47% at 10 years. This relationship between carcinogenesis and the immune response has provoked a considerable number of studies in which the early effects of exposure to chemical carcinogens on the immune response have been examined. While these studies have not proven that immune alterations induced by chemical carcinogens are responsible for the progression of carcinogenesis, they have demonstrated that particular chemical carcinogens such as diethylstilbestrol, polycyclic aromatic hydrocarbons, polyhalogenated aromatic hydrocarbons and cyclophosphamide alter immune functions and, in fact, are capable of inhibiting cell-mediated immunity and/or natural killer cell activity (rev. in Dean, et al., 1982).

Benzidine is a carcinogen associated with urinary bladder tumors in humans and with hepatomas, mammary tumors, and to a lesser extent lymphomas in rodents (rev. by Haley, 1975; IARC, 1982a, b). Of particular relevance to the present studies is a recent report which showed a direct relationship between immuno-suppression and neoplasia in workers engaged in the manufacture of benzidine (Gorodilova and Mandrik, 1978). The present studies indicate that benzidine exposure results in suppression of a variety of immune functions at tumorigenic and subtumorigenic dose levels in mice. This was evidenced by suppressed proliferation of bone marrow progenitor cells, delayed hypersensitivity responses and lymphoproliferative responses to mitogens and allogeneic leukocytes as well as suppressed natural killer cell activity in chemically-treated mice. The dose levels at which immunosuppression were observed are similar to those reported to induce tumors in rats and mice. For example, a dose of 60 mg/kg in rats over a 30 day period has been reported to elicit a mammary tumor incidence of 50% (Grieswold, et al., 1968), while similar doses in mice have been reported to elicit a 60% incidence of liver tumors (Vesselinovitch, et al., 1975). These data, while not definitive, are consistent with the hypothesis that immuno-suppression may serve as a cofactor in benzidine-induced neoplasia.

Benzidine was immunosuppressive at dose levels which did not induce signs of overt toxicity, such as organ weight changes or histopathological effects. The immunosuppression appears to be due to inhibition of early events in cell activation and not because of a cytolytic process as indicated by the fact that lymphocyte cell viability was not affected following incubation with benzidine (data not shown). Unlike other immune functions, the antibody PFC response to SRBCs was not compromised by benzidine exposure despite the fact that LPS mitogen responses were suppressed. LPS-induced activation may occur through a non-specific mitogen signal provided to the cell at an unidentified recepetor (Coutinho, et al., 1974). In contrast, specific antigen binding is required prior to antibody formation suggesting that benzidine may affect non-specific signals occurring at the cell membrane and not specific immunoglobulin receptors. Suppression of immune functions induced by benzidine exposure also was manifested by increased susceptibility following challenge with infectious agents or transplantable tumor cells.

The ability to resist Listeria infection and tumor development was severely altered following chemical exposure. The ability to resist Listeria infection (rev. by Hahn and Kaufman, 1981) evokes host resistance mechanisms which primarily involve cell mediated immunity. In contrast, altered resistance to Plasmodium infection, which only occurred in the high dose group, is dependent on both cellular and humoral immunity (Playfair, 1982).

The addition of benzidine in vitro to mitogen-activated lymphocytes mimicked the suppression of lymphocyte responsiveness to mitogens observed following in vivo exposure. Benzidine in its parent form is relatively innocuous and it is believed that metabolic products are primarily responsible for its carcinogenicity and toxicity. Thus, we assumed that metabolism of the parent compound to reactive metabolites via lymphocyte-derived enzymatic conversion was a pre-requisite for the obsrved in vitro immunotoxicity. Benzidine is metabolized in the liver to reactive hydroxylated intermediates by the cytochrome P-450 system; the majority of these products ultimately found as glucuronide or glutathione conjugates (Lynn, et al., 1984). The intermediates in this pathway include mono- and diacetylbenzidine and highly reactive 3-OH diacetylbenzidine and N-OH-diacetylbenzidine, the latter metabolite being mutagenic (Lynn, et al., 1984). Benzidine can also be metabolized to reactive products capable of macro-molecular binding through oxidative mechanisms by serving as a co-oxidative substrate for peroxidase reactions required in the conversion of arachidonic acid to prostaglandins or hydroxy-fatty acids (rev. in Eling, 1983). Mononuclear cells are capable of producing cytochrome P-450 drug metabolizing enzyme in the presence of mitogen and an appropriate chemical inducer. The present studies, however, indicate that hydroxylated metabolites, as occur in the liver, are probably not responsible for suppression of proliferation since acetylated or hydroxylated metabolites were not nearly as effective in inhibiting lymphoproliferative response as the parent compound. In contrast, a number of compounds which, like benzidine, serve as cooxidative substrates for peroxidases in the conversion of arachidonic acid to prostaglandins and hydroxyfatty acids demonstrate a similar potency to that of benzidine in suppressing blastogenesis. This would suggest that qualitative and/or quantitative products in the metabolism of arachidonic acid to hydroxy-fatty acids and prostaglandins may be responsible for the observed effects. The importance of such products including prostaglandins, hydroxy fatty-acids, leukotrienes and guanylate cyclase for lymphocytic activation has been described (Suzuki, et al., 1980; Coffee and Hadden, 1984; Coffee, et al., 1981; Bailey, et al., 1982). We are presently further exploring these observations by quantitating the production of arachidonic acid products in lymphocyte cultures exposed to benzidine.

Table 1

The Effects of Benzidine Exposure on Selected Organ Weights
and Hematological Values

Parameter[a]	Daily Exposure Level (mg/kg)[a]			
	0	11	22	44
Body and Organ Weights				
Body (g)	19.0 ± 0.8	19.1 ± 0.2	22.3 ± 0.5	20.1 ± 0.4
Liver (mg)	985 ± 35	1094 ± 29	1258 ± 37[b]	1048 ± 44
Spleen (mg)	63 ± 2	78 ± 4	119 ± 7[b]	127 ± 7[b]
Kidney (mg)	150 ± 8	156 ± 6	182 ± 5	170 ± 6
Thymus (mg)	55 ± 3	49 ± 3	53 ± 5	53 ± 2
Peripheral Blood				
WBC ($10^3/mm^3$)	4.9 ± 0.1	4.1 ± 0.4	4.2 ± 0.3	4.6 ± 0.3
RBC ($10^6/mm^3$)	6.3 ± 0.2	6.3 ± 0.2	7.1 ± 0.3	7.1 ± 0.2
Lymphocytes (%)	79 ± 2	78 ± 2	71 ± 4	82 ± 2
Monocytes (%)	3.6 ± 0.8	2.6 ± 0.5	4.5 ± 1.0	2.6 ± 0.3

[a]Each value represents the mean ± SE of at least 5 mice per group. Mice were exposed by gavage in water for 5 consecutive days.

[b]Significantly different from controls at $P<0.01$.

Table 2

Bone Marrow Cellularity and Progenitor Cell Proliferation
In Benzidine Exposed Mice

Benzidine Treatment[a] (mg/kg)	Nucleated Cells/ Femur (x10^6)	CFU-GM/ 10^5 Cells	CFU-S/5x10^4 Cells
Vehicle	24 ± 1.2	78 ± 1.6	17.0 ± 0.1
11	21 ± 0.4	73 ± 1.2[b]	16.3 ± 0.3
22	22 ± 1.4	65 ± 1.7[c]	15.9 ± 0.2[c]
44	22 ± 0.6	61 ± 1.9[c]	14.8 ± 0.4[c]

[a]Each value represents the mean ± SE of at least 6 mice per group.

[b]Significantly different from control values at $P<0.05$.

[c]Significantly different from control values at $P<0.01$.

Table 3

The Effects of Benzidine Exposure on Immune Parameters

Parameter		Exposure Level[a]			
		0	11	22	44
Antibody Response to SRBC[b]					
IgM-PFC/10^6 Cells		2332 ± 295	1953 ± 299	2101 ± 224	1751 ± 181
IgG-PFC/10^6 Cells		4485 ± 708	4234 ± 492	4127 ± 650	3731 ± 412
NK Cell Activity[c]	100:1	16	17	19	9[e]
% cytolysis	50:1	10	12	13	3[e]
Lymphoproliferative Response (^{3}H-TdR Incorp. [CPM x 10^{-3}])					
PHA Activated		70 ± 5	69 ± 5	62 ± 3	37 ± 4[e]
LPS Activated		39 ± 3	25 ± 2[e]	23 ± 2[e]	26 ± 2[e]
Mixed Leukocyte Culture		106 ± 10	81 ± 7	68 ± 7[e]	54 ± 2[e]
Delayed Hypersensitivity Response (DHR) Index[d]		3.6 ± 0.4	3.6 ± 0.3	3.0 ± 0.2	2.4 ± 0.3[e]

[a] All values represent a mean ± SE of at least 5 mice per group.

[b] IgM antibody response was determined 4 days following immunization with SRBCs. IgG antibody responses were determined 5 days following immunization by adding an appropriate dilution of γ-chain specific antiserum to the culture.

[c] YAC-1 tumor cells were used at the indicated effector to target cell ratios in a 4 hr ^{51}CR release assay.

[d] The DHR index was calculated by dividing cpm of challenged ear by the cpm of the control ear.

[e] Significantly different from control values at P<0.05.

Table 4

Susceptibility to Listeria, Plasmodium yoelii and PYB6 Tumor Cell
Challenges Following Benzidine Exposure

Dosage (mg/kg)	L. monocytogenes Mortality/No. Challenged (%)[a]	Plasmodium Infection (% Parasitemia)[b]	PYB6 Tumors [No. with Tumors/ No. Challenged (%)[c]]
0	3/13 (23)	11.1 ± 2.2	3/25 (12)
11	8/13 (62)[d]	13.7 ± 3.2	3/15 (20)
22	9/15 (60)[d]	17.9 ± 3.3	4/15 (27)
44	13/13 (100)[d]	27.9 ± 3.3[d]	7/13[d](57)

[a]Mortality to L. monocytogenes recorded at 14 days following an iv injection with 5×10^4 viable bacteria per mouse.

[b]Percent parasitemia determined 12 days (peak infection) following an iv injection of 1×10^6 parasitized mouse erythrocytes.

[c]Mice were injected subcutaneously with 1×10^4 viable PYB6 tumor cells and monitored for 60 days.

[d]Significantly different from controls at $P<0.05$.

Table 5

Inhibition of LPS-Induced B Cell Activation by Hydroxylated (P-450)
Metabolites of Benzidine or Other Co-oxidative Substrates

Compound Tested	Percent Suppression	
	10^{-5} M	5×10^{-6} M
Benzidine	64[b]	40[b]
Metabolites in Liver		
Monoacetylbenzidine	34[b]	7
Diacetylbenzidine	11[b]	3
N-OH-Diacetylbenzidine	29[b]	4
Co-oxidized Substrates		
3,3',5,5'-Tetramethylbenzidine	41[b]	36[b]
Nafazatrom	35[b]	19[b]
4-Aminophenol	87[b]	23[b]
4-Aminobiphenyl	15[b]	9

[a]All compounds were added to lymphocyte cultures stimulated with LPS at a concentration of 10^{-5} M or 5×10^{-6} in EtOH so as not to exceed a final concentration of 0.1% EtOH. Control represented LPS-stimulated cultures to which 0.1% EtOH was added.

[b]Significantly different from controls at $P<0.01$.

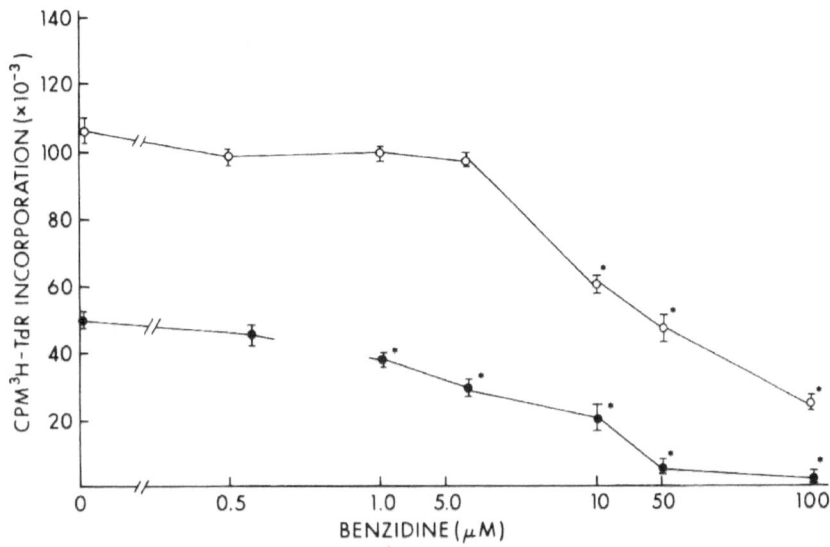

Figure 1: In vitro suppression of mitogen-stimulated lymphocyte proliferation by benzidine. Mouse splenic lymphocytes were cultured with Con A (o) or LPS (•) and the indicated concentrations of benzidine. The results are expressed as CPM ^{3}H-TdR incorporation ± SEM. The asterisk represents statistical significance at P<0.01.

REFERENCES

BAILEY, J.M. BRYANT, R.W. LOW, C.E. PUPILLO, M.B. & VANDERHOEK, J.Y. (1982). Regulation of T-lymphocyte mitogenesis by the leukocyte product of 15-hydroxy-eicosatetraenoic acid (15-HETE). Cell. Immunol., 67: 112-120.

BAKER, R.K. (1953). The carcinogenic activity of dihydroxybenzidine: Further investigations. Cancer Res., 13: 137-140.

BOORMAN, G.A., HONG, H.L., DIETER, M.P., HAYES, H.T., POHLAND, A.E. STACK, M. & LUSTER, M.I. (1984). Myelotoxicity and macrophage alterations in mice exposed to ochratoxin A. Toxicol. Appl. Pharmacol., 72: 304-312.

BRADLEY, T.R. & METCALF, D. (1966). The growth of mouse bone marrow in vitro. Aust. J. Exp. Biol. Med. Sci. 44: 287-300.

COFFEY, R.G., HADDEN, E.M. & HADDEN, J.W. (1981). Phyto-hemagglutinin stimulation of guanylate cyclase in human lymphocytes. J. Biol. Chem., 256: 4418-4424.

COFFEE, R.G. & HADDEN, J.W. 1984. Stimulation of lymphocyte guanylate cyclase by arachidonic acid and ketes. In Prostaglandins and Leukotrienes, in press.

COUTINHO, A., GRONOWICZ, E., BULLOCK, W.W. & MOLLER, G. (1974). Mechanisms of thymus-independent immunocyte triggering mitogenic activation of B cells results in specific immune response. J. Exp. Med., 139 74-85.

DEAN, J.H. LUSTER, M.I. & BOORMAN, G.A. (1982). Immunotoxicology. In Immunology-Toxicology, (ed. Sirois, P.). pp. 349-397. Elsevier/North Holland, New York.

ELING, T., BOYD, J., REED, G., MASON, R. & SIVARAJAH, K. (1983). Xenobiotic metabolism by prostaglandin endo-peroxide synthetase. Drug Metab. Rev., 14: 1023-1053.

GORODILOVA, V.V. & MANDRIK, E.V. (1978). The use of some immunological reactions for studying the immune response in persons presenting a high oncological risk. Sov. Med., 8: 50-53.

GRIESWOLD, D.P., CASEY, A.E., WEISBURGER, E.K. & WEISBURGER, J.H. (1968). The carcinogenicity of multiple intra-gastric doses of aromatic and heterocyclic nitro or amino derivatives in young female Sprague-Dawley rats. Cancer Res., 28: 924-937.

HAHN, H. & KAUFMAN, S.H.E. (1981). The role of cell-mediated immunity in bacterial infections. Rev. Infect. Dis., 3 1221-1280.

HALEY, T.J. (1975). Benzidine revisted: a review of the literature and problems associated with the use of benzidine and its congeners. Clin. Toxicol. ,8: 13-42.

HOLSAPPLE, M.P., PAGE, D.G. & SHOPP, G.M. (1984). Characterization of the delayed hypersensitivity response to a protein antigen in the mouse: I. Kinetics of reactivity and sensitivity to classical immunosuppressants. Int. J. Immunopharmacol., 6: 399-406.

IARC. (1982a). IARC Monographs on the Evaluation of the Carcinogenic Risk of Chemicals to Humans. Vol.29, Lyon, France, pp. 149-183.

IARC. (1982b). IARC Monographs on the Evaluation of the Carcinogenic Risk of Chemicals to Humans. Supplement 4, Lyon, France.

KALLAND, T. & FORSBERG, J.G. (1981). Natural killer cell activity and tumor susceptibility in female mice treated neonatally with diethylstilbestrol. Cancer Res., 41: 5134-5140.

LUSTER, M.I., DEAN, J.D. & MOORE, J.A. (1982). Evaluation of immune functions in toxicology. In Methods in Toxicology, (ed. Hayes, W.) pp 561-586. Raven Press, New York.

LUSTER, M.I., HAYES, H.T. KORACH, K., TUCKER, A.N., DEAN, J.H. GREENLEE, W.F. & BOORMAN, G.A. (1984). Estrogen immunosuppression is regulated through estrogenic responses in the thymus. J. Immunol., 133: 110-116.

LYNN, R.K., GARVIE-GOULD, C.T., MILAM, D.F., SCOTT, K.F., EASTMAN, C.L., ILIAS, A.M. & RODGERS, R.M. (1984). Disposition of the aromatic amine, benzidine, in the rat: characterization of mutagenic urinary and biliary metabolites. Toxicol. Appl. Pharmacol., 72: 1-14.

ORTALDO, J.R., BONNARD, G.D. & HERBERMAN, R.B. (1977). Cytotoxic reactivity of human lymphocytes cultured in vitro. J. Immunol., 119: 1351-1359.

OUTZEN, H.C. (1980). Development of carcinogen-induced skin tumors in mice with varied states of immune capacity. Int. J. Cancer, 260: 87-94.

PENN, I. (1984). Consequences of immunosuppression. In Toxicology of the Immune System, (eds. Dean, J.H. Munson, A.E. and Luster, M.I.) in press. Raven Press New York.

PLAYFAIR, J.H.L. (1982). Immunity to malaria. Br. Med. Bull., 38: 153-159.

292

STJENSWARD, J. (1966). Effect of noncarcinogenic and carcinogenic hydrocarbons on antibody-forming cells measured
at the cellular level in vitro. J. Natl. Cancer Inst.,
36: 1189-1194.

STUTMAN, O. (1975). Immunodepression and malignancy. Adv.
in Cancer Res., 22: 261.

SUZUKI, T., SADASIVAN, J., SAITO-TAKI, T., STECHSCHULTE, D.J.,
BALENTINE, L. & HELMSAMP, G.M. (1980). Studies of Fc
receptors of human B lymphocytes: Phospholipase Az
activity of Fc receptors. Biochem., 19: 6037-6044.

TEVETHIA, S.S., ZARLING, J.M. & FLAX, M.H. (1976). Macrophages and the destruction of syngeneic virus-induced
tumors. In Immunobiology of the Macrophage, (ed.
Nelson, O.S.) pp. 509-523. Academic Press, New York.

TILL, J.E. & MCCULLOCH, E.A. (1961). A direct measurement
on the radiation sensitivity of normal mouse bone marrow
cells. Radiat. Res., 14: 213-222.

VESSELINOVITCH, S.D., RAO, K.V.N. & MIHAILOVICH, N. (1975).
Factors modulating benzidine carcinogenicity bioassay.
Cancer Res., 35: 2814-2819.

MECHANISMS OF METAL-INDUCED IMMUNOTOXICITY

D. Lawrence, S.Mudzinski, U.Rudosfsky, & Warner

Department of Microbiology/Immunology, Albany Medical College,
Albany, NY 122208 U.S.A.

Metals such as lead (Pb) and mercury (Hg) have definite cytotoxic effects on numerous cell types including the cellular components of the immune system, but only posited mechanisms of pathology due to the influences of subtoxic doses of Pb and Hg on lymphocyte will be discussed. In vitro, Pb and Hg were not toxic to lymphocytes at doses $<5 \times 10^{-4}M$ and $5 \times 10^{-7}M$, respectively, and actually enhanced some immune reactivities (1,2). This augmentation of immune responsiveness has the potential to produce pathologic results. Heavy metals may modulate immune reactivites by directly altering lymphocyte (T cell and B cell) and/or accessory "antigen presenting" cell (macrophage) physiology and/or altering the antigenicity of self antigens involved in immunoregulation. The main cell surface antigens known to be involved in immune recognitions are the products of the major histocompatibility complex (MHC; 3). Figure 1 depicts the typical interaction of T cells, B cells and "antigen processing/presenting" cells. Any alteration of a cell's physiology or surface markers could modulate the interactions. Preliminary studies in our laboratory suggest that ^{210}Pb and [203]Hg do associate selectively with somme cellular proteins. Immunomodulation of the immune system by Pb and Hg will be elaborated on in this report in terms of its possible role in autoimmune diseases.

Divergence from the normal balance achieved by immunoregulation could result in a pathologic disorder, Immunopotentiation could lead to hyperimmunity to self (autoimmunity) which is the result of increased helper T cell activity, decreased suppressor T cell activity, and/or hyperactive B cells. Immunosuppression could lead to increased susceptibility to infectious diseases and loss of immune surveillance, resulting in increased incidence of tumors. Since metals such as Pb and Hg can induce allergic hypersentitivities (4-7), we already know that they probably are capable of making immunogens by binding to self constituents. Any metal known to produce an allergic response could be a promoter of autoimmunity.

Although previous studies had indicated that Pb suppressed in vivo humoral immune responses to sheep erythrocytes (SRBC; 8,9) we have been unable to confirm this point. Since our in vitro data with Pb indicated that Pb enhanced humoral immunity (1,10), it was important to evaluate the in vivo effects. We have examined the in vivo effects of Pb on numerous strains of mice and some of the strains (inbred and outbred) are reported. As apparent in Table 1, no strain has been found to be suppressed by a 3- or 4-week exposure to a high dose of Pb (10mM). Although not reported in Table 1, this is also true for mitogen-induced responses. To date, the only apparent significant effects were enhanced responses in Balb/c mice.

The enhancement is modest but significant. Similar results are observed with Pb in other mouse strains, but only after a single injected dose (11,12). Hg in limited strains of rats also has been reported to enhance antibody production (13). Thus, Pb (and Hg) could produce some pathologic effects _in vivo_ by enhancing, not inhibiting, the immune response. _In vitro_ studies have suggested that Pb enhances by direct effects on B cells and possibly inhibition of suppressor T cell activity (10); whereas, Hg appeared to enhance via a T cell and/or macrophage effect only (2). A bypass of T cell immunoregulation by unregulated B cells could give rise to autoimmune problems. In this light, it is interesting to note that the only strain (Table 1) enhanced by Pb was the Balb/c strain is extremely sensitive to radiation (possibly relating to cellular thiol differences - heavy metals have high affinities for thiols) and very susceptible to the induction of plasma cell (B cell) tumors.

The hypothesis we would like considered is that heavy metal-induced immunomodulation could cause autoimmune diseases. Therefore, the effects of Pb on mouse strains with a high incidence or susceptibility to autoimmunity was investigated. Heavy metal concentrations can accumulate with age, and with aging, the incidence of tumors and autoimmunity increase (14). Since Pb had no apparent _in vivo_ immunosuppressive effect, its influences on pathology in a lupus strain (B/W) and the SJL/J strain were of interest. No Pb effects on humoral immune (PFC) responses to SRBC were apparent in B/W and SJL/J mice, but these strains did have enhanced mortality due to Pb. The B/W strain is a lupus strain, that is 100% of the mice develop autoimmunity similar to systemic lupus erythematosus (SLE) in man. By 34 and 54 weeks of age, respectively 50% of female and male B/W mice have died as an outcome of this autoimmune disease. We have studied the effects of Pb in these mice. The results provide the first data (known to us) in which one reagent produced opposite effects in female and male mice. A 10mM oral dose enhanced mortality in males and decreased mortality in females (Table 2.) Usually, the disease is considered similar in the females and males, with the exception of the kinetics of onset of the disease. Our results with Pb suggest that the mechanisms of disease process may be different in the sexes. This may be useful in the delineation of the pathogenesis of SLE, as well as the immunopathology of Pb. Only mortality data has been generated with the female B/W mice, but other parameters already have been assessed with Pb-treated male B/W mice. As expected for 60 week-old mice, their immune reactivity (mitogen response, PFC response) was low. Pb did not alter significantly the mitogen responses but polyclonal activation of PFC responses differed significantly (Table 3). The 2mM dose enhanced the polyclonal PFC response induced by LPS, but the 10mM dose significantly suppressed the response. The other strain in which Pb increased mortality was SJL/J (Table 4). The Pb-treated SJL/J mice had reduced MLC responses and mitogen responses induced by Con A and PHA, but not LPS, which suggests that T cell reactivity was inhibited more than B cell reactivity in these mice. SJL/J mice do not develop spontaneous autoimmune problems like B/W mice, but they are very susceptible to the induction of some experimental autoimmune diseases. SJL mice also have a high incidence (>90%) of reticulum cell sarcoma by 13 months of age. It has been reported that immune reactivities enhance the growth of these tumors, in that, an intact immune system is required to support tumor growth (15). Thus, in both B/W and SJL mice, Pb may accelerate and/or exacerbate the pathology by enhancing immune responses. Pb appears to have increased renal pathology in these mice, and we are in the process of determining if this is due to immunopathologic mechanisms. Both Pb and Hg have been implicated in the immunopathology of renal disease in man (16-18). Our preliminary studies on Hg-poisoned individuals suggest that their mitogen-induced responses are not significantly altered, but there was an increase in their percentage of T11, but not T3, positive cells and a decrease in B cells in their peripheral blood (Table 5). The significance of these differences is unknown at present.

The mechanisms involved in the immunomodulation by Pb and Hg still are unknown. Information gathered on the cellular requirements and sensitivities of the lymphocyte subpopulations will help to delineate how heavy metals can modify "immune homeostasis" which, if altered, could lead to the development of immunopatholgy. Both suppressor and cytolytic murine T cells are Lyt-2,3 T cells and it should be noted that Lyt-2,3 T cells re more sensitive to thiol blockers and oxidants than Lyt-1 helper T cell (19;Table 6).Some doses of permeant (N-ethylmaleimide) and impermeant (BESA) thiol-reactive compounds enhance net help. Incubation of T cells with Pb also increased net help (10). The recognition phase of cytolytic T Cells has been shown to be thio-dependent (20); therefore, contact between cytolytic T cells and tumors could be inhibited by heavy metals which have high affinities for sulfhydryls. Pb may not react well with cell surface thiols. It has been reported that the binding of Pb to cells is entirely different from that of sulfhhydryl seeking metals such as Hg (23). The differences in Hg and Pb association with cell surface sulfhydryls may help to explain the different mechanisms involved in their immunomodulatory capabilities. Although membrane thiols may have low reactivities with Pb, Pb has been reported to modulate intracellular glutathione (24,25). Glutathione does decrease with age (26), and the incidence of autoimmune dieases may increase as the thiol content (intra-and extra-cellular) of an individual declines. Interestingly, Pb enhanced mortality in male B/W mice and significantly lowered glutathione levels in peritoneal cells but not lymphocytes (Table 7).

We have initiated studies to assess the effects of Pb on the subcellular triggering of events involved in T cell activation. In vivo Pb treatments do appear to enhance thymocyte proliferation induced by Con A and IL2. These results may reflect an enhancement of T cell ontogeny due to Pb. The thymocyte responses enhanced by Pb were not altered significantly by BESA, a thiol-specific impermeant probe; however, BESA enhanced the response of non-Pb-treated thymocytes (Fig.2). In vitro Pb exposures inhibited slightly the proliferation of an IL2-dependent cell line (HT-2) in the presence of IL2(Fig. 3). These results suggest that Pb modulates T cell activities, as well as B cell activities (10).

The subcellular mechanisms of heavy metal alteration of lymphocyte physiology may involve thiol-related constituents. Some drugs, hormones, and immunologic factors such as cytochalasin B, insulin, and interferon, respectively, have the ability to affect lymphocyte reactivities. Although their biologic reactivities may be diverse, they have common biochemical reactivities, in that, cytochalasin B (27), insulin (28), and interferon (29) interact with cellular thiols. Some complex immunomodulating reagents including heavy metals may have relatively simple biochemical effects on the cell biology of lymphocytes. Cellular thiols are an obvious subcellular parameter to consider for heavy metal modulation because of the high affinity of heavy metals for sulfhydryl groups. Cellular thiols have been known for 50 years to be involved in cell proliferation (75). Cellular thiols are intimately involved in cell transport, DNA synthesis, and movement. The release of immunoregulatory factors, as well as the receptors for these factors, may involve common biochemical parameters such as the need for free sulfhydryl as posited (19) or specific thiol disulfide interchanges as supported by the folowing evidence:

1. A microsomal enzyme is involved in a "disulfide-shuffling" process (31), and proteins including immunoglobulin molecules have been found with low molecular weight thiols attached (32).

2. Some polypeptide interactions on the T cell surface utilize their interacting thiols, such as the complex formed between the Lyt-2 and Lyt-3 molecules (33).

3. Even a T cell regulatory factor has been reported to require thiol interactions as indicated by the necessary disulfide linkage of an Ia-like polypeptide with an antigen-binding polypeptide (34).

4. Cell surface thiols are intimately involved in numerous membrane phenomena including transport, hormonal interactions, and secretion (35), and T cell activation has been shown to be dependent on free surface thiols (36).

Two recent reviews (37,38) have discussed the effects of exogenous thiols on lymphocytes and both concluded that exogenous thiols have been shown to be consistently capable of enhancing various immunological responses of lymphocytes, although the mechanism of such enhancement has received little attention thus far. Numerous immunomodulating agents used clinically (levamisole, penicillamine, interferon, and thiouracil - to name a few) have thiol reactivity. In addition, the modulation of T cells by helper (thiol-protective) and suppressor (oxidants) factors from macrophages has been suggested (19) to involve cellular redox potentials. The immunotoxic effects of thiol-related components recently has been reviewed (39).

Heavy metals may directly modify cell thiols. However, they also can indirectly influence cellular thiols by modulating oxidative products. Heavy metals are known to affect lipid peroxidation, and lipid peroxidation can lead to an altered redox state of the cell and/or a modulation of synthesis of immuno-regulatory products such as prostaglandins (40). Heavy metal interference with cellular oxidases, peroxidases, reductases, and glutathione may lead to dysregulation of immunity due to differential effects on the lymphoid subsets (19). Such interference could be a reason for heavy metal suppression of macrophage phagocytosis (41) and macrophage-mediated tumoricidal activity (42). Most likely, Hg modulates lymphocyte functions via interactions with cellular thiols; however, Pb may not. As discussed above, Pb has a significantly lower association with surface sulhydryls than Hg (23), and it has been suggested that Pb has a better association with cellular phosphoryl groups than sulfhydryls (43). Pb has been reported to bind to phosphatidylcholine (44). Therefore, Pb may activate lymphocytes via a cellular phosphoryl group. Modulation of membrane phospholipids has been implicated in lymphocyte activation, probably involving a protooncogene product or protein kinase C (45).

The actual mechanisms by which metals alter lymphocyte and monocyte functions remain to be delineated. The ability of heavy metals to immunomodulate is clear, and their ability to be immunotoxic in some strains and species is evident. Investigation of the genetics and biochemistry of heavy metal toxicity on the multiple components of the immune system will enhance our understanding of the basis for susceptibility to heavy metal immunotoxicity.

ACKNOWLEDGEMENT

The authors would like to thank Paul Ginouves and Kathy L. Smith for their assistance in various aspects ot the reported experiments, and Kathleen Cavanagh for her assistance in the preparation of the manuscript. Our presented studies have been supported by grants from the Environmental Protection Agency No R809349 and the National Institutes of Health No ES03179.

Table 1

In Vivo and In Vitro Anti-SRBC PFC Responses of Various
Lead-treated Mouse Strains

Strain	Exposure[a] Duration	Pb	Blood Pb (μg/dl)	In Vivo[c] PFC/Spleen	In Vitro[d] PFC/Culture
C57B1/6	8 wk	-	4 ± 1	298,651 ± 66,140	-
		+	76 ± 9	351,144 ± 63,017	-
A/J[b]	8 wk+5 d	-	4 ± 1	281,994 ± 125,241	2,579 ± 712
		+	132 ± 28	226,976 ± 68,588	3,687 ± 958 *
DBA/1J	8 wk	-	3 ± 1	102,401 ± 38,046	1,755 ± 663
		+	59 ± 8	117,758 ± 45,792	1,846 ± 796
Balb/C Cumb	3 wk	-	2 ± 1	682,510 ± 188,639	-
		+	ND	922,361 ± 175,156 **	-
Balb/C Cumb	8 wk	-	3 ± 1	345,342 ± 66,643	12,278 ± 7,068
		+	69 ± 7	408,300 ± 100,451 **	15,224 ± 7,103
CBA/J	4 wk	-	ND	32,720 ± 17,169	
		+	ND	28,062 ± 8,513	
	10 wk	-	ND	16,759 ± 6,733	
		+	ND	25,740 ± 4,107	
Swiss Webster	8 wk	-	2 ± 1	95,042 ± 38,934	13,833 ± 6,878
		+	97 ± 60	110,142 ± 47,507	11,004 ± 7,102
SJL/J	8 wk	-	3 ± 1	60,731 ± 81,652	38,251 ± 20,815
		+	202 ± 251	55,155 ± 43,817	28,768 ± 24,366

[a] Mice were given either 0 or 10mM lead acetate in the water for the indicated times and were placed on distilled water at SRBC immunization.
[b] A/J mice were treated with lead water until sacrifice.
[c] Mice were injected with 10^8 SRBC i.p. and sacrificed 5 days later for PFC/spleen determination.
[d] Splenocytes obtained at sacrifice were set up in culture with 0.1% SRBC and harvested 5 days later for direct PFC determination.
* Significant difference at $p < 0.05$.
** There was a significant increase in the number of $PFC/10^6$ cells ($p > 0.05$) but not PFC/spleen.

Table 2

Pb Effects on Female and Male B/W Mice[a]

Pb Dose (mM)	Mortality (%, Age)			
	Female		Male	
0	50%	34 wk	0%	60 wk
2	50%	40 wk	50%	60 wk
10	30%	44 wk	50%	58 wk

[a]   Mice were started on 0, 2, or 10 mM Pb acetate in their drinking water at 10 weeks of age.

Table 3

Pb Effects on Mitogen, Mixed Lymphocyte Culture (MLC), and PFC Responses
of Surviving Male B/W Mice

Pb Dose[a] (mM)	Blood Pb (µg/dl)	Mitogen Response[b]		MLC[c]	PFC[d]
		Con A	LPS		
0	2 ± 0	2,389	8,896	2,026	80 ± 48
		± 3,912	± 2,820	± 966	
2	39 ± 13	2,965	4,694	1,741	899 ± 1,923
		± 2,770	± 3,425	± 1,216	
10	377 ± 174	1,566	9,920	1,740	4 ± 7
		± 1,365	± 8,963	± 769	

[a]   Mice were exposed to Pb for 50 weeks prior to in vitro analysis.
[b]   CPM/culture.
[c]   CPM/culture.
[d]   PFC/culture.

Table 4

Pb Effects on SJL/J Mice

Pb Dose[a] (mM)	% Mortality (58 wk)	Tumor Incidence in Surviving Mice[b]
0	30%	+
0.08	10%	±
0.4	20%	+
2	20%	+
10	80%	++

[a] Mice were given Pb in their drinking water starting at 10 weeks of age.
[b] The mice still alive after 48 weeks of exposure to Pb were assessed for tumor in spleen and liver.

Table 5

Lymphoid Subset Analysis of Peripheral Blood Lymphocytes

from Hg-poisoned Humans

(> 20ng Hg/ml blood)

Subset	Percent	Normal Range
T3	57.5 ± 2.2 [a]	52–74
T4	40.5 ± 2.1	33–51
T8	29.5 ± 2.5	15–37
T11	77.2 ± 1.8	50–79
sIg	5.5 ± 0.8	6–24

[a] Mean ± S.E. (n=13).

Table 6

Thiol Characteristics of Lymphocytes Subsets[a]

Thiol Characteristic	CELL TYPE			
	B Cell	Th Cell Lyt-1	Ts/c Cell Lyt-2,3	MØ
Proliferation (2-ME)[a]	+++	+	++	ND
Number surface sulfhydryls	++	+	+++	ND
Intracellular glutathione	+	+	+	++
Sensitivity to permeant thiol blockers	+++	+	++	ND
Sensitivity to impermeant thiol blockers	-	-	+	ND
Sensitivity to impermeant oxidant	++	-	+	ND
Radiosensitivity	+++	+	++	-

[a]   Similar information reported in reference 19.

Table 7

Glutathione Levels in Cells From Surviving

Pb-treated Male B/W Mice

Pb Dose[a] (mM)	Glutathione Level (attomole/cell)	
	Peritoneal Cells	Spleen Cells
0	899 ± 267	318 ± 15
2	925 ± 236	329 ± 66
10	439 ± 5	345 ± 35

[a]   Mice were exposed to Pb in their drinking water for 50 weeks before sacrifice at 60 weeks of age.

302

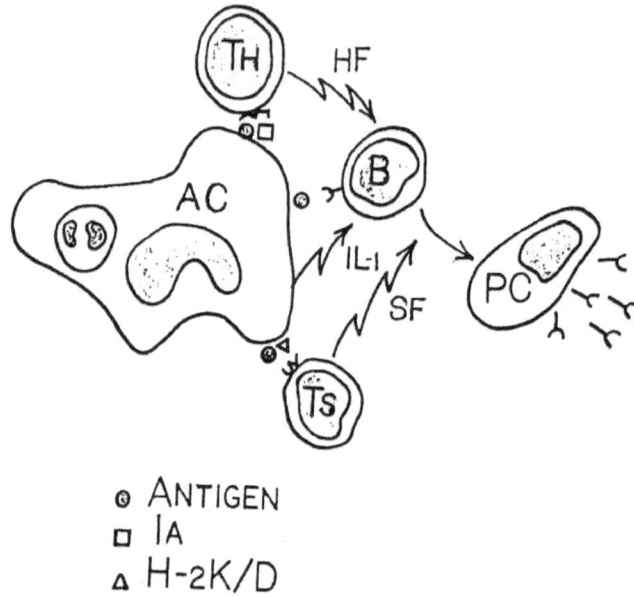

○ ANTIGEN
□ IA
△ H-2K/D

Figure 1.   The antigenic interactions of T cells, B cells, and accessory cells in the development of humoral immune responses. Th = Lyt-1, helper T cells; Ts = Lyt-2,3, suppressor T cells; B = B cells; AC = accessory "antigen processing/ presenting" cells; HF = helper factors (IL2; TRF; BCGF; BCDF); SF = suppressor factors.

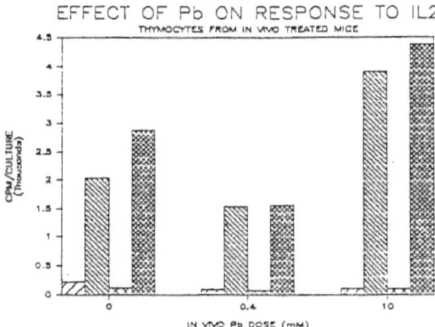

Figure 2. The in vivo effect of Pb on the ability of thymocytes to proliferate in response to IL-2. Thymocytes were obtained from animals that were maintained for 6.5 wks on 0, 0.4, or 10.0 mM Pb in their drinking water. Thymocytes were aliquoted into 96 well plates at 1×10^5 cells/0.1 ml/well. Media (RPMI-1640,▨), Con A (2.0 µg/ml,▧), BESA (10^{-5}M,▨), or Con A + BESA (2.0 µg/ml + 10^{-5}M,▨), was added to the appropriate wells. Partially purified IL-2 (40-80% ammonium sulfate cut), derived from the FS613.14 cell line, was added such that the final in well dilution was 1:100. Plates were incubated at 37°C, in special gas, pulsed with 0.5 µCi [^{3}H]-thymidine/0.025 ml/well at 66 hrs and harvested at 72 hrs. The results represent the arithmetic mean of triplicate cultures.

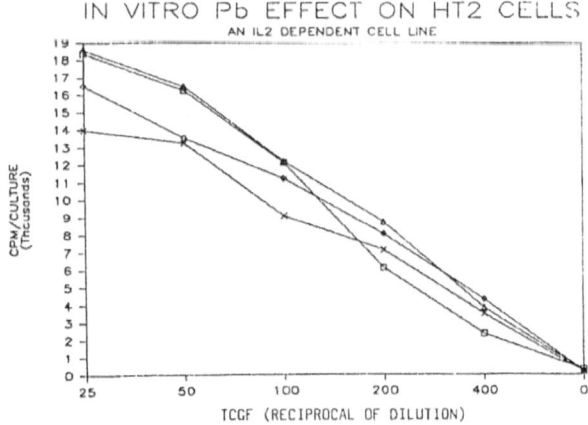

Figure 3. The in vitro effect of Pb on TCGF-induced proliferation of HT2 cells. HT2 cells were harvested, washed 3X with BSS + 5% FBS and resuspended in RPMI-1640, 5% FBS at 5×10^4 cells/ml.

REFERENCES

1. Lawrence, D.A. (1981): Heavy metal modulation of lymphocyte activities. I. In vitro effects of heavy metals on primary humoral immune responses. Toxicol. Appl. Pharmacol. 57: 439-451.

2. Hirsch, F., Couderc, J., Sapin, C., Fournie, G., & Druet, P. (1982): Polyclonal effect of HgCl2 in the rat, its possible role in an experimental autoimmune disease. Eur.J.Immunol. 12: 620-625.

3. Dorf, M.E., editor (1981): The Role of the Major Histocompatibility Complex in Immunobiology. Garland Press, NY.

4. Edwards, F.K., & Edwards, E.K. (1982): Allergic contact dermatitis to lead acetate in a hair dye. Cutis 30: 629-630.

5. Fregert, S. (1973): Allergic contact dermatitis from lead. Contact Dermatitis Newsletter 13 (Jan.).

6. Feuerman. E.J. (1975): Recurrent contact dermatitis caused by mercury in amalgam dental fillings. Int'l. J. Dermatol. 14: 657-660.

7. North American Contact Dermatitis Group (1983): Epidemiology of contact dermatitis in North America. Arch. Dermatol. 108: 537-540.

8. Koller, L.D., & Kovacic, S. (1974): Decreased antibody formation in mice exposed to lead. Nature (London) 250: 148-150.

9. Koller, L.D., & Roan, J.G. (1980): Effects of lead, dadmium and methylmercury on immunological memory. J. Environ. Pathol. Toxicol. 4(4): 47-52.

10. Lawrence, D.A. (1981): Heavy metal modulation of lymphocyte activities. II. Lead, an in vitro mediator of B-cell activation. Int'l. J. Immunopharmacol. 3: 153-161.

11. Koller, L.D., Roan, J.G., & Exon, J.H. (1976): Humoral antibody response in mice after single dose exposure to lead or cadmium. Proc. Soc. Exp. Biol. Med. 151: 339-342.

12. Lawrence, D.A., Mitchell, D., & Rudofsky, U. (1983): Heavy metal modulation of lymphocyte and macrophage activity. In "Proceedings of the 13th Annual Conference on Environmental Toxicology"., AFAMRL-TR-82-1o1,pp.63-79.

13. Sapin, C., Mandet, C., Druet, E., Gunther, G., & Druet, P. (1981): Immune complex type disease induced by HgCl2: genetic control of susceptibility. Transplant. Proc. 13: 1404-14o6. 14. Makinodan, T., & Kay, M.M.B. (1980): Age influence on the immune system. Adv. Immunol. 29:287-330.

15. Bonvida, B. (1983). The SJL/J spontaneous reticulum cell sarcoma:New insights in the fields of neoantigens, host-tumor interactions, and regulation of tumor growth. Adv. Concer Res. 38:1.

16. Tubbs, R.R., Gephardt, G.N. McMahon, J.T. Pohl, M.C., Vidt, D.G., Barenberg, S.A., & Valenzuela, R. (1982): Membranous glomerulonephritis associated with industrial mercury exposure. Study of pathogenetic mechanisms. Am.J.Clin. Pathol. 77: 409-413.

17. Lindquist, K.J. (1974): Immunofluorescence and electron microscopic studies of kidney biopsies from patients with nephrotic syndrome, possibly induced by skin lightening cream containing mercury. East Afr. Med. J. 51: 168.

18. Wedeen, R.P., Mallik, D.K., & Betuman, V. (1979): Detection and treatment of occupational lead nephropathy. Arch. Intern. Med. 139: 53-57.

19. Lawrence, D.A. (1981): Antigen activation of T-cells. In "Handbook of Cancer Immunology", edited by H. Waters, pp. 257-32o. Garland Press, NY.

20. Redelman, D., & Hudig, D. (1980): The mechanism of cell-mediated cytoxocity. I. Killing by murine cells requires cell surface thiols and activated proteases. J. Immunol. 124: 870-878.

21. Lawrence, D.A. (1984): Immunotoxicity of heavey metals. In "Toxicology of the Immune System", edited by J.H.Dean, A. Munson, & M. Luster, Chapter 27. Raven Press, NY (in press).

22. Kerkvliet, N.I., & Baecher-Steppan. L. (1982): Immuno-toxicology studies on lead: effects of exposure on tumor growth and cell-mediated tumor immunity after syngeneic or allogeneic stimulation. Immunopharmacology 4: 213-224.

23. Passow, H., Rothstein, A., & Clarkson, T.W. (1961): The general pharmacology of the heavy metals. Pharmacol. Rev. 13: 185-224.

24. Dalvi, R.R., & Robbins, T.J. (1979): Effect of Cd, Co, Pb, and Se on hepatic microsomal monoxygenase enzyme system and glutathione in mice. Toxicol. Appl. Pharmacol. 48: A110.

25. Hager-Malecka, B., Szczepanski, Z., & Romanska, K. (1982): Zachowanie sie nietorych bialek osocza oraz glutationu zredukowanego erytrocytow w przebiegu prezew-leklego zatrucia olowiem u dzieci. Pe. Pol. 57: 309-313.

26. Abraham, E.C., Taylor, J.F., & Lang, C.A. (1978): Influence of mouse age and erythrocyte age on glutathione metabolism. Biochem. J. 174: 819-825.

27. Noelle, R.J., & Lawrence, D.A. (1981): Modulation of T-cell functions. II. Chemical basis for the involvement of cell surface thiol-reactive sites in control of T-cell proliferation. Cell. Immunol. 60: 453-469.

28. Caeh, M.P., Lawrence, J.C., & Lynn, W.S. (1974): Evidence for the involvement of sulfhydryl oxidation in regulation of fat cell hexose transport by insulin. Proc. Natl. Acad. Sci. USA 71: 4173-4177.

29. Johnson, H.M. (1980): Similarities in the suppression of the immune response by interferon and by a thiol-oxidizing agent (40882). Proc. Soc. Exptl. Biol. Med. 164: 380-385.

3o. Hammett, F.S. (1929): The chemical stimulus essential for growth by increase in cell numbers. Protoplasma 7: 297-322.

31. Goldberger, R.F., Epstein, C.J., & Anfinsen, C.B. (1963): Acceleration of reactivation of reduced bovine pancreatic ribonuclease by a microsomal system from rat liver. J. Biol.Chem. 238: 628-635.

32. Askonas, B.A., & Parkhouse, R.M.E. (1971): Assembly of immunoglobulin M-blocked thiol groups of intracellular 7S subunits. Biochem. J. 123: 629-634.

33. Ledbetter, J.A., Seaman, W.E., Tsu, T.T., & Herzenberg, L.A. (1981): Lyt-2 and Lyt-2 antigens are on two different polypeptide subunits linked by disulfide bonds. Relationship of subunits to T-cell cytolytic activity. J. Exp. Med. 153: 1503-1516.

34. Taniguchi, M., Saito, T., Takei, I., & Tokushisa, T. (1981): Presence of interchain disulfide bonds between two gene products that compose the secreted form of an antigen-specific suppressor factor. J.Exp. Med. 153: 1672-1677.

35. Rothstein, A. (1970): Sulfhydryl groups in membrane structure and function. Curr. Topics Membrane Transport. 1: 135-176.

36. Noelle, R.J., & Lawrence, D.A. (1981): Modulation of T-cell functions. II. Chemical basis for the involvment of cell surface thiol-reactive sites in control of T-cell proliferation. Cell. Immunol. 60: 453-469.

37. Loor, F. (1980). Plasma membrane and cell cortex interactions in lymphocyte functions. Adv. Immunol. 30: 1-120.

38. Unanue, E. (1981): The regulatory role of macrophages in antigenic stimulation. Symbiotic relationship between lymphocytes and macrophages. Adv. Immunol. 31: 1-136.

39. Irons, R.D. & Pfeifer, R.W. (1984): In "Toxicology" of the Immune System", edited by J.H.Dean, A. Munson, and M. Luster). Raven Press, NY (in press).

40. Cunnane, S.C. (1982): Differential regulation of essential fatty acid metabolism to the prostaglandins: possible basis for the interaction of zinc and copper in biological systems. Prog. Lipid Res. 21: 73-90.

41. Graham, J.A., Gardner, D.E. Waters, M.D., & Coffin, D.C. (1975): Effect of trace metals on phagocytosis by alveolar macrophages. Infect. Immunity 11: 278-1283.

42. Nelson, D.J., Kiremidjian-Schumacher, L., & Stotzky, G. (1982): Effects of cadmium, lead and zinc on macrophage-mediated cytotoxicity toward tumor cells. Environ. Res. 28: 154-163.

43. Passow, H. (1970): The red blood cell: penetration, distribution, and toxic actions of heavy metals. In "Effects of Metals on Cells, Subcellular Elements, and Macromolecules", edited by J. Maniloff, J.R. Coleman, and M. Miller), p. 291. C.C.Thomas, IL.

44. Vallee, B.L., & Ulmer, D.D. (1972): Biochemical effects of mercury, cadmium an lead. Ann. Rev. Biochem. 41: 91.

45. Nishizuka, Y. (1984): The role of protein kinase C in cell surface signal transduction and tumor promotion. Nature 308: 693.

SOME ASPECTS OF IMMUNE ALTERATIONS INDUCED BY CHLORO-DIBENZO-p-DIOXINS AND CHLORODIBENZOFURANS

A. Vecchi

Instituto di Ricerche Farmacologiche, Mario Negri; Milano, Italy

INTRODUCTION

Polychlorinated dibenzo-p-dioxins (PCDDs) and polychlorinated dibenzofurans (PCDFs) are two series of tricyclic aromatic compounds that exhibit similar physical, chemical and biological properties. The number of chlorine atoms in these compounds can vary between one and eight to produce up to 75 PCDD and 135 PCDF positional isomers. The interest in these compounds comes from the fact that these two classes of aromatic compounds have been detected as contaminants of different commercial products (phenoxy-herbicides, hexachlorophene, chlorophenols, polychlorinated biphenyls, diphenyl ether herbicides) and thus they can enter the environment as inadvertant contaminants (1). PCDD und PCDF have also been reported to occur in fly ask from industrial facilities (1) and in fly ash and flue gas condensate from municipal incinerators (2). In addition, these compounds have been involved in at least seven serious incidents in the last fifteen years: the poisoning of horse arenas in Missouri, in 1971; the chemical plant accident in Seveso, Italy, in 1976; the Love Canal incident in Niagara Falls N.Y., in 1979; the fire in the Binghampton N.Y. State Office Building in 1981; the street contamination of the entire town of Times Beach, Mo. in 1982-1983 and the "Yusho" disease in Japan in 1968 and in Taiwan in 1979.

From the toxicity studies performed in the past, it appears that the 2.3.7.8-tetrachloro substituted dibenzo-p-dioxin (TCDD) and the 2.3.7.8-tetra (TCDF), 1.2.3.7.8- and 2.3.4.7.8-pentachloro substituted dibenzofurans represent the most toxic isomers. A sign of toxicity common to PCDDs and PCDFs in all the species investigated is thymus atrophy, while involvement of other organs (as for example liver, stomach, skin, eyelids ecc.) varies in the different animal species studied. Thymus toxicity suggests PCDDs and PCDFs could affect immune responses: however only the most toxic isomers, TCDD and TCDF, have been studied. While TCDD effects have been investigated for at least ten years in different species and different experimental conditions (3-6), studies on TCDF effects are still limited (7,8).

2.3.7.8.- TETRACHLORODIBENZO-P-DIOXIN

After the initial studies of Vos et al. (5) and Zinkl et al. (4) where effects on thymus and peripheral lymphocytes were detected after administration of fairly high doeses of TCDD, subsequent investigations have shown that immune responses can be very sensitive to exposure at doses of TCDD that are <

1/100 the LD 50 (9). Humoral as well as cell mediated immune
responses can be depressed by TCDD exposure. Preferential
sensitivity of immune reactivities differs in the various
species investigated: delayed hypersensitivity reaction to
tuberculin is depressed in guinea pigs by 40 ng/kg of TCDD
given for 8 weeks, while secondary, but not primary, antibody
response to tetanus toxoid is suppressed only at higher doses
(3). Similarly, repeated weekly treatments (8 doses) as low
as 0.1 μg/kg decrease the blastogenic response to phytomitogens
in rabbits and CD1 mice (10), while doses of at least 1 g/kg
are needed to induce a significant decrease in serum immunoglobulins in both species. Subsequent experiences in inbred
mice have shown that primary and secondary humoral antibody
production can be significantly depressed for more than 40
days by single doses of 1 μg/kg, when specific antibodies
against a T-dependent antigen (sheep erythrocytes) rather than
the total serum immunoglobulin levels are evaluated (11). The
same study shows that antibody production against a
T-independent antigen (pneumococcal polysaccharide type III)
is also significantly reduced, suggesting that the ihibition
of antibody production is not limited to TCDD effects on T
cells, as was initially suggested by the preferential toxicity
for the thymus. The same single dose does not modify the
blastogenic response of splenocytes to Concanavallin A (Con A)
and Lipopolysaccharide (LPS). However, a preferential sensitivity of T cells to TCDD exposure has been repeatedly
reported in experiments with chronic exposure (3,12), at least
in adult mice, adult rats being less susceptible to TCDD
immunotoxicity. Blastogenic responses to specific mitogens,
delayed hypersensitivity and graft versus host reactions, skin
allograft rejection are significantly depressed, though some
of these reactivities are reduced only at nearly toxic doses
(4 weekly treatments with 25 μg/kg).

Natural resistance mechanisms, usually evaluated in terms of
activity of NK cells and macrophages are not significantly
affected when adult mice are exposed to single or repeated
doses of TCDD (4 treatments up to 50 μg/kg) (13,14). Macrophage activity is not modified when evaluated as ability to
non specifically kill or phagocytize Listeria monocytogenes,
reduction of nitro-blue tetrazolium and basal or
endotoxin-stimulated cytotoxicity against tumor target cells
in vitro (13,14). Increased endotoxin sensitivity has been
observed in TCDD treated adult mice and macrophage impairment
has been suspected, these cells being considered of primary
importance in endotoxin detoxification (5). Moreover, susceptibility to bacterial (Salmonella bern), but not to viral
infection (Herpes suis) gave further support to the hypothesis
that increased sensitivity to endotoxin from gram-negative
bacteria was relevant in resistance to infections. However,
TCDD increases mortality also in mice infected with the
non-endotoxin-producing bacterium Listeria monocytogenes,
suggesting that decreased resistance to bacterial infection is
not merely related to an increase in endotoxin sensitivity
(5,15).

From the extensive data reported in the literature, it can be
concluded that thymus atrophy is a constant finding in animals

given TCDD as adults, and that humoral and cell-mediated immune responses are relatively more sensitive than natural resistance mechanisms (11,13).

If, however, TCDD is given during the developmental phase of the immune system, that is during the perinatal period through maternal feeding, it causes severe effects in mice and rats that can persist for up to 4 months of age (12.16). In addition to the effects observed in adults, suppression of humoral and cell mediated reactivities, TCDD administered in the perinatal period to mice depresses splenic NK cell acti- vity evaluated at 5 weeks of age, decreases the lympho- prolipherative response to the B cell mitogen LPS, alters bone marrow stem cell maturation, increases the incidence of mortality after Listeria monocytogenes infection and the percentage of syngeneic tumor takes (17). Macrophage functions, phagocytosis and response to colony stimulating factor, are not affected, but they decrease, in percentage as well as in number, in the peritoneal cavity after perinatal exposure to doses that do not alter macrophage functions (18). Sensitivity to endotoxin is further increased, doses 5 times lower than those used in adults being fully active.

Studies performed in perinatally exposed rats show that humoral immune functions are relatively resistant, while cell mediated reactivities, delayed hypersensitivity responses and responses to mitogens Con A and Phytohaemagglutinin (PHA) are suppressed. Impairment of T-cell function is selective in that helper function is not suppressed (16). Perinatal exposure increased the sensitivity of the immune system to TCDD effects in either mice and rats, but the subsets of immunocytes can be differentially affected in the various species investigated.

The depressed responses observed in perinatal exposed mice seem not to be obtained throught activation of suppressor cells, either lymphocytes or macrophages, as shown by co-cultures or adherence depletion experiments (5,17). Only in adult exposed mice is there a suggestion that TCDD can activate suppressor cells (19): This conclusion is based on the observation that in vitro cytotoxic T-cell (CTL) genera- tion is depressed in lymphocytes from TCDD treated mice, without decrease in the frequency of CTL precursors. This situation has been explained as a consequence of suppressor cells activation.

To elucidate the mechanism(s) responsible for TCDD-induced immunosuppression many hypothesis have been considered. No alterations in zinc and circulating corticosteroid levels have been observed in TCDD treated mice and guinea pigs (3,14); thymus atrophy is not an indirect effect mediated through adrenals or pituitary (20), nor can be related to alterations of serum α-fetoprotein or reduced food intake (5). Interestingly, thymosin does not reduce TCDD suppression of lymphoproliferative response or thymic involution, suggesting that lymphoid cells are severely damaged and are no longer sensitive to the thymic hormone. No restoration of humoral antibody production is obtained by <u>Corynebacterium parvum</u> administration to TCDD treated mice, while splenomegaly occurs in control as well as in treated mice (21).

<u>In vitro</u> studies with lectin-stimulated lymphocytes, though limited by the insolubility of TCDD in physiological buffers and by the use of DMSO as a solubilizing agent, suggest that immunosuppression is not due to an alteration in lymphocyte ability to bind lectins, rather to a direct alteration of lymphocyte activity. However the mechanism(s) of TCDD induced immunosuppression are still to be discovered. Some effects, including thymus athrophy, have been reported to segregate in mice with the Ah locus, which regulate the expression of a cytosolic binding protein with high affinity for TCDD (Ah receptor). This receptor can be detected in different tissues of mice and rats and its presence, genetically determined, is associated with high susceptibility to aryl hydrocarbon hydroxylase (AHH) enzyme induction. The Ah receptor has been detected in thymus, in rats this organ shows the highest concentration, and in mice it is about one fourth the concen-tration of liver, where it is maximally expressed (22). TCDD induced toxic effects such as malformations, thymus athrophy and porphyria are more severe in mouse strains where the Ah receptor is detectable (responsive strains), while the same effects are modest or absent in non-responsive strains, where the receptor is not detectable unless mice have been pretrea-ted with suitable doses of TCDD (22). Studies on TCDD immuno-suppression performed in responsive and nonresponsive mouse strains have shown that the genetic background is of relevance for the effects being observed (9). Humoral antibody produc-tion was more markedly depressed in responsive strains (C57B1/6 - C3H/He) and the degree of inhibition paralleled well what expected for the presence of Ah receptor in F1 and backcross generations between responsive and non-responsive strains (DBA/2 - AKR). The relevance of the Ah receptor presence has been similarly reported in subsequent experiments by Clark and coworkers (23), who descdribed a more marked depression of <u>in vitro</u> CTL generation in C57B1/6 than DBA/2 treated mice.

Data obtained in responsive and non-responsive strains, though highly suggestive of an involvement of the Ah receptor in the expression of TCDD immunodepressive potential, do not clarify whether the effects on immune responses are directly related to an interaction with the receptor at lymphoid organ level(thymus)or are secondary to a sequence of events evoked in different organs (for example the strong and long lasting induction of AHH enzyme in liver with metabolic alterations). One suggestion in favour of the hypothesis that the entire "environment" rather than lymphoid tissues only is relevant for TCDD effects comes from Nargakatti's study (24). Using chimeric mice, it was shown that TCDD affects <u>in vitro</u> CTL generation if given to responsive mice, irrespective whether they were transfused, after lethal irradiation, with bone marrow from responsive or non-responsive strains; no effects were seen if bone marrow recipient chimeras were non-responsive mice. Unfortunatly, we do not know yet whether the Ah receptor is present in bone marrow cells, while being expressed in thymus.

That the Ah receptor plays a role in immunotoxicity is further supported by the results obtained with 3.4.3'.4'.-tetrachloro biphenyl, 2.3.7.8-tetrachlorodibenzofuran, 3-methylcholan-threne and β-naphthoflavone (18). These polycyclic aromatic hydrocarbons, which are the most potent in vitro inhibitors of TCDD binding to the Ah receptor, significantly depress antibody prduction when given to C57B1/6 or C3H/He mice, but not when given to DBA/2 mice. Very recently it has been reported that the Ah receptor has associations with fertility, fitness and longevity (25), suggesting a physiological role for this binding specificity that till now had been considered relevant only for foreign compounds. A better knowledge of the physiological role of Ah receptors will probably help in understanding, at least partially, the mechanism(s) of TCDD induced toxicity.

2..3.7.8.- TETRACHLORODIBENZOFURAN

Few studies have been directed at finding possible alterations of the immune system by PCDFs in laboratory animals. Toxic doses of 2.3.7.8.-tetra- and 2.3.4.7.8.-penta-CDF have been shown to cause severe thymus atrophy in guinea pigs and mice (26). Lymphopenia, atrophy of the thymic cortex and reduction in the number of germinal centers in the spleen are produced in chicks dosed with 1 to 5 μg/kg for 21 days (27). Studies on the immune system of female guinea pigs show that the effects of 2.3.7.8. tetrachlorodibenzofuran (TCDF) resemble those of TCDD (7). Depression of cell-mediated responses are seen only at high dose levels (0.5 to 1 μg/kg weekly for six weeks); humoral immunity is only slightly depressed.

Experiments with single doses of TCDF in mice have shown reduction in thymus weight and splenocyte numbers after oral or intraperitoneal adminsitration of relatively low doses (100 μg/kg in C57B1/6 mice with an LD 50 of more than 6000 μg/kg) (8,9). Humoral antibody production is significantly inhibited. The dose-response curve is similar to that of TCDD, but shifted to right, TCDF being about thirty times less active than TCDD in terms of ug/kg. The time course of immunosuppression differs from that of TCDD, the latter being highly suppressive for up to six weeks, while TCDF effects recover completely by that time (8). Increased susceptibility to endotoxin has been described in mice treated with a mixture of tetra-and penta-CDFs for 4 weeks (18).

TCDF induced thymus athrophy and immunosuppression are more marked in responsive than in non responsive mouse strains, suggesting that the individual genetic background plays a role in TCDF immunotoxity, analogous with what reported for TCDD (9). Recent data have shown a positive correlation between AHH inducing ability of different dibenzofurans given at single doses and thymic involution (29), showing that dibenzo-furans toxicity to the immune system can be in some way linked to their inducing potential.

Data on other PCDFs are still very limited. One group (30) reported that, in female monkeys, commercial PCB preparations specifically treated to elimate contaminant PCDFs were more immunosuppressive on humoral antibody production than the commercial PCBs with PCDFs impurities. However reduction in red and white cells in blood was the same for PCDFs-free or commercial preparations. Other reports suggest that the simultaneous presence of PCDF and PCDD can induce, in different experimental conditions, synergistic effects as regards toxicity in guinea pigs (31) and antagonistic effects as regards immunosuppression and enzyme inducibility in mice (32). The data on PCDFs effects on the immune system are at present still limited: however the results obtained with pure isomers show that the pattern of immunotoxicity for active PCDF isomers is very similar to that displayed by the corresponding PCDD isomers, provided that higher doses are used.

Acknowledgment This work was partially supported by contract no. 82.02031.56 from CNR (Consiglio Nazionale delle Ricerche), Rome, Italy.

REFERENCES

1) Rappe C., *Analysis of polychlorinated dioxins and furans*, *Environ. Sci. Techno.*, 18 (1984) 78A - 90A

2) Olie, K., P.L. Vermeulen, O. Hutzinger, *Chlorodibenzo-p-dioxins and chlorobidenzofurans are trace components of fly ash and flue gas of some municipal incinerators in the Netherlands*, *Chemosphere*, 6 (1977) 455-459.

3) Vos, J.G., J.A. Moore & J.G. Zinkl, *Effects of 2.3.7.8-tetrachlorodibenzo-p-dioxin on the immune system of laboratory animals*, *Environ. Health Perspect.*, 5 (1973) 149-162.

4) Zinkl, J.G., J.G. Vos, J.A. Moore & B.N. Gupta, *Hematologic and clinical chemistry effects of 2.3.7.8-tetrachlorodibenzo-p-dioxins in laboratory animals*, *Environ. Health Perspect.*, 5 (1973) 111-118.

5) Vos, J.g. R.E. Faith & M.I. Luster, *Immune alterations*, in *"Halogenated Biphenyls, Terphenyls, Napthalenes, Dibenzodioxins and Related Products"* R.D. Kimbrough ed. *Elsevier North Holland Biomedical Press*, Amsterdam, (1980).

6) Dean, J.H. M.I. Luster & G.A. Boorman, *Immunotoxicology*, in *"Immunopharmacology"* P. Sirois and M. Rola-Pleszcynski eds., *Elsevier Biomedical Press*, Amsterdam (1982) 349-397.

7) Luster, M.I., R.E. Faith & L.D. Lawson, *Effects of 2.3.7.8-tetrachlorodibenzofuran (TCDF) on the immune system in guinea pigs*, *Drug Chem. Toxicol.* 2 (1979) 49-60.

314

8) Vecchi, A., M. Sironi, M.A. Canegrati & S. Garattini,
    Comparison of the immunosuppressive effects in mice of
    2.3.7.8-tetrachlorodibenzo-p-dioxin and 2.3.7.8.-tetra-
    chlorodibenzofuran, in "Chlorinated Dioxins and Dibenzo-
    furans in the Total Environment" G. Choudhary et al.
    eds. Ann Arbor Science (Butterworths), Boston, Mass.
    (1983) 397-405.

9) Vecchi, A., M. Sironi, M.A. Canegrati, M. Recchia & S.
    Garattini, Immunosuppressive effects of 2.3.7.8-tetra-
    chlorodibenzo-p-dioxin in strains of mice with different
    susceptibility to induction of aryl hydrocarbon hydro-
    xylase, Toxicol. Appl. Pharmacol. 68 (1983) 434-441.

10) Sharma, R.P., R.J. Kociba & P.J. Gerhing., Immunotoxi-
    colocogical effects of 2.3.7.8-tetrachlorodiben zo-p-
    dioxin in laboratory animals, Toxicol. Appl. Pharmacol.
    45 (1978) 333.

11) Vecchi, A., A. Mantovani, M. Sironi, W. Luini, M.
    Cairo & S. Garattini, Effect of acute exposure to
    2.3.7.8.-tetrachlorodibenzo-p-dioxin on humoral antibody
    production in mice. Chem-Biol. Interact. 30 (1980)
    337-342.

12) Vos, J.G. & J.A. Moore, Suppression of cellular im-
    munity in rats and mice by maternal treatment with
    2.3.7.8-tetrachlorodibenzo-p-dioxin. Int. Arch.
    Allergy Appl. Immunol. 47 (1974) 777-794.

13) Mantovani, A., A. Vecchi, W. Luini, M. Sironi, G.P.
    Candiani, F. Spreafico & S. Garattini, Effect of
    2.3.7.8.-tetrachloridbenzo-p-dioxin on macrophage and
    natural killer cell-mediated cytotoxicity in mice.
    Biomedicine 32 (1980) 200-204.

14) Vos, J.G., J.G. Kreeftenberg, H.W.B. Engel, A. Minder-
    houd & L.M. van Noorle Jansen, Studies on
    2.3.7.8.-tetrachlorodibenzo-p-dioxin induced immune
    suppression and decreased resistance to infection:
    endotoxin hypersensitivity, serum zinc concentrations and
    effect of thymosin treatment. Toxicology 9 (1978) 75-86.

15) Thigpen, J.E., R.E. Faith, E.E. Mc Connell & J.A.
    Moore, Increased susceptibility to bacterial infection as
    a sequela of exposure to 2.3.7.8.-tetrachlorodibenzo-p-
    dioxin. Infection Immun. 12 (1975) 1319-1324.

16) Faith, R.E., M. I. Luster & J.A. Moore, Chemical
    separation of helper cell function and delayed hypersen-
    sitivity responses. Cell. Immuno. 40 (1978) 275-284.

17) Luster, M.I., G.A. Boorman, J.H. Dean, M.W. Harris,
    R.W. Luebke, M.L. Padarathsingh & J.A. Moore, Exami-
    nation of bone marrow immunological parameters and host
    susceptibility following pre- and postnatal exposure to
    2.3.7.8.-tetrachlorodibenzo-p-dioxin. Int. J.
    Immunopharmacol. 2 (1980) 301-310.

18) Silkworth, J.B. & A. Vecchi. Role of the Ah receptor in halogenated aromatic hydrocarbon immunotoxicity. in " Toxicology of the Immune System" J.H. Dean et al. eds. Raven Press, (1984) in press.

19) Clark, D.A., J. Gauldie, M.R. Szewczuk, G. Sweeney. Enhanced suppressor cell activity as a mechanism of immunosuppression by 2.3.7.8.-tetrachlorodibenzo-p-dioxin. Proc. Soc. Exp. Biol. Med. 168 (1981) 290-299.

20) Van Logten, M.G., B.N. Gupta, E.E. Mc Connell & J.A. Moore. Role of the endocrine system in the action of 2.3.7.8.-tetrachlorodibenzo-p-dioxin (TCDD) on the thymus. Toxicology 15 (1980) 135-144.

21) Garattini, S., A. Vecchi, M. Sironi & A. Mantovani. Immunosuppressant activity of TCDD in mice. in "Chlorinated Dioxins and Related Compounds. Impact on the Environment" O. Hutzinger et al. eds. Pergamon Press; Oxford (1982) 403-409.

22) Mason, M.E. & A.B. Okey. Cytosolic and nuclear binding of 2.3.7.8.-tetrachlorodibenzo-p-dioxin to the Ah receptor in extra hepatic tissues of rats and mice. Eur. J. Biochem. 123 (1982) 209-215.

23) Clark, D.A., G. Sweeney, S. Safe, E. Hancock, D.G. Kilburn & J. Gauldie, Cellular and genetic basis for suppression of cytotoxic T cell generation by haloaromatic hydrocarbons. Immunopharmacology 6 (1983) 143-153.

24) Nargakatti, P.s., G.D. Sweeney, J. Gauldie & D.A. Clark. Sensitivity to suppression of cytotoxic T cell generation by 2.3.7.8.-tetrachlorodibenzo-p-dioxin (TCDD) is dependent on the Ah genotype of the murine host. Toxicol. Appl. Pharmacol. 72 (1984) 169-176.

25) Nebert, D.W., H.J. Eisen & O. Hankinson. The Ah receptor: binding specificity only for foreign chemicals? Biochemical Pharmacology 33 (1984) 917-924.

26) Moore, J.A., E.E. Mc Connell, D.W. Dalgard & H.W. Harris Comparative toxicity of three halogenated dibenzo-furans in guinea pigs, mice and Thesus monkeys. Ann. N.Y. Acad. Sci. 320 (1979) 151-163.

27) Mc Kinney, J.D., K. Chae & B.N. Gupta. Toxicological assessment of hexachlorobiphenyl isomers and 2.3.7.8.-tetrachlorodibenzofuran in chicks. I. Relationship of chemical parameters. Toxicol. Appl. Pharmacol. 36 (1976) 65-80.

28) Oishi, S & K. Hiraga. Effect of polychlorinated biphenyl, dibenzofuran and dibenzo-p-dioxin on the susceptibility of male mice to endotoxin. J. Environ. Sci. Health B 15 (1) (1980) 77-85.

316

29) *Yoshihara, S., K. Nagata, H. Yoshimura, H. Kuroki & Y. Masuda. Inductive effects on hepatic enzymes and acute toxicity of individual polychlorinated dibenzofuran congeners in rats. Toxicol. Appl. Pharmacol. 59 (1981) 580-588.*

30) *Hori, S., H. Obana, T. Kashimoto, T. Otake, H. Nashimura, N. Ikegami, N. Kunita, Y. Fukuda & H. Uda. Biological effects of the compounds related to yusho on female cynomolgus (Macaca fascicularis). II. Studies on biochemical findin of blood, hepatic microsomal enzyme, immune response and histopathology. Osaka-furitsu Koshu Eisei Kenkyusho Kenkyu Hokoku, Shokuhin Eisei Hen. 12 (1981) 925.*

31) *Silkworth, J.B., D. Mc Martin, A. De Caprio, R. Rej, P. O'Keefe & L. Kaimusky. Acute toxicity in guinea pig and rabbit of soot from a polychlorinated biphenyl-containing transformer fire. Toxicol. Appl. Pharmacol. 65(1982) 425-439.*

32) *Rizzardini, M., M. Romano, F. Tursi. M. Salmona, A. Vecchi, M. Sironi, F. Gizzi, E. Benfenati, S. Garattini & R. Fanelli. Toxicological evaluation of urban waste incinerator emissions. Chemosphere 12 (1983) 559-564.*

IMMUNOTOXICOLOGICAL EFFECTS OF ASBESTOS

Klara Miller.

Immunotoxicology Department
The British Industrial Biological Research Association,
Woodmansterne Road,
Carshalton, Surrey, SM5 4DS (U.K.)

INTRODUCTION

Exposure to asbestos dust may stimulate a severe reaction in the lungs leading to parechymal and pleural fibrosis. There is also an association between exposure to asbestos and the development of bronchogenic carcinomas and mesotheliomas. While the pathogenesis of these disorders is unknown, altered immunoregulatory mechanisms may be important and it also becomes increasingly important to know whether select individuals may react in an immunologically hyperactive way to inhalation of asbestos. This was recognized in 1973 when the Report of the Advisory Committee on Asbestos Cancer to the Director of the International Agency for Research on Cancer (Report 1973) recommended enquiring into the immunocompetence of asbestosis with regard to the role of immunity in the subsequent development of neoplasms. Since then there have been several clinical studies indicating definitive alterations in the immune profile of asbestos workers (Section I).

It has been suggested that early events in the development of asbestos induced injury are fundamentally different to those caused by inhalation of other inorganic dusts(1) and tissue and cell culture techniques have been used to study the biological effects of asbestos at the cellular level (Section II). In particular asbestos toxicity to macrophages has been the subject of many studies as the location and function of alveolar macrophages means that they are one of the first cell types to encounter inhaled mineral fibres. A number of in vitro and short term studies have demonstrated alterations in macrophage function including stimulation of oxidant production and release of immunological mediators. Whilst much more work is needed to identify effects specific to asbestos fibres, these findings demonstrate the potential of asbestos to modify macrophage function.

In order to study in vivo participation of macrophages with the immune system experimental animals have been exposed to asbestos for prolonged periods (see Section III). In vivo observations support the hypothesis that phagocytosed asbestos persists and is relatively non-toxic to macrophages. The alveolar macrophages were shown to have altered surface morphology and to evoke humoral immune responses directed against surface membrane determinants. In vivo exposure also resulted in macrophages that were perceived by lymphocytes as if they had mitogenic or antigenic products expressed on their membrane. These investigations may lead to a greater understanding of the complex function of the macrophage and its role in the pathogenesis of asbestos associated disease.

I. IMMUNOLOGICAL STUDIES IN ASBESTOS EXPOSED POPULATIONS

Studies of workers with long-term occupational exposure to asbestos have shown alterations of cellular and humoral immune reponses in the individuals (Table 1). Impaired expression of several parameters of cell-mediated immunity and hyperactive humoral immunity has been described using both in vivo and in vitro procedures. Delayed hypersensitivity skin tests on patients with interstitial fibrosis show significantly fewer positive responses to standard test antigens such as strepto-kinase - streptodornase (SKSD) and Candida albicans, commonly used to assess immunological recall (2,3,4,5,) Studies of total circulating T lymphocyte numbers and function have yielded conflicting results (6,7,8,9,5) but all data indicate an association between asbestos exposure and diminished numbers of T lymphocytes. Analysis of T-cell subpopulations has shown decreases in cells expressing phenotypes for both helper-inducer (OKT4) and suppressor-cytoxic (OKT8) activity (10). These authors also stipulate that the immunological pertubations are epiphenomena, unrelated to the pathogenesis of asbestosis itself. The observation of a diminished ability to generate suppressor activity by lymphocytes obtained from asbestos - exposed subjects, however, (5) supports the concept of a qualitative alteration of T lymphocyte function. That a qualitative T-cell defect may occur in patients with asbes-tosis has also been demonstrated in vitro phytohaemagglutinin (PHA) -induced lymphocyte proliferative assays which show a significant impairment of lymphocyte responsiveness (7,11), although normal responsiveness has been reported in asbestos-exposed heavy smokers (9).

Differences in T lymphocyte function have also been found in subjects with occupational asbestos exposure associated with pleural plaques compared to those with similar exposures but no evidence of pleural reactions. A significant depression of lymphocyte responsiveness to PHA was demonstrated in the group with pleural plaques compared to the control group, whilst no difference was found in the response pattern by lymphocytes obtained from subjects without a pleural reaction (12). Another parameter of cellular immunity, PHA-induced cytotoxic cell function, was found to be consistently reduced in the group with pleural plaques with lymphocytes obtained from 16 out of 18 patients causing less than 9% Cr rerelease from labelled target cells (Fig 1). PHA-induced cytotoxic effector cell function has also been found to be significantly reduced amongst abestosis patients when compared to controls (7). The majority of studies, therefore, suggest a link between impai-red T lymphocyte function and the group of subjects that develop asbestosis or pleural plaques after exposure to asbestos. There is little evidence, however, that impaired T-cell function, as measured by these in vitro assays, is defective in asbestos-associated malignancy. In studies on patients with pleural mesothelioma (13,11) the majority of patients have been reported to have normal T lymphocyte responses both in vitro and in vivo depite relatively reduced numbers of circulating lymphocytes.

In contrast to impaired expressions of cellular immunity, subjects with asbestosis often manifest hyperactivity of humoral immune responses, suggesting an imbalance between the cellular and humoral components of the immune response. Significantly increased levels of the serum immunoglobulins IgA IgM & IgG have been reported in several studies when compared with corresponding values of control groups (2,15,16,17,18,1,19) although not all of these studies found increases in all the classes of immunoglobulins. The reason for the polyclonal increase of serum immunoglobulins is not evident and could be related to the adjuvant-like action ascribed to asbestos by Miller & Kagan, (20) which might augment the helper role of T-lymphocytes in a non-antigen-specific fashion (21). Alternatively, reduction of suppressor T-cell function, which can exert specific feedback control on antibody synthesis by B lymphocytes (22) could explain the general increase in immunoglobulin production. Increased prevelance of non-specific auto-antibodies and elevated levels of IC has also been reported in workers exposed to asbestos (23,3,19).

It has been suggested that unchecked B lymphocyte activity resulting in increased production of immunoglobulins, and auto-antibody production could be the cause of lympho-proliferative disorders which have been reported in patients with asbestos-exposure (5,24). In this context it is well to remember that whilst there is no association between exposure to silica and the development of neoplasms, silicosis is associated with increased levels of immunoglobulins, a greatly increased prevalance of autoantibodies and a high incidence of "autoimmune" disease. (19,25). However only minor differences have been found between cell-mediated immune responses in patients with silicosis and control subjects (26). The differing _in vivo_ effects of silica and asbestos on the alveolar macrophage (27) could result in different responses to asbestos and silica particularly as regards the breakdown of conventional immune surveillance mechanisms mediated by macrophages (28). The participation of macrophages in both cell-mediated and humoral reactions clearly focuses attention on the important role of the macrophage as an immunoregulatory cell and the effect of asbestos on macrophages has been studied in a number of _in vitro_ and _in vivo_ systems.

II. FUNDAMENTAL EARLY CELLULARL EVENTS

While the macrophage plays a crucial role in the pathogenesis of asbestosis and silicosis little is known of the sequence of events following phagocytosis. Clearly the location and function of alveolar macrophages means that they are one of the first cell types to encounter inhaled mineral fibres and these fibres are then phagocytosed. Although not usually taken into account the intersittial macrophages are also important in the pulmonary reaction to inhaled asbestos (29).

Many studies have made use of tissue and cell culture techniques to understand the biological affects of asbestos at a cellular level (30,31). The fibrogenic factor reported to be produced by macrophages exposed to silica (32,33) has not been found in asbestos treated cultures (34). Rather Davies et al. (35) demonstrated that asbestos could apparently cause the release of lysosomal enzymes to a greater degree than cell death (as measured by the release of lactic dehydrogenase). This "selective release" could be caused by the increased permeability of the cell membrane during phagocytosis (36) or by the partial ingestion of long fibres. Such enzyme release could be merely one sign of sublethal cell damage. The released enzymes as well as neutral proteases, free radicals and inflammatory mediators could themselves damage tissue and thus be causally related to fibrosis through some inflammatory process. There have been several studies on the release of neutral proteases, oxygen derived radicals and prostaglandins (PC) from both mononuclear and plymorphonuclear cells.

A number of studies (37) have demonstrated that cells treated with asbestos secrete plasminogen activator and this can be inhibited by anti-inflammatory steroids (ibid). White & Kuhn (38) have reported that peritoneal and alveolar macrophages exposed to a variety of particles release increased amounts of elastase. However, the effects of fibrogenic dusts including two types of asbestos, was less than that of latex. This illustrates a common problem in in vitro studies, that while stimulating one activity, asbestos can also damage the cells thus reducing the overall effect obtained and making inter-pretation of the results extremely difficult.

A large number of stimuli are known to result in the release of so called free radicals from immunocompetent phagocytic cells and are extremely imporant in determining the micro-biocidal and tumouricidal activities of macrophages. A number of authors have examined the effects of asbestos on phagocytic cells using free radical formation as an endpoint (39). Hatch et al, (40) using guinea-pig alveolar macrophages found that amphibole asbestos samples produced the most chemiluminescence; however silica, zymosan and polymethyl methacrylate produced more effect than chrysotile asbestos. Doll et al, (41,42) investigated the effect of incubation with various types of asbestos on the release of oxygen metabolites from PMN and peripheral monocytes and on the exposed cells' subsequent response to zymosan. The overall effect of the asbestos was small and the significance of the released radicals difficult to assess. Considerably more work on radical formation using a whole range of cells and detection methods is necessary before any firm conclusions on the role of these phenomena in pathogenesis can be reached.

A large number of stimuli are known to cause the release of arachidonic acid metabolites from macrophages (43). Using the macrophage like cell line P388DI Brown & Poole (in press, 12) have found that crocidolite and chrysotile caused the release of PGE2 and F2 alpha. It is of great interest in this context to note the well known effect of PG on suppressor cell ac-tivity (44). There have been no studies published on the release of other arachidonic acid metabolites such as the leukotrienes; these could be important given the role of some lipoxygenase products in chemotaxis.

In addition to pure in vitro experiments some studies have involved the administration of asbestos by the intraperitoneal and other routes prior to an in vitro evaluation of macrophage structure and function. Adminsitration of both chrysotile and crocidolite asbestos fibres has demonstrated changes in the membrane topography of peritoneal macrophages. These changes were indicative not only of activation (20) but also showed an alteration in surface glycoprotein organisation (45); such alterations could lead to modification of the immunobiology of these cells.

III. IMMUNOREGULATORY EFFECTS IN EXPERIMENTAL ANIMALS.

Several animal species have been used successfully in the study of histological reactions to inhaled asbestos particles. The alveolar macrophage is intimately involved in a variety of immunological events and may leave the lung by migration into the lymphatic system as well as by mucociliary transport (46,47,48). It seems pertinent therefore to study the in vivo interaction of macrophages and lymphocytes in considering immunological mechanisms in the pathogenesis of dust diseases.

In a number of investigations, Miller and colleagues exposed rats to asbestos by inhalation over prolonged periods. In vivo studies have demonstrated that both chrysotile and crocidolite asbestos were non-toxic to macrophages and stimulate the cells to develop into mature non-specifically activated cells (20,49,50) (Table 2). Significant differences in Fc receptor activity was shown in one study, (20) when macrophages from exposed animals were compared to control cells both in the percentage of cells forming EA rosettes and in the avidity of the receptor. It was postulated that these surface-related changes could be paralleled by changes in surface antigenicity. This hypothesis was supported when alveolar macrophages from exposed animals were found to exhibit significantly increased immune adherence as compared with control cells, indicating that deposition of complement components on alveolar macrophages had occurred in vivo (51). This was thought to be a manifestation of a humoral immune response directed against surface membrane determinants of macrophages altered by the ingestion of asbestos fibres in vivo. (Further evidence of systemic B cell activation has recently been reported by Bozelka et al (52) in mice.

Miller et al (53) used two model systems to investigate whether asbestos inhalation could lead to systemically sensitised T lymphocytes. The first was based on that devised by Rosenthal and his co-workers (54,55) for studying the recognition of macrophage-associated antigens by T cells. In their studies they showed that T cells bind reversibly to macrophages in the absence of antigen. When the macrophages were pulsed with soluble antigen, however, T lymphocytes sensitised to the antigen clustered around the macrophages in a sustained fashion. The second model used the chemical alteration of cell membranes by $NaIO_4$ and other agents, which act through the oxidation and cleavage of cell surface glycoproteins with the generation of surface aldehyde moieties. Such alterations also induce macrophage-dependent lymphocyte binding (56) which can be blocked or reduced by agents such as borohydride and L-cysteine (57).

When these models were used to study the effects of asbestos inhalation, two separate asbestos-related effects, both dependent on plasma membrane changes were observed (53,27,58). The first phenomenon, which was analogous to that produced after control alveolar macrophages were pulsed with $NaIO_4$, was observed in co-cultures of exposed macrophages with control lymphocytes. In these cultures binding of lymphocytes to macrophages occurred followed by a blastogenic response. Both the binding and proliferation of lymphocytes could be abolished by treatment of the asbestos-exposed or $NaIO_4$-treated macrophages with L-cysteine. This effect is similar to alveolar macrophage membrane peroxidation, and provides a functional correlate of the adjuvant-like morphological response described previously (20). Reports that adjuvant-activated macrophages interact with immunocompetent T lymphocytes in a fashion that render them incapable of responding to a further stimulant (59) may thus provide an explanation for the depressed cellular immune responses noted in asbestosis subjects.

The second asbestos-related phenomenon, an antigen-like effect, was noted in cocultures of macrophages and lymphocytes obtained from exposed animals. Sustained lymphocyte clustering was observed which was maximal after 24 hours incubation and was followed by a peak proliferation response after 96 hours incubation. These effects were not abrogated by L-cysteine and required major histocompatibility complex-linked restriction between the interacting macrophages and lymphocytes. Since splenic lymphocytes were used, these findings are consistent with a systemic immune recognition and lymphoid activation. The recent report (60) that macrophage-lymphocyte co-culture supernants, when obtained from immunized, asbestos exposed rats, contained greater interleukin-1 and interleukin-2 activity than supernatants from untreated controls, provides additional evidence for the antigen-like elaboration of lymphocyte stimulating factors after asbestos inhalation (Table 3). Thus the pathological changes in the lung following asbestos inhalation may be accompanied and amplified by macrophages whose altered immuno-biology could result in an imbalance between cellular and humoral immunity (Fig. 2). It is interesting that no evidence of sensitised lymphocytes or humoral activation was found where animals were exposed to silica instead of asbestos (27). Whether there is any relationship between the lack of altered immunobiology of the macrophage and lack of association between silicosis and the development of carcinomas can at present only be a matter of speculation.

CONCLUSION

The possible mechanisms of the immunological abberations noted in clinical studies on asbestotics, has been investigated in a number of animal studies. In vitro tests and short term animal assays have demonstrated that exposure of macrophages to asbestos fibres causes the release of various chemical mediators. When macrophage accumulation due to asbestos inhalation occurs in the lung (61), there could be persistent secretion of enzymes which cause tissue damage as well as arachidonic acid metabolites and factors that stimulate fibroblast production (62). Such reactions would depend on the composition, surface area and durability of the asbestosis fibre (63).

Prolonged inhalation of asbestos by experimental animals has a profound effect on several different surface-related membrane characteristics of macrophages, all of which could lead to an altered immune response. The in vivo deposition of complement components on the surface of macrophages could indicate a humoral immune response against an "altered" cell. This concept provides some explanation towards the distrubances of humoral immunity found in subjects with asbestoses (64), although a loss of suppressor T-cell modulation would also explain increased production of immunoglobules.

The inbalance between cellular and humoral functions noted in clinical studies could have their origin in the altered immunobiology of the alveolar macrophage demonstrated in animal studies. In these investigations specific effects of asbestos on T lymphocytes was found after prolonged inhalation and lymphocyte proliferation was induced by both an aldehyde-like alteration of asbestos-exposed macrophage membranes and by an association between macrophages with antigen-like molecules and immunospecific T lymphocytes. Whilst the nature of the proliferating T lymphocytes has not been determined they may have been rendered incapable of respending to further stimulation. These findings may explain the depressed cell-mediated responses found in asbestos exposed subjects. Asbestos-mediated macrophage induction of lymphocyte blastogenesis may also have initiated changes in T cell subsets.

Whilst it is not possible to extrapolate directly from laboratory studies to the human situation, both in vitro and in vivo investigations into the immunotoxic effects of asbestos has demonstrated that asbestos has an impact on the immune system which may figure importantly in the primary or secondary pathogenic events of lung injury. In this context, it might also be important to point out that inhaltation of fibre-glass fibres has been shown to produce changes in alveolar macrophage membrane characteristics similar to those demonstrated following prolonged asbestos inhaltation (64) (Table 4).

Further fundamental studies, particularly of lymphocyte functions, are needed to elucidate the immunological mechanisms involved and to help differentiate between those effect that relate to fibrosis only and those that may be involved in the development of neoplasms.

TABLE 1. *Immunological Perturbation in asbestos-exposed Populations.*

IMMUNOLOGICAL PERTURBATIONS IN ASBESTOS – EXPOSED POPULATIONS

DEPRESSED SKIN DTH RESPONSES

DIMINISHED NUMBERS OF CIRCULATING T LYMPHOCYTES

REDUCED PHA-INDUCED BLASTOGENESIS IN VITRO

REDUCED PHA-INDUCED IN VITRO CYTOTOXIC CELL FUNCTION

DIMINISHED ABILITY TO GENERATE SUPPRESSOR ACTIVITY IN VITRO

INCREASED LEVELS OF SERUM IMMUNOGLOBULINS

INCREASED PREVALANCE OF SERUM AUTOANTIBODIES

TABLE 2. *Non-specific effects of asbestos-inhalation on aveolar macrophages in animals.*

NON-SPECIFIC EFFECTS OF ASBESTOS INHALATION ON ALVEOLAR MACROPHAGES IN ANIMALS

ALTERED SURFACE MORPHOLOGY

ENHANCED ABILITY TO SPREAD ACROSS A GLASS SUBSTRATE

MORE EXTENSIVE CYTOPLASMIC PROCESSES

SIGNIFICANT INCREASE IN IgG RECEPTOR SITES

DECREASED CHEMOTACTIC ACTIVITY

TABLE 3. *Immunoregulatory effects of asbestos-inhalation on alveolar macrophages in animals.*

IMMUNOREGULATORY EFFECTS OF ASBESTOS INHALATION ON
ALVEOLAR MACROPHAGES IN ANIMALS

SIGNIFICANT INCREASE IN IMMUNE
ADHERENCE ACTIVITY

INCREASED PRODUCTION OF 1L-1

PROLONGED MACROPHAGE – LYMPHOCYTE
BINDING

MACROPHAGE-INDUCED LYMPHOCYTE
BLASTOGENESIS

TABLE 4. *Effects of crocidolite or fibre-glass fibres on IgG receptor activity of rat alveolar macrophages as measured by increased ability to bind sensitised sheep erythocytes ("EA" rosette formation).*

"EA" ROSETTE FORMATION BY ALVEOLAR MACROPHAGES AFTER
4 HR IN CULTURE

MACROPHAGES	% ROSETTES	No. OF ERYTHROCYTES/ROSETTE
CONTROL CELLS	62±12	4.5±2.2 (3-9)[*]
CROCIDOLITE-DUSTED CELLS	75±10	9.1±4.8 (3-18)[*]
GLASS-FIBRE-DUSTED CELLS	91±8	14.5±7.9 (3-32)[*]

MEAN OF 12 EXPERIMENTS PERFORMED IN TRIPLICATE ± S.E.
[*] P 0.001

326

PHA-INDUCED (10ug) LYMPHOCYTE CYTOTOXICITY

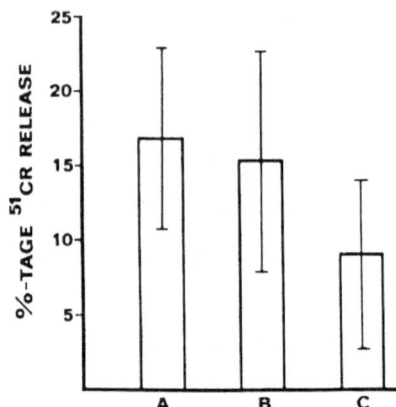

Fig.1. <u>In vitro</u> *PHA-induced cytotoxic lymphocyte function in peripheral blood lymphocytes in normal subject (A), subjects with past occupational asbestos exposure and pleural plaques (C). P 0.05 when differences between C and B were tested using the Mann Whitney U test.*

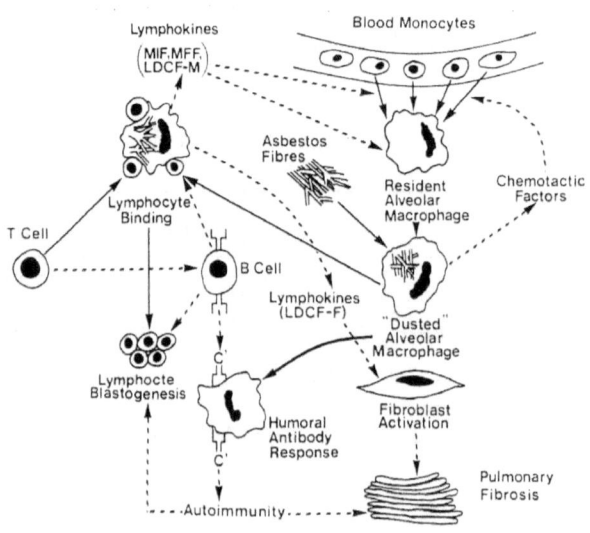

Fig.2. *Immunological mechanisms which could act in asbestos-related diseases. MIF = migration inhibition factor; MFF = macrophage fusion factor; LDCF-F = lymphocyte derived chemotatic factor for fibroblasts; LDCF-M = lymphocyte derived chemotatic factor for macrophages.*

REFERENCES

1. *Turner-Warwick, M. A perspective view on widespread pulmonary fibrosis. Br. Med. J., 2 (1974) 371-376.*

2. *Kagan, E., Solomon, A., Cochrane, J.C., Kuba, P., Rocks, P.H. & Webster, I. Immunological studies of patients with asbestosis. II Studies of circulating lymphoid numbers and humoral immunity. Clin. exp. Immunol. 28 (1977) 268-275.*

3. *Lange, A., Sibinski, G., & Garncarek, D. The follow-up study of skin reactivity to recall antigens and E-and EAC-RFC profiles in blood in asbestos workers. Immunobiol. 157 (1980) 1-11.*

4. *Lange, A. Anergy and autoimmunity in asbestos-exposed people. Arch. Immunol. Ther. Exp. 30 (1982) 211-218.*

5. *Gaumer, H.R., Doll, N.Y., Kaimmal, Y., Schuyer, M.& J.E. Salvaggio. Diminshed suppressor cell function in patients with asbestosis. Clin. exp. Immunol. 44 (1981) 108-116.*

6. *Kang, K-Y., Sera, Y., Okochi, T., & Yamamura, Y.T lymphocytes in asbestosis. N. Engl. J. Med. 291 (1974) 735-736.*

7. *Kagan, E., Solomon, A., Cochrane, J.C., Beissner, E.K., Gluckman, J., Rocks, P.H. & Webster, I. Immunological studies of patients with asbestosis. I Studies of cell mediated immunity. Clin. Exp. Immunol. 28 (1977) 261-267.*

8. *Wagner, M.M.F., Brown, D.G., Campbell, M.J., Coles, R.M., Edwards, R.E. & Scott, M.P. Immunological monitoring of an asbestos-exposed population. Arch. Immunol. Ther. Exp. 30 (1982) 201-205.*

9. *Campbell, M.J., Wagner, M.M.F., Scott, M.P. & Brown, D.G. Sequential immunological studies in an asbestos exposed population. II. Factors affecting lymphocyte function. Clin. exp. Immunol. 39 (1980) 176-181.*

10. *DeShazo, R.D., Nordberg, B.A., Baser, Y., Bozelka, B. Weill, H. & Salvaggio, J. Analysis of depressed cell-mediated immunity in asbestos workers. J. Allergy Clin. Immunol. 71 (1983) 418-424.*

11. *Haslam, P.L., Lukoszek, A., Merchant, J.A. & Turner-Warwick, M. Lymphocyte responses to phytohaemagglutinin in patients with asbestois and pleural mesothelioma. Clin. exp. Immunol. 31 (1978) 178-188.*

12. *Miller, K. & Brown, R.C. The Immune System and asbestos disease. In: Toxicology of the Immune System (J.H. Dean, A. Munson & M. Luster, eds). Raven Press, New York. (In press).*

328

13. Ramachandar, K., Schechlev, R., Phelps, B. Immuno
competence in patients with pleura mesothelioma. Am
Assoc. Cancer Res. 16 (1975) 142 (Abst. No. 567).

14. Wagner, M.M.F., Campbell, M.J. & Edwards, R.E. Sequential immunological studies on an asbestos-exposed
population. I. Factors affecting peripheral blood
leucocytes and T lymphocytes. Clin. exp. Immunol. 38
(1979) 323-331.

15. El/Sewefy, A.Z., & Hassan, F. Immunoelectrophoretic
pattern changes in abestosis. Ann. occup. Hyg. 14
(1971) 25-28.

16 Lange, A., Smolik R., Zatonski, W., Szymanska, Y.
Autoantibodies and serum immunoglobulin levels in asbestos workers. Int. Arch-Arbeitsmed. 32 (1974) 313-325.

17. Huuskonen, M.S., Rasanen, Y.A. Harkonen, H. & Asp., S.
Asbestos exposure as a cause of immunological
stimulation. Scand. J. Resp. Dis. 59 (1978) 326-332.

18. Lange, A. An epidemiological survey of immunological
abnormalities in asbestos workers. II. Serum immunoglobulin levels. Environ. Res. 22 (1980) 176-183.

19. Doll, N.J., Stankus, R.P., Hughes, Y., Weill, H., Guptar,
R.C., Rodriguez, M., Jones, R.N., Alspangli, M.A. &
Salvaggio, Y.E. Immune complexes and autoantibodies in
silicosis. J. Allergy Clin. Immunol. 68 (1981)
281-285.

20. Miller, K. & Kagan, E. The in vivo effects of asbestos
on macrophage membrane structure and population characteristics of macrophages. A scanning electron microscope
study. J. Reticuloendothel. Soc. 20 (1976) 159-171.

21. Allison, A.C., Denman, A.M. & Barnes, R.D. Co-operating
and controlling functions of thymus-derived lymphocytes
in relation to autoimmunity. Lancet, 2 (1971), 135-140.

22. Basten, A. Specific suppression of the immune response
by T cells. In: Immunological Tolerance - Mechanisms
and Potential Therapeutic Applications. Edited by D.H.
Katz and B. Benacerraf, pp 107-129. Academic Press, New
York (1974).

23. Turner-Warwick M. & Parkes, W.R. Circulating rheumatoid
and anti-nuclear factors in asbestos workers. Br. Med.
J. 3 (1970) 492-495.

24. Kagan, E. the alveolar macrophage: Immune derangement
and asbestos-related malignancy. Sem. Oncol. 8 (1981)
258-267.

25. Jones, R.N., Turner-Warwick, M., Ziskind, M., & Weill, H.
High prevalence of antinuclear antibodies in sandblasters
silicosis. Amer. Rev. Resp. Dis 113 (1976) 393-395.

26. Schuyler, M., Ziskind, M. & Salvaggio, J. Cell mediated immunity in silicosis. Amer. Rev. Resp. Dis. 116: 147-151.

27. Miller, K. Alterations in the surface-related phenomena of alveolar macrophages following inhalation of crocidolite asbestos and quartz dust. An overview. Environ. Res. 20 (1979) 162-182.

28. Normann, S.J. & Sorkin, E. (1982). Editors: Macrophages and Natural Killer Cells. Regulation and Function. Adv. Exp. Med. Biol. 155. Plenum Press, New York.

29. Barry, B.E., Wong, K.C., Brody, A.r. & Crapo, J.D. Reaction of rat lungs to inhaled chrysotile asbestos following acute and subchronic exposures. Exp. Lung Res. 5 (1983) 1-22.

30. Brown, R.C., Gormley, I.P., Chamberlain, M. & Davies, R. The In vitro effects of mineral dusts. Academic Press, London, (1980).

31. Miller, K. The effects of asbestos on macrophages. CRC Crit. Rev. Toxicol. 5 (1978) 319-354.

32. Heppleston, A.G. & Styles, J.A. Activity of a macrophage factor in collagen formation by silica. Nature (London) 241 (1967) 521-522.

33. Aalto, M Potila, M & Kulonen, E.. The effect of silica-treated macrophages on the synthesis of collagen and other proteins in vitro. Exptl. Cell Res. 97 (1976) 193-202.

34. Goldstein, R.H., Miller, K., Glassroth, J., Linscott, R., Snider, G.L., Franzblau, C & Polgar, P. Influence of asbestos fibers on collagen and prostaglandin production in fibroblast and macrophage co-cultures. J. Lab. clin. Med. 100 (1982) 778-785.

36. Koshi, K., Hayashi, H., Hanada, A. & Sakabe, H. The toxiceffect of various dusts on the intraperitoneal monocyte in rat. Bull. Nat. Inst. Health (Japan) 6 (1969) 10-27.

37. Hamilton, J.A., Vassalli, J.D., & Reich, E. Macrophage-plaminogen activator induction by asbestos in blocked by anti-inflammatory steroids. J. Exp. Med. 144 (1976) 169-189.

38. White, R. & Kuhn, C. Effects of phagocytosis of mineral dusts on elastase secretion by alveolar and peritoneal exudative macrophages. Arch. Environ. Health 35 (1980) 106-109.

39. Donaldson, K. & Cullen, R.T. Chemiluminescence of asbestos-activated macrophages. Br. J. exp. Path. 65 (1984) 81-96.

40. Hatch, G.E., Gardner, D.E. & Menzel, D.B. *Stimulation of oxidant production in alveolar macrophages by pollutant and latex particles. Environ. Res. 23 (1980) 121-136.*

41. Doll, N.J., Stankus, R.P., Goldbach, S. & Salvaggio, J.E. In vivo Doll, N.J., Stankus, R.P., Goldbach, S. & Salvaggio, J.E. In vitro *effect of asbestos fibres on polymorphonuclear leukocyte function. Int. Archs. Allergy appl. Immunol. 68 (1982a) 17-21.*

42. Doll, N.J., Bozelka, B.E., Goldbach, S., Anorve-Lopez, E. & Salvaggio, J.E. *Asbestos-induced alteration of human peripheral blood monocyte activity. Int. Archs. Allergy appl. Immunol. 69 (1982b) 302-305.*

43. Gemsa, D., Seiz, M., Kramer, W., Thill, G. & Resch, K. *The effects of phagocytosis, dextran sulfate, and cell damage on PGE1 sensitivity and PGE1 production of macrophages. J. Immunol 120 (1978) 1187-1194.*

43a. Doll, N.J., Dicon, J.E., Jones, R.N., Rodriguez, M., Bozelka, B.E., Stankus, R.P., Weill, H., & Salvaggio, J.E. *Humoral immunologic abnormalities in workers exposed to asbestos cement dust. J. Allergy. Clin. Immunol. 72 (1983) 509-519.*

44. Nicklin, S. & Shand, F.L. *Abrogation of suppressor cell function by inhibitors of prostaglandin synthesis. Int. J. Immunopharmacol. 4 (1982) 407-414.*

45. Donaldson, K. *The effect of asbestos on the paeritoneal macrophage population of the mouse. PhD.thesis, Faculty of Medicine University of Edinburgh, (1983).*

46. Myrvik, Q.N. *The role of the alveolar macrophage. J. Occup. Med. 15 (1973) 190-193.*

47. Brody, A.R., Hill, L.H., Adkins, B. & O'Connor, R.W. *Chrysotile Asbestos Inhalation in rats. Deposition pattern and reaction of alveolar epithelium and pulmonary macrophages. Amer. Rev. Resp. Dis. 123 (1981) 670-679.*

48. Holt, P.F. *Translocation of asbestos dust through the bronchiolar wall. Environ. Res. 27 (1981) 255-260.*

49. Miller, K., Webster, I., Handfield, R.I.M. & Skine, M.I. *Ultrastructure of the lung in the rat following exposure to crocidolite asbestos and quartz. J. Pathol. 124 (1978) 39-44.*

50. Kagan, E., Oghiso, Y. & Hartmann, D.P. *The effects of chrysitile and crocidolite asbestos on the lower respiratory tract. Analysis of bronchoalveolar lavage constituents. Environ. Res. 32 (1983) 382-397.*

51. Miller, K. & Kagan, E. Immune adherence reactivity of rat alveolar macrophages following inhalation of crocidolite asbestos. Clin. exp. Immunol. 29 (1977) 152-158.

52. Bozelka, B.E., Gaumer, H.R., Nordberg, Y & Salvaggio, J.E. Asbestos induced alterations of human lymphoid cell mutagenic responses. Environ. Res. 30, (1983), 281-290.

53. Miller, K., Weintraub, Z. & Kagan, E. Manifestations of cellular immunity in the rat after prolonged asbestos inhalation. In Physical interaction between alveolar macrophages and splenci lymphocytes. J. Immunol. 123. (1979) 1029-1038.

54. Rosenthal, A.S. & Shevach, E.M. Function of macrophages in antigen recognition by guinea pig T lymphocytes. I. Requirement for histocompatible macrophages and lymphocytes. J. Esp. Med. 138. (1973) 1194-1212.

55. Rosenthal, A.S., Blake, J.T., Ellner, J.J., Creineder, D.K. & Lipsky, P.E. Macrophage function in antigen recognition by T lymphocytes. In: Immunobiology of the Macrophage edited by D.S. Nelson, pp 131-160. Academic Press, new York (1976),

56. Greineder, D.K. & Rosenthal, A.S. The requirement for macrophage - lymphocyte interaction in T lymphocyte proliferation induced by generation of aldehydes on cell membranes. J. Immunol. 115 (1975) 932-938.

57. Novogrodsky, A. Lymphocyte activation induced by modifications of surface membrane saccharides. In: Immune Recognition, edited by A.S. Rosenthal, pp. 43-61. Academic Press, New York (1975).

58. Miller, K. & Kagan, E. Manifestations of cellular immunity in the rat after prolonged asbestos inhalation. II Alveolar macrophage - induced splenic lymphocyte proliferation. Environ Res. 26 (1981) 182-194.

59. Florentin, I., Bruley-Rosset, M., & Davigny, M. Lymphocyte-macrophage interactions in BCG-treated mice. In: Lymphocytes, Macrophages and Cancer, edited by G. Mathe, I. Floretin and M.C. Simmlev, pp. 49-57. Springer, Berlin, (1976).

60. Hartmann, D.P., Georgian, H.M., Oghiso, Y. & Kagan, E. Enchanced interleukin activity following asbestos inhalation. Clin. exp. Immunol 55 (1984) 643-650.

61. Warheit, D.B., George, G., Hill, L.H. & Brody, A.R. Inhaled asbestos fibres activate chemotactic factor for macrophages on lung surfaces. In: In vitro effect of Mineral Dusts, 1984. (J. Bignon & A. Scharmann eds). In Press.

332

62. Sirois, P. Rola-Pleszczynski, M. & Begin, R. Phospholipase A activity and protaglandin synthesis from alveolar macrophages exposed to asbestos. Prostasglandis and
medicine: 5 (1980) 31-37.

63. Brown, R.C., Chamberlain, M., Griffiths, M., & Timbrell,
V. The effect of fibre size on the in vitro biological
activity of three types of amphibole asbestos. Int. J.
Cancer 22 (1978) 721-727.

64. Miller, K. The in vivo effects of glass fibres on
alveolar macrophage membrane characteristics. In:
Biological Effects of Mineral Fibres (Ed. J.C. Wagner)
IARC Scientific Publ. No. 30. 1980, pp 459-466.

EFFECTS OF DIMETHYLNITROSAMINE

A.E. Munson, M. P. Holsapple & S.S. Duke

Department of Pharmacology, Medical College of Virginia,
Richmond VA, 23298 U.S.A.

I. INTRODUCTION

The possibility that chemicals found in the environment can
suppress certain immune responses is one of the cornerstones
of immunotoxicology. The nitrosamines represent an environ-
mentally important group of compounds that includes dimethylnitrosamine (DMN, N-Nitrosodimethylamine). DMN is a potent
carcinogen in several rodents (Magee and Barnes, 1967) and is
a suspected carcinogen in man (Craddock, 1983). N-nitroso
compounds are formed when primary, secondary, or tertiary
amines react with nitrogen oxides or nitrite (Ember, 1980).
Studies have shown that the generation of nitrosamines occurs
not only in the external environment, but may also occur in
the human stomach (Sander, 1967). Later investigations showed
that several species of bacteria, including Escherichia coli,
were capable of forming nitrosamines from secondary amines and
nitrites (Montesano and Magee, 1970). Therefore, the possibility of nitrosamine formation in the digestive tract coupled
with the possibily for direct exposure to the preformed
nitrosamines in the environment via ingestion, inhalation, or
dermal contact suggest a potential hazard for the population
at large.

Toxicological interest in the N-nitroso compounds was first
aroused in 1954 when dimethylnitrosamine (DMN) was introduced
into the laboratory as a solvent (Barnes and Magee, 1954).
Barnes and Magee reported that two laboratory technicians
developed cirrhosis of the liver after handling DMN. Subsequent experiments conducted by Barnes and Magee indicated
that DMN readily produced severe liver injury in rats,
rabbits, mice, guinea pigs, and dogs. Centrolobular and
midzonal necrosis, depletion of glycogen, fat deposition,
dilution of sinusoidal spaces, hemorrhagic peritoneal exudate
and bleeding into the lumen of the gut were striking features
following acute exposure to DMN. Prolonged administration of
relatively low doses of DMN (100, 50 or 25 ppm in the diet)
resulted in fibrosis and gross nodular cirrhosis of the liver
(LePage and Christie, 1969). Besides the hepatotoxic effects,
primary tumors were detected in the liver, kidney, esophagus,
stomach, and central nervous system following exposure to DMN
and related nitrosamines (Magee and Barnes, 1956, Craddock,
1971). subsequent studies by Craddoch indicated that the
tumors could be induced following a single dose of DMN if
given during liver regeneration following a partial hepatectomy (Craddock, 1971, 1973,1975).

From a mechanistic point of view, most of the toxicity which
characterizes DMN and the nitrosamines is thought to be
mediated by a metabolite generated in the enzymatic oxidative

334

demethylation of DMN (Health, 1962, Magee and Barnes, 1967, Gol-Winkler and Goutier, 1977, Kroeger-Koepke and Michejda, 1979). This metabolic activation of DMN, which occurs predo-minantly in the liver, results in the intracellular formation of a methylating agent which alkylates nucleic acids, prima-rily at the N-7 position of guanine (Gol-Winkler and Goutier, 1977). While there are many papers which describe the immuno-suppressant effects of such alkylating agents as cyclo-phosphamide (Diamantstein et al., 1981), few studies have defined the relationships between the administration of DMN and the immune response. The studies summarized in this chapter provide evidence that DMN can suppress immune respon-siveness in some animal species.

II. EFFECTS OF DMN ON HEMATOPOIETIC AND LYMPHOID TISSUE

Magee and Barnes (1967) reported that DMN had hepatotoxic and carcinogenic properties in several animal species. In their studies and their reports of other studies, nitrosamines given orally, subcutaneously, or intraperitoneally were cited as causing damage to liver, kidney, lung, nasal sinus, esophagus, stomach, bronchi, bladder, brain, nerves, and colon. Historically, the primary targets for DMN-induced toxicity have been those organs possessing the necessary enzymes to generate the alkylating intermediates, i.e., the liver, and sometimes the kidney, but generally not the hematopoietic or lymphoid tissue. Waynforth and Magee (1974) studied the effect of a single oral or intrapentonal dose of DMN to rats and mice.They reported an apparent leukostasis in DMN treated rats(p.o.,40mg DMN/kg,single dose), but not in mice (i.p., 14 or 7 mg DMN/kg, single dose). Any effects of DMN on lymphoid tissue were not reported and were, presumably, unobserved.

More recent studies have investigated the alterations in immune response following subchronic (14 day) DMN treatment in mice (Holsapple et al., 1984a). The results of the subchronic DMN exposure (i.p. 1.5, 3.0, or 5.0 mg DMN/kg, 14 daily single doses) confirm the lack of direct effect by DMN on the spleen as evidenced by the histopathology, although DMN exposure did produce a slight splenomegaly which was not dose-related (Holsapple et al., 1984a). Subchronic DMN exposure also affected the hematology as there was a shift in the relative peripheral blood differentials without an effect on the number of leukocytes (Holsapple et al., 1984b). The percentage of lymphocytes was decreased (33%) while those of neutrophils and monocytes were increased (240% and 60%, respectively) in mice exposed to the highest concentration (5 mg/kg/day for 14 days).

In the investigation by Holsapple et al., (1984b), the effects of exposure to DMN on bone marrow were also determined. These results indicated a profile of activity which parallels the hematological effects discussed above. There was no effect on bone marrow cell number. However, the number of granulocyte/monocyte stem cells measured with CFU/GM was increased in a dose-related fashion with a 62% increase noted at the highest dose.

With the exception of the effects on hematology and bone marrow, DMN apparently exhibited minimal direct toxic effects on lymphoid tissue. Immunotoxic effects however, may not always be demonstrated as gross or histological changes in lymphoid tissue. Oftentimes, changes may occur in immune function which are not correlated with histopathological changes. This may be the case with DMN, as the next two sections suggest that exposure to DMN does alter both humoral and cell-mediated immune responses.

III. EFFECTS OF DMN ON THE HUMORAL IMMUNE RESPONSE (Table 1)

One of the earliest reports of the immunosuppressive effects of a nitrosamine was reproted by Waynforth and Magee (1974). In this systematic study, Wistar rats were administered a single dose (p.o) of 40 mg D MN/kg body weight (the approximate LD_{80} dose) and mice were administered a single dose (i.p.) of either 14 mg (the approximate LD_{60}) or 7 mg DMN/kg body weight. An inhibition in hemolytic plaque formation and in the circulating hemagglutinin antibody titre was observed only in the mice receiving the higher dose of DMN. An increase in plaque formation was observed in rats, while the circulating hemagglutinin antibody titres was decreased.

A more recent study was reported by G.C. Hard (1981). The objective of this investigation was to determine the effects of exposure to a relatively high single dose of DMN (60 mg/kg, i.p.) on antibody responses to both a T-independent antigen (Brucella abortus) and a T-dependent antigen (sheep erythrocytes) relative to the development of a DMN-induced tumor of the kidney in rats. The T-dependent response, but not the T-independent response, was suppressed as soon as 24 hours after exposure to DMN and the magnitude of the suppression was constant for 10 days. From 2 weeks, there was a gradual recovery with full restoration occurring by 8 weeks at the time of emergence of the neoplastic foci in the kidney. The observation that the first recognizable tumor aggregations became manifest when the immune responsiveness had fully recovered prompted Hard (1981) to conclude that the immune suppression by DMN was not associated with the carcinogenic event. It is important to emphasize that the presence of the renal tumors was determined by conventional histological procedures. Therefore, one could argue that the immune suppression by DMN did contribute to the tumor formation by allowing the initial carcinogenic event to go undetected which would be expected to occur soon after exposure to the chemical. The tumor growth would then proceed until being capable of detection by histology, at a time when the immune response could have recovered.

The most recent study on the effects of DMN on humoral immunity reported that subchronic doses of DMN also caused a suppression in mice (Holsapple, et al., 1984a). Spleen cells obtained from mice administered 1.5, 3.0, or 5.0 mg DMN/kg for 14 days (i.p., daily doses) exhibited a dose-dependent reduction of the IgM antibody-forming cell response to a T-dependent antigen (SRBC) on days 4 and 5. The IgG response was only affected at the high dose of DMN and only on the peak day of the response (day 5). A comparable exposure regimen did not affect the response to a T-independent antigen (DNP-Ficoll) on any of the days tested. When recovery from the effects of DMN exposure was studied, it was observed that the IgM response to SRBC remained significantly suppressed (48%) 34 days after DMN exposure was ended, reflecting a persistent immuno-suppressive effect. The most sensitive indicator of the suppression of antibody production following exposure to DMN was the in vitro response of DMN-treated spleen cell suspensions to lipopolysaccharide (LPS) and sheep red blood cells (SRBC). Both the day 2 polyclonal response to LPS and the day 4 response to the T-dependent antigen, SRBC, were completely (>90%) suppressed by all doses of DMN. In addition to the suppression of antibody production, the proliferative response to the B-cell mitogen, LPS, was also suppressed in a dose-dependent manner, with a range of suppression from 15 to 32%.

The duration of the immunosuppressive effects of DMN on humoral immunity has not been determined. One could speculate that the mechanism for this long-lasting suppression is not due to the persistence of free, reactive metabolites of DMN as these have been shown by whole body autoradiography to be produced and to bind within minutes after the administration of ^{14}C-DMN (Johansson and Tjalve, 1978). As described in the preceeding section, DMN produced hematological changes, most notably a decrease in the percentage of lymphocytes in the differential count (Holsapple et al. 1984b). These

results further indicated that DMN has an effect on the bone marrow which was manifested as an increase in the number of granulocyte/monocyte stem cells. This effect could have occurred at the expense of lymphocyte differential, since the number of bone marrow cells was not changed. Such an effect could explain the persistence, if the ability of the bone marrow to repopulate the immunocompetent organs with func-tional (i.e., immunocompetent) lymphocytes and/or macrophages/monocytes is altered.

The investigation by Holsapple et al. (1984a) was also the first time that DMN was added directly to cultured spleen cells. The results indicated that the ability of lymphocytes to respond in an in vitro antibody assay was not affected by concentrations up to 100mM. In addition, DMN plus either plenobarbital-induced liver proteins or 3-methylcholanthrene-induced liver proteins, which were capable of metabolizing DMN, also did not have an effect. The lack of direct effect in vitro compared to the potent effects in vivo suggests that the reactive metabolites of DMN, which contribute to the toxicity of the liver, mutagenicity, and carcinogenicity by DMN, may not play a role in mediating the humoral immunosuppression produced by subchronic exposure to this compound.

IV. EFFECTS OF DMN ON THE CELL-MEDIATED RESPONSE (Table 2)

In general, the studies which employed large single injections of DMN have failed to demonstrate effects on cell-mediated immune parameters. Waynforth and Magee (1974) reported that the survival time of skin allografts was not affected by exposure to 40 mg/kg (p.o.) in rats or to 7 or 14 mg/kg (i.p.) in mice. Similar results were also reported by Hard (1975) who again measured an immune response at various times after exposure to 60 mg/kg (i.p.) relative to the development of DMN/induced renal tumors in rats. The blastogenic response of lymhocytes to phytohemagglutinin (PHA) was not affected at any time after exposure to DMN.

Studies have also been done which investigated the alterations in cell-mediated immune response following subchronic (14 days) DMN treatment (Holsapple et al., 1984b). The results from these studies demonstrate that the cell-mediated immuno-competence of the B6C3F1 mouse could be either significantly suppressed or enhanced, indicating that effects of DMN on cell-mediated immunity may be somewhat more complex than the effects on humoral immunity.

In contrast with the earlier results by Hard (1975) with acute exposure to DMN, the lymphoproliferative responses to the T-cell mitogens, Con A and PHA, were suppressed by subchronic exposure to DMN, although the effects were only marginally dose-related. DMN-treated animals did, however, exhibit a dose-related decrease in the mixed lymphocyte response. The optimal response (day 4) was suppressed by 41% in mice treated with the high dose of DMN (5.0 mg/kg). The mixed lymphocyte response is more specific than mitogenicity, as the former requires the cell to be able to recognize alloantigens and to proliferate. Both tests indicate that the T-lympocytes from DMN-treated mice have an impaired ability to respond.

The delayed hypersensitivity response (DHR) represents a holistic in vivo correlate for cell-mediated immunity. The investigation by Holsapple et al. (1984b) utilized several models of the DHR to characterize the effects of DMN on cell-mediated immunity. The magnitudes of these responses were measured by radioisotopic procedures which reflected the release of lymphokines by the sensitized T-lymphocytes, namely an increase in the vascular permeability of a radiolabelled protein, or an increase in the influx of radiolabelled monocytes. The initial model tested was a DHR to keyhole limpet hemocyanin (KLH) in which the monocytes were labelled endogenously by pretreating the mice with ^{125}I-iododeoxyuridene 24 hours prior to challenge. Suprisingly, this reponse was increased in a dose-related manner with a 300 % increase noted at the highest dose (5 mg/kg/day). In contrast, when the DHR was measured by extra-vasation of ^{125}I-human serum albumin, adminsitered 18 hours after challenge, there was a 54% decrease in mice exposed to the highest dose. In parallel experiments, the DHR to shepp erythrocytes, a particulate antigen, was decreased by 60% when measured with ^{125}I-HSA in mice exposed to 5.0 mg/kg. DMN was not found to have an effect on the increase in vascular permeability associated with the acute inflammatory response

to carrageenin. Therefore, the effects on the latter DHR
models can be attributed to immunosuppression and not to
nonspecific anti-inflammatory activity.

However, if these results (i.e., DHR models measuring vascular
permeability and the lymphoproliferative responses) reflect an
overall suppression of cell-mediated immunocompetence in
agreement with the effects on humoral immunocompetence
(Holsapple et al., 1984a), then the enhancement of the KLH DHR
model measured by the influx of endogenously labelled monocytes becomes an enigma. The possibility that exposure to DMN
produced a differential effect on specific lymphokines (i.e.,
decrease those mediating vascular permeability and increase
those mediating chemotaxis) was considered unlikely1. As
described previously, experiments measuring bone marrow showed
that DMN caused a dose-dependent increase in CFU-GM (Holsapple
et al., 1984b). These results may help explain the puzzling
dichotomy. One hypothetical explanation for the divergent DHR
results is that DMN treatment caused the number of bone marrow
cells differentiating to form granulocyte-moncytes to increase
resulting in a larger pool of cells available to be called
into the challenge site. This hypothesis was corroborated by
adoptive transfer studies which were performed by exogenously
labelling bone marrow by incubation with chromium 51 and using
these cells to measure the cellular influx in a DHR to KLH.
Bone marrow cells derived from either control (vehicle) or
DMN-treated donor mice could comparably respond in a DHR in
recipient mice exposed to the vehicle. However, the DHR in
recipient mice exposed to 5.0 mg DMN/kg was suppressed by more
than 65% regardless of the source of bone marrow cells.
Therefore, the ability of DMN-treated mice to elicit a monocyte (exogenously-labelled) influx in response to KLH was
impaired, in agreement with the DMN-induced suppression of the
DHR to either KLH or SRBC as measured by vascular permeability
and the suppression of the lymphoproliferative responses.

In summary, exposure to DMN suppresses many aspects of cellular immune function (Holsapple et al., 1984b), including
T-lymphocyte function in the lumphoproliferative response to
T-cell mitogens, in the mixed lymphocyte response, and in
selected models of the DHR. As described in the preceeding
section, these DMN-induced alterations may be mediated via an
effect on bone marrow differentiation. Regardless of the
mechanism, changes in humoral and cell-mediated immunocompetence may ultimately be manifested as functional changes
in host resistance. This possibility is explored in the next
section.

V. EFFECTS OF DMN ON HOST RESISTANCE (Table 3)

Recognizing that changes in humoral and cell-mediated immunity
may potentially alter the course of susceptibility of animals
to infectious agents, studies have been done to assess the
effects of DMN on host resistance (Bradley and Jessee, 1984,
and Duke et al., 1984, and Holsapple et al., 1984b). Subchronic exposure (14 days) to 1.5, 3.0, or 5.0 mg DMN/kg body
weight had little effect on most of the host resistance models

used in this study: encephalomyocarditis virus (resistance to this virus generally involves interferon, neutralizing anti-body and antibody dependent cell mediated immunity) Herpes simplex virus type 2 (T-lymphocytes, B-lymphocytes, NK cells, macrophages, and interferon), Naegleria fowleri (complement) and Plasmodium berghei (T-cell dependent antibody, B-lymphocytes, macrophages) (Bradley and Jessee, 1984). Those infections for which host resistance depends predominantly upon macrophages and cell mediated immunity, e.g. Listeria monocytogenes (Holsapple et al., 1984b) and Cryptococcus neoformans (Bradley and Jessee, 1984), exhibited a trend toward a decreased mortality (i.e., increased resistance). In light of the effects on cell-mediated immunity, particularly the DHR, these results were somewhat unexpected and may be more related to the increased (48% at the high dose) phago-cytic capacity of macrophages (peritoneal exudate cells) from DMN treated animals as reported by Duke et al. (1984).

Another host resistance model in which DMN-treated mice were more resistant was the B16F10 (tumor) melanoma model (Duke et al., 1984). Following 14 days of exposure to 1.5, 3.0, or 5.0 mg DMN/kg, an increase in host resistance to B16F10 melanoma was observed. There was a reduction in both the incidence and the number of pulmonary tumor nodules in DMN-treated mice given 1×10^5 tumor cells and a reduction in the number of pulmonary tumor nodules in mice given 3×10^5 tumor cells. Results from this study suggested that the increase in resis-tance to the B16F10 melanoma may be mediated by a combination of a significant increase in the activity of macrophages and a slight increase in the activity of NK cells.

Of the host resistance studies reported, DMN appeared to decrease the host resistance to only one infectious agent, Steptococcus pneumoniae (Bradley and Jessee, 1984). DMN administered intraperitoneally at 3.0 mg/kg for 14 days prior to challenge impaired host resistance. The ability for a host to resist S. pneumoniae depends primarily upon opsonizing antibody, complement, and phagocytosis by PMNs. Preliminary results have indicated that exposure to DMN does not alter complement (K.L. White, Jr., Medical College of Virginia, personal communication). The effects of DMN on the phagocytic capability of PMNs has not been determined. Therefore, while the suppression of humoral immunocompetence may contribute to the increased mortality with S. pneumoniae, a nonspecific impairment of innate host resistance cannot be ruled out at this time.

Host resistance to infection is often mechanistically complex and may be determined by several different components of the immune system. Although the in vivo studies with DMN did not definitively identify the site of immunotoxic action of DMN, the assessment of host resistance to select pathogens comple-ments the profile of effects on immunologic competence.

VI. SUMMARY

The overall effect of DMN on immune responsiveness was a depression of humoral and cell-mediated immune responses. These effects appeared to be greatest with subchronic (repeated) exposure compared to an acute (single) injection. Concomitant with these effects on immune function, exposure to DMN produced an alteration in the bone marrow stem cell population. An increase in both the number and phagocytic activity of macrophages and the number of neutrophils from DMN treated mice was observed. Ultimately, these changes appeared to alter the course of susceptibility of animals to some infectious agents (B16F10 melanoma, Listeria monocytogenes, Cryptococcus neoformans, and Streptoccos pneumoniae.)

VII. FUTURE DIRECTION

While the aforementioned effects on the bone marrow may contribute to the observed profile of immunotixity, the effects on other organs may also indirectly modulate the immune response. As stated at the outset, the primary target organ for DMN toxicity is the liver. In all of the subchronic studies with DMN, a dose-related increase in damage to the liver, measured by histopathology and clinical chemistry, was obsrved (Holsapple et al., 1984a, Holsapple et al., 1984b, and Duke et al., 1984). The livers of animals exposed to the highest dose (5 mg/kg/day) were described as precirrhotic, and between 25% and 50% of these animals developed ascites. The earlier studies by Hard (1975 and 1981) stated that only 50% of the rats exposed to 60 mg/kg DMN survived and were used to determine the subsequent effects on immuno-competence. Therefore, dose-regimens which are capable of perturbing immune function, are also clearly hepatotoxic. A preliminary investigation has demonstrated that the two events may be related. Munson et al. (1984) showed that liver homogenates, but not spleen homogenates, from DMN (5 mg/kg/day)/treated mice, but not vehicle-treated mice, were directly suppressive when added to cultures of spleen cells from untreated mice which were then stimulated with SRBCs to make antibody. The greatest effects were observed with serum, as 0.031 microgram protein of DMN-serum produced 50% suppression while 27 micrograms protein of vehicle-serum was without effect. The conclusion from these studies was that the effects of DMN on the liver result in the production of a factor which is capable of producing a potent suppression of immunity. Investigations are currently underway to isolate and characterize this factor. One area receiving a great deal of consideration involves the acute phase reactant (APR) proteins which are primarily produced in the liver. Feldman (1982) demonstrated that the production of APR proteins was markedly increased by a combined regimen of carbon tetrachloride and phenobarbital which induced cirrhosis. One of the principle APR proteins of the mouse, serum amyloid A (SAA) has been demonstrated to be immunosuppressive when added to cultures of spleen cells from untreated mice (Benson and Aldo-Benson, 1979 and 1982).

Interestingly, another series of papers have demonstrated that other   APR proteins, the isoferritans and transferrin, can
affect the differentiation of the granulocyte/monocyte population (Broxmeyer, 1982 and Broxmeyer et al., 1983). These results are important because they indicate that one of the most important probes for chemical carcinogenicity can also be used to investigate the possible modulation of immuno-competence by the liver.

TABLE 1. Summary of the Effects of Dimethylnitrosamine on Humoral Immunity

Strain/Species	Dose of DMN (mg/kg)	Route and Duration of Exposure	Parameter	Effect	Ref.
Wistar rats	40	p.o., single	Hemolytic plaque assay	(41%)*	a
Wistar rats	40	p.o., single	Hemagglutinin titres	(54%)	a
(C57BLxBALB/C) F1 mice	14	i.p., single	Hemolytic plaque assay	(88%)	a
(C57 BALB/C)F1 mice	14	i.p., single	Hemagglutinin titres	(68%)	a
Wistar rats	60	i.p., single	Hemolytic plaque assay (T-dep)	(98%)	b
Wistar rats	60	i.p., single	Hemagglutinin titre (T-ind)	NE	b
B6C3F1 mice	5	i.p., 14 daily	Day 4 IgM Ab response to T-dep	(81%)	c
B6C3F1 mice	5	i.p., 14 daily	Day 5 IgG Ab response to T-dep	(60%)	c
B6C3F1 mice	5	i.p., 14 daily	IgM Ab response to T-ind	NE	c
B6C3F1 mice	5	i.p., 14 daily	In vitro poly-clonal Ab response to LPS	(96%)	c
B6C3F1 mice	5	i.p., 14 daily	In vitro T-dep Ab response	(97%)	c
B6C3F1 mice	5	i.p., 14 daily	Mitogen response to LPS	(32%)	c

a Waynforth and Magee, 1974   b Hard, 1981   c Holsapple et al., 1984a

T-dep = T-dependent antigen
T-ind = T-independent antigen
 Ab = antibody

LPS = lipopolysaccharide
NE = no observed effect

The numbers in parentheses represent the % decrease in the experimental value in comparison to the control, with the exception of * which is the % increase.

TABLE 2. Summary of the Effects of Dimethylnitrosamine on
Cell-mediated Immunity

Strain/Species	Dose of DMN (mg/kg)	Route and Duration of Exposure	Parameter	Effect	Ref.
Wistar rats	40	p.o., single	Allograft rejection	NE	a
(C57BLxBALB/C)F1 Mice	14	i.p., single	Allograft rejection	NE	a
Wistar rats	60	i.p., single	Mitogen response to PHA	NE	b
B6C3F1 mice	5	i.p., 14 daily	Mitogen response to PHA	(32%)	c
B6C3F1 mice	5	i.p., 14 daily	Mitogen response to Con A	(28%)	c
B6C3F1 mice	5	i.p., 14 daily	Mixed Lymphocyte Response	(41%)	c
B6C3F1 mice	5	i.p., 14 daily	DHR to KLH: monocyte influx (labelled endogenously)	(339%)	c
B6C3F1 mice	5	i.p., 14 daily	DHR to KLH: vascular permeability	(54%)	c
B6C3F1 mice	5	i.p., 14 daily	DHR to SRBC: vascular permeability	(69%)	c
B6C3F1 mice	5	i.p., 14 daily	DHR to KLH: monocyte influx (labelled exogenously)	(69%)	c
B6C3F1 mice	5	i.p., 14 daily	Acute Inflammation: vascular permeability	NE	c
B6C3F1 mice	5	i.p., 14 daily	Macrophage (PEC) phagocytosis	(48%)*	c
B6C3F1 mice	5	i.p., 14 daily	Natural Killer	NE	d

a Waynforth and Magee, 1974   b Hard, 1975
c Holsapple et al., 1984b   d Duke et al., 1984

PHA   = phytohemagglutinin   DHR = delayed hypersensitivity response
Con A = Concanavalin A   PEC = peritoneal exudate cells
SRBC = sheep erythrocytes   NE = no observed effect
KLH   = keyhole limpet hemocyanin

The numbers in parentheses represent the % decrease in the experimental value
in comparison to the control, with the exception of * which is the % increase.

TABLE 3. Summary of the Effects of Dimethylnitrosamine* on Host Resistance

Infectious Agent	Route of Infection	Inoculum (per mouse)	Effect	Reference
EMC	i.p.	1.1×10^{-7}	NE	a
HSV-2	i.v.	3×10^3 PFU	NE	a
Naegleria fowleri	i.v.	5×10^3 cells	NE	a
Plasmodium berghei	i.v.	1×10^6	NE	a
Listeria monocytogenes	i.p.	7.7×10^3 CFU	↓ mortality	b
Cryptococcus neoformans	i.v.	1.2×10^5 cells	↓ mortality	a
B16F10 melanoma	i.v.	1.2×10^5 cells	↓ tumor of nodules	c
Streptococcus pneumoniae	i.p.	1.7×10^6	↑ mortality	a

a Bradley and Jessee, 1984
b Holsapple et al., 1984b
c Duke et al., 1984

EMC = encephalomyocarditis virus
HSV = Herpes Simplex Virus
PFU = plaque forming units
CFU = colony forming units
NE = no observed effect

*5 mg/kg/day, i.p., for 14 days

VIII. **REFERENCES**

Barnes, J.N. & Magee, P.N. (1954). Some toxic properties of dimethylnitrosamine. Br. J. Ind. Med., 11: 167-174.

Benson, M.D. & Aldo-Benson, M. (1979). Effect of purified protein SAA on immune responses in vitro: Mechanisms of suppression. J. Immunol., 122: 2077-2082.

Benson, M.D. & Aldo-Benson, M. (1982). SAA suppression of in vitro antibody response. Ann. N.Y. Acad. Sci., 381: 121-125.

Bradley, S.G. & Jessee, E. (1984). Effects of N-Nitrosodimethylamine on immunocompetence. Susceptibility of mice to selected infectious agents. NIH Immunotoxicology Workshop. Research Triangle Park, N.D. (Oct. 17-18, 1983). (in press).

Broxmeyer, H.E. (1982). Relationship of cell-cycle expression of Ia-like antigenic determinants on normal and leukemia human granulocyte-macrophage progenitor cells to regulation in vitro by acidic isoferritans. J. Clin. Invest., 69: 632-642.

Broxmeyer, H.E., Gentik, P., Bognacki, J. & Ralph, P. (1983). Lactoferrin, transferrin, and acidic isoferritans: regulatory molecules with potential therapeutic value in leukemia. Blood Cells, 9: 83-87.

Craddock, V.M. (1971). Liver carcinomas induced in rats by single administration of dimethylnitrosamine after partial hepatectomy. J. Nat. Cancer Inst., 47: 889-905.

Craddock, V.M. (1973). Induction of liver tumors in rats by a single treatment with nitroso compounds given after partial hepatectomy. Nature (Lond.), 245: 386-388.

Craddock, V.M. (1975). Effects of single treatment with the alkylating carcinogens, dimethylnitrosamine, diethylnitrosamine and methylmethanesulfonate, on liver regenerating after partial hepatectomy. I. Test for induction of liver carcinomas. Chem-biol. Interact., 10: 313-321.

Craddock, V.M. (1983). Nitrosamines and human cancer: proof of an association? Nature, 306: 638.

Diamantstein, T., Klos, M., Hahn, H., & Kaufmann, S.H.E. (1981). Direct in vitro evidence for different susceptibilities to 4-Hydroperoxy-cyclophosphamide of antigen-primed T cells regulating humoral and cell-mediated immune responses to sheep erythrocytes: a possible explanation for the inverse action of cyclophosphamide on humoral and cell-mediated immune responses. J. Immunol., 126: 1717-1719.

Duke, S.S., Schook, L.B., & Holsapple, M.P. (1984). Effects on N-Nitrosodimethylamine on tumor susceptibility. J. Leukocyte Biol. (in press).

Ember, L.R. (1980). Nitrosamines: assessing the relative risk. Chem. Eng. News, 58: 20-26.

Feldman, G. (1982). Synthesis and secretion of acute phase proteins by the hepatocytes from rats with normal liver or cirrhosis during the inflammatory reaction. Ann. N.Y. Acad. Sci., 381: 446-447.

Gol-Winkler, R. & Goutier, R. (1977). DNA synthesis inhibition by dimethylnitrosamine in regenerating rat liver. Eur. J. Cancer, 13: 1081-1087.

Hard, G.C., (1975). Thymus-dependent lymphocyte function in dimethylnitrosamine-induced renal carcinogenesis is not depressed. Oncology, 31: 139-146.

Hard, G.C. (1981). Effect of a single carcinogenic dose of Dimethylnitrosamine on antibody responses in the rat. Oncology, 38: 47-52.

Heath, D.F. (1962). The decomposition and toxicity of dialkylnitrosamines, Biochem. J., 85: 72-91.

Holsapple, M.P., Tucker, A.T., McNerney, P.J. & White, K.L., Jr. (1984a). Effects of N-Nitrosodimethylamine on Humoral Immunity. J. Pharmacol. Exp. Ther., 229: 493-500.

Holsapple, M.P., Bick, P.H., & Duke, S.S., (1984b). Effects of N-Nitrosodimethylamine on cell-mediated immunity. J. Leukocyte Biol. (in press).

Johansson, E.B., & Tjalve, H. (1978). The distribution of °14C§-dimethylnitrosamine in mice. Autoradiographic studies in mice with inhibited and noninhibited dimethylnitrosamine metabolism and a comparison with the distribution of °14C§-formaldehyde. Toxicol. appl. Pharmacol., 45: 565-575.

Kroeger-Koepke, M.D. & Michejda, C.J. (1979). Evidence for several demethylase enzymes in the oxidation of dimethylnitrosamine and phenylmethylnitrosamine by rat liver fractions. Cancer Res., 39: 1587-1591.

LePage, R.N. & Christie, G.S. (1969). Induction of liver tumors in the rabbit by feeding dimethylnitrosamine. Br. J. Cancer, 23 125-131.

Magee, P.N. & Barnes, M.D. (1956). The production of malignant primary hepatic tumours in the rat by feeding dimethylnitrosamine. Br. J. Cancer, 10: 114-122.

Magee, P.N. & Barnes, J.N. (1967). Carcinogenic Nitroso Compounds Adv. Cancer Res., 10: 163-246.

Montesano, R. & Magee, P.N. (1970). Metabolism of dimethylnitrosamine by human liver slices in vitro. Nature (Lond.), 228: 173-174.

CLINICAL IMMUNOLOGY STUDIES IN INDIVIDUALS EXPOSED TO ENVIRONMENTAL CHEMICALS

J. George Bekesi*, J.P. Roboz*,
A. Fischbein** & I.J. Selikoff**

*Department of Neoplastic Diseases
The Mount Sinai School of Medicine
New York, New York 10029

**Environmental Sciences Laboratory
The Mount Sinai School of Medicine
New York, New York 10029

With the recognition that chemicals can have direct effect on the immune system the relatively new field of immunotoxicology is gaining wide support and interest, Gibson, Hubbard and Parke (1983). The objective of this article is to review some of our work on the immunotoxicology of asbestos and poly-brominated biphenyls (PBB).

IMMUNE STATUS OF PATIENTS WITH MALIGNANT MESOTHELIOMA

The possibility has been raised that the apparent immuno-suppression or the lack of it observed in asbestos exposed indiviuals might directly relate to the course of the disease and the ultimate development of mesothelioma or other asbestos related neoplasms, Lange et al. (1978) and Wagner et al. (1979). The risk of developing cancer peaks 20-38 years after the onset of exposure to asbestos. Then one third of all deaths among asbestos workers are due to some form of lung cancer.

In 1965, the first indication appeared that autoimmune mecha-nisms might be involved in asbestos-related disease in studies of rheumatoid factor in the serum of asbestos workers, Turner-Warwick and Parkes (1970). This was later confirmed, together with the finding of increased frequency of non-organ specific antibodies (antinuclear factor) and the possibility was raised that ANA production in asbestos-exposed workers might be under genetic control, since HLA-B8 antigen was more frequently seen among ANA positive workers than in negative controls, Turner-Warwick (1973), Lange et al. (1974), Matez et al. (1978).

There have also been a few earlier reports concerning immuno-logical changes in patients with asbestosrelated mesothelioma, particularly quantitative deficiency of circulating T-cells, Kagan et al. (1977), Haslan et al. (1978), Fischbein et al. (1978), Wagner et al. (1979). There is therefore at least suggestive evidence that immune dysfunction might play a role in the development of malignancy in asbestos exposed individuals.

We have studied the immunological status of 57 untreated mesothelioma patients who have been referred to us for the evaluation of their immunological status. Not surprisingly,

moderate to severe immunosuppression was observed among these patients. The in vivo cell mediated immunity as measured by delayed cutaneous hypersenitivity response to recall antigens (PPB, mumps, candida, varidase and dermatophytin) showed that 26% of the 57 patients were anergic (responding to < 2 recall antigens) compared to 10.4 % of control industrial workers who have not been exposed to asbestos. The high frequency (45%) of positive responses to PPD among the mesothelioma patients appears to be characteristic, since only 11.5% of patients with other types of cancer were PPD positive. Also, in these patients, the markedly lower response to mumps antigen as compared to a control population (Figure 1) might be a significant finding.

Analysis of various subclasses of lymphocytes (T and B) and monocytes revealed that the majority of the patients had significantly reduced T-lymphocyte subsets (Figure 2), normal distribution of B-cells and an increase of lymphocytes without surface marker property (null cells). Study of the functional integrity of T-lymphocytes revealed that only 30 % of the patients exhiibited lymphocyte responses within the normal range to PHA in autologous plasma (Figure 3). This was correctable in some cases by substituting with normal AB plasma, indicating the possible presence of serum blocking factor(s). Most patients with mesothelioma ultimately received some form of therapy including surgery, radiation or chemotherapy.

Our findings concerning unexpected longevity in a group of untreated patients with malignant mesothelioma with a normal immunological status is suggestive of participation of the host immune system in the control of the disease. All such patients who have decided not no receive treatment have been monitored longitudinally for their clinical and immunological status. Representative data on four patients are summarized in Table 1. They had normal or near normal distribution of various subpopulations of lymphocytes which remained unchanged during the observation period of 5 to 8 years. The functional intergrity of the lymphocytes as measured by lymphoblasto-genesis appeared to be at the lower range of the normal values and showed no evidence of serum blocking factor in these patients. Also, there was no measurable progression of disease during that period. The question, however, remains to be answered whether the longevity of patients with mesothelioma with normal or near normal immune function represents those individuals whose tumor is more antigenic thus provokes stronger immunological response which can adequately control the diseases and/or is a reflection of the satisfactory immunobiological status of the patient at the onset and/or during the course of the disease.

IMMUNE STATUS OF HIGH RISK ASBESTOS WORKERS

The immunological status was also assessed of 104 asbestos workers at 20+ years after the initial exposure. These workers were clinically well at the time of examination and had shown no evidence of serious disease of any kind.

The in vivo cell mediated immunity was determined by measuring the delayed cutaneous hypersentitivity response 48 hours after exposure to a battery of bacterial, viral and fungal antigens (PPD, mumps, candida, varidase and dermatophytin). The asbestos workers exhibited a similar pattern of response to recall antigens to patients with malignant mesothelioma. Twenty-two percent of the workers were anergic, 38% of the responders gave positive reactioon to PPD as compared to 45% of the mesothelioma patients and 10% of the control (Figure 1). Also similarly to the mesothelioma patients, the asbestos workers yielded markedly lower responses to mumps. Thus, the in vivo cell mediated immune response in asbestos workers reflects an altered immunological status even in the absence of malignancy.

The in vitro immunocompetence of asbestos workers was evaluated by phenotyping the peripherial blood lymphocytes and by measuring their functional integrity via blastogenic transformation assays. The total T lymphocytes (T11) fell below the normal range in 30% of the asbestos workers (Figure 2). Significant reduction was also observed in their helper T cells (T4) with a concomitant increase in the suppressor T cell (T8) population (Figure 4). Here, unlike in acquired immunodeficiency syndrome where the T4 is reduced but the T8 is essentially unchanged, the T4/T8 ratio becomes inverted due to abnormalities in both helper and suppressor lymphocyte numbers. In terms of function, 40% of the tested group showed decreased lymphoblastogenesis both in autologous and normal AB plasma thus excluding the possibility of a blocking factor such as was found in the serum of patients with mesothelioma (Figure 3).

In summary, based on both the in vivo and in vitro assessment of the immune status of asbestos workers there is suggestive evidence that exposure to asbestos adversely effects the human immune response by contributing to anergy, heightened PPD reaction without tuberculosis, numerical reduction in circulating T lymphocytes, inverted T helper/T suppressor ratio and lowered function. Since no evidence of malignancy was found in the examined asbestos workers, it is highly possible that exposure to asbestos may contribute to an immunodeficiency state potentially rendering the host susceptible to neoplasms.

CONSEQUENCES OF ENVIRONMENTAL CONTAMINATION BY POLYBROMINATED BIPHENYLS IN MICHIGAN

A commercial preparation containing polybrominated biphenyls (PBB) was inadvertently used in 1973 in place of magnesium oxide in the preparation of a special feed supplement for lactating cows, Dunckle (1975), Carter (1976). The contaminating agent a was mixture of brominated biphenyls consisting of two penta-, four hexa-, and two octabromobiphenyl isomers which had been developed as a flame retardant (Firemaster FF-1), Sundstrom et al. (1976).

Adverse effects of PBB in lactating cows were first reported in animals by Jackson and Halbert in 1974. They described anorexia and decrease in milk production a few weeks after ingestion of the contaminated feed. Some animals developed hematomas, abscesses, abnormal hoof growth, alopecia and thickening of the skin, developed cachexia followed by death within six months. Consequently, more than 500 dairy and poultry farms were quarantined in Michigan in 1973 and 1974. More than 30,000 cattle and 1.5 million chickens died and 5 million eggs had to be destroyed. Unfortunately, dairy products (beef, poultry, eggs, milk, cheese, butter) containing PBB were widely consumed in Michigan until 1978. PBB was subsequently found in the serum and/or adipose tissue of dairy farm residents, workers employed by the chemical company which manufactured the PBB containing fire retardant, and in most Michigan residents (Kay, 1977).

Polybrominated biphenyls, which have a chemical structure similar to that of polychlorinated biphenyls (PCB), are fat soluble and are stored in the thymus, liver, brain and adipose tissues, where they persist for long periods of time (Kay, 1977). Effects on the liver, kidney, thyroid, thymus and lymph nodes have been reported. The effects include intrahepatic bile duct hyperplasia, skin changes and preneoplastic changes, and in addition, microsomal enzyme induction has been demonstrated following PBB exposure in animals. Polybrominated biphenyls have been shown to be tumor promoters. PBB and several (purified) congeners were shown to inhibit the metalbolic cooperation between 6-thioguanine sensitive and resistant Chinese hamster V79 cells in a manner similar to known tumor promoters, such as the phorbol esters, Torosko et al. (1981) and Tsushimoto et al. (1982).

CLINICAL MANIFESTATIONS

To determine the long-term consequences of PBB exposure, investigation was undertaken first in 1976-77 and in 1981-83 of 332 adult dairy farmers from Michigan, 29 chemical workers who were involved in the manufacturing of PBB and 156 individuals from the general populations of Michigan. A group of 150 Wisconsin dairy farm residents served as controls.

A high prevalence of clinical signs and symptoms was found in the examination of adult Michigan subjects. Four major categories of symptoms were recognized: neurological, musculoskeletal, dermatological and gastrointestinal, Anderson et al. (1978). The neurological symptoms were the most prominent and included fatigue, decrement in the individual's capacity for physical and intellectual work, increase in the number of hours of sleep, memory impairment, headaches, dizziness and irritability, The musculoskeletal findings consisted of arthritis-like abnormalities including swelling of joints with deformities in some cases, joint pain and various degrees of limitation of movement. Knees and ankles were most frequently affected, but small joints such as fingers and hands were also often involved. The prevalence of symptoms among consumers of dairy farm products was similar to that found among the dairy farmers, Lilis et al. (1978). The frequency of clinical symptoms observed in the Michigan dairy farmer population were compared to a control population consisting of dairy farmers from Wisconsin. Significant differences were found in the prevalence of most symptoms. This investigation identified for the first time the presence of a "human toxic PBB syndrome" primarily characterized by effects on the neurological and musculoskeletal organ systems in a large segment of Michigan residents.

IMMUNOLOGICAL FINDINGS

Significant deviations from normal in both percent and absolute number of T-lymphocytes were observed in PBB exposed Michigan dairy farm residents and chemical workers, Bekesi et al. (1978), (1983a), (1983b). Thirty-four percent of the Michigan farm residents and 59% of the chemical workers manifested reduced T cell and increased null cell values. The percent and absolute number of T, B and null cells measured in the Michigan general population group in most cases were within the normal range. Direct (chemical workers) and indirect exposure (Michigan farm residents and consumers) to PBB resulted in various degrees of abnormalities in cell mediated immunity. Marked decrease in lymphocyte response to T and B cell specific mitogens as well as the proliferative T lymphocyte responses in the MLC reaction were observed. An attempt was made to establish a toxic PBB syndrome profile in the exposed Michigan population, by examining the prevalence of multiple clinical symptoms between Michigan farm residents with multiple immune dysfunction and those with no or one abnormal immune function, (subgroup I in Table 2). Subgroup 2 consisted of individuals with significantly reduced lymphocyte function, both for T and B cells. There was prevalence of multiple clinical symptoms among these 52 subjects particularly neurological and musculoskeletal symptoms. Subgroup 3 had numerical (T and Null-cells) and function (T and B cells) defects in addition to multiple clinical symptoms.

Subgroup 4 reflected increased levels of IgG and IgA (with prominent monospecific peak) as well as elevated C_3 but reduced C_4 values. This aberration in serological profile was not accompanied by numerical or functional alterations in lymphocytes. Subgroup 5 included 25 Michigan dairy farm residents with the most serious multiple immune dysfunctions i.e. polyclonal hypergammaglobulinaemia, reduced T-cell population and function and increased null cell population (Table 3). The abnormalities found in subgroup 4 were also accompanied by significantly heightened in vivo reponse to recall antigens mumps and varidase and multiple neurological and musculoskeletal symptoms. The plasma levels of PBB in the subgroups ranged between 0.6-70 ppb and in 25% of the subjects an increase was found as compared to the 1976 and 1978 values, Wolf et al. (1979, 1982). There was no apparent relationship between serum PBB levels and the prevalence of clinical symptoms and/or immunobiological findings. On the other hand,

the PBB content of white blood cells particularly the apolipo-
protein B fraction of the affected individuals appears to
correlate with the most severe immune dysfunctions(s) (Roboz
et al., 1979, 1982).

FAMILY CLUSTERING OF IMMUNE DYSFUNCTION AND CLINICAL SYMPTOMS

The immunobiological abnormalities and clinical symptoms were
examined with respect to family units in order to establish
whether the observed effects may be genetically determined
rather than related to the potential exposure. Cluster
analysis of clinical data and various immunological
parameters, i.e. T and Null cell surface markers T and B
lymphocyte function (PHA, ConA PWM) and levels of immunoglobulins (IgG, IgA and IgM), were performed for husbands and
wives in the 101 family units. A summary of the findings is
presented in Table 4. Strong family clustering abnormalities
in the immunological neurological and musculoskeletal systems,
for husbands and wives was positively established. Moreover,
there were significant correlations between multiple symptoms
and immune dysfunctions for husbands and wives independent of
age and serum or fat PBB levels, Bekesi et al. (1983).
Similarly, intrafamily clustering was observed for serum and
adipose PBB levels of quarantined and non-quarantined families
suggesting the importance of common dietary source, rather
than a genetic factor for the prevalence of multiple clinical
symptoms and immune dysfunctions observed in Michigan dairy
farm populations exposed to PBB (Wolf et al., 1978).

In summary, based on longitudinal studies of Michigan farmers
who have been exposed to PBB, the presence of a toxic syndrome
related to this exposure has been established. The symptoms
and immunological manifestations persist and it is now known,
that PBB is transmitted via breast milk. The long-term health
effects of PBB exposure in both adults and children can only
be a matter for a speculation at present because of the long
latency associated with potential carcinogens.

TABLE 1

IMMUNOLOGICAL PROFILE OF UNTREATED LONGTERM SURVIVORS WITH MALIGNANT MESOTHELIOMA

SUBJECTS	Lymphocyte Subsets in Absolute Number			Lymphocyte Function cpm X 10^3	
	T lymphocytes	B lymphocytes	Null Cells		
Normal Controls	1702±98	495±23	180±19	105.2±11	97.5±6
Patients with Malignant Mesothelioma	741±88	342±36	553±56	25.2±3.2	50.5±12.6
Untreated Longterm Malignant Mesothelioma Cases					
(a)[1]	1308	436	151	73.5	59.3
(b)[2]	1269	393	125	70.2	99.6
(c)[3]	1390	325	90	64.5	83.1
(d)[4]	1127	439	344	66.3	62.4

(1) Diagnosed in 1972; (2) Diagnosed in 1976; (3) Diagnosed in 1974 and (4) Diagnosed in 1975.

TABLE 2

PBB INDUCED IMMUNE DYSFUNCTION PROFILE

IN THE EXPOSED MICHIGAN POPULATION

	Michigan Farm Residents	
SUBGROUPS	No	%
1. No or only one abnormal immune parameter	199	60.0
2. Low lymphocyte stimulation induced by PHA, ConA, PWM with normal surface markers (T, B, and Null-cells)	52	15.7
3. Low lymphocyte stimulation induced by PHA, ConA, PWM with abnormal surface markers (T and Null-cells)	30	9.0
4. Increased levels of IgG, IgA, C_3, LOW C_4 with normal surface markers (T, B, and Null-cell) and lymphocyte function (PHA, ConA, PWM)	26	7.8
5. Increased levels of IgG, IgA, C_3 with abnormal surface markers T and Null-cells and lymphocyte function (PHA, ConA)	25	7.5
T O T A L	332	100

TABLE 3

ELEVATED IgG, IgA, C_3 AND N-CELLS WITH LOW T-CELLS AND FUNCTIONS (PHA and ConA)

AMONG PBB EXPOSED MICHIGAN FARM SUBJECTS

SUBJECTS	No. of SUBJECTS	IgG mg/dl*	IgA mg/dl*	C_3	T-CELLS Percent*	NULL-CELLS Percent*	PHA c.p.m.X10$^-$	ConA c.p.m.X10$^-$
Control	150	924±264	174±80	76.9±21	69.1±4.6	11.4±1.2	99±18	94.0±13
Dairy farm residents	25 (7.5%)	2409**	543**	158**	49.2*	30.7**	51.4**	41.8*
(Range)		(1809-4085)	(471-490)	(123-206)	(18-59)	(21-59)	(31-69)	(19-55)

* Mean ± S.D.

** Difference is statistically significant at p < .001 between control and the study group.

355

TABLE 4

ANALYSIS OF IMMUNOLOGICAL PARAMETERS FOR HUSBANDS

AND WIVES IN PBB-EXPOSED MICHIGAN DAIRY FARMERS

Immune Parameter	Means ± S.D.		Absolute Mean Difference (S.D.)	Spearman Correlation Coefficient (RHO)
	Husband	Wife		
Surface Markers: T-Cells (%)	59.17±10.9	60.93±10.8	1.80 (11.88)	0.298**
Null Cells (%)	22.14±13	20.59±11.7	1.56 (13.57)	0.337**
Lymphocyte Functions: T-Cell by PHA (c.p.m. X 1000)	77.83±23	73.30±17.9	4.30 (24.33)	0.303**
B-cells By PWM (c.p.m. X 1000)	72.84±24.9	73.91±24.8	0.241 (29.63)	0.282**
Immunoglobulins: IgG (mg/dl)	1637.24±491.9	1616.55±510.6	27.34 (564.76)	0.324**
IgA (mg/dl)	323.24±140.3	280.98±133.6	41.09 (197.11)	0.053
IgM (mg/dl)	121.09±69.6	147.40±84.9	27.80 (102.62)	0.150

* $p < 0.05$ ** $p < 0.01$

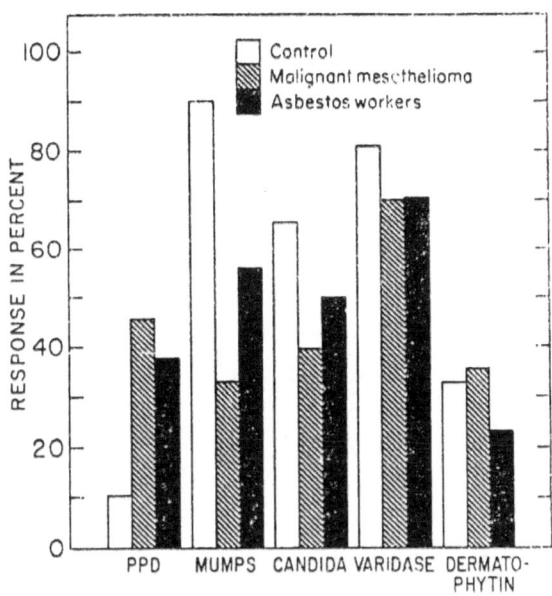

Figure 1. Response to Recall Antigens in Asbestos Workers and

Patients with Malignant Mesothelioma.

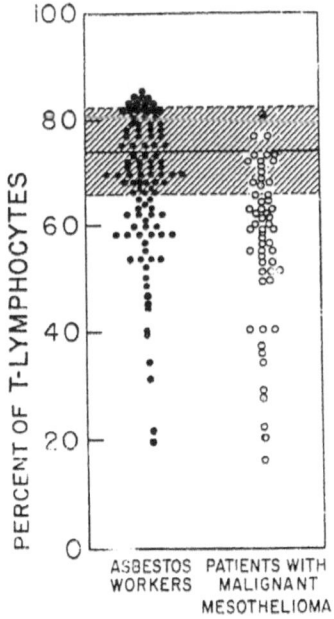

Figure 2. Total circulating T lymphocytes in Asbestos Workers

and Patients with Malignant Mesothelioma.

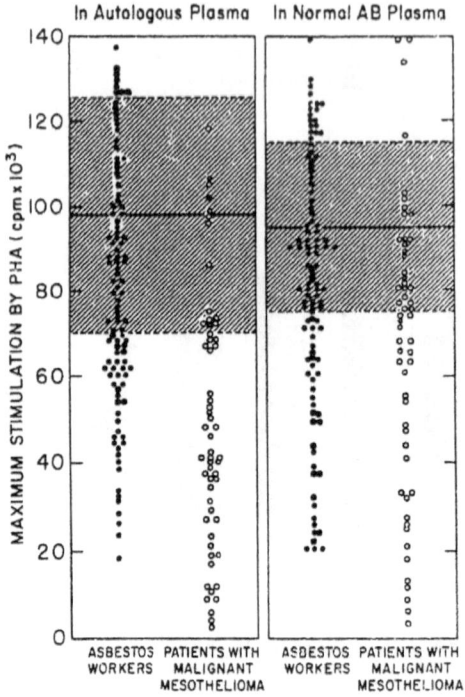

Figure 3. PHA Induced Lymphoblastogenesis in Asbestos Workers and Patients with Malignant Mesothelioma.

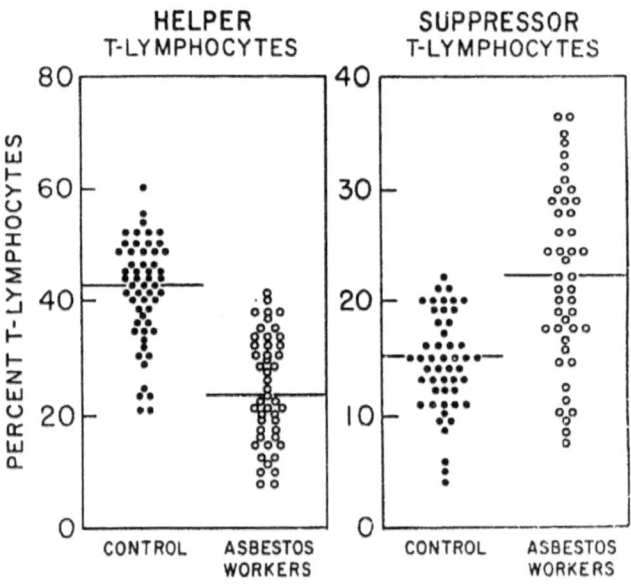

Figure 4. Helper and Suppressor Lymphocytes in Asbestos Workers and Healthy Subjects.

REFERENCES

1. ANDERSON, H.A.R., LILIS, R., SELIKOFF, I.J., ROSENMAN, K.D., VALCIUKAS, J.A., & FREEDMAN, S. (1978). Unanticipated prevalence of symptoms among dairy farmers in Michigan and Wisconsin. Environ. Health Perspect., 23: 217-226.

2. BEKESI, J.G., HOLLAND, J.F., ANDERSON, H.A., FISCHBEIN, A.S., ROM, W., WOLFF, M.S., & SELIKOFF, I.J. (1978). Lymphocyte function of Michigan dairy farmers exposed to polybrominated biphenyls. Science 199: 1207-1209.

3. BEKESI, J.G., ROBOZ, J.P., SOLOMON, J., FISCHBEIN, A., ROBOZ, J., & SELIKOFF, I.J. (1983). Persistent immune dysfunction in Michigan dairy farm residents exposed to polybrominated biphenyls. In Advances in Immunopharmacology, 2, (eds. Hadden, J.W., Chadid, L., Ducor, P., Spreafiro, S. and Willoughby, D.) pp. 33-39. Pergamon Press, New York.

4. BEKESI, J.G. ROBOZ, J.P., SOLOMON, S., FISCHBEIN, A.S. & SELIKOFF, I.J. (1983). Altered immune function in Michigan residents exposed to polybrominated biphenyls. In Immunotoxicology, (eds. Gibson, G.G., Hubbard, R. & Parke D.V.) pp. 181-191. Academic Press, New York.

5. CARTER, L.T. (1976). Michigan's PBB incident: chemical mix-up leads to disaster. Science, 192: 240-243.

6. DUNCKEL, A.E. (1975). An updating on the polybrominated biphenyl disaster in Michigan. J. Amer. Vet. Med. Assoc., 167: 838-841.

7. FISCHBEIN, A., SUZUKI, Y. SELIKOFF, I.J. & BEKESI, J.G. (1978). Unexpected Longevity of a Patient with Malignant Pleural Mesothelioma. Cancer, 42: 1999-2004.

8. GIBSON, G.G. HUBBARD, R. & PARKE, D.V. (1983). Immunotoxicology, pp. 1-505. Academic Press, New York.

9. HASLAM, P.L., LUROSZEK, A. MERCHANT, J.A. & TURNER-WARWICK, M. (1978). Lymphocyte responses to phytohaemagglutinin in patients with asbestosis and pleural mesothelioma. Clin Exp Immunol., 31: 178-188.

10. JACKSON, T.F. & HALBERT, F.L. (1974). A toxic syndrome associated with the feeding of polybrominated biphenyls-contaminated concentrate to dairy cattle. J.Amer. Vet. Med. Assoc., 165: 437-439.

11. KAGAN, E., SOLOMON, A., COCHRANE, J.C., KUBA, P., ROCKS, P.H. & WEBSTER, I. (1977). Immunological studies of patients with asbestosis. II. Studies of circulating lymphoid cell numbers and humoral immunity. Clin Exp Immunol., 28: 208-275.

360

12. KANG, K.V., SERA, Y., OKOCHI, T. & YAMAMURA, Y., (1974).
    T lymphocytes in asbestosis. New Eng J Med., 291:
    735-736.

13. KAY, K. (1977). Polybrominated,biphenyls (PBB) environ-
    mental contamination in Michigan, 1973-1976. Environ.
    Res., 13: 74-93.

14. LANGE, A., SMOLIK, R., CHMIELARCZYK, W., GARNCAREK, D., &
    GIELGIER, Z. (1978). Cellular immunity in asbestosis.
    Arch Immuno Ther Exp.,26: 899-903.

15. LANGE, A., SMOLIK, R., ZATONSKI, W. & SZYMANSKA, J.
    (1974). Autoantibodies and serum immunoglobulin levels
    in asbestos workers. Int Arch Arbeitmed, 32: 313-325.

16. LILIS, R., ANDERSON, H.A. VALCIUKAS, J.A., FREEDMAN, S.
    & SELIKOFF, I.J. (1978). Comparison of findings among
    residents on Michigan dairy farms and consumers of
    produce purchased from these farms. Environ. Health
    Perspect., 23: 105-109.

17. MATEZ, H., LANGE, A., GARNCAREK, D., SMOLIK, R., ROSZAK,
    E. (1978). HLA and antinuclear antibody incidence in
    asbestos workers. Arch Immunol Ther Exp., 26: 201-205.

18. ROBOZ, J., SUZUKI, R.K., BEKESI, J.G., HOLLAND, J.F.,
    ROSENMAN, K. & SELIKOFF, I.J. (1979). Mass spectral
    identification and quantification of polybrominated
    biphenyls in blood compartments of exposed Michigan
    chemical workers. J. Environ. Pathol. Toxicol., 3:
    363-378.

19. ROBOZ, J., GREAVES, J., HOLLAND, J.F. & BEKESI, J.G.
    (1982). Determination of polybrominated biphenyls in
    serum by negative chemical ionization mass spectrometry.
    Anal. Chem., 54: 1104-1108.

20. SUNDSTROM, G., HUNTZINGER, O. & SAFE, S. (1976).
    Environmental chemistry of flame retardants. Part II.
    Identification of 2, 2',4,4', 5, 5'-hexabromobiphenyl as
    the major constituent of flame retardant Firemaster BP-6.
    Chemosphere, 5: 11-14.

21. TROSKO, J.E., DAWSON, B. & CHANG, C.C. (1981). PBB
    inhibits metabolic cooperation in Chinese hamster cells
    in vitro: Its potential as a tumor promotor. Environ.
    Health Perspect., 37: 179-182.

22. TSUSHIMOTO, G., TROSKO, J.E., CHANGE, C.C. & AUST. S.D.
    (1982). Inhibition of metabolic cooperation in Chinese
    hamster V79 cells in culture by various polybrominated
    biphenyl (PBB) congeners. Carcinogenesis, 3: 181-186.

23. TURNER-WARWICK, M.& PARKES, W.L. (1970). Circulating
    rheumatoid and antinuclear factors in asbestos workers.
    Br Med J., 3: 492-495.

24. *TURNER-WARWICK, M. (1973). Immunologic mechanisms in occupational disorders. Immunolgy and asbestosis.* <u>Proc Roy Soc Mes.</u>, *66: 927-930.*

25. *WAGNER, A.M., CAMPBELL, M.J. & EDWARDS, R.E. (1979). Sequential immunological studies on an asbestos-exposed population. I. Factors affecting peripheral blood leukocytes and T lymphocytes.* <u>Clin exp. Immunol.</u>, *38: 323-331.*

26. *WOLFF, M.S., HAYMES, N., ANDERSON, H.A. & SELIKOFF, I.J. (1978). Family clustering of PBB and DDE values among Michigan dairy farmers.*<u>Environ. Health Perspect.</u>, *23: 315-319.*

27. *WOLFF, M.S. , ANDERSON, H.A., CAMPER, E., NIKAIDO, M.N., DAUM, S.M., HAYNES, N., SELIKOFF, I.J. & AUBREY, B. (1979a). Analysis of adipose tissue and serum from PBB (polybrominated biphenyl) exposed workers.* <u>J. Environ. Pathol. Toxicol.</u>, *2: 1397-1411.*

28. *WOLFF, M.S., ANDERSON, H.A. & SELIKOFF, I.J. (1982). Human tissue burdens of halogenated aromatic chemicals in Michigan.* <u>J.Amer.Med. Assoc.</u> *247: 2112-2116.*

IMMUNOLOGICAL EFFECTS OF DIETHYLSTILBESTROL IN THE HUMAN

T. Kalland [1] & R. Hofman [2]

[1] Lunds Universitet Institute of Anatomy,
Lund, Sweden
[2] Institute of Toxicology, E. Merck,
Darmstadt, F.R. Germany

INTRODUCTION

Diethylstilbestrol (DES) is a synthetic non-steriodal compound that possesses estrogenic activity (Fig. 1). DES has been widely used as a therpeutic estrogen in humans since it is inexpensive and effective after oral administration (1). The major clinical application of DES has been estrogen replacement therapy (hormonal dysgenesis, postmenopausal symptoms), treatment of prostatic cancer, postcoital contraception and suppression of lactation. From the late 1940's DES became accepted as useful for the prevention of threatened abortion. This treatment was in 1971 shown to lead to cervical and vaginal carcinomas in female offspring of treated mothers and is the first example of transplacental carcinogenesis of humans (2,3). Exposure to DES may also be a question of environmental concern. Recently, several reports have appeared indicating that the use of anabolic agents, mainly DES, for growth promotion in poultry and meat production, was responsible for episodes of epidemic breast enlargement in Puerto Rico and Italy (4,5).

Estrogens, including DES, have well documented effects on the immune system of rodents (6,8). Clinical observations such as the prevalence of certain autoimmune diseases among females and their increased susceptibility to infectious agents during pregancy indicate a possible influence of female sex steroids on the human immune system as well. In spite of the wide use of DES in humans, studies on the immune effects in man have not been extensive

T LYMPHOCYTE ASSOCIATED FUNCTIONS

Mitogens polyclonally activate lymphoid cells to proliferate and to express various lymphocyte regulatory and effector functions in a manner analogous to specific antigens. These substances have been used for the characterization of functional lymphocyte subclasses and as a measure of general immunocompetence (9). The effect of treatment with DES on lectin activation of T lymphocytes has been investigated in patients with prostatic cancer. Ablin et al. (10) found a profound inhibition of Phytohaemagglutinin (PHA) stimulated lymphocyte proliferation after 5 days of treatment with DES. Lymphocyte activation, expressed as a proliferation stimulatory index, was reduced to 35 % of pretherapy levels when patients were compared on an individual basis. The effect was not related to an increase in serum a_2-globulin level which is known to affect PHA responsiveness in lymphocyte cultures due to binding of the lectin (11). The depressed PHA responsiveness was reversible and abrogated within two weeks after cessation of therapy. Unfortunately, no details on the treatment regimen used was given making comparisons to similar studies difficult. The importance of the drug regimen in the immunotoxic effects of DES was emphasized by a recent study of Haukaas et al. (12). They investigated the effect of conventional oral low dose (10 mg per day for 2 weeks, later 2 mg daily) as well as acute high dose intravenous (1000 mg daily for one week) DES therapy on lymphoproliferative responses. No effect by DES on responsiveness to either PHA or Concanavalin A (Con A) was observed during one month of oral low dose treatment. However, high dose intravenous DES therapy significantly reduced T cell activation by PHA after one week of treatment althought it had no effect on the response to Con A (Table I). The effect was observed irrespective of whether autologous or pooled AB serum was used, indicating that DES was not acting by bringing about alterations in serum factors. The significance of the difference in effects on PHA and Con A induced responses is not clear. The patient sample was small, and the difference, although statistically significant, is not convincing. T cells with receptors for IgM-Fc (T helper cells) respond preferentially to PHA while Con A activates the whole T cell population (13). When peripheral blood lymphocytes from healthy young men or patients with prostatic cancer were stimulated with Con A in the presence of DES, a dose dependent inhibition of the proliferative response was observed (12). However, concentrations equal to or above $10^{-5}M$ was necessary to induce significant inhibition. It should be noted that the in vitro inhibition curves were identical in patients before and during treatment with DES indicating that DES treatment per se does not alter the distribution of lymphocyte populations with putative different sensitivity towards DES (12). A single i.v. injection of DES has been reported to reversibly alter the proportion of Fc-alpha receptor positive cells in peripheral blood (14).

In a series of papers, Ablin and coworkers investigated the effect of DES on tumor associated immunity against prostatic tumor antigens using the leukocyte adherence inhition test (15-17). Patients receiving DES therapy had lower levels of tumor associated immunity than patients receiving no or non-hormonal therapy, irrespective of tumor grade or stage (15). The reduction mounted to about 40% as judged by the leukocyte adherence inhibition assay. A significant inhibition of reactivity was also observed after exposure of lymphocytes from the patients to $10^{-4}M$ DES in vitro. The effect of DES was specific for reactivity against prostatic tumor antigens and was not seen against extracts of other tumors of the genitourinary tract, indicating a specific effect on anti-tumor reactivity.

Five day treatment with 1000 mg DES i.v. daily had no effect on either the responder or stimulator capacity in mixed lymphocyte reactions (18). However, addition of DES to the MLR in vitro inhibited proliferation at concentrations great that $10^{-4}M$. After activation of the MLR for 24 hours, which perhaps more accurately reflects an already stimulated immune response in the patients, DES was only partially suppressive at concentrations of 7×10^{-3}M. We have recently confirmed these observations and also shown that the presence of DES during MLR prevents the develoment of alloantigen specific cytotoxic T lymphocytes (19). Moreover, differentiated CTL's are also sensitive to DES since cytotoxic activity agains allogenic blast cells are reduced in a dose dependent manner when DES is included in the assay (Fig. 2).

B LYMPHOCYTE ASSOCIATED FUNCTIONS

No data are available concerning the effects of DES on humoral immunity in the human. Observations from murine studies indicated that B lymphocyte associated functions were somewhat less prone to the inhibitory effect of DES than T cell functions. The lymphoproliferative response to B cell mitogens, serum titer of antibody as well as the number of antibody producing cells in spleen, after immunization with T-independent antigens, were all reduced after treatment with DES, but the doses required to impair B cell respnses was generally higher than those affecting T cell functions.

NATURAL KILLER CELL ACTIVITY

In a study comparing DES with another commonly used drug for treatment of of prostatic cancer, estramustine phosphate (Estracyt ®), DES in contrast to the latter was found to severely impair the activity of natural killer (NK) cells (20). Conventional oral doses (10 mg daily for 2 weeks, thereafter 2 mg daily as well as high dose i.v. (1000 mg daily for one week) therapy profoundly reduced NK activity after one week of treatment (Fig. 3). The effect persisted for at least the 4 weeks of treatment covered by the study but did not decrease further after the first week of treatment (20). Recently, Hofman and coworkers studied patients treated with estramustine phosphate or DES for prolonged times (mean 1.1 and 2.3 years respectively) (21). They confirmed the observation that estramustine had no adverse effect on the NK cell system, but found a slight decrease of NK activity in patients exposed to DES. It should be noted, however, that these patients were treated with a low dose of 2 mg of DES daily, and also that comparisons were made on a treatment group base, not on an individual base comparing treatment NK levels with pretherapy levels. Pertubation of the NK cell system in these patients however, was indicated from the fact that lymphocytes from DES treated patients responded less well to stimulation with interferon in vitro than lymphocytes from patients treated with estramustine phosphate or following orchidectomy (Fig. 4).

The mechanism of action of DES was not adressed in the above patient studies. DES is not directly cytotoxic to human lymphocytes or the NK cell containing large granular lymphocyte population (22,14). Acute i.v. administration of DES has been reported to reduce NK activity in parallell with depletion of Fc-receptor positive cells (14). Since the majority of NK cells in the human have Fc receptors, this finding was interpretated as a redistributing effect of DES to other compartments than peripheral blood. However, the recent observation that NK cells are the lymphocyte population in peripheral blood most susceptible to DES in vitro (22,23), argue against a simple redistribution as a cause of the reduced NK cell activity in DES treated patients. When human peripheral blood lymphocytes were incubated with DES for 18 hours, a profound dose and time dependent inhibition of NK activity, was found down to $1\mu M$ concentration(23) (Fig. 5). Since estradiol 17 had no effect even at the highest concentrations tested, $100\mu M$, estrogenicity per see is apparently not the main property of DES responsible for the inhibition of NK activity. The effect of DES was fully reversible when the cells were further incubated for 24 hours without DES. DES was shown to selectively interfere with the lytic activity of NK cells without affecting the number of NK cells or their target recognizing ability (Fig. 6). Lymphoid cells exposed to DES for 18 hours were able to suppress NK activity of fresh lymphocytes when cocultured during the NK assay. The suppression was not prevented by separation of the DES precultured cells and indicator NK cells with a membrane with a cut-off value of 10kD, indicating that a soluble product with molecular weight less than 10,000 was responsible for the suppression (24). When indomethacin or aspirin were included together with DES during the 18 hours preculture time, the DES induced inhibition of NK activity was completely reversed (Table II). Taken together, these data indicate that DES inhibits NK activity by induction of a suppressive product of the cyclooxygenase system. Whether this product belongs to the prostaglandin series which is known to inhibit NK activity (25), or an oxidative metabolite of DES following cooxidation by cyclooxygenase (26) is not known.

BONE MARROW AND RETICULOENDOTHELIAL SYSTEM

Very few observations are available concerning the effects of DES on human bone marrow structure or function. A myelodyspoietic syndrome has been associated with prolonged therapy with massive doses of DES in a case of prostatic cancer (27). It is not known whether this case of myelodyspoiesis was preceeded by hypocellularity as is the case with other forms of drug-induced myelodyspoiesis (28). In three patients with concurrent chronic lymphatic leukemia and cancer of the prostate, treatment with DES for the latter condition also induced remission of the leukemia. Moreover, previously noted lymphocytic infiltration of the bone marrow in one patient was not evident after three months of DES therapy (29). Although some cases of thrombocytopenia have been observed following DES therapy (30), no common bone marrow related side effects of DES have been reported during treatment for prostatic cancer. However, only general parameters such as peripheral white blood cell and platelet counts have been studied. The apparent lack of effect on human bone marrow is in sharp contrast to murine studies. Prolonged treatment with high doses of estrogens, including DES, induced endosteal bone formation and concomitant loss of bone marrow function (31). Short-term DES treatment, in doses relevant to the therapeutic situation in man, caused hypocellularity of the bone marrow and a decrease of pluripotent hemopoietic stem cells and macrophage-granulocyte progenitors (32). Recently, the myelotoxic effects of DES have been examined mechanistically and have been found to be directly influenced by regulatory factors produced from thymic eipthelium (33). Estrogens, including DES, have consistently been reported to stimulate the phagocytic capacity of cells in the mouse and rat reticuloendothelial system (34). In fact, DES is one of the most potent stimulators of the reticuloendothelial system known, as judged by its ability to increase phagocytosis. It is not known whether this is true in the human or if this property has any relevance for the observed immunomodulatory effects of DES in man.

GENERAL CONSIDERATIONS

DES has been shown to exert immunotoxic effect on some components of the human immune system both during treatment of patients with the drug and in vitro. Comparison of the sensitivity of the various immunological functions tested clearly indicate that the NK cell system is the most susceptible to DES, both during patient treatment and after exposure in vitro (Fig. 2). The proliferative response to lectins, to alloantigens in MLR, the generation of CTL in MLR as well as the cytotoxic activity of CTL's were affected by DES at considerably higher concentrations. Estimates of serum DES levels after oral administration are available but differ considerably between studies as well as between individuals (35-37). Abraham et al. (35) have reported peak serum levels of DES in the range of 10^{-8}M after ingestion of a 10 mg dose, while Guinan et al estimated a serum level of 10^{-4}M following an equivalent dose (36). Serum levels of DES during treatment of patients with prostatic cancer may thus reach levels shown to affect human lymphoid functions in vitro.

Estrogen receptors have recently been demonstrated in human thymus, in OKT8 positive lymphocytes as well as in certain fresh or cultured leukemic cell lines (38-40). Compared to physiological estrogen levels, however, the concentrations of DES affecting the immune response are extremely high, strongly arguing against a receptor-mediated mechanism of action. Evidence has been presented that the DES-induced inhibition of NK activity is mediated by prostaglandins although this has not been directly shown. It is tempting to speculate that administration of cyclooxygenase inhibitors during DES treatment may abolish the effect of DES on NK cells. T lymphocyte associated functions shown to be impaired by suprapharmacological concentrations of DES have the common feature of being dependent on cytoskeletal activity. DES have colchicin like effects in fibroblasts (41). Moreover, DES has also been reported to affect capping in mouse lymphocytes (42) and effects of estrogen metabolites in vitro on PHA-induced blastogenesis directly correlate with the lectin-stimulated agglutination response of cells occurring within minutes. (43). This suggests a role for estrogens in modulating events of lymphocyte activation at the cell surface or cytoskeletal level independent of cytosolic receptor mediated events.

The relevance of the above effects of DES on the immune system in the human is unclear. Impairment of NK cell activity during treatment of patients with prostatic cancer may influence the surveillance of metastasizing tumor cells. Evidence from murine studies supports this assumption since DES treated mice have an increased susceptibility to transplanted and primary carcinogen-induced tumors as well as an impaired ability to prevent metastasis formation after intravenous injection of tumor cells (44-46). It is also important to point out that the developing immune system is clearly more susceptible to toxic effects in general (47-48) and that this holds true also for the effects of DES (7). In the mouse, exposure of the immature immune system to DES leads to persistent pertubations of the immune system, in particular a decreased NK activity (7,47). Similar studies are not available in humans, but potential immunotoxic effects of DES should be a matter of special concern in the exposed fetus and in children.

TABLE 1

Effect of treatment of patients with prostatic cancer on lymphoproliferative response to T cell mitogens

^{3}H-thymidine incorporation(cpm x 10^{-3}±SE)

Treatment	n	Con A		n	PHA	
		pretherapy	posttherapy		pretherapy	posttherapy
Estracyt	7	45 ± 4	41 ± 9	3	34 ± 12	40 ± 8
Diethylstilbestrol-Estradurin	8	39 ± 14	47 ± 10	5	54 ± 13	61 ±20
Honvan	4	28 ± 7	33 ± 12	5	62 ± 11	40 ± 9*

* indicate statistical difference from pretherapy level, p<0.05.

For details of treatment regimen, see text.

TABLE 2   EFFECT OF ESTROGENS AND CYCLOOXYGENASE INHIBITORS ON NK ACTIVITY

Drug exposure	Drug concentration (µM)	Cyclooxygenase inhibitor	$V_{max} \times 10^{-3}$
vehicle	-	-	23.5 ± 3.5
vehicle	-	Indomethacin	35.0 ± 5.8
vehicle	-	Aspirin	31.2 ± 5.0
DES	10	-	12.8 ± 1.5 [1]
DES	10	Indomethacin	32.9 ± 4.9
DES	10	Aspirin	27.4 ± 3.6
estradiol-17β	10	-	21.7 ± 3.3
estradiol-17β	50	-	24.3 ± 3.5
estradiol-17β	100	-	21.7 ± 3.6
transstilbene	10	-	25.5 ± 2.9
transstilbene	100	-	22.1 ± 3.4
dienestrol	10	-	15.2 ± 2.6 [1]
dienestrol	100	-	6.7 ± 1.3 [1]
dienestrol	10	Indomethacin	28.0 ± 4.7
dienestrol	10	Aspirin	25.6 ± 3.5

Peripheral blood mononuclear cells were cultured for 18 hours as described in materials and methods section in the presence of various test substances and tested for NK activity against K-562 target cells. The effect of cyclooxygenase inhibitors on inhibition was tested by inclusion of Indomethacin (10^{-6}M) or Aspirin (10^{-5}M) in the cultures. Mean ± SE of 2-5 experiments. [1] statistically different from control value, $p < 0.01$.

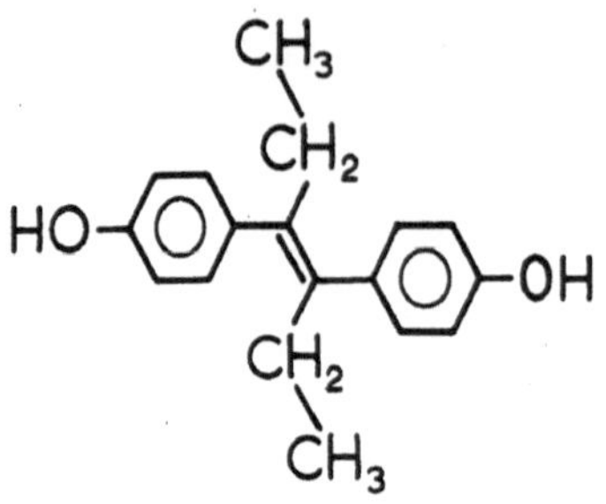

370

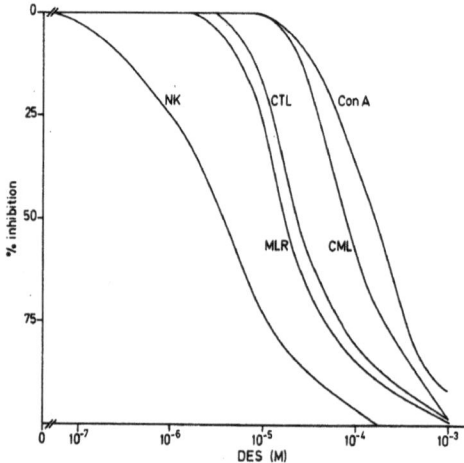

Figure 1:Structure of DES.

Figure 2:Inhibitory effects of DES on some immunological parameters
in vitro.The data are presented as percent inhibition in the
presence of DES related to unexposed values and are summarized
from ref.12,18,19,23,and 24.
NK,natural killer cell activity ;MLR,proliferative response
to alloantigens in a mixed leukocyte reaction;CTL,cytotoxic
activity of alloantigen-specific T lymphocytes generated in
a mixed leukocyte reaction in the presence of DES;CTL,cytotoxic
activity of T lymphocytes generated in a an untreated mixed
leukocyte reaction and assayed in the presence of DES;Con A,
proliferative response to Concanavalin A.

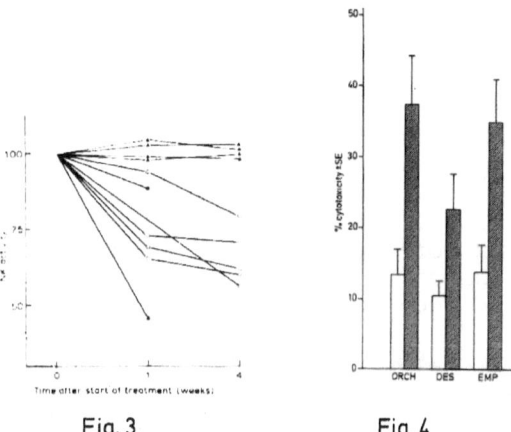

Fig. 3   Fig. 4

Figure 3:Natural killer cell activity in peripheral blood of patients
treated for prostatic cancer with estramustine phosphate(▲),
diethylstilbestrol-polyestradiol phosphate(○) or high dose
diethylstilbestrol(●).The activity after 1 and 4 weeks of
treatment is related to pretherapy level.For details on treatmen
regimen,see text.

Figure 4:Natural killer cell activity against K-562 target cells of
patients with prostatic cancer treated with orchidectomy(ORCH),
DES(Honvan[r] ,2mg daily) or estramustine phosphate(Estracyt[r],
840 mg daily).Basal (□) and interferon activated (▨) natural
killer cell activity is shown.

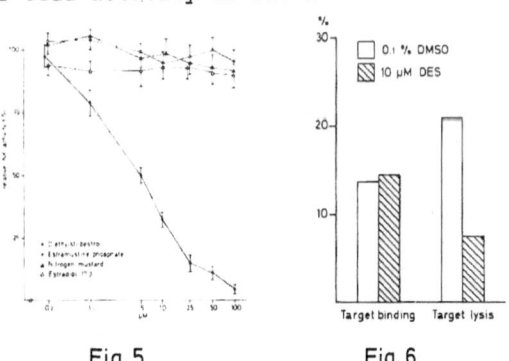

Fig. 5   Fig. 6

Figure 5:Natural killer cell activity   of
peripheral blood lymphocytes incubated for 18 hours in the
presence of various concentrations of DES,estradiol-17b,
estramustine or nitrogen mustard,washed and tested for cytotoxic
activity against k-562 target cells .

Figure 6:Effect of culture of peripheral blood mononuclear cells
in the presence of 10 uM DES or vehicle(0.1% dimethylsulphoxid,
DMSO) on the percenatge of target binding lymphocytes and
the percentage of conjugated cells lysing their target.For
details on the methods, see ref. 23

REFERENCES

1. McLachlan, J.A. & Dixon, R.L. 1976. Transplacental toxicity of diethylstilbestrol: A specific problem in safety evaluation. In: Advances in modern toxicology (eds M.A. Mehlman) p. 423, Hemisphere Publishing Co. Washington.

2. Herbst, A.L., Ulfelder, H. & Poskanzer, D.C., 1971. Adenocarcinoma of the vagina: Association of maternal stilbestrol therapy with tumor appearance in young women. N. Engl. J. Med, 284:878.

3. Herbst, A.L., 1981. The epidemiology of vaginal and cervical clear cell adenocarcinoma. In: Developmental effects of diethylstilbestrol in pregnancy. (eds A.L. Herbst and H.A. Bern) p. 63, Thieme-Stratton Inc., New York.

4. Comas, A.P., 1982. Precocious sexual development in Puerto Rico. Lancet i: 1299.

5. Pasquino, A.M., Balducci, R., Manca Bitti, M.L., Spadoni, G.L., & Boscherini, B. 1982. Transient pseudo-precocious puberty by probable oestrogen intake in 3 girls. Arch. Dis. Child. 57:954.

6. Ahlquist, J. 1976. Endocrine influences on lymphatic organs, immune responses, inflammation and autoimmunity. Acta Endocrinol. 83:1.

7. Kalland, T. 1982. Long-term effects on the immune system of an early life exposure to diethylstilbestrol. Banbury Report 11. In: Environmental factors in human growth and development (eds V.R. Hunt, M.K. Smith and D. Worth) p. 217, Cold Spring Harbor Laboratory.

8. Luster, M.I. Pfeifer, R.W. & Tucker, A.N. The immuno-toxicity of natural and environmental estrogens. In: Toxicology of the immune system (eds J.H. Dean, R. Munson, and M.I. Luster) Raven Press, New York,in press.

9. Hume, D.A. & Weideman. 1980. Mitogenic lymphocyte transformation. Research monographs in immunology, vol. 2 Elsevier/North Holland, Amsterdam.

10. Ablin, R.J., Bruns, G.R., Guinan, P.D., Sheik, A.L. & Bush, I.M., 1976. Hormonal therapy and alteration of lymphocyte proliferation. J. Lab. Clini. Med. 87:227.

11. Musa, B.U., Seal, U.S. & Doe, R.P., 1965. Elevations of certain plasma proteins in man following estrogen administration. A dose-response relationship. J. Clin. Endocrinol. 25:1163.

12. Haukaas, S.A., Huisater, P.A. & Kalland, T. 1982. In vitro and in vivo effects of diethylstilbestrol and estramustine phosphate (Estracyt ʀ) on the mitogen responsiveness of human peripheral blood lymphocytes. The Prostate. 3:405.

13. Moretta, L., Ferrarini, M. Mingari, M.C., Moretta, A. & Webb, S.R. 1976. Subpopulations of human T lymphocytes identified by receptors for immunoglobulins and mitogen responsiveness. J. Immunol.-17:2171.

14. Onsrud, M., & Sander, S. 1982. Influence of in vivo diethylstilbestrol phosphate on some human blood lymphocyte subpopulations. Acta path, Microbiol. Scand. Sect. C 90:271.

15. Ablin, R.J., Bhatti, R.A. & Guinan, P.D. 1978. Effect of estrogen on tumor associated immunity in patients with adenocarcinoma of the prostate. Cancer Res. 38:3702.

16. Ablin, R.J., Bhatti, R.A., Guinan, P.D. & Khin, W. 1979. Modulatory effects of estrogen on immunological responsiveness. II. Suppression of tumorassociated immunity in patients with prostatic cancer. Clin. Exp. Immunol. 38:8391.

17. Ablin, R.J., Guinan, P.D. & Bhatti, R.A. 1983. Cell mediated immunity in prostatic cancer and its diagnostic relevance. Eur. J. Cancer Oncol. 19:467.

18. Herr, H.W. 1982. Effect of estrogen on the mixed leukocyte reaction in normal individuals and prostatic cancer patients. The Prostate 3:17.

19. Campbell, T. & Kalland, T. The effect of DES on generation and activity of cytotoxic T lymphocytes. In preparation..

20. Kalland, T. & Haukaas, S.A. 1981. Effect of treatment with diethylstilbestrolpolyestradiol phosphate or estramustine phosphate (Estracyt ʀ) on natural killer cell activity in patients with prostatic cancer, Invest. Urol. 18:437.

21. Hofman, R., Lehmer, A., Reidel, G., Schwemmer, B., Schuetz, W. & Braun, J. Natural killer cell activity in patients with prostatic carcinoma. Abstract........

22. Djeu, J., Stocks, N. & Ramsey, K.M. 1982. Inhibition of human natural killer (NK) cell activity by immunopharmacological agents and time-dependent reversal of inhibition by interferon (Abstract) Immunobiol. 163:213.

23. Kalland, T. & Campbell, T. Effects of diethylstilbestrol on human natural killer cells in vitro. Immunopharmacol., in press.

24. Kalland, T. & Campbel, T. unpublished observation.

374

25. Bankhurst, A.D. 1982. The modulation of human natural killer cell activity by prostaglandins. J. Clin. Lab, Immunol. 7:85.

26. Degen, G.H., Eling, T.E. & McLachlan, J.A. 1982. Oxidative metabolism of diethylstilbestrol by prostaglandin synthetase. Cancer Res, 42:919.

27. Andersson, A.L. & Lynch, E.C. 1980. Myelodyspoietic syndrome associated with diethylstilbestrol therapy. Arch. Int. Med, 140:976.

28. Pierre, R.V. 1974. Preleukemic states. Sem. Hemato. 11:73.

29. Narasimhan, P. & Amaral, L. 1980. Lymphopenic response of patients presenting with chronic lymphatic leukemia associated with carcinoma of the prostate to diethylstilbestrol. Am. J. Hemato.. 8:369.

30. Nachtsheim, D.A., McPershon, R.A., Pollen, J.J. & Schmidt, J.D. 1980. Trombocytopenia during diethylstilbestrol diphosphate (Tilphostrol) infusion for carcinoma of the prostate. The Prostate 1:105.

31. Urist, M.R., Buddy, A.M. & McLean, F.C., 1950. Endosteal bone formation in estrogen treated mice. J. Bone and Joint surg, 32:143.

32. Boorman, G.A., Luster, M.I., Dean, J.H. & Wilson, R.E. 1980. The effect of adult exposure to diethylstilbestrol in the mouse on macrophage function and number. J. Reticuloend. Soc, 28:547.

33. Luster, M.I., Boorman, G.A., Korach, K.S., Dieter, M.P. & Hong, L. Myelotoxicity resulting from exogenous estrogens: evidence for bimodal mechanism of action. Submitted for publication.

34. Loos, L.D. & Di Luzio, N.R. 1976. Dose-related reticuloendothelial system stimulation by diethylstilbestrol. J, Reticuloend. Soc. 20:457.

35. Abraham, G.E., Reifman, E.M. Buster, J.E., Distepha, J. & Marshall, J.P. 1972. Production of specific antibodies against diethylstilbestrol. Anal. Lett. 5:449.

36. Guinan, P.D., Ablin, R.J., Al Sheik, H. & Bush, I.M. 1975. Diethylstilbestrol levels in patients with carcinoma of the prostate. Clin. Res. 23:338.

37. Kemp, H.A., Read, G.G., Riad-Famv, D., Pike, A.W., Gaskell, S.J., Queen, K., Harper, M.E. & Griffiths, K. 1981. Measurement of diethylstilbestrol in plasma from patients with cancer of the prostate. Cancer Res. 41:4693.

38. Danel, L., Souweine, G., Monier, J.C. & Saez, S. 1983. Specific estrogen binding sites in human lymphoid cells and thymic cells. J. Steriod Biochem. 18:559.

39. Danel, L., Cordier, G., Revillard, J.P. & Saez, S. 1982. Presence of estrogen binding sites and growth stimulating effect of estradiol in the human myelogenous cell line HL-60. Cancer Res. 42:4701.

40. Cohen, J.H.M., Danel, L., Cordier, G., Saez, S. & Revillard, J.P. 1983. Sex steroid receptors in peripheral T cells: Absence of androgen receptors and restriction of estrogen receptors to OKT-8 positive cells. J. Immunol. 131:2767.

41. Sawada, M. & Ishidate, M. 1978. Colchicine like effects of diethylstilbestrol on mammalian cells in vitro. Mutat. Res. 57:175.

42. Kalland, T. & Forsberg, J.-G. 1980. Permanent inhibition of capping of spleen lymphocytes from neonatally estrogen treated female mice. Immunol. 39:281.

43. Pfeifer, R.W. & Patterson, R.M. Modulation of lectin-stimulated lymphocyte agglutination and mitogenesis by estrogen metabolites: Effects on early events of lymphocyte activation. Submitted for publication.

44. Dean, J.H., Boorman, G.A., Luster, M.I., Luebke, R.W. & Lauer, R.D. 1980. The effect of adult exposure to diethylstilbestrol in the mouse: alterations in tumor susceptibility and host resistance parameters. J. Reticuloend. Soc. 28:571.

45. Kalland, T. & Forsberg, J.-G. 1981. Natural killer cell activity and tumor susceptibility in female mice treated neonatally with diethylstilbestrol. Cancer Res. 41:5134.

46. Kalland, T. & Haukaas, S.A. Effects of diethylstilbestrol and estramustine phosphate (Estracyt (R)) on natural killer cell activity and tumor susceptibility in male mice. The Prostate, in press.

47. Faith, R.A. & Moore, J.A. 1977. Impairment of thymus-dependent immune functions by exposure of the developing immune system 2,3,7,8,-tetrachlorodibenzo-p-dioxin (TCDD). J. Toxicol. Environm. Health 3:451.

48. Luster, M.I., Boorman, G.A., Harris, M.W. & Moore, J.A. 1980. Laboratory studies on polybrominated biphenyl-induced immune alterations following low-level chronic or pre/postnatal exposure. Int. Immunopharmacol. 2:69.

IMMUNE SYSTEM DISORDERS ASSOCIATED WITH ADULTERATED COOKING OIL

J.J. Gomez-Reino

Ministerio de Sanidad y Consumo,
Instituto Nacional de la Salva,
Hospital "1st de october", Section Thematology.
Madrid, Spain.

EPIDEMOLOGY, CLINICAL DESCRIPTION AND PATHOLOGY OF TOXIC OIL SYNDROME.

The Toxic Oil Syndrome (TOS) is a new disease that appeared in Spain in 1981 following the consumption of adulterated rapeseed oil. The disease is characterized by an acute onset of pleurocarditis, fever, rashes and eosinophilia. In a number of cases it had a chronic outcome, characterized by an evolution through different phases: acute, intermediate and chronic, with an overlapping of a neuromuscular syndrome, a scleroderma-like picture, Raynauds phenomenon, pulmonary hypertension and Sjogren syndrome.

Epidemology.

Rapeseed oil denaturated with anilines was imported to Spain for industrial use only, however because of its low price some companies illegally removed the anilines and sold the oil for human use. The association between TOS and denaturated oil was discovered in June 1981. Following the official announcement of the association, the number of new cases with the disease dropped sharply, and no new cases were seen after August 1981. Several epidemological studies have confirmed this association (1-4). The number of individuals exposed to the toxic oil, but unaffected is unknown, but close to 20,000 are known to have been affected. In spite of extensive work in a number of centers and, many analytical studies of suspected oil and numerous animal experiments, no single substance has been identified as the cause of the disease.

Clinical description (Figure 1)

Some 2-3 weeks after the ingestion of toxic oil patients developed fever, rashes, interstitial pneumonitis, pleuropericarditis, gastro-intestinal symptoms and marked eosinophilia. A few died from acute respiratory insufficiency. By two months the picture changed to myalgias, arthralgias, edema of the face, numbness of the limbs and thrombocytopenia (4-8) while the other symptoms gradually disappeared. Around 5% of the patients had thromboembolic accidents and a quarter of them died as a consequence. In 4 months, 15% of the patients developed a new set of symptoms which seemed to be the definitive ones. The rest of the patients showed a tendency to improve and became asymtomatic. The chronic phase was characterized by the overlapping of a neuromuscular syndrome, an scleroderma-like picture, Raynauds

FIGURE 1

Acute Phase	Intermediate Phase	Chronic Phase
Neumonitis	Myalgias	Neuromuscular S.
Fever	Edema	Scleroderma-like S.
Rash	Numbness	Raynaud's phenomenom
Arthralgias	Thromboembolism	Pulmonary hypertension
Eosinophilia	Thrombopenia	Sjogren S.

May 1981------------July 1981----------------October 1981----

Clinical spectrum of TOS.

phenomenon Sjogren syndrome and pulmonary hypertension. The spectrum of the disease varied from the presence of one of the above syndromes, in a mild form, to the overlapping of all of them with different degrees of intensity. The patients with the more severe disease had, also,the further complication of a superimposed malnutrition (7). The neuromuscular syndrome consisted of a sensory and, on occasions, motor deficit predominantly of the lower extremities (6-9). The skin of the entire body was affected by areas of infiltration and/or atrophy. Apart from Raynauds phenomenon, pulmonary hypertension and dysphagia no other organs, commonly involved in clasic scleroderma, were affected (6-8).

Severly affected patients developed a characteristic deformity of limbs with the elbows in flexion and the forearms in pronation. The hands showed thickening of the palmar fascia, extension of the metacarpophalangeal joints and flexion of proximal and distal interphalangeal joints. Flexion-contractures were also present in ankles, knees and wrist (7). Deaths in the chronic phase were due to respiratory insufficiency and complications of mechanical ventilation.

Pathology (Figure 2)

Although the clinical picture has shown a changing pattern as the different phases developed, the pathology has been characterized by a uniform non-necrotizing vasculitis in all the tissues studied and in all stages of evolution (6,7,10). The vascular lesion involved all the structures and all types of vessels. The endothelium showed, initially, swelling followed by proliferation and, in some cases, intimal fibrosis. There was also perivascular, medial and intimal infiltration with mononuclear cells and eosinophils. Fibrinoid necrosis was never seen (6,7,10) In the early phases, the lungs showed septal and alveolar edema, mild interstitial infiltration with mononuclear cells, and cuboidal metaplasia of type II pneumocytes. No pulmonary fibrosis was seen (10). The study of peripheral nerves from patients in the chronic phase showed epineural and perineural infiltration with mononuclear cells. In severe cases a profound perineural fibrosis followed the infiltration. The muscle presented superficial (fascial and epimysial) infiltration with mononuclear cells and neutrophils. In advanced stages a denervation atrophy took place (6,10). In The skin, in the acute phase, a mononuclear infiltration was present around both superficial and deep blood vessels. These changes were followed by interstitial infiltration and, later, fibrosis (6,7,10). The lesions described above were not all present in every patient, and those in the chronic phase were usually confined to the more severely affected cases. Nevertheless, random skin biopsies taken from asymptomatic patients have shown a significant increase in fibrous tissue (10).

IMMUNE DISORDERS ASSOCIATED WITH THE TOXIC OIL SYNDROME

The clinical and pathological similarities between TOS and certain collagen diseases had led several groups to investigate the possibility that autoimmune mediated mechanisms, triggered off by a toxic agent, were involved in the pathogenesis of the disease. Most of the available information has been obtained by in vivo and clinical studies. Animal and in vitro studies have been limited by the fact in that no etilogical agent has been identified.

Sex and HLA system

The sex ratio (F/M) in affected adults changed from the acute to the chronic phase. In the acute phase a ratio almost 1:1 was found, whereas in the chronic phase it was 6-10:1 (6,7). In a recent report no difference between the sexes was reported, however the definition of chronicity in this study was different from the one used in earliest work (4). In children the F/M ratio in the acute phase was, also, 1:1 but it did not change as the disease evolved (8). HLA A,B,C and DR studies were conducted on chronic patients. DR3 and/or DR4 were found to be significantly associated with the disease in females, but not in males. No relation between the presence of defined clinical or serological manifestations and HLA antigens could be seen (11).

Eosinophilia

A significant increase in the eosinophil count ($500/mm^3$) was present in 50-98% of the patients up until Novewmber 1981. Thereafter the incidence decreased and by April 1982 the majority had a normal count (Table.1, ref. 6,12). Platelets Between April and August 1981 about 20% of the patients presented thrombocytopenia (<150.000/mm3). In one third of them evidence of platelet activation was found in the acute phase (12). A year later 5 out of 8 patients studied with chronic symptoms still showed evidence of activation (13). There was no correlation between this activation and the severity of the disease or the presence of defined clinical syndromes. In the acute phase, the platelets had functional defects (12)., namely a decrease in ADP induced aggregation and absence of the second phase of aggregation. From September 1981 to April 1982, 10-12% of the patients had thrombocytosis (Fig. 3).

FIGURE 3

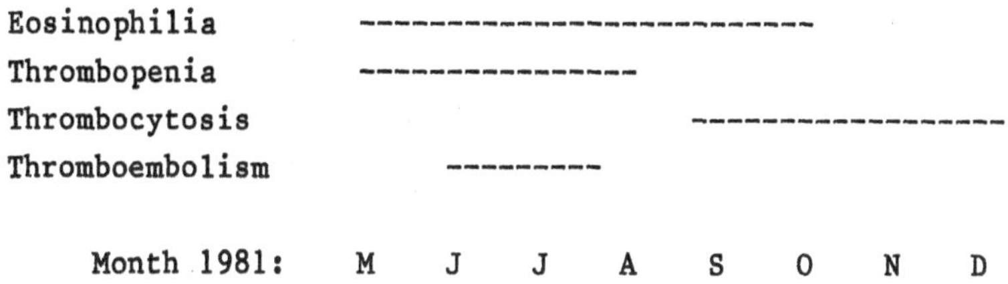

```
Eosinophilia        --------------------------
Thrombopenia        ----------------
Thrombocytosis                          ------------------
Thromboembolism        ---------

Month 1981:    M    J    J    A    S    O    N    D
```

Eosinophil and platelet changes in TOS

Their relation to thromboembolism

Lymphocytes

The total number of lymphocytes was normal in the acute phase. However alterations of the T cell count and T cell subpopulations were detected. In one study 75% of the patients had normal T-helper but low T-suppresor cells (12). In the early chronic phase we found low T-suppresors (Table 2). B and T cell cytotoxic autoantibodies were also detected (11). We found a serum factor that selectively decreased the number of the suppresors, by incubation of lymphocytes with patients sera followed by the use of monoclonal antibodies (OK3,OK4 and OK8). This factor seemed to be complement dependent (Table 1). "In vitro" the responses of the lymphocytes to mitogens and antigens were within normal limits (14).

Unstimulated and allogeneic stimulated lymphocytes from chronic patients released a factor in the culture media that produced changes in fibroblast cultures (see below).

Immunoglobulins

The initial picture of the disease (i.e. rash, pneumonitis and eosinophilia) was suggestiver of an IgE mediated type of reaction. Therefore several groups investigated the prsence of elevated levels of IgE or specific IgE antibodies. In our hospital a study conducted in 561 patients and 357 exposed but unaffected individuals demonstrated a significant elevation of IgE in both groups. A comparison between the levels of both showed no difference (15). In an other study, 70% of the patients were found to have raised IgE during the first few weeks of the disease, and 6 months later 20% still had this alteration (14). Brostoff et al. failed to demonstrated the existence of specific IgE antibodies against the potencial oil contaminants (16,17) Other immunoglobulins were not altered.

Autoantibodies

Different types of autoantibodies were identified during the course of the disease. Antinuclear antibodies (ANA) were found in all the studies (Table 3). In the first few months

96% of our patients had positive ANA, and in 50% of them the titre was 1:40 (7). Two years later this was followed up in 96 chronic patients. Seventeen still had a titer 1:40 (Table 4). In our experience, anti extractable nuclear antigen, anti human spleen extract and anti DNA were negative or seldom positive. In a multicentric study, in the acute phase, 50% of the patients were found to have positive ANA (14). Antilymphocyte antibodies were detected. Arnaiz-Villena et al. reported a cytotoxic antibody to T and B cells in 10% of the chronic phase patients. We also found a serum factor that selectively depleted T-suppresor cells (Table 2)). Other groups had similar findings (14,18) Anticollagen antibodies were present in the acute and chronic phases. However they were differences between them (23). Patients in the acute phase had higher incidence than those in the chronic. It seemed that the presence or absence of antibodies did not predict the evolution to chronicity. In the chronic phase, there was a lack of relation between the severity of the disease and the presence of antibodies (Table 5).

Immunocomplexes and complement

The complement levels were always in the normal range (6,7). Immunocomplexes (IC), detected by different methods, were found in a small number of patients (14). Indirect evidence of IC mediated damage was, in general, absent. The widespread non-necrotizing vasculitis, when studied with immunofluorescen techniques, did not reveal deposits of immunoglobulins or complement in a consistent pattern (10). Only in 4 cases (out of 842), with proliferative glomerulonepritis, we found deposits of IgG and complement in the basal menbrane and capilary loops of the glomeruli. In those cases the electron microscopic examination showed subepithelial, subendothelial and mesangial dense deposits (19).

Fibroblasts and fibroblast related changes

In the early phases, skin biopsies demonstrated fibroblast activitity similar to the reparative myofibroblasts found in other conditions (10). Cultures of 25 skin biopsies taken from the infiltrated skin of chronic patients yielded only 3 stable fibroblast lines (20). The morphology and distribution of cells in cultures was abnormal. The biosynthesis of collagen by those cells in culture was substantially decreased (Table 6). Moreover, electrophoretic analysis of the cultures showed an increase in the fibronectin band and a decrease in the collagen bands (20). Supernatants of the non-stimulated and allogeneic stimulated lymphocytes from chronic patients produced a significant increase in collagen synthesis by normal fibroblasts (21). The supernatants of stimulated cultures did not further increase the production caused by non-stimulated cultures, suggesting a preactivation of the cells (Table 7). When stimulated and non-stimulated supernatants were added to normal fibroblast cultures they produced changes also in cell morphology (22). Cultures of normal fibroblast in the presence of control oil and suspected toxic oils containing media demonstrated a increase in collagen synthesis by the latter. (Table 8). Electrophoretic analysis of medium and cells revealed a decrease in the fibronection band and increase in the collage bands (2).

Animal experiments and in vitro studies

Animal experiments and vitro studies have been of limited value and the results obtained inconclusive. Frequently in vitro studies have produced contradictory results (24-26). Every attempt to reproduce the TOS in different animal species has been unsuccessful (27-28). Several reasons have been advanced to explain this state of affairs: (1) Analysis of different oil types have yielded inconsistent results. Many toxic sustances have been identified (2). Collection of toxic oil definitively associated with the illness was not achieved owing to the emergency of the situation. Some batches could well have had no related to the TOS (3). The details of how the oil was actually denatured and refined (illigally)were only made available recently.Consequently it is now improbable that the original toxic oil will ever be reproduced and thus the source of the industrial "rape seed oil" involved in the disaster remains a mistery.

Comments

The epidemology and genetic studies suggest that sex, or sex hormones, and factors related to the chromosome 6 (HLA region) might have determined the evolution to chronicity. HLA studies in patients who did not have the chronic disease may reveal whether the susceptibility to the disease was also genetically determined. Hypereosinophilia, low platelet and endothelial damage might have been related phenomena. They could also be the result of a direct toxic effect.

The transient presence of anti-lymphocyte antibodies could explain the presence of other antibodies. There was evidence that antibodies were directed against T-cell (possibly T-suppresor) and caused T-supressor depletion. The initial insult could have damaged a T-cell population and generated the production of antibodies against them. The selective depletion of an autoregulatory population could result in the production of autoantibodies.

Positive ANA is a complication of ingestion of aromatic amine and hydrazine class chemicals. TOS is related to the consumption of oil denatured with aromatic amines. This could explain the finding of positive ANA in TOS. The study of the specificity of the nuclear antibodies might clarify whether they are disease markers or related to its pathogenesis.

The fibroblast and fibroblast related changes could have several explanations. A toxin might have stimulated the fibroblast, directly or through the activation of other cells (mononuclear?, endothelial?), to produce collagen. This, in turn, may have exhausted the cells. Cultures taken at this point (chronic phase) could reflect this alteration. On the other hand, the skin biopsies showed activated cells similar to the reparative myofibroblast. Studies of these skin biopsies could have reflected the difference in protein synthesis between the skin fibroblast and the myoblast.

Some of the information included in this report is preliminary. Much more work is clearly called for to explain this dramatic and baffling new disease. Finding an animal model would greatly facilitate progress in this direction.

This unprecedent experience should alert all authorities against the uncontrolled widespread and indiscriminate use of chemicals in industrial countries.

FIGURE 2.

	Acute Phase	Intermediate Phase	Chronic Phase
LUNG:	Edema Mononuclear infiltration Alteration pneumocytes type II	Diffuse infiltration	Fibrosis
SKIN:	Perivascular infiltration		
NERVE:		Epineuritis Perineuritis	Perineural fibrosis Axonal degeneration
MUSCLE:		Superficial Infiltration	Denervation atrophy, Fibrosis
VESSEL:	Endothelial swelling	Endothelial Proliferation Vasculitis	Intimal fibrosis

The pathology of TOS.

TABLE 1

Eosinophilia	-------------------------
Thrombopenia	-----------------
Thrombocytosis	------------------
Thromboembolism	----------

Month 1981   M   J   J   A   S   O   N   D

Eosinophil and platelet changes in TOS

Their relation to thromboembolism

TABLE 2

| | A | | B | | C | |
	HE	SU	HE	SU	HE	SU
N	55	31	50	7	–	–
P1	82	13	–	0	–	–
P2	90	3	91	0	–	–
P3	74	26	72	4	–	–
P4	58	32	50	14	57	34
P5	64	30	64	16	63	23
P6	64	37	64	3	58	28

Effect of TOS patients sera on the
T-helper and T-suppressor count (%)
A : preincubation values
B : after incubation with patients sera
C : after incubation with normal serum
N : normal control, P: patients
HE: helper, SU: suppressor

TABLE 3

	Acute Phase	Chromic Phase
Antinuclear Antibodies	++	+
Antilymphocyte Antibodies	++	–
Anticollagen Antibodies	++	+

Presence of autoantibodies in the acute and chronic TOS

TABLE 4

	Acute Phase n=50	Chronic Phase n=96
Negative	8.0	61.9
Titer 1:40	46.0	22.9
Titer 1:40	46.0	17.7

Percent of patients with antinuclear antibodies in TOS.

TABLE 5

	Acute Phase n=44	Chronic Phase n=51
Type I	29.5	11.7
II	18.1	3.9
III	31.8	3.9
IV	31.8	1.9
V	31.8	1.9
Total	52.0	19.5

Percent of patients with collagen antibodies in TOS.

TABLE 6

	A	B	C
N	9.5	7.5	5.6
S1	-	-	12.7
S2	-	-	15.5
P1	4.7	3.0	1.4
P2	4.9	2.5	1.3

Collagen production by fibroblast of TOS
patients obtained from skin biopsies (% Collagen)

N: normal control
S: scleroderma patients
P: TOS patients
A: before confluency
B: at confluency
C: 48 hrs of confluency

TABLE 7

	Non-stimulated cells	Allogenic stimulated cells
C1	1.8	–
C2	2.0	–
C3	4.0	4.0
C4	1.6	1.0
P1	8.7	8.8
P2	9.6	9.5
P3	10.1	7.5
P4	6.9	6.1

Increase in collagen synthesis (percent of maximum) produced by peripheral mononuclear cells of TOS patients (C:controls, P:patients) acting on normal fibroblast culture

TABLE 8

	A	B	C
M	7.4	–	–
0	11.2	7.4	8.4
01	13.0	11.3	10.0
02	14.8	11.8	7.7
03	14.3	9.5	9.1
04	12.4	10.0	7.3

Effect of toxic oil on collagen production by normal fibroblast (% of collagen synthetized)

M: culture with medium
0: culture with control oil
01-04: culture with potential toxic oils
A, B, C: different oil concentrations

REFERENCES

1- Catala FJ, Mata de la Torre JN.: Epidemologia del Sindrome Toxico In: Simposium Nacional Sindrome Toxico. Minsiterio de Sanidad y Consumo, Madrid 1982: 143-67.

2- Casado J. Casquero J. Garcia R, et al.: Encuesta alimentacion a ninos con Sindrome toxico. In: Simposium Nacional Sindrome Toxico. Ministeriode Sandidad y Consumo. Madrid 1982: 224-5.

3- Working Group on Denaturated Rapeseed Oil Toxicology Sindrome. WHO Regional Office for Europe. Meeting. Madrid, March 1983.

4- Kilbourne EM, Rigau-Perez J, Health CW, et al.: Clinical epidemology of Toxic-oil Syndrome. Manifestations of a new illness. N. Eng J. Med. 309: 1408 1983.

5- Tabuenca JM.: Toxic allergic syndrome caused by ingestion of rapeseed oil denaturated with aniline. Lancet 2:567. 1981.

6- Noriega A, Gomez-Reino J. Lopez-Encuenta A, et al.: Toxic Epidemic Syndrome. Spain 1981. Lancet 2: 697 1982.

7- Mateo I, Izquierdo M, Fernandez MP, et al.: Toxic Epidemic Syndrome: Musculoskeletal manifestations. J Rheumatol (in press)

8- Izquierdo M, Mateo I, Rodrigo M, et al.: Chronic Juvenile Toxic Epidemic Syndrome (submitted).

9- Portera A, Franch O, Del Ser.: Neuromuscular manifestations of Toxic Oil Syndrome: A recent outbreak in Spain. In : Clinical and biological aspects of peripheral nervous system diseases. Edited by Battistin, Hashim and Lajtha. Alan R. Uss. Inc. Scientific Medical and Scolarly Publications. New York (in press).

10- Martinez-Tello F, Navas-Palacios J, Ricoy JR, et al.: Pathology of a new toxic syndrome caused by adulterated oil in Spain. Virchow Arch (Pathol Anat) 397:261 1982.

11- Vicario JL, Serrano-Rios M, San Andres T, et al.: HLADR3 DR4 increase in chronic stage of spanish oil syndrome. Lancet 1: 276. 1982

12- Ribera C, Calero A, Toledo T, et al.: Patologia hematologica en el STE. In: Simposiun Nacional Sindrome Toxico. Ministerio de Sanidad y Consumo Madrid 1982: 346-51

13- Kahaleh B, LeRoy EC, Gomez-Reino J. Unpublished

388

14- *Estudios Inmunologicos en el Sindrome Toxico. (Resumen).In: Simposium Nacional Sindrome Toxico. Ministerio de Sanidad y Consumo. Madrid 1982: 132-37.*

15- *Bensabat Z, Vives R, Canto G., et al.: Niveles de IgE en poblacion consumidora de aceite de colza denaturalizado. Presented at XIII Congreso de la Sociedad Espanola de alergia. Sevilla 1982.*

16- *Brostoff J, Blanca M, Boulton P, Serrano S.: Absence of specific IgE antibodies in Toxic Oil Syndrome. Lancet 1:277 1982.*

17- *Blanca M, Boulton P, Brostoff J.: Toxic Oil Syndrome, clinical and immunological characteristics: a review. Clin Allerg 14: 68 1984.*

18- *LaHoz C, Garcia R, Tricas L.: Immunological aspects of Toxic Syndrome induced ingestion of adulterated oil in humans. Presented at the British Society of Immunology Meeting. London November 1981.*

19- *Gutierrez V, Navas J. Gomez-Reino J, Fernandez JL.: Renal involvement in Toxic Oil Syndrome. Lancet 1:1120 1982.*

20- *Lizarbe MA: Unpublished*

21- *Krakauer R, Gomez-Reino J. Unpublished*

22- *Lizarbe MA, Gomez-Reino J. Unpublished*

23- *Pereira RS, Bailey A, Black CM, Duance V, Holden AJ, Welsh K, Arnaiz A, Gomez-Reino J, Vicario JL. In preparation.*

24- *Murphy RB, Vodyanoy V.: Fatty acid anilines and the Toxic Oil Syndrome. Lancet 1:98 1982.*

25. *Tena G.: Fatty acid anilines and the Toxic Oil Syndrome Lancet 1:98 1982.*

26- *Kemper F, Luepke N, Renhof M, et al.: Fatty acid anilines and the Toxic Oil Syndrome. Lancet 1:98 1982.*

27- *Fernandez P, Martinez Cabruja R, Borregon A, et al: Anatomia Patologica experimental en modelo animal. In : Simposium Nacional Sindrome Toxico Ministerio de Sanidad y Consumo, Madrid 1982: 482-86.*

28- *Rojo J, Fueyo A, Marin P: Ingesta de aceite de colza en ratas: Estudio patologico. In : Simposium Nacional Sindrome Toxico. Ministerio de Sanidad y Consumo Madrid 1982: 487-93.*

VULNERABILITY TO TOXIC OR THERAPEUTIC IMMUNOMODULATION - AS TWO COMPLEMENTARY ASPECTS OF AGE AND NUTRITION DEPENDENT IMMUNODEFICIENCY

J. Shoham

Department of Life Sciences,
Bar Ilan University, II -
52000 Ramat Can, Israel.

I. INTRODUCTION

The aim of this communication is to increase awareness to specific problems of certain population sectors whose immunological system may be more sensitive to toxic damage than the normally functioning system. Indeed, the title of the presentation was selected with three considerations in mind: (a) It is possible and instructive to compare therapeutic immunomodulation, with which there is relatively more experience, and immunotoxicity, and by doing so to gain better insight into the general rules and potential mechanisms of toxic effects on the immune system. Moreover, therapeutic immunomodulatory agents are known to cause immunotoxicity under certain circumstances (Shoham, 1984a) and, in principle, the reversed situation is also possible. (b) Conditions of "deficiency","in sufficiency" or "failure" of the immune system may amplify or modify the effect of either type of agents. Accordingly, these conditions call for more caution and specific attention to potential adverse effects of such agents, which could cause further deterioration of the deficient immune system. Moreover, conditions of immunodeficiency are important targets for the therapeutic use of immunomodulating agents and these conditions may give rise to toxicity rather than benefit as as an outcome of this therapeutic manipulation. (c) There are certain similarities between the effect of age (either too young or too old) and malnutrition on the immune system, which justify considering them together in connection with potential toxic damage.

The field of immunopharmacology (and more so - immunotoxicology) is in its infancy and, therefore, data bearing directly on the questions to be discussed here are virtually non-existent. Accordingly, in preparing this communication I have relied upon circumstantial, indirect data in order to point out some of the unique features of the conditions under discussion which may guide us in analysing the vulnerability of the immune system to toxic damage under these conditions. The features to be discussed are related to the age and nutrition dependent changes in the pharmacokinetics (or more generally "chemobiokinetics", WHO report, 1978) (Section III) and the changes in the target organ, which may modify the response (pharmacodynamics) to either the therapeutic or toxic agents (Section IV). These sections of the communication will be preceded by a short description and classification of known agents of both types (Section II) and will be followed by a discussion on the mechanisms which may cause the increased vulnerability to immunopharmacological and immunotoxic agents in age and nutrition dependent immunodeficiencies.

II. CLASSIFICATION OF IMMUNOMODULATORY AND IMMUNOTOXIC AGENTS

Table 1 classifies the various agents which act with some degree of selectivity on the immune system. The selectivity is generally quantitative, i.e., effect on the immune system is seen at doses lower than those causing general or other specific toxicological or pharmacological effects. The classification is based on clinical-pharmacological criteria and reflects a certain conceptual approach:

(a) Immunotoxicity is related not only to immunosuppression but also to immunoenhancement, i.e., any clinically significant undesirable deviation from the homeostatic control of normal functioning immune system caused by a foreigns substance can be regarded as an immunotoxic effect.

(b) Immunotherapeutic agents may also be immunotix when the effect is exaggerated or when it is "paradoxical" (see below). The definition used in the classification here is operational, namely, an immunotoxic agent does not have an exploitable therapeutic potential.

(c) Included in Table 1 are agents that have a direct effect on the immune system, and not via an effect on other body systems.

The substances mentioned in Table 1 are heterogenous in their source strucutre, type of effect, mechanism and target cells (Fig. 1). Indeed, the ideal classification of immunoactive agents should be based on attributes like those generally illustrated in Fig. 1 (target cells, type and mechanism of effect). Unfortunately, such knowledge is extremely limited and we must rely on a formal classification of the type used in Table 1. More detailed discussion of the immunopharmacology and immunotoxicology of the various agents listed here can be found in several recent reviews (Vos, 1977; Spreafico and Anaclerio, 1977; Hadden et al., 1977; Koller, 1980; Spreafico et al., 1981; Rees and Lackwood, 1982; Bach, 1982; Dean et al., 1982; Shoham, 1984 a,b). Here we will confine ourselves to the more general questions of the impact of immunoactive agents on certain immunodeficient conditions. Discussion of some specific agents will serve only as example to illustrate general principles.

III. AGE AND NUTRITION DEPENDENT CHANGES IN CHEMOBIOKINETICS

Chemobiokinetic studies have the same scope and aims as pharmacokinetic studies and the new term was introduced (WHO report, 1978) in order to generalize the evaluation of biological effects of all chemicals, toxic or therapeutic, which are collectively called xenobiotics (Spreafico and Vecchi, 1984). Age and nutrition are strong modifying factors of the disposition of drugs and xenobiotics. The effect of these modifying factors has been observed in virtually every aspect of chemobiokinetics, as summarized in Table 2 and discussed in more detail below. The comparison will include the young (primarily, neonatal period), the old (>70 year) and the malnurished (protein-caloric malnutrition, PCM).

A. Absorption

Absorption of a chemical into the body can take place potentially by all routes of exposure, e.g., oral, dermal or inhalation and for drugs - by injection. The route of administration can greatly influence the rate at which the foreign chemical is distributed in the body and may cause modification of its structure and consequently its biological activity. The following discussion will be limited to absorption through the gastrointestinal tract (GIT) as an example of age and nutrition effects on the process. Three processes are involved in absorption of xenobiotics from the GIT lumen: (1) passive diffusion, (2) active transport and (3) pinocytosis. The rate and extent of absorption are dependent on physico-chemical properties of the drug (e.g., polarity, ionization), on the one hand, and on biological factors of the exposed individual (e.g., rate of stomach emptying, transit time in small intestine, surface area available for absorption and vascularity and blood flow in GIT), on the other hand.

The mechanism of gastrointestinal absorption in infants is reasonably comparable to that in adults. There are, however, some factors which cause a certain delay in absorption in the infant, including gastric pH, bacterial flora of the intestine and motility (Jusko, 1972; Morselli, 1976).

In the aged, a general involution of the GIT takes place, resulting in reduced surface area available for absorption, as well as reduced motility and blood flow. These changes make absorption of drug from GIT, a slow, less complete and less reliable process as aging occurs (Bender, 1964f; Geokas and Haverback, 1969).

In patients with PCM, oral administration of drugs presents a problem as diarrhea and vomiting are common. This means that the drug may not be retained and if it is, the transit time through the bowel may be such that absorption of drugs, particularly poorly soluble ones, may be impaired. Even in the absence of diarrhea and vomiting atrophy of the intestinal mucosa, which occur in severe PCM, may impair drug absorption (Buchanan et al., 1976).

B. Distribution and binding

Once absorbed, the distribution of a chemical is determined by the relative plasma concentration, the rate of blood flow through various organs and tissues, the rate by which the chemical penetrates cell membranes and the binding sites that are available in the plasma and tissues. In the bloodstream most chemicals are bound to plasma proteins (mainly albumin).

It should be noted that for drugs that are strongly bound to albumin, a small decrease in albumin concentration can virtually double or triple the concentration of free drug available to the effector organs. Thus, in essence we are dealing with 2 main parameters: total volume of distribution (Vd) and concentration of plasma proteins, both undergo age and nutrition related changes.

In the infant, especially the neonate, the apparent volume of distribution of several drugs was shown to be increased, whereas the binding capacity of plasma proteins is diminished. The last effect is generally of larger magnitude. The reasons for the lower binding in the infant, in spite of adequate albumin levels, may be related to: (a) a high concentration of endogenous compounds that bind to albumin (e.g., bilirubin); (b) possible qualitative differences between neonatal and adult albumin and (c) lower pH in neonatal plasma (Friis-Hansen, 1961; Jusko, 1972; Kurz et al., 1977).

In the elderly, the distribution of many drugs is likely to be altered in view of the changes in apparent volume of distribution (which differ with several individual drugs that were tested), decrease in blood flow through various vital organs, reduction in total body water and lean body mass, relative malnutrition and reduced plasma albumin (Wallace et al., 1976; Vestal, 1978).

Malnutrition has a profound effect on distribution and binding of drugs (and obviously, xenobiotics, in general). Plasma volume is increased in kwashiorkor (Cohen and Hansen, 1962); most of it is related to a decrease in hematocrit values (Alleyne, 1966). In addition, total body water is increased, mainly because of an expansion of the extracellular fluid, lowering plasma concentration of water soluble drugs. Concentration of albumin is diminshed in PCM, leaving a high proportion of unbound drugs in the plasma (Leonard and McWilliam, 1965)

C. Biotransformation

This process converts a foreign chemical to a derivative which is usually more polar and water soluble and can be more readily excreted from the body. The derivative is frequently less toxic than the parent compound. However, in many cases the biotransformation causes activation and the metabolite becomes more toxic (McLean, 1971). The liver is the major site of biotransformation. The enzymes involved in this process are found in the soluble, mitochondrial and microsomal fractions of the cell. Four main types of biotransformation processes are known: 1) oxidation, the most important reaction exerted primarily by microsomal mixed function oxidases, 2) reduction, 3) hydrolysis and 4) synthetic, or conjugation reactions (i.e., the addition of polar groups such as glucoronic acid, acetylation, etc.). Single or multiple reactions of these types may be involved.

Diminished drug metabolising capacity in young animals as well as human neonates has been well documented. The attainment of values approaching those of adults takes varying periods of time after birth (Rane and Sjowist, 1972). Indeed, the rate of acquisition of normal level of drug metabolising capacity is a function of the degree of maturity of the newborn and his liver (Pitlik et al., 1978), although some types of reaction (e.g., conjugation by sulphation) are reasonably well developed even in the newborn (Levy et al., 1975).

On the other extreme of life, changes in liver structure and function occur with increasing age, including decrease in weight, disintegration of hepatocytes, increase in vacuolization and fat components and decrease in the activity and inducibility of drug metablising enzymes (Vink, 1959; Kato et al., 1970; Vestal, 1978).

As far as malnutrition is concerned, most of the information has been derived from animal experiments, which indicate that starvation depresses hepatic microsomal drug metabolism, in vitro and in vivo (affecting oxidative more than reductive pathways), reduces the capability of drugs to induce the synthesis of drug metabolising enzymes and diminishes the maximum reaction rate (Vmax) of microsomal enzymes. Studies in experimental animals cannot be directly extrapolated to man because of large species variations in drug metabolising enzymes. However, studies in human subjects with varying grades of malnutrition do indicate that the mixed function oxidase system may be affected in severe malnutrition (Campbell, 1977). One has to add to it the general evidence for liver damage in malnutrition, including fatty infiltration and vacuolization and impairment of liver functions caused by other insults which frequently occur in the malnourished patient particularly in the tropics, including parastic infestation, cirrhosis and liver damage due to mycotoxins (Krishnaswamy, 1978).

E. Excretion

Chemicals are excreted as the parent chemical, as metabolites or as conjugates of the parent chemical or its metabolites. The kidneys are the most important route of excretion of foreign compounds and this is accomplished by either glomerular filtration or tubular transport, passive or active. Biliary excretion is secondary, but still a major route for the excretion of some foreign chemicals.

There are important differences in the rate of elimination of drugs (or chemicals) in neonates, infants and children, differences which can be related to the different developmental physiological states of the various age groups (Morselli, 1976). This is reflected in a successive increase in the rate of elimination with increasing age. A decreased capacity to eliminate drugs is most marked in the newborn, particularly premature infants. As the age dependent rate of elimination varies with the particular drug and the individual patient, no general rule can apply to the calculation of dosage for all drugs.

In old age, renal function diminishes even in the absence of apparent renal disease. Accordingly, even when blood urea or creatinine are normal, elderly patients have a smaller renal reserve than do younger people. Indeed, glomerular filtration rate may fall as much as 50% between the ages of 20 and 90 years (Rowe et al., 1976). Renal plasma flow declines about 1.9% per year after the age of 30. Similarly, tubular function deteriorates with age (Hansen et al., 1970). In addition to the physiological decline in glomerular and tubular function, the geriatric patient is particularly liable to renal impairment due to dehydration, congestive heart failure, hypertension, urinary retention, diabetic nephropathy, pyelonephritis, etc.

In PCM, there is marked diminution in cardiac output, resulting in decrease in renal plasma flow (Alloeyne, 1966). Glomerular filtration rate and tubular function have also been shown to be inadequate.

The summation of these effects decreases the rate of excretion of drugs or chemicals and elevates serum concentrations of those drugs which are eliminated mainly by the kidneys. In addition, kidney involvement by tropical diseases (e.g., Schistosoma hematobium infection) may further complicate the situation and interfere with kidney mechanisms of excretion.

Biliary excretion can also be affected in all the above-mentioned conditions, mainly as a result of liver damage that may accompany these conditions, as mentioned before.

In conclusion, most of the important parameters of chemobio-kinetics are imapired in the 3 conditions analysed here (Table 2). Obviously, there are widely scattered individual differences in each group and for different drugs or chemicals. However, as a general rule it is apparent that people belonging to these population sectors are much more vulnerable to toxic damage of any xenobiotic even if only the various parameters of chemobiokinetics are taken into consideration. Changes in the immune system, the target organ, that are encountered in these conditions, amplify its vulnerability to toxic damage as will be explained below.

IV. AGE AND NUTRITION DEPENDENT CHANGES IN THE IMMUNE SYSTEM

The immune response at the cellular level represents an intricate system of inductive and regulatory cell circuits which, in turn, affect the various activities of the effector cells. Both humoral and cell-mediated immune responses to most antigens are the result of a complex series of well-balanced interactions among cells (T, B, macrophages) and regulatory factors (lymphokines, monokines, thymic factors). The level of complexity of the immune system is comparable only to that of the central nervous system. However, the latter is more protected ("blood brain barrier") and its cells, being non-dividing resting cells, are less vulnerable to toxic damage. Accordingly, the immune system may suffer more than any other organ the toll of toxic injury.

Furthermore, the specific deviations or derangements in the immune system in the very young, the aged and the malnourished (Table 3) pose specific complicating safety problems.

A. Changes in the Immune Response During the Neonatal Period

The prenatal and neonatal periods are characterized by immuno-imcompetence in comparison to the adult. However, while the immunological immaturity of the fetus and newborn does extend to both humoral (Playfair, 1978) and cell-mediated reactions (Howe and Manziello, 1977), ontogenetic studies frequently fail to reveal any obvious quantitative deficiency in the cellular constituents considered necessary to initiate an immune response (Spear et al., 1973). Thus, it was shown that immune cells of either neonatal or adult rabbits do not function well when transferred to neonatal recipients, but did so, to a comparable degree, when transferred to irradiated adult recipients (Dixon and Weigle, 1957, 1959). In another study (Press et al., 1973) it was shown that adoptive transfer of neonatal spleen cells to adult, lethally-irradiated, carrier-primed recipients, maximizes the responsiveness of neonatal B cells. Moreover, there is good evidence that the repertoire of antigen binding cells in adult and young animals is similar (Klinman and Press, 1978) and that these cells arise early in development, at a time which may precede the ability of the animal to mount a specific immune response (Decker and Sercarz, 1974). Indeed, some qualitative changes do occur in the lymphoid cells subsequent to the appearance of recognizable B and T cells, with their apparent full range of antigen-binding specificities. Thus, all the immune cells undergo time-dependent maturational events expressed as phenotypic shifts in B and T surface markers (Cooper et al., 1980; Cantor and Gershon, 1980), as well as maturational changes in antigen presenting mechanisms mediated by sub-populations of macrophages (Niederhaber et al., 1979). All these data taken together indicate that the relative immuno-deficiency in the newborn may not be primarily due to an inadequate population of responding B cells, neither can it be solely attributed to an underdeveloped antigen processing system or the lack of helper T cell function (Peak et al., 1979). Neonatal incompetence is, at least in part, a manifestation of overriding active humoral and cellular suppression. Thus, we can look at the development of the immune system during the prenatal and neonatal periods as representing a precisely coordinated sequence of reaction patterns to achieve an optimal situation at any given time during development. Before birth the fetal immune system must function sufficiently to protect against invading microorganisms as well as against maternal lymphocytes sensitized to paternal alloantigens. At the same time there must be appropriate controls to prevent potentially damaging autoreactive processes. Indeeed, the immune system develops this restricted, well-controlled capacity during gestation. This is followed by quite dramatic changes in reactivity profiles subsequent to delivery. The maturation of the immune system after birth can be shown to closely parallel the normal physiological decay of strong elements of regulatory suppressor cells and inhibitory humoral factors, the factors being of both endogenous and exogenous origin. It is obvious, therefore, that any interference with the delicately balanced immune system during prenatal or neonatal periods may have major consequences, much more than in the adult.

B. Changes in the Immune Response in the Elderly

Aging is known to be accompanied by progressive decline in immune functions (Makinodan and Yunis, 1977). The morphological hallmark of immune senescence is the involution in the cellular mass of the thymus, which begins at sexual maturity and is complete by 45 to 50 years of age in man. At this time the thymus retains only 5 to 10 percent of its maximal mass (Kendall, 1981). The involution of the thymus gland during the first half of life is conceivably the main cause of the altered function of the immune system during the second half of life. This alteration is not manifested in the total number of lymphocytes or in the number of T or B lymphocytes in the peripheral blood.However, the distribution of sub-population of T lymphocytes does change with age - the number of helper or inducer cells, identified by OKT4 monoclonal antibody, increases, while the number of suppressor or cyto-toxic T lymphocytes, identified by the OKT8 monoclonal antibody, decreases (Moody et al., 1981). Although the changes in the proportion of T-lymphocyte subsets are modest, they may be important to the regulation of immune reactivity. In addition, some enzymes found in lymphocytes change with age in a way that may be associated with altered and deficient immune reactivity (Boss et al. 1980). Lymphocytes from the elderly are more susceptible to damage induced by ionizing radiation, ultraviolet light and mutagenic drugs and their recovery from such damage, e.g., radiation, is impaired, suggesting defective activity of DNA repair enzymes (Walford and Bergmann, 1979).

Analysis of the functional activity of the immune system in the aged animal or human indicates that T cell functions are much more impaired than B cell ones. There is altered balance among regulatory T lymphocytes as well as impairment of effector functions of cell-mediated immunity, including reduced delayed type hypersensitivity, graft versus host reaction, ability to mount cytotoxic response and to respond to antigens or T cell mitogens by cell proliferation (Hefton et al., 1980). The cellular basis of the impaired response of lymphocytes, which may be related to a decreased number of responsive T lymphocytes, which may be attributed to the involution of the thymus. In addition, the proliferative capacity of the remaining T cells is impaired and this defect may be related to reduced response and increased dependency on calcium ions (Kennes et al., 1981) as well as decreased capacity to produce and to bind interleukin-2 (Thoman and Weigle, 1982). Impairment in humoral immunity was also detected (e.g., decline in natural antibodies, increase in auto-antibodies and monoclonal immunoglobulins and decrease in response to new foreign antigens), but it reflects a disordered immune regulation mediated by T cells and not a primary defect of B cells. Indeed, thymectomized mice show the same derangements in humoral immunity as aged mice (Radl et al., 1980). The function of macrophages is not significantly altered with age.

C.   Changes in the Immune Response in Malnutrition

Most of the information in this connection is related to protein-calorie malnutrition (PCM). In referring to the changes in immune response in PCM, one should remember that PCM is not a discrete all or none phenomenon, but it rather spans an entire spectrum, ranging from subclinical malnutrition compatible with adequate life, to extreme lethal stages of nutritional deficiency. Also, vitamin and mineral deficiencies exist along with those of protein and calories, each of these deficiencies and their interacting effects may have important consequences on the immune response. Moreover, the vast majority of people suffering from PCM, also suffer heavy burdens of infection and both interfere with normal immune responses; infections also deplete the host's metabolic energy.

Among all the aspects of immune response it is the T cell functions that have been shown to be the most profoundly affected by nutritional factors . The thymus is the most vulnerable organ and the effect can be so severe that the term "nutritional thymectomy" can be justified (Watts, 1969). In patients with severe PCM, the effect can be as great as that to occuring in primary cellular immunodeficiencies. In lymphnodes thymus-dependent areas are depleted (Smythe et al., 1971), while plasma cells and germinal centers remain relatively intact. Other lymphoid organs are also grossly atrophied. The absolute number of lymphocytes in peripheral blood is moderately reduced, but the number of T lymphocytes is markedly reduced (15-25% of lymphoid cells forming rosettes with sheep red blood cells, E-rosettes, as compared to normal percentage of 60-75%, Chandra, 1974).The percentage of null cells and the activity of terminal transferase (an enzyme marker of T cells in early maturational stages) were both shown to be increased (Chandra, 1979a). The percentage of E-rosette forming cells is increased, in vitro, by incubation with thymic hormones (Chandra, 1980). Levels of serum thymic hormone activity have been found to be low in PCM, in both clinical and experimental studies (Chandra, 1979b). These data suggest maturational arrest of T-lymphocytes, which is at least partially related to thymic factor deficiency and can be corrected by it. T lymphocyte functions are also markedly impaired, including reduced or negative delayed-type hypersensitivity skin reactions (both recall reactions and primary sensitization) reduced proliferative response to mitogens (Newmann et al., 1975) and reduced interferon production (Woodruff, 1970).

On the other hand, humoral responses appear to be little affected by malnutrition. The number of B cells is normal and the cells are able to mount adequate antibody response after immunization. Also, the basic functions of the phagocytic system appear normal.

Intrauterine malnutrition may affect T cell functions and such abnormality may persist for prolonged periods (Chandra, 1974). Thus, the fetal immune system is particularly susceptible to nutritional deprivation (Beach et al., 1982). Indeed, nutritional therapy restores all the changes in cell-mediated immunity except in the case of malnutrition occurring during fetal life. Among isolated nutritional deficiencies, zinc, vitamin A and pyridoxin deficiency were shown to be consistently associated with impairment of immune functions and, once more, the T cell system is the most afflicted one (Prasad, 1983).

In summary, the impairments in the immune system which accompany the 3 conditions discussed here have certain formal similarities (Table 3). The main derangement is in T cells, with minimal or no change in B cell or macrophage functions. Although differences do exist in the fine details of the changes and their mechanisms, the specific purpose of the present communication is to show that a broad comparative discussion can be helpful.

V. AGE AND NUTRITION DEPENDENT VULNERABILITY TO IMMUNOMODULATION

The interaction of a chemical with a complex biological system such as the human body cannot be easily defined and analysed. The outcome of such an event is dependent on the nature of the chemical and the conditions of exposure to it (route, dose, duration), on the one hand, and on factors related to the exposed biological system ("host factors"), on the other hand. The host factors relate to: a) handling and disposition of the chemical determining the ultimate real exposure at the cellular level, and b) the condition of the target organ(s) and its responsiveness to the chemical effect. As more is known about drugs than toxic chemicals and since the mechanisms operating in both are, at least formally, similar, I will refer to the therapeutic and toxic effects as representing two complementary aspects of the same problem.

The three conditions discussed here are associated with significant changes in the handling and disposition of xenobiotics, with certain similarities in the direction of most of the observed changes (Table 2). The net result of all these changes is to increase the concentration of the chemical and the duration of exposure to it, at the cellular level. This obviously increases the risk of damage. It is difficult to quantitate the different factors contributing to the increased tissue exposure to the chemical. Accordingly, the magnitude of the net effect may vary widely even in the same group and sometimes in the same individual in different times. We can thus speak only in general terms on the increased susceptibility of such individuals to toxic damage caused by many xenobiotics, including those acting on the immune system.

In contrast to the general pharmacokinetic mechanisms which are operating to a comparable degree for all xenobiotics, the unique characteristics of the immune system make the pharmacodynamic aspect of the problem a more specific and complex one.

In essence, the uniqueness of the system relates to its extreme inhomogeneity. In most of the body systems all the basic elements (e.g., heart muscle cells, hepatocytes, lung alveoli) are similar and the functional reserve of the organ is essentially homogenous. A toxic chemical cuts down a certain fraction of the reserve and the clinical significance of such damage is a function of the size of the reserve. Thus damage to say 10% of hepatocytes will not be apparent clinically because there is a large reserve, but may be critical if this reserve is greatly reduced e.g.in cirrhosis. This simple relationship does not hold for the immune system. The various subsets of effector and regulatory cells of the immune system exhibit different sensitivities to toxic effects and as a result the activity of the immune system may be modified both quantitatively and qualitatively, namely, not only the intensity of the response will be changed (diminished or increased), but there may also be a change in the direction of the response and the relationships among the different components of it. By the same token, age and nutritionally dependent changes in the immune system may predispose to a quite different profile of chemically induced modifications in the immune response.

The main changes in the immune system in the 3 conditions discussed here (Table 3) are confined mostly to T cells and are minimal for B cells or macrophages. Thymus atrophy is the main source of the changes occurring in the elderly and the malnourished, whereas in the neonate it is related to programmed immaturity and overriding suppressor activity. On the other hand, T cells are also the most susceptible to exogenous, xenobiotic effects (Dean et al., 1982). Moreover, the different T cell subsets may exhibit selective sensitivity to different chemical agents (Faith et al., 1978). As T cells contribute to central regulatory functions (Cantor and Gershon, 1980) and are responsible for several key effector functions in the whole immune response profile, it is clear that damage to one of their components can be of considerable significance. The selectivity of the effects of xenobiotics is related not only to structural differences among them. A remarkable degree of differential effect on different lymphoid cell subsets can be achieved by modifying the concentration and/or duration of exposure to a given chemical. This brings us to another complicating feature of the immune system - the type of dose-effect relationships that occur. In general, dose-effect relationships are not necessarily linear, but using various transformations most of them can be expressed as such (Finney, 1952). This is not the case for effects exerted on the imune system; they are usually in the form of a bell-shaped curve (Shoham and Eshel, 1980; Shoham et al., 1980; Klein and Shoham, 1981; Shoham, 1984a,b), i.e., when a peak of effect is achieved, higher doses may be without effect or even have the opposite effect. This holds true for both immunotherapeutic and immunotoxic agents (Toyama and Kolmer, 1918; Gainer, 1972; Koller et al., 1976; Spreafico et al., 1981; Dean et al., 1982; Shoham, 1984a,b).

In conclusion, composite sets of changes occur in the three conditions discussed here - changes in pharmacokinetics which may modify (genrally increase) the local concentration of the chemical, on the one hand, and changes in components of the immune system which may modify its response quantitatively and qualitatively, as compared to a population of young healthy adults. The final vector of the effect cannot be predicted on general, theoretical grounds and must be tested directly. Moreover, we have discussed the three age and nutrition modified conditions collectively. It should be remembered, however, that these conditions are entirely different from each other, in spite of the apparent similarities among them. Accordingly, inference from one situation to the other may be completely misleading. These conditions were brought together here in order to emphasize certain common problems which are unique to the immune system and to the attempts at its manipulation and to its exposure to toxic chemicals.

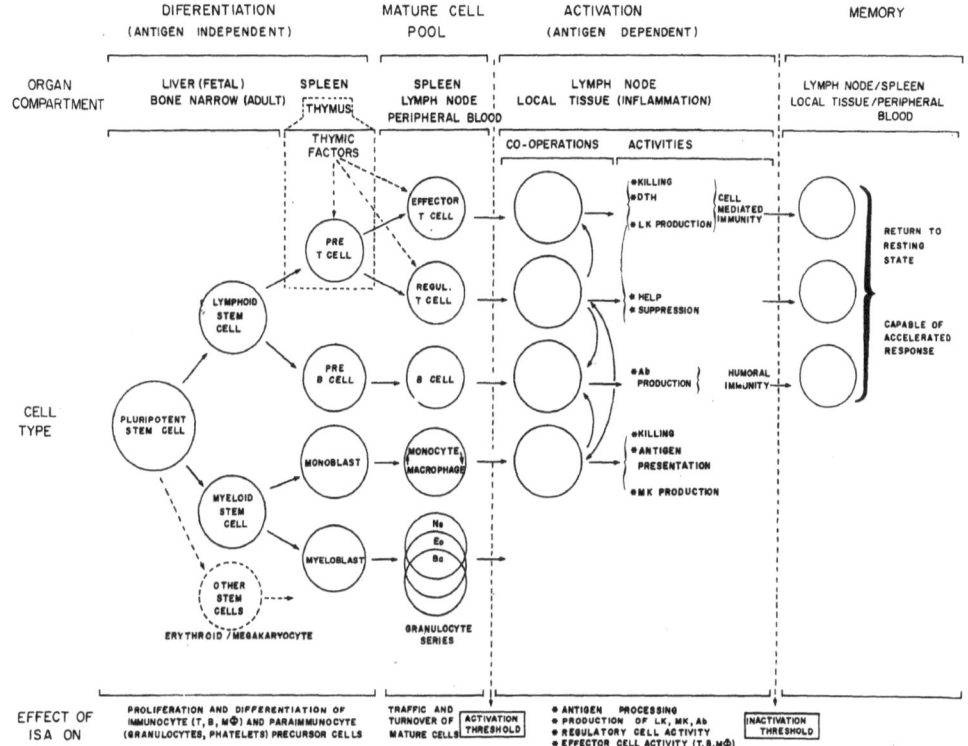

Figure 1. Main differentiation and activity features of the immune system and
their relationships with presumed sites of immunopharmacological and immunotoxicological effects of Immuno-Stimulating or Immuno-Suppressive Agents
(ISAs). A simplified schematic diagram.

Abbreviations: LK, Lmphokines; Ab, antibody; MK, monokines; DTH, delayed type
hypersensitivity; T,b, respective subpopulations of lymphocytes; MФ,
macrophages; Ne, neutrophil; Eo, eosinophil; Ba, basophil (of the granulocyte series).

Table 1. Classification of agents acting on the immune system

Category	Examples
I. Therapeutic agents with primarily immunostimulating effect	
A. Chemical (synthetic) agents	Levamisole, tilorone, polynucleotides, isoprinosine, azimexon
B. Microbial and plant products	Mycobacteria (BCG and derivatives) Corynbacteria, lipopolysaccharides, polysaccharides (Glucans, mannans) Bestatin, Cyclomunine, Krestin
C. Physiologically relevant substances	Lymphokines, thymic factors, tuftsin, Interferons, transfer factor
II. Therapeutic agents with primarily immunosuppressive effect	
A. Chemical (synthetic) agents	Alkylating agents, thiopurines
B. Microbial products (antibiotics)	Cyclosporin A, Adriamycin
C. Physiologically relevant substances	Steroids, diethylstilbsterol
III. Toxic agents with primarily immunostimulating effect	
A. Chemicals	Phrobol esters, vinyl chloride, propyleneglycol, α-thioglycerol, hexachlorobenzene
B. Microbial products	T-2 toxin (Fusarium)
IV. Toxic agents with primarily immunosuppressive effect	
A. Chemicals:	
1. Halogenated aromatic hydrocarbons	Polyhalogenated (Cl,Br) benzenes, phenols, biphenyls
2. Polycyclic aromatic hydrocarbons (carinogens)	3-methylcholanthrene, benz(a)pyrene
3. Pesticides	DDT, organophosphors (parathion, metathion, etc.)
4. Metals and salts	Lead, cadmium, mercury, arsenicals, zinc, organotins
B. Microbial and plant products	Ricin, aflatoxins, abrin, ochratoxins, fusarenon

Table 2. Comparison of age and nutrition dependent changes in chemobiokinetics (pharmacokinetics) of drugs and chemicals

	Neonatal (0-4 wks)	Aged (>70 y)	Malnourished (severe PCM)
Absorption (oral route)	=,↓	↓	↓
Distribution (apparent Vd)	↑	↓	↑
Binding (albumin concentration)	↓	↓	↓
Biotransformation (oxidative enzymes)	↓	↓	↓
Elimination (via kidneys)	↓	↓	↓

See text for more details

↓ , decrease; ↑ , increase; = No change. All compared to young healthy

adults.

Table 3. Comparison of age and nutrition dependent changes in the immune system

Organ or cell	Criterion of evaluation	Neonatal (0-4 wks)	Aged (>70 y)	Malnourished (severe PCM)
Thymus	Weight/body weight	↑	↓	↓↓
	Thymocytes	↑	↓	↓↓
	Thymic hormones	↑	↓	↓
Lymph nodes	Germinal centers	≈	≈	≈
	Thymus dependent areas	↓≈	↓	↓↓
Peripheral blood				
T cells	Number	↓≈	≈	↓
	Function: DTH response	↓	↓	↓
	PR	↓	↓	↓
	Cytotoxicity	↓	↓	↓
B cells	Number	≈	≈	≈
	Function: PFC	≈	≈	≈
Null cells	Number	↑	↑	↑
	Responsiveness to thymic hormones	↑	↑	↑
Monocytes	Number	≈	≈	≈
	Function: Phagocytosis	≈	≈	≈

Abbreviations: DTH, delayed type hypersensitivity; PR, proliferative response; PFC, plaque forming cells

↑ , increase; ↓ , decrease; ↓↓ , severe decrease; ≈ , about the same. All compared to young healthy adults.

405

VI. REFERENCES

ALLEYNE, G.A.O. (1966). Cardiac function in severely malnourished Jamaican children. Clin. Sci. 30. 553-562.

BACH, J.F. (1982). Immunopotentiation. In Clinical Aspects
of Immunology, (eds. Lachmann, P.J. and Peters, D.K.)
pp. 565-578. Blackwell Scientific Public., Oxford.

BEACH, R.S., GERSHWIN, M.E. & HURLEY, L.S. (1982). Gesta-
tional zinc deprivation in mice. Persistence of immunodeficiency for three generations. Science 218. 469-471.

BENDER, A.D. (1964). Pharmacologic aspects of aging. A
survey of the effect of increasing age on drug activity
in adults. J. Am. Geriatr. Soc., 12: 114-139.

BOSS, G.R., THOMPSON, R.F., SPEIGELBERG, H.L., PICHLER, W.J.
& SEEGMILLER, E. (1980). Age dependency of lymphocyte
ecto-5'-nucleotidase activity. J. Immunol., 125:
679-682.

BUCHANAN, N., HANSEN, J.D.L., VAN DER WALT, L.A., ROBINSON, R.
& KOORNHOF, H.J. (1976). Chloramphenicol metabolism in
children with PCM. Am. J. Clin. Nutr., 29: 327-328.

CAMPBELL, T.C. (1977). Nutrition and drug metabolising
enzymes. Clin. Pharmacol. Ther., 22: 699-706.

CANTOR, H. & GERSHON, R.K. (1980). T-cell sets: the role
of their genetic programme in immunoregulation. In The
Immune System: Functions and Therapy of Dysfunction
(eds. Doria, G. & Eshkol, A.) pp. 13-26. Academic
Press, London.

CHANDRA, R.K. (1974). Rosette forming T-lymphocytes and cell
mediated immunity in malnutrition. Br. Med. J., 3:
608-609.

CHANDRA, R.K. (1979a). T and B lymphocyte subpopulations and
leukocyte terminal deoxynucleotidyl transferase in
malnutritiion. Acta Paediat. Scan., 68: 841-845.

CHANDRA, R.K. (1979b). Serum thymic activity in protein
energy malnutrition. Clin. Exp. Immunol., 38:
228-230.

CHANDRA, R.K. (1980). Cell mediated immunity in nutritional
imbalance. Fed. Proc, 39: 3088-3092.

COHEN, S. & HANSEN, J.D.L. (1962). Metabolism of albumin
and -globulin in kwashiorkor. Clin. Sci., 23: 351-359.

COOPER, M.O., BURROWS, P.D. & LAWTON, A.R. (1980). Generation of B cell diversity. In The Immune System: Functions and Therapy of Dysfunction (eds. Doria, G. &
Eshkol, A.) pp. 1-12. Academic Press, London.

406

DEAN,J.H., LUSTER, M.I. & BOORMAN, G.A. (1982). Immunotoxicology. In Immunopharmacology (eds. Sirois, P. and Rola-Pleszczynski, M.) pp. 349-397. Elsevier Biomedical Press, North Holland.

DECKER, J.M. & SERCARZ, E.E. (1974). Early simultaneous appearance of antigen binding cells in fetal sheep. Nature 252: 416-418.

DIXON, F.J. & WEIGLE, W.O. (1957). The nature of the immunologic inadequacy of neonatal rabbits by cell transfer studies. J. Exp.Med.,105: 75-83.

DIXON, F.J. & WEIGLE, W.O. (1959). The nature of the immunologic inadequacy of neonatal rabbits. II. Antibody formation by neonatal spleen cells transferred to adult recipients. J. Exp. Med., 110: 139-146.

FAITH, R.E., LUSTER, M.I. & MOORE, J.A. (1978). Chemical separation of helper cell function and delayed hypersensitivity responses. Cell. Immunol., 40: 275-284.

FINNEY, D.G. (1952). Statistical Methods in Biological Assays. pp. 661. Charles Griffin Ltd., London.

FRIIS-HANSEN, B. (1961). Body water compartments in children: changes during growth and related changes in body composition. Pediatrics 28: 169-181.

GAINER, J.H. (1972). Effects of arsenicals on interferon formation Band action. Am. J. Vet. Res., 33: 2579-2583.

GEOKAS, M.C. & HAVERBACK, B.J. (1969). The aging gastrointestinal tract. Am. J. Surg., 117: 881-892.

HADDEN, J.W., DELMONTE, L. & OETTGEN, H.F. (1977). Mechanisms of immunopotentiation. In Immunopharmacology (eds. Hadden, J.W. Coffey, R.G. and Spreafico, F.) pp. 279-314. Plenum Publishing Corp., New York.

HANSEN, J.M., KAMPMANN, J. & LAURSEN, H. (1970). Renal excretion of drugs in the elderly. Lancet i: 1170.

HEFTON, J.M., DARLINGTON, G.J., CASAZZA, B.A. & WEKSLER, M.E. (1980). Immunologic studies of aging. V. Impaired proliferation of PHA responsive human lymphocytes in culture. J. Immunol., 125: 1007-1010.

HOWE, M.L. & MANZIELLO, B. (1972). Ontogenesis of the in vitro response of murine lymphoid cells to cellular antigens and phytomitogens. J. Immunol., 109: 534-539.

JUSKO, W.J. (1972). Pharmacokinetic principles in pediatric pharmacology. Pediatric Clinics N.Am., 19: 81-100.

KATOM R., TAKANAKA, A. & ONODA, K.I. (1970). Studies on age differences in mice for the activity of drug metabolising enzymes of liver microsomes.Japan J. Pharmacol., 20: 572-576.

KENDALL, M.D. (1981). Age and seasonal changes in the thymus. In The Thymus Gland (ed. Kendal, M.D.) pp. 21-36. Academic Press, London.

KENNES, B., HUBERT, C. & NEVE, P. (1981). Early biochemical events associated with lymphocyte activation in aging. I. Evidence that Ca_{2+} dependent processes induced by PHA are impaired. Immunology 42: 119-126.

KLEIN, A.S. & SHOHAM, J. (1981). The effect of the thymic extract TP-1 (thymostimulin) on the survival rate of tumor bearing mice. Cancer Res., 41: 3217-3221. KLINMAN, N.R. & PRESS, J.L. (1978). The characterization of the

B-cell repertoire specific for 2,4-dinitrophenyl and 2,4,6-trinitrophenyl determinants in neonatal Balb/c mice. J.Exp.Med., 141: 1133-1146.

KOLLER, L.D. (1980). Immunotoxicology of heavy metals. Int. J. Immunopharmac., 2: 269-279.

KOLLER, L.D., EXON, J.H. & ROAN, J.G. (1976). Humoral antibody response in mice after single dose exposure to lead or cadmium. Proc. Soc. Exp. Biol. Med., 151: 339-342.

KRISHNASWAMY, K. (1978). Drug metabolism and pharmacokinetics in malnutrition. Clin. Pharmacokinetics, 3: 216-229.

KURZ, H., MICHELS, H. & STICKEL, H.H. (1977). Differences in the binding of drugs to plasma proteins from newborn and adult man. Eur. J. Clin. Pharmacol. 11: 469-478.

LEONARD, P.J. & McWILLIAM, K.M. (1965). The binding of aldosterone in the serum of kwashiorkor. Am. J. Clin. Nutr., 16: 360-363.

LEVY, G., KHANNA, N.N., SODA, D.M., TSUZUKI, O. & STERN, L. (1975). Pharmacokinetics of acetaminophen in the human neonate. Pediatrics 55: 818-825.

MAKINODAN, T. & YUNIS, E. (1977). Immunology and Aging. Plenum Publishing Corp., New York.

McLEAN, A.E.M. (1971). Conversion by the liver of inactive molecules into toxic molecules. In Mechanism of Toxicity (ed. Aldridge, W.N.) pp. 219-228. MacMillan, London.

MOODY, C.E. INNES, J.B., STAIANO-COIOCO, INCEFY, G.S. THALER, H.T. & WEKSLER, M.E. (1981). Lymphocyte transformation induced by autologous cells. XI. The effect of age on the autologous mixed lymphocyte reaction. Immunology 44: 431-438.

MORSELLI, P.L. (1976). Clinical pharmacokinetics in neonates. Clinical Pharmacokinetics 1: 81-95.

NEWMANN, C.G., LAWLER, G.J., STIEHM, E.R., SWENDSEID, M.E. NEWTON, C., HERBERT, J., AMMANN, A.J. & JACOB, M. (1975) Immunologic responses in malnourished children. Am. J. Clin. Nutr., 28: 89-104.

NIEDERHUBER, J.E., ALLEN, P. & MAYO, L. (1979). The expression of Ia antigenic determinants on macrophages required for the in vitro antibody. J. Immunol., 122: 1342-1349.

PITLICK, W., PAINTER, M. & PIPPENGER, C. (1978). Phenobarbital pharmacokinetics in neonates. Clin. Pharmacol. Therap., 23: 346-350.

PLAYFAIR, J.H.L. (1978). Strain differences in the immune response of mice. I.The neonatal response to sheep red blood cells. Immunology 15: 35-50.

PRASAD, A.S. (1983). Clinical, biochemical and nutritional spectrum of zinc deficiency in human subjects: an update. Nutrition Rev., 41: 197-208.

PRESS, J.L. & KLINMAN, N.R. (1973). Enumeration and analysis of antibody forming precursors in the neonatal mouse. J. Immunol., 111: 829-835.

PTAK, W., NAIDORF, K.F., STRZYZEWSKA, J. & GERSHON, R.K. (1979). Ontogeny of cells involved in the suppressor circuit of the immune response. Eur. J. Immunol., 9: 495-500.

RADL, J., DEGLOPPER, E., VANDENBERG, P. & JANZWIETEN, M.J. (1980). Idiopathic paraproteinemia. III. Increased frequency of rare proteinemia in thymectomized aging C57Bl/KalwRij and CBA/BrARij mice. J. Immunol., 125: 31-35.

RANE, A. & SJOQVIST, F. (1972). Drug metabolism in the human fetus and newborn infant. Pediatr. Clin. N.Am., 19: 37-50.

REES, A.J. & LOCKWOOD, C.M. (1982). Immunosuppressive drugs in clinical practice. In Clinical Aspects of Immunology (eds. Lachmann, P.J. and Peters, D.K.) pp. 5o7-564. Blackwell Scientific Public., Oxford.

ROWE, J.W., ANDRES, R. & TOBIN, J.D. (1976). The effect of age on creatinine clearance in man: a cross-sectional and longitudinal study. J. Gerontol., 31: 155-163.

SHOHAM, J. (1984a). Specific safety problems of inappropriate immune responses to immunostimulating agents. Trends Pharmacol. Sci. (in press).

SHOHAM, J. (1984b). Clinical assessment of the safety of immunostimulating drugs - past experience and guidelines for the future. In Present Problems and Future Trends in Drug Toxicology (ed. Zbinden, G.) (in press).

SHOHAM, J. & ESHEL, I. (1980). Thymic hormonal effect on human peripheral blood lymphocytes. III. Conditions for mixed lymphocyte tumor culture assay. J. Immunol. Methods 37: 261-273.

SHOHAM, J., COHEN, M., CHANDALI, Y. & AVNI, A. (1980). Thymic hormonal effect on human peripheral blood lymphocytes. I. Reciprocal effect on T and B lymphocytes. Immunology 41: 353-359.

SMYTHE, P.M., SCHONLAND, M., BRERETON-STILES, G.C. (1971). Thymolymphatic deficiency and depression of cell mediated immunity in protein-caloric malnutrition. Lancet 2 : 939-940.

SPEAR, P.G., WANG, A.-L., RUTISHAUSER, U. & EDELMAN, G.M. (1973). Characterization of splenic lymphoid cells in fetal and newborn mice. J. Exp. Med., 138: 557-573.

SPREAFICO, F. & ANACLERIO, A. (1977). Immunosuppressive agents. In Immunopharmacology (eds. Hadden, J.W., Coffey, R.G. and Spreafico, F.) pp. 245-278. Plenum Publishing Corp., New York.

SPREAFICO, F. & VECCHI, A. (1984). Immunomodulation by xenobiotics: The open field of immunotoxicology. In Immunomodulation: New Frontiers and Advances. (eds. Fudenberg, H.H., Whitten, H.D. and Ambrogi, F.) pp. 311-330. Plenum Publishing Corp., New York.

SPREAFICO, F., VECCHI, A., CONTI, G. & SIRONI, M. (1981). On the heterogeneity of immunotherapeutic agents. In Advances in Immunopharmacology (ed. Hadden, J.W.) pp. 51-63. Pergamon Press, Oxford.

THOMAN, M.L. & WEIGLE, W.O. (1982). Cell mediated immunity in aged mice: an underlying lesion in IL2 synthesis. J. Immunol., 128: 2358-2361.

TOYAMA, I. & KOLMER, J.A. (1918). The influence of arsphenamine and mercuric chloride on complement and antibody production. J. Immunol., 3: 301-312.

VESTAL, R.E. (1978). Drug use in the elderly: A review of problems and special considerations. Pract. Ther., 16: 358-382.

VINK, C.L.J. (1959). Liver function and age. Clin. Chim. Actas 4: 674-682.

410

VOS, J.G. (1979). *Immune suppression as related to toxicology.* CRC Crit. Rev. Toxicol., 5: *67-101.*

WALFORD, R.L. & BERGMANN, K. (1979). *Influence of genes associated with the main histocompatibility complex on deoxyribonucleic acid excision repair capacity and bleomycin sensitivity in mouse lymphocytes.* Tissue Antigens 14: *336-342.*

WALLACE,, S., WHITING, B. & RUNCIE, J. (1976). *Factors affecting drug binding in plasma of elderly patient.* Br. J. Clin. Pharmacol., 3: *327-330.*

WATTS, T. (1969). *Thymus weights in malnourished children.* J. Trop.Pediatr., 15: *155-158. WHO Report (1978). ""Principles and Methods for Evaluating the Toxicity of Chemicals, Part I".* Environmental Health Criteria 6. *p.116. World Health Organization, Geneva.*

WOODRUFF, J.F. (1970). *The influence of quantitated post-weaning undernutrition on Coxsackie-virus B3 infection of adult mice. II. Alteration oh host defense mechanisms.* J. Infec. Dis., 121: *164 181.*

BASIC MECHANISMS OF HYPERSENSITIVITY : AN UPDATE

G.L. Asherson.

Division of Immunological Medicine,
Clinical Research Centre,
Harrow, U.K.

INTRODUCTION

In discussing immunology with an audience interested in immuno-toxicology it may be useful to focus on a specific problem such as contact dermatitis while recognizing that factors similar in principle but differing in detail will apply to other immunological diseases such as asthma. Because this is not a formal review many of the references are based on work with which I am closely familiar from which further references to the literature may be found. To begin with it may help to consider a particular manifestation and then to see how our experimental knowledge of contact sensitivity bears on this.

Nickel dermatitis is a common disease and is acquired by contact with nickel mainly through costume jewellry and earrings (sleepers) which contain nickel. Nickel has the chemical reactivity which is a common feature of contact sensitizers. It dissolves under slightly acid conditions in sweat and its salts have a high affinity for a number of proteins including albumin (Dolovich et al, 1984) which has a metal binding site and for C3b, B in which bivalent nickel can replace magnesium and actually generates an unusually stable C3 convertase (Fishelson et al, 1983). This interaction with protein is due to the ability of nickel to form coordination compounds with the amino groups of lysine and the N terminal amino acids and the imino group of histidine.

It is not clear why the immune system regards nickel as a good contact sensitizer. However the ability of nickel suphate to cause blast transformation in unimmunized animals and newborn humans (Al Tawil et at, 1981; Nordlind, 1983) raises the question whether it has a direct effect on macrophages and other antigen presenting cells and causes them to release IL-1 (see below).

Nickel dermatitis poses several problems

a) If nickel were a new agent, could its ability to sensitize be predicted and would there be a serious alternative to testing in man?

b) Is the incidence of nickel dermatitis a direct reflection of the level of exposure or are there individual factors which explain why under similar environmental conditions some individuals have no lesions, other minors lesions around the point of exposure while yet others have intermittent or chronic eczema of the hands (Hansen et al, 1982)?

c) What is the mechanism of the skin lesion ?

MECHANISM OF THE CONTACT SENSITIVITY REACTION

The classical view is that following exposure to antigen, proliferation occurs in the regional lymph nodes and gives rise to effector cells. These effector cells leave the lymph node and circulate in the blood and move to the skin test site as the result of the minor degree of inflammation caused by challenge. There is argument whether there is any antigen specificity in this arrival, i.e. whether cells clonally committed to the antigen show greater arrival than other cells. The lymphocytes then interact with antigen, probably on the surface of antigen presenting cells which provide class II major histocompatibility products (MHC) which are otherwise known as transplantation antigens. The lymphocytes then release various lymphokines which cause the local inflammation and in particular lead to the futher influx of cells and to fibrin deposition in the more severe lesions.

Recently it has been realized that basophils enter some lesions in the guinea pig and man. It is thought that a subset of lymphocytes and in some situations circulating antibody is responsible, see Mitchell and Askenase, (1982). However in general antibody only plays a subsidiary role in augmenting certain delayed hypersensitisity (but not apparently contact sensitivity) skin reactions, while the essential reaction is transferred by T lymphocytes (Asherson, 1967).

Askenase and his coworkers have described a futher mechanism which probably serves to amplify the contact sensitivity reaction (Askenase et al, 1983; Askenase and Loveren, 1983). Mice with established contact sensitivity have T lymphocytes which liberate an antigen specific T cell factor. This factor is reminiscent of IgE in that it arms mast cells. These then release mediators, of which serotonin may be the main one, which increase the permeability of the local capillaries to protein and to cells. The increased permeability then facilitates the passage of the classical effector T cells which liberate lymphokines and are responsible for the bulk of the reaction. It is not yet critically clear whether these two functions are due to different sets of T lympphocytes.

CONTROL OF THE SIZE AND DURATION OF THE CONTACT SENSITIVITY REACTION

Generalities

Some of the main factors which influence contact sensitivity are listed in table 1. It is outside the scope of this article to discuss physiological and pharmacological factors such as skin permeability and the dermal equivalent of the bronchial hyperreactivity seen is asthma, although these are clearly important and skin permeability in particular will influence the dose of antigen received by an individual. This increase in permeability may explain in part the greater ease with which contact dermatitis is induced when agents are applied to damaged skin and the adverse effect of irritants and detergents. However it is possible that immuno-toxicological factors such as the ability of certain irritants to activate macrophages and other antigen presentings cells may be involved.

TABLE 1

Factors which may influence the contact sensitivity reaction

Permeability of skin which affects dose.

Production of IL-1 by antigen presenting cells.

Production of IL-2 (T cell growth factor) .

Helper cell circuits.

Suppressor cell circuits.

Contra- suppressor cell circuits.

Genetic factors

The antigen presenting cell

Classically the macrophage was regarded as the only antigen presenting cell. It is now realized the several different cells have this property, including the Langerhans cell in the skin, and its equivalent in the afferent lymph (veiled cell) and lymph node (dendritic cell). It is possible that the epithelial cell (the keratinocyte) can present antigen when the skin is inflammed as under these condition the keratino-cytes acquire class II major histocompatibility complex products (which in humans are called HLA-D and in mouse I-A) and are able produce an IL-1 like factor called epidermal thymus activating factor (ETAF).

TABLE 2

Antigen presentation

Partial proteolsis by enzymes.

Association of antigen with MHC. Production of IL-1

One of the key questions is : what activates the macrophage to present antigen or more colloquially: how does the macro-phage know when to present antigen? (See Raff, 1982) Enzyma-tic digestion (processing or fragmentation) is required for most antigens probably to allow incorporation into the mem-brane and association with class II MHC products. There is also a requirement for IL-1 production. Chemically reactive contact sensitizing agents may bypass this requirement for processing by combining directly with membrane components. However processing may be important when the immune response is directed against a derivatized skin protein and not against a derivatized antigen presenting cell.

The two other factors in antigen presentation are the presence of class II major histocompatibility complex products on the surface of the antigen presenting cell and the production of IL-1. Some of the cues for the appearance of class II MHC products and the production of IL-1 are shown in Table 3.

TABLE 3

Factors which influence the activation of the antigen presenting cell

Bacterial endotoxin (lipopolysaccharide).

Bacterial cell wall (muramyl dipeptide).

Gamma interferon.

Activited C5 and hence immune complexes and polysaccharides which activate the alternate complement pathway ?

antigen specific T helper factor ?

chemically reactive haptenes

It will be seen that bacteria can activate antigen presenting cells directly by their cell walls and endotoxin, and indirectly by activating the complement system. Viruses can cause activation through gamma interferon, although it is puzzling that this is an immune interferon produced by lymphocytes and not the alpha or beta interferon which arises directly as a result of viral infection of cells. It is less clear how other antigens activate the antigen presenting cell. One possibility is that there are naturally occurring antibodies or antigen specific T cell products which are cytophilic for the antigen presenting cell and provide it which a receptor for binding and recognizing antigen which then leads to activation. In the case of the antigen specific T helper factor which bears class II MHC determinants it is possible that the factor itself provides some of the I-A needed for the lymphocytes to respond to antigen. (See Colizzi et al., 1984). Another possibility is that the contact sensitizing agents, by virtue of their chemical reactivity, modify the surface of cells and hence activate (or lead to the liberation of factors which activate) the antigen presenting cell. In this connection it is interesting that many immunological adjuvants are surface active compounds and this raises the question whether the clinical observation that the surfactant detergents and other irritants favour the development of contact sensitivity is due in part to activation of the antigen presenting cells.

The role of IL-1 and IL-2 in influencing the outcome of the immune response

The induction of the immune response is summarized in Fig. 1. The antigen presenting cell provides antigen and class II MHC product together with the nonspecific signal, interleukin-1, to a T lymphocyte. This causes the T lymphocyte to produce interleukin-2 (IL-2) which was formerly called T cell growth factor. At the same time the antigen presenting cell provides antigen and class II MHC product to a second T cell which acquires a receptor for IL-2. This cell then proliferates in the presence of IL-2. Futher downstream there are nonspecific differentiation factors (at least in the cytotoxic system) required to convert the proliferating cell into the final effector cell. This diagram suggests that IL-1 and hence IL-2 play a critical role in determining whether a conventional immune response occure.

Three lines of experimental evidence suggest that IL-2 may play a role in determining the balance between immunity and tolerance. The first series of experiments studied the neonatal induction of tolerance by the injection of semiallogeneic cells which is a classical system based on the early work of Medawar.It was found that the injection of supernatants containing IL-2 one day after the injection of the tolerogenic stimulus prevented the induction of tolerance as judged by skin graft rejection. This is an example of IL-2 converting a tolerogenic stimulus into a neutral stimulus (Merkovsky et al, 1984), although the actual mechanism may be the stimulation of an early immune response which causes the rejection of the lymphoid cells used to induce tolerance. It is thought that the continued presence of the cells used to induce tolerance is required for the maintenance of tolerance.

In the second series of experiments the effects of IL-2 on the induction of unresponsivenss to contact sensitizer was assessed. Normally the intravenous injection of picrylated cells lead to unresponsivenss and it is easy to demonstrate suppressor cells (Colizzi et al,1983). In particular the mice do not develop contact sensitivity when formally immunized by painting the skin with picryl chloride. However mice develop contact sensitivity, when recombinant IL-2 is given 24 hours after the injection of the picrylated cels (Colizzi et al, 1984). In this situation IL-2 converts a net tolerogenic stimulus into a net immunogenic stimulus.

The third series of experiments explored the hypothesis that exposure of cells to antigen in the relative absence of IL-2 leads to clonal anergy or deletion in short term (8 day) experiments. Advantage was taken of the fact that the nonspecific inhibitor produced by a suppressor T cell circuit (see below) suppresses IL-2 production. A mixed lymphocyte reaction was undertaken in the presence of the inhibitor and the lymphocytes then reexposed at 4 days to the same mouse alloantigen as they met in the primary. It was found that they failed to respond on the second occasion to an antigen which they had first met in the presence of the inhibitor.

This short term anergy did not occur when IL-2 was added to the primary culture. As no suppressor cells could be demonstrated it was assumed that short term clonal anergy had occured. The key question is whether transient exposure to antigen in the relative absence of IL-2 can lead to long term clonal deletion and immunological unresponsiveness.

Suppressor T cell circuits

The size of an immune response is also influenced by the existence of suppressor cell circuits. These have been extensively studied in the picryl contact sensitivity system and several reviews are available (Dorf and Benacerraf, 1984; Green et al, 1984; Claman et al, 1980; Asherson et al, 1980; Task and Okui 1978; Tada and Okurmura, 1979 and Asherson et al, 1985). The foEowing generalizations may be made.

1. T and B suppressor cell circuits arise under routine conditions for producing contact sensitivy. For this reason they should be seen as a normal concomitant of the immune response and not as an anusual feature which only occurs after special modes of immunization (Zembala et al, 1982).

2. In the case of the T suppressor cell, commonly called T suppressor efferent (Ts-eff or Ts_3) the induction signal for the cell is the presentation of antigen together with a MHC-related product called I-J. The implication is that the availability of I-J on the surface of antigen presenting cells is one of the determinants of the activation of suppressor cell circuits and hence of the size and duration of the contact hypersensitivity response.

3. The T suppressor efferent circuit has two distinct T cells the Ts-eff which is equivalent to the Ts_3 of Dorf (Asherson et al, 1984) and the T acceptor cell otherwise called the T suppressor auxiliary cell (Sy et al, 1979). The circuit is illustrated in Fig.

4. Exposure of the mouse to haptenated cells bearing I-J induces the Ts-eff by a process of immunization (Colizzi et al, 1983). This cell then produces antigen specific T suppressor factor. This factor by itself does not supress the cell that mediates contact sensitivity directly. Instead it arms the nonspecific T acceptor cell, i.e. a cell which lacks relevant immunological specificity but acquires it passively when armed with an antigen specific factor, The IgE mast cell system provides a simple analogy. In this system the antigen specific IgE antibody arms the mast cell. This then releases the final mediator nonspecific inhibitior when exposed to antigen. In fact this triggering event requires both antigen and the MHC-related product I-J, and is an example of associative recognition.

5. The nonspecific inhibitor(s) has two properties. On the one hand it blocks the passive transfer of contact sensitivity (Zembala et al, 1982). On the other hand it limits cell proliferation by blocking IL-2 production (Malkovsky et al, 1983). It is this nonspecific inhibitor which was used in the experiment on clonal anergy in vitro.

6. In describing T suppressor cell circuits it is important to recognize the different linkages which occur between the cells. Five types of linkages are listed below.

Type I The Link of immunization. This linkage occurs when an antigen presenting cell with an appropriate MHC-related product such as I-J gives rise to a suppressor cell by a process of immunization. A good example is the generation of Ts_3 by immunization with picrylated I-J$^+$ cells. Similarly, an I-J$^+$ antigen-specific product, TsF$_1$, from an I-J$^+$ antigen-directed Ts$_1$ cell generates an anti-idiotypic T suppressor cell (Ts$_2$) by a process of immunization (Okuda et al, 1981).

Type II The link of triggering. This linkage occurs when antigen, characteristically on an I-J$^+$ cell or an I-J$^+$ anti-idiotypic T suppressor factor, triggers a cell to release its product. One example is the triggering of the antigen-directed Ts of DCorf to release TsF$_3$ when triggered by the I-J$^+$ antiidiotypic TsF$_2$ (Minami et al, 1983). Another example is the triggering of the T acceptor cell armed with TsF by antigen on the surface of an I-J$^+$ cell (Zembala et al, 1982).

Type III The link of arming. This involves a cytophilic factor and a nonspecific acceptor cell which is armed by it. An acceptor cell is defined as a cell lacking relevant immunological specificity which acquires specificity when it binds an antigen specific factor. One example is the binding of antigen specific TsF to an acceptor cell such as the T acceptor cell or the macrophage which then releases a nonspecific inhibition when triggered with antigen on the surface of an I-J$^+$ cell (Zembala et al, 1982: Ptak et al, 1981).

Type IV The link of help. In effector responses the development of the effector cell may require IL-1 and IL-2 and nonspecific differentiation factors and may be facilitated by antigen specific factors. Similar phenomenon have been described affecting suppressor cells. For instance the ability of antigen specific T suppressor factor to augment the suppressor cell response to antigen should probably be interpreted as antigen specific help for the generation of T suppressor cells (Tsurufuji et al, 1983). As the factor is I-J$^+$ this may be a further example of the rule that the presentation of antigen together with I-J favours the induction of suppressor cells. Factors favouring the differentiation of suppressor cells have also been described (Rich et al, 1984).

Type V The link of complementation. An interesting link is provided by the finding that T suppressor factor may be produced as two separate chains both of which are required for activity. In this case the chains are described as complementing each other and this is one of the ways in which distinct cells may collaborate in causing suppression. For instance in the picryl system in addition to the high molecular weight disulphide bonded TsF presumably made by one cell, there is also low moleculare weight factor. This factor occurs as two separate chains. Both of these chains are needed for biological activity. Moreover these chains may be made by distinct cells with different Lyt phenotypes. This requirement for two cells for the arming of the nonspecific T acceptor cell may be termed complementation.

7. In addition to the present T suppressor circuit, there is a T suppressor cell which blocks the induction of contact sensitivity and of antigen specific T helper factor. It does not act through the Ts-efferent (Asherson et al, 1985; Thomas et al, 1981).

8. Finally there are B suppressor circuits some probably based on antibody to the antigen and others anti-idiotypic which influence contact sensitivity (Zembala et al, 1976; Sy et al, 1979 and Moorhead, 1982).

Contrasuppressor cells

Several workers have described cells which negate the effect of a suppressor circuit. There are several possible mechanisms. In some cases an anti-idiotypic B cell blocks the action and possibly the development of the Ts-eff described above (Asherson et al, 1981). This is an example of a sup-pressor of a suppressor cell. In other cases the contra-suppressor cell is thought to stimulate the target cell and render it refractory to the suppressive stimulus. This is the mechanism suggested by the data of Lehner (1983) and Ptak et al (1984). Finally suppression due to inhibition of IL-2 production may be overcome by cells which produce IL-2 and hence circumnavigate the block. This may explain some of the situations in which tolerance is broken by an allogeneic reaction (McCullagh, 1970).

Genetic factors

In mice there are clear strain difference in the response to antigen. These are usually due to Ir genes which are iden-tical to the genes determining class II MHC products. In some cases low responsiveness is due to the disproportionate production of supressor cells. In these case inactivation of suppressor cells by cyclophosphamide or other methods allows a response in low responder strains (Benacerraf and Germain, 1979). In other cases the Ir genes act directly and not via a suppressor cell system. Similar genetic effects due to suppressor cells may occur in man (Nishimura and Sasazuki, 1983).

CONCLUSIONS

The outcome of exposure to a contact sentitizing agent depends on several factors. Empirically it has been found that dosage is important both unduly high or low doses causing unrespo-niveness and there is a window of immunization in between (See Asherson et al, 1979). Lehner (1983) has raised the interes-ting question whether in humans this window is caused by the activity of contrasuppressor cells whose preferred antigen concentration for activation is related to class II MHC products (HLA-D). Dosage is affected by irritants and surfactants which damage the skin and facilitate absorption. These agents may possibly activitate the antigen presenting cell. We can also consider the role of antigen. We must also consider suppressor and contrasuppressor circuits and finally the role of genetic factors, some of which act through the suppressor cell circuit, but others of which may affect contrasuppressor circuits and antigen presentation. Against his background it is _a priori_ unlikely that testing in guinea pigs and mice will do more than detect the most potent contact sensitizers. One possible alternative is that the more potent contact sensitizers may have two properties, first they may induce antigen presenting cells to make IL-1 and second lymphocytes able to react with them may be well represented in the clonal repertoire. The ability to stimulate IL-1 production can be measured directly, while the presence of relatively large numbers of clonally committed cells might be detected by the ability to give a primary _in vitro_ blast transformation response. This is true for good contact sensitizers such as the dinitro and trinitrophenyl (picryl) compounds and metals such as nickel and mercury. Hence careful research may increase our ability to suspect potential contact sensitizers using a human _in vitro_ system. Nevertheless there is no current substitute for cautious testing of new agents in man.

420

*Diagram of the role of the antigen presenting cell, IL-1 and
IL-2 in the induction of the immune response.*

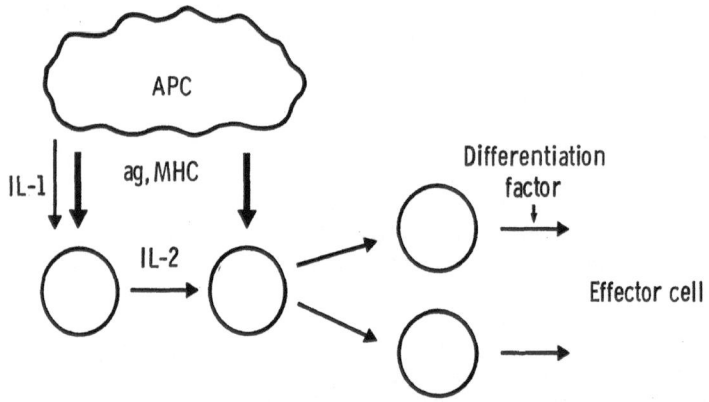

Figure 1. The figure shows an antigen presenting cell (APC). On the left, the heavy
errow shows the APC presenting antigen together with major histocompatibility complex
product (MHC) to a T lymphocyte. The light arrow shows that the APC secretes IL-1 (or
has IL-1 on its surface). As a result of this double stimulation the T lymphocyte
produces IL-2. The heavy right hand arrow shows the APC presenting antigen and MHC to
a second T lymphocyte. As a result the lymphocyte develops receptors for IL-2 and is
stimulated to divide by IL-2. However differentiation factors may be needed before
the final effector cell is generated.

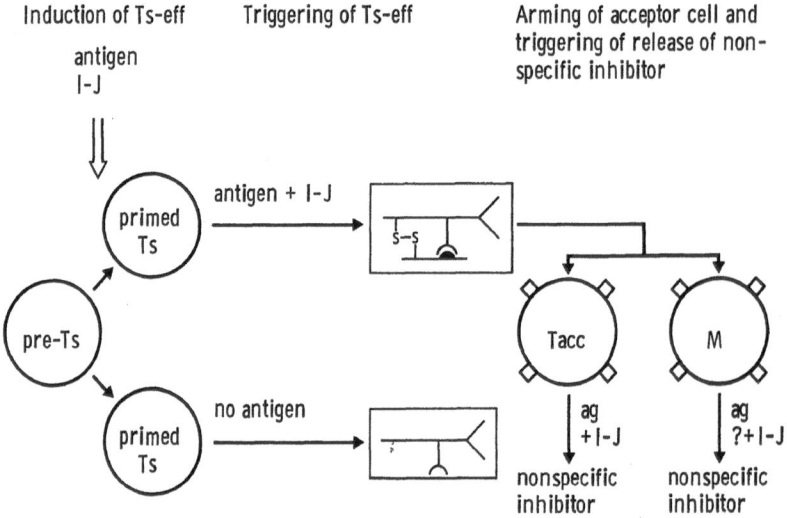

This circuit leads to the production of nonspecific inhibitor which blocks the passive
transfer of contact sensitivity and IL-2 production. It can be divided into three
stages: the induction of the Ts-eff, the triggering of the TS-eff to release T
suppressor factor and the arming of the acceptor cell and triggering of the release of
nonspecific inhibitor.

On the left, antigen on the surface of an I-J$^+$ cell induces the resting or pre-Ts to
become a primed Ts by a process of immunization   LINK 1 in text

REFERENCES

Al-Tawil, N.G., Marcusson, J.A. & Moller, E. 1981 *Lymphocyte transformation test in patients with nickel sensitivity: an aid to diagnosis.* Acta Dermatoven (Stock.) 61: 511-515.

Asherson, G.L. 1967 *The passive transfer of delayed hypersensitivity in the guinea pig. II. The ability of passively transferred antibody to cause local inflammation and retention of antigen and the role of these phenomena in the passive transfer of delayed hypersensitivity.* Immunology, 13: 441-451.

Asherson, G.L. & Zembala, M. 1974 *Suppression of contact sensitivity by T cells in the mouse. I. Demonstration that suppressor cells act at the effector stage of contact sensitivity and their induction following in vitro exposure to antigen.* Proc. R. Soc. Lond. B. 187: 329-348.

Asherson, G.L., Perera, M.A.C.C. & Thomas, W.R. 1979 *Contact sensitivity and the DNA response in mice to high and low doses of oxazolone: Low dose unresponsiveness following painting and feeding and its prevention by pretreatment with cyclophosphamide.* Immunology. 36: 449-459.

Asherson, G.L., Zembala, M., Thomas, W.R. & Perera, M.A.C.C. 1980 *Suppressor cells and the handling of antigen.* Immunol. Rev. 50: 3-45.

Asherson, G.L. Zembala, M., Gautam, S. & Watkins, M. 1982 *Control of suppressor cell activity: autoanti-idiotypic B cells produced by painting with picryl chlorid inhibit the T suppressor cells which block the efferent stage of contact sensitivity.* Cell. Immunol. 70: 160-169.

Asherson, G.L., Colizzi, V. & James, B.M.B. *The control of the contact sensitivity skin reaction: T suppressor afferent cell blocks the production of antigen specific T helper factor.* Immunology. In press.

Asherson, G.L., Dorf, M.E., Colizzi, V., Zembala, M. & James, B.M.B. 1984. *Equivalence of conventional anti-picryl T suppressor factor in the contact sensitivity system and monoclonal anti-NP TsF3 : their final nonspecific effect via the T acceptor cell.* Immunology. 53: 491-499.

Asherson, G.L., Watkins, M.C., Zembala, M.A. & Colizzi, V. 1984. *Two chain structure of T suppressor factor: antigen specific T suppressor factor occurs as a single molecule and as separate antigen binding and I-J+ chains both of which are required for biological activity.* Cell. Immunol. 86: 448-459.

Asherson, G.L., Zembala, M. & Colizzi, V. 1986. *The role of I-J determinants in suppressor cell circuits.* Ann. Rev. Immunol. 4: 37-68.

Askenase, P.W., Rosenstein, R.W. & Ptak, W. 1983. T cells produce an antigen binding factor with in vivo activity analogous to IgE antibody. J. Exp. Med. 157: 862-873.

Askenase, P.W. & Van Loveren, M. 1983. Delayed type hypersensitivity: activation of mast cells by antigen-specific T cell factors initiates the cascade of cellular interactions. Immunol. Today. 4: 259-264.

Braley-Mullen, H. 1983. Activation of type III pneumococcal polysaccharide-specific suppressor T cells in cyclophosphamide-treated mice: requirement for recognition of antigen and I-J determinants on antigen coupled to syngeneic spleen cells. J. Immunol. 131: 2190-2263.

Claman, H.N., Miller, S.D. Conlon, P.J. & Moorhead, J.W. 1980. Control of experimental contact sensitivity. Adv. Immunol. 30: 121-153.

Colizzi, V., Asherson, G.L. & James, B.M.B. 1983. The role of I-J in the suppressor T-cell circuit which influences the effector stage of the contact sensitivity reaction: antigen together with syngeneic I-J region determinants induces and activates T suppressor cells. Immunology. 49: 191-199.

Colizzi, V., Asherson, G.L., James, B.M.B. & Malkovsky, M. 1984. T helper factor in contact sensitivity: antigen-specific I-A+ helper factor is made by an Lyt-1+ 2- , I-A+ , I-J- T cell. Immunology. 52: 261-267.

Colizzi, V., Malkovsky, M., Lang, G. & Asherson, G.L. Conversion of a tolerogenic stimulus into an immunogenic stimulus by the administration of interleukin-2 in vivo. Submitted for publication.

Dolovich, J., Evans, S.L. & Niebor, E. 1984. Occupational asthma from nickel sensitivity: I. Human serum albumin in the antigenic determinant. Brit. J. Ind. Med. 41: 51-55.

Dorf, M.E. & Benacerraf, B. Suppressor cells and immunoregulation. Ann. Rev. Immunol. 2: 127-158.

Fishelson, Z., Pangburn, M.K. & Muller-Eberhard, H.J. 1983. C3 convertase of the alternative complement pathway. J. Biol. Chem. 258: 7411-7415.

Green, D.R., Flood, P.M. & Gershon, R.K. 1983. Immunoregulatory T-cell pathways. Ann. Rev. Immunol. 1: 439-464.

Hansen, H.E., Menne, T. & Larsen, S.O. 1982 HLA antigens in nickel sensitive females. Tissue Antigens. 19: 306-310.

Lehner, T. Antigen-binding human T suppressor cells and their association with the HLA-DR locus. Eur. J. Immunol. 13: 370-378.

Malkovsky, M., Asherson, G.L., Chandler, P., Colizzi, V., Watkins, M.C. & Zembala, M. 1983. Nonspecific inhibitor of DNA synthesis elaborated by T acceptor cells. I. Specific hapten- and I-J-driven liberation of an inhibitor of cell proliferation by Lyt-1+ 2- cyclophosphamide-sensitive T acceptor cell armed with a product of Lyt-1+ 2- specific suppressor cells. J. Immunol. 130: 785-796.

Malkovsky, M., Medawar, P., Hunt, R., Palmer, L. & Dore, C.1984 A diet enriched in vitamin A acetate or in vivo administration of interleukin-2 can counteract a tolerogenic stimulus. Proc. Roy. Soc. Lond. B. 220: 439-445.

Minami, M., Okuda, K., Furusawa, S. & Dorf, M.E. 1983. Analysis of T cell hybridomas. IV. Characterization of inducible suppressor cell hybridomas. J. Exp. Med. 157: 1379-1395.

Mitchell, E.B., Crow, J., Chapman, M.D., Jouhal, S.S., Pope, F.M. & Platts_mills, T.A.E. 1982 Basophils in allergen-induced patch test sites in atopic dermatitis. Lancet.i: 127-130.

Mitchell, E.B. & Askenase, P.W. 1982 . Suppression of T cell mediated cutaneous basophil hypersensitivity by serum from guinea pigs immunized with mycobaterial adjuvant. J. Exp. Med. 156: 159-172.

Moorhead, J.W. 1982. Antigen receptors on murine T lymphocytes in contact sensitivity. III. Mechanism of negative feedback regulation by auto-anti-idiotype antibody. J. Exp. Med. 155: 820-830.

Nishimura, Y. & Sasazuki, T. 1983 Suppressor T cells control the HLA-linked low responsiveness to streptococcal antigen in man. Nature. 302 : 67-69.

Nordlind, K. 1983. Stimulating effect of mercuric chloride and nickel sulfate on DNA synthesis of thymocytes and peripheral lymphoid cells from new born guinea pigs. Int. Arch. Allergy 72: 177-179.

Okuda, K., Minami,M., Sherr, D.M. & Dorf, M.E. 1981. Hapten-specific T cell responses to 4-hydroxy-3-nitrophenylacetayl. XI. Pseudogenetic restrictions of hybridoma suppressor factors. J. Exp. Med. 154: 468-479.

424

Ptak, W., Zembala, M., Asherson, G.L. & Marcinkiewicz,, J. 1981. Inhibition of contact sensitivity by macrophages: The separate phenomena of the production of nonspecific macrophage suppressor factor by macrophages armed with specific T suppressor factor, and the nonspecific inhibition of passive transfer by high density macrophages. Int. Arch. Allergy 65: 121-128.

Ptak, W., Bereta, M., Ptak, M., Gershon, R.K. & Green, D.R. 1984. Antigen-specific contrasuppressor factor in cell-mediated immunity: interactions leading to eradication of the tolerant state. J. Immunol. 133: 1124-1131.

Raff, M.C. 1982. Do antigen-presenting cells distinghuish self from non-self? Nature 298: 791-792.

Rich, G., Carpino, M.R. & Arhelger, C. 1979. Suppressor T cell growth and differentiation. Identification of a cofactor required for suppressor T cell function and distinct from interleukin-2. J. Exp. Med. 159: 1473-1490.

Sy, M.S., Miller, S.D., Moorhead, J.W. & Claman, H.N. 1979. Active suppression of 1-fluoro-2, 4-dinitrobenzene-immune T cells: requirement of an auxiliary T cell induced by antigen. J. Exp. Med. 149:1197-1207.

Sy, M.S., Moorhead, J.W. & Claman, H.N. 1979. Regulation of cell mediated immunity by antibodies: possible role of anti-receptor antibodies in the regulation of contact sensitivity to DNFB in mice. J. Immunol. 123: 2593-2598.

Tada, T. & Okumura, K. 1979. The role of antigen specific T cell factors in the immune response. Adv. Immunol. 28: 1-87.

Thomas, W.R., Watkins, M.C. & Asherson, G.L. 1981. Differences in the ability of T cells to suppress the induction and expression of contact sensitivity. Immunology, 42: 53-59.

Tsurufuji, M., Benacerraf, B. & Sy, M.S. 1983. An antigen-specific signal required for the activation of second-order suppressor T cells in the regulation of delayed hyperreactivity to 2,4,6-trinitrobenzenesulfonic acid. J. Exp. Med. 158: 932-935.

Zembala, M., Asherson, G.L., Noworolski, J. & Mayhew, B. 1976. Contact sensitivity to picryl chloride: the occurrence of B suppresssor cells in the lymph nodes and spleen of immunized mice. Cell. Immunol. 25: 266-278.

425

Zembala, M., Asherson, G.L., Colizzi, V. & Watkins, M.C. 1982. Desensitization in vitro: the role of T-suppressor cells, T-suppressor factor and T acceptor cells in the inhibition of the passive transfer of contact sensitivity to picryl chloride by exposure to antigen in vitro. Immunology. 47: 605-615.

Zembala, M., Asherson, G.L., James, B.M.B., Stein, V. & Watkins, M.C. 1982. Anti-hapten T suppressor factor acts through an I-J+ , Lyt-1- 2+ , T acceptor cell which releases a nonspecific inhibitor of the transfer of contact sensitivity when exposed to antigen. J. Immunol. 129: 1823-1829.

Zembala, M., Colizzi, V., Asherson, G.L. & Watkins, M.C. 1984. Nonspecific inhibitor made by T acceptor cells inhibits both the afferent and efferent stage of the contact sensitivity reaction. Immunology. 52: 599-606.

Zembala, M., Watkins, M., Colizzi, V. & Asherson, G.L. 1984. T suppressor factor activity is due to two separate molecules: Lyt-1- 2+, I-J+ cells of mice primed with antigen made by an antigen binding molecule which is only active when complemented by cofactor made by Lyt-1+ 2- , I-J+ cells. Cell. Immunol. 87: 240-251.

MECHANISMS OF PSEUDO-ALLERGY

D.R. Stanworth

Rheumatology and Allergy Research Unit,
Department of Immunology,
The University of Birmingham
The Medical School Birmingham
U.K.

1. INTRODUCTION

The application of modern immunological methodology to the field of allergy over the last 20 years has attributed a central role to reaginic (IgE) antibodies in the mediation of immediate-type hypersensitivity responses. Indeed, the involvement of this class of immunoglobulin has come to be regarded as an essential feature of allergies of the asthma-hay-fever-urticaria type. Although (see Stanworth, 1983A), there are some clinical allergy situations in which anaphylactic antibodies of the IgG4 (rather than IgE) class appear to be implicated (Stanworth, 1983B).

Work undertaken in my laboratory in recent years is beginning to suggest a mechanism whereby IgE antibody-antigen (allergen) interaction on target mast cell (or basophil) membranes initiates the release of histamine, and other mediators of immediate-type hypersensitivity reactions. Hopefully, this will lead eventually to the design of more effective anti-allergy compounds. But, it also offers an explanation of the basis of clinically similar allergic reactions, the socalled "pseudo-allergic" responses, in which there is no evidence of the involvement of anaphylactic antibodies.

As will be indicated, these include adverse reactivity to polypeptide antibiotics and amino glycosides: and compounds like intravenous anaesthetics and radiographic contrast media, which appear to act by eleciting the formation of the his-tamine releasing complement C3a and C5a subcomponents (the "anaphylatoxins"). Other types of pharmaceutical agent that have been placed in this category are colloid plasma substitutes, where however there is evidence in some cases of the involvement of antibodies of the IgG class: and aggregate-contaminated preparations of IgG used for clinical infusion, as will also be discussed.

2. MOLECULAR BASIS OF IGE ANTIBODY-MEDIATED HYPERSENSITIVITY REACTIONS.

Our long term study of the molecular basis of the immuno-logical triggering of mast cells (and basophils) has pointed to a dual role of IgE antibodies (as has been discussed in detail elsewhere; eg. Stanworth, 1973). As our early passive sensitisation-inhibition studies, using proteolytic and chemical cleavage fragments of human myeloma IgE, (Stanworth et al. 1968) were the first to demonstrate, anaphylactic antibodies of this class bind to mast cells via

Fc receptors. Owing to the relatively high association constant of this non-covalent interaction, transferred anti-body will persist at such local transfer sites (eg. in the skin of normal recipients) for long periods (up to several weeks); this being a "null" event as far as the target mast cell is concerned.

It is the subsequent presentation of specific antigen (allergen) to such sensitised cells which sets in train a complex series of biochemical events culminating in the energy and calcium ion-dependent, non-lytic, release of histamine and other mediators of immediate-type hypersensitivity responses (depicted diagrammatically in Figure (1).

Although some investigators maintain that the immunological triggering event responsible for initiating this mediator release process merely involves the cross-linking of Fc receptors on the mast cell plasma membrane, indirectly through the bridging of IgE antibody bound to those receptors by allergen, we have always contended that the latter process results in antibody providing a direct triggering signal to the target mast cell as a result of a conformational change brought about by the antigen cross-linking (as is depicted diagrammatically in Figure 2). Furthermore, extensive studies using synthetic peptides, which have been carried out in my laboratory over the last fifteen years (Jasani et al. 1973, 1979; Stanworth et al. 1984) have delineated that part of the IgE antibody Fc region (within the C 4 domain), which appears to be responsible for providing such a signal, as has been discussed in detail recently elsewhere (Stanworth, 1984). Moreover, recent collaborative studies undertaken with R. Cherry and colleagues of Essex University based on the mea-surement of basic peptides capacity to immobilise band 3 protein in a model (erythrocyte) membrane system (Dufton et al. 1984), have begun to suggest how such as cytophilic antibody Fc effector site could initiate the mast cell mem-brane changes culminating in mediator release.

It seems likely that a sequence of around 10 amino acids within that part of the ϵ chain comprising this effector site (see Figure 3) insert (via the C-terminal hydrophobic region) into the mast cell plasma membrane: the cationic N-terminal region then bringing about the aggregation of protein compo-nents within the membrane which provides the primary stimulus ultimately resulting in mediator release. Obviously, such a form of triggering would be facilitated if the interaction of mast cell bound IgE antibody with allergen were to lead to the activation of a membrane peptidase, which selectively cleaves such a histamine releasing -peptide from the antibody C-ϵ 4 domain. (This is a possibility which is now receiving serious attention in our laboratory).

In this connection, it is interesting to note that substance P, an undecapeptide released from primary afferent neurones (in response to antidromic impulses) where it is thought to act indirectly on neighbouring mast cells (to release histamine), shows remarkably similar structural features to

the histamine releasingε-chain peptide (as will be seen from
Figure 3). Thus, basic ligands other than that comprising the
IgE antibody Fc effector site are capable of similarly eliciting non-cytolytic mediator release from mast cells; the
essential structural requirement being a cationic "head"
separated by a suitable number of "inert" amino acid residue
from a "hydrophobic" tail (as our recent detailed studies on
the histamine releasing capacity of a range of synthetic
chain analogues indicated: Stanworth et al. 1984). In
other words, absolute amino acid specificity does not appear
to be necessary for the primary triggering of mast cells; in
contrast to the structural requirements for polypeptide
hormone-agonist recepttor interaction.

As will be discussed below, this offers scope for certain
drugs and other low molecular weight substances to initiate
the non-cytolytic release of mediators from mast cells by a
process closely resembling the immunologically stimulated one;
and which results in the same clinical manifestations of an
immediate-type allergic response.

Scope for non-immunological mast cell triggering.

According to the mechanism of immunological (ie. IgE antibody
mediated) mast cell triggering just described, there ought to
be scope for the direct mediator releasing action of other
basic peptides (and related compounds) besides the neuropeptide substance P already mentioned. Indeed, as discussed
at length elsewhere (Stanworth, 1980A), this would seem to
offer an explanation of the severe anaphylactic-like reactions
occcationally seen to the ACTH (1-24) peptide, Synacthen; and
to basic polypeptide antibiotics (such as polymyxin B, colis-
tin and bacitracin) and the basic aminoglycosides (discussed
by Dewdney, 1980).

Studies undertaken on sera from a group of patients, who had
reacted adversely to the administration of Synacthen, failed
to reveal any evidence of the formation of anaphylactic IgE
antibodies directed against this synthetic polypeptide hormone
(which, incidentally, possesses the same amino acid sequence
as the first 24 amino acid residues of human ACTH). On the
other hand, we have in the past obtained substantial experimental evidence (eg. see Jasani et al. 1973; 1979) that
such polypeptides are capable of eliciting the non-cytolytic
release of histamine from normal rat mast cells in vitro, at
relatively low doses (ie. 10^{-6} M effects of the order of 50%
release of the total available histamine). We assume that
such polypeptides act directly on the mast cell plasma
membrane, in a similar manner to that ascribed earlier to the
synthetic ε-chain peptide; thereby "short circuiting" the
regular two stage IgE antibody mediated trigger process.

As shown in Figure 4, the whole 39 amino acid residue native
ACTH molecule is a much less effective histamine releasing
agent. Intriguingly, as our structure-activity studies
(Jasani et al. 1973; 1979) have indicated, this can be
attributed to the presence of the amino acid residues in the

25-39 region of the whole ACTH molecule. Omission of these (which were thought to comprise the foreign antigenic determinant in porcine ACTH, against which some patients appeared to mount antibody responses) in the synthetic 1-24 residue poly peptide (Synacthen), has resulted in a much more basic structure (comprising a cluster of basic amino acids spanning positions 15-18) as will be seen from Figure 5; and, therefore, a much more potent histamine liberator.

3. ROLE OF C3 RECEPTORS IN MAST CELL TRIGGERING.

It has been recognised for many years that incubation of serum with insoluble high molecular weight substances (such as starch, dextran, yeast and bacterial endotoxic lypopolysaccharides), as well as with certain antigen-antibody complexes, results in the formation of a toxic product termed "anaphylatoxin"; because of its capacity to produce anaphylaxis-like (ie. smooth muscle contraction, peripheral vasodilation, increase vascular permeability and oedema) effects in vivo. Such activities have since been associated with the complement compoment C3 cleavage products C3a andC5a (Osler et al. 1959). Not only do such fragments, which are produced during activation of the alternative complement pathway (as indicated in Figure 6), show chemotactic activity for polymorphonuclear leucocytes. It can also be demonstrated (Johnson et al. 1975) that they are capable of initiating histamine release from isolated normal rat peritoneal mast cells (as will be seen from Figure 7). This, therefore, provides another means by which certain drugs and other low molecular weight substances could be capable of eliciting the clinical symptoms of immediate-type hypersentivity (as has been discussed in more detail in Stanworth, 1980); without recourse to the classical IgE antibody mediated histamine release process (outlined in Section 2); and so such responses can also be regarded as pseudo-allergic reactions. On the other hand, although C3b receptors have also been demonstrated on mast cells and basophils, there is no evidence that their activation plays any primary role in the triggering of mediator release (as has been discussed elsewhere: Stanworth, 1980B); in contrast to their active involvement in the stimulation of phagocytic cells (eg. macrophages and polymorphonuclear leucocytes, discussed in Stanworth, 1984C).

Examples of the apparent activation of the alternative complement pathway by pharmaceutical agents, as a basis of adverse clinical reactivity.

a. Action of radiographic contrast media (RCM)

Adverse reactions of an allergic symptomatology (urticaria, angiodema, asthma etc.) have been reported in as many as 2% of patients receiving these radio-opaque triiodinated benzoic acid derivatives (some of which are illustrated, structurally,in Figure 8) prior to x-ray analysis (Witten, 1975)

It is conceivable that such compounds promote adverse IgE antibody-metiated reactions in those patients who react adversely to their administration; particularly as there have been reports that patients with a history of allergy, or a prior history of anaphylactoid reactions to RCM, pertain to a greater risk of adverse reactivity to this type of compound. But, in extensive experimental sensitisation studies performed recently in my laboratory, using a range of RCM in rats and mice, IgE antibody responses could not be demonstrated when the free RCM was adminstered in doses equivalent to those employed clinically (Al Ani et al. 1984). Although, the formation of RCM specific IgE antibodies in rats (as revealed by subsequent in vitro challenge studies on their isolated peritoneal mast cells) was achieved by sensitising the animals with RCM which had been chemically coupled to a protein carrier (eg. ovalbumin or β-lactoglobulin). Another possibility was that RCM effected mediator release by acting directly on certain (susceptible) individuals' mast cells. But in vitro studies undertaken in our laboratory, of the direct effect of a series of RCM on rat peritoneal mast cells, showed that such compounds were capable only of eliciting cytolytic histamine release, and even then only at high dose levels.

On the other hand, we found that all of the four contrast media examined (ie. methylglucamine acetrizoate methylglucamine diatrizoate, methylglucamine ioxithalamate and ioglunide) consumed comple ment from normal human serum via the alternative pathway in vitro (see Figure 9), when we applied a simple haemolytic assay developed in our laboratory (Riches and Stanworth, 1980) to the measurement of this parameter. However, in subsequent in vitro studies undertaken in our laboratory, inclubation of RCM with rat mast cells or human peripheral blood leucocytes in the presence of fresh rat or human serum, respectively, failed to obtain any direct evidence that RCM are capable of effecting histamine release in vivo as a result of anaphylatoxin formation.

In contrast, we have obtained indirect evidence that RCM interact with the complement C3 component via mechanisms which differ from either the established classical or alternative pathways, when incubated with fresh human serum in vitro. These observations are consistent with those of other investigators (eg. Lasser et al. 1979; Hasselbacker and Hahn, 1980) whose findings also point to an atypical mode of activation of the complement C3 component by RCM.

In this connection, it is conceivable that some of the adverse reaction to RCM could perhaps be attributable to the initiation of release of lysosomal enzymes and other mediators from phagocytic cells, because our recent studies on immunological (and other) mechanisms of triggering of such target cells have demonstrated a relationship between the capacities of insoluble immune complexes and other secretagogues (including several primary aliphatic monoamines) to activate the alternative complement pathway, and to effect the non-cytolytic release of these ezymes from mouse peritoneal macrophages _in vitro_ (Riches and Stanworth, 1981). Moreover, such an effect is also shown by other weak bases, such as ammonium chloride (Riches and Stanworth, 1980), which has been used as a solvent in some RCM preparation. But studies performed in my laboratory on the direct effect of the four RCM referred to earlier (eg. inFigure 9) on isolated mouse peritoneal macrophages failed to reveal any evidence of the initiation of non lytic acid hydrolase release by physiologically significant doses.

b. Action of intravenous anaesthetics

There have been various reports in the literature (reviewed in Watkins, 1979) of anaphylactoid reactions to intravenous anaesthetics such as: alphaxalone and alphadolone (Althesin) and propanidid (Eportol). Furthermore there have been claims that such adverse responses are attributable to activation of the alternative complement pathway, with the formation of anaphylatoxic C3a and C5a sub-components. But, here too, convincing direct experimental evidence has not been provided in support of this contention. There is, however, agreement that many such adverse reactions are attributable to the solvent cremphor E.L. (a surfactant produced by epoxylation of castor oil) used in the formulation of intravenous anaesthetics. Moreover, a high frequency of adverse responses to injection of this agent has been observed in the mini-pig, 7 days following an initial injection (Glen et al. 1979). The responses noted in the pigs differed from those associated with adverse reactions to cremophor in man, in that bronchospasm was not a feature of the reaction in the pig, whereas marked hypertension rather than hypotention was a consistent finding. But, the release of histamine in some of the _in vivo_ reactions observed, as well as marked changes in polymorph count, are features common to the reactions seen in both man and pig.

With one exception, the reactions observed inpigs occurred following prior exposure to a particular agent or solvent. But, the short time interval required to induce sensitivity, and the disappearance of this sensitivity after 3 weeks, has been interpreted that it is unlikely that classical IgE mediated hypersensitivity is involved; a conclusion which was supported by the failure to demonstrate specific IgE antibodies in the animals' circulations, by PCA testing.

The pioneering work of Lorenz and associates (reviewed in Lorenz et al. 1981); involving the application of a highly refined fluorometric assay to the measurement of histamine levels in serial plasma samples, has provided direct evidence of the in vivo release of this mediator in response to the administration of anaesthetic and hypnotic drugs as well as Cremophor E.L. But, it is not easy to distinguish between "reactive" and "non-reactive" individuals on this basis; particularly as the injection of saline alone was found to elicit an elevation in plasma histamine levels in some subjects (Lorenz and Doenicke, 1978).

4. ADVERSE REACTIONS TO PLASMA PRODUCTS AND PLASMA SUBSTITUTES.

The administration of plasma proteins (immunoglobulin, coaglulation factors etc.) and plasma (ie. colloid volume) substitutes, is another form of treatment which can elicit adverse reactions in some individuals. But here, as in the case of types of response discussed in earlier sections, it is not always easy to establish whether allergic responses of the classical or pseuo type have occurred.

a. Pseudo-allergic reactions to human ɣ-globulin preparations

It has long been recognised that there is a danger in administering human IgG preparations intravenously, because of the possible presence of some aggregated material capable of eliciting a pseudo-allergic response. Consequently, great efforts have been made in recent years to free commercial IgG preparations of such undesirable polymer forms; in some cases by employing a mild enzyme treatment to digest them (Janeway et al. 1968). It would seem most likely that the adverse reactivity of aggregated forms of human IgG are attributable to their capacity to activate the classical complement pathway. Work undertaken in our laboratory (Evans and Stanworth, unpublished) has revealed that human IgG trimers are the smallest polymer forms capable of this biological activity. Whilst collaborative studies which we undertook with Holborrow and colleagues (Embling et al. 1978) revealed that similar structural requirements appear to be necessary for aggregated forms of human IgG to localise in the germinal centres of mice.

The supposition that complement activation is involved in adverse reactivity to such pharmaceutical agents is supported by observations that all compounds of the complement system were found to be reduced following an IgG infusion, whereas, there was no evidence of raised levels of histamine or serotonin in the circulations of such patients.

Such adverse reactions appear to be more prominent in immunodeficient patients who, of course, are major recipients of this form of treatment; and there is evidence that severe clinical symptoms associated with intravenous human IgG infusion are more often seen in immunodeficient patients (Barandin et al. 1968). Yet, in a study which we undertook some years ago (McLaughlan et al. 1974) involving the measurement of serum IgE levels in 48 such patients, we found no evidence that those patients experiencing anaphylactic-type reactions following IgG infusion had higher circulating levels of this immunoglobulin.

b. Pseudo-allergic reactions to colloid volume substitutes.

Of the adverse reactions encountered to various materials (plasma protein constituents, gelatin, starch, dextran employed as colloid volume substitutes, those initiated by dextran preparations have been investigated in most detail from the immunological stand point.

Anaphylactoid reactions elicited by this polysaccharide are most frequently observed in the initial phase of its infusion. Furthermore, a relatively high incidence (ie.40%) of atopy has been observed in patients showing mild incompatibility to dextran, but not in patients who react severely to its administration. But, none of the laboratory investigations undertaken on this form of human adverse reactivity have produced evidence that IgE antibodies directed against dextran were responsible for the sensitivity exhibited by certain strains of rats (West, 1977); whose mast cells release vasoactive amines in response to dextran challenge, by a non IgE antibody dependent process. On the other hand, high titres of dextran-reactive haemagglutinating antibodies of the IgG class have been detected in the sera of patients reacting adversely to dextran infusion; their levels showing a strong correlation with the severity of the clinical response (Richter and Hadin, 1982). The complement profiles of such patients have revealed decreases in the levels of Clq suggestive of the activation of the classical pathway. This is attributed to immune complexes comprising dextran and the IgG anti-bodies (of the IgG2 sub-class).In other words, it seems likely that the anaphylactoid reactions initiated by this colloid volume substitute are of Type III (ie. immune complex mediated).

Interestingly, the observation that hapten inhibition can prevent lethal experimentally-induced dextran anaphylaxis in guinea pigs has been exploited to reduce the incidence of dextran induced anaphylactoid reactions in patients, by the administration of a monovalent low molecular weight (ie. 1000) polyglucose preparation two minutes prior to the infusion of clinical dextran (Messmer et al. 1980).

5. CONCLUDING COMMENTS

As has been indicated, there is still much to be learnt about the mechanisms of the so-called pseudo-allergic reactions. But, even at this stage it is apparent that these are quite varied; despite the similarities in the clinical manifestations.

In the limited time available, the major types of non-anaphylactic antibody mediated allergic response have been outlined; and their probable mechanisms have been discussed. Some would question the inclusion of allergic reactions to dextran in this category; although the attribution of immune complexes as the cause of the severe adverse reactions to this colloid volume substitute has yet to be established unequivocally. There is growing evidence that pseudo-allergic reactions to, at least, some of the other pharmaceutical agents considered here, such as radiographic contrast media and intravenous anaesthetics, result from an effect on the alternative complement pathway. However, direct evidence that such reactions lead to the formation of anaphylatoxic complement sub-components (C3a and C5a) in vivo has yet to be obtained.

On the other hand, as has been discussed at some length, it seems likely that polypeptide drugs like ACTH and certain antibiotics initiate vasoactive amine release as the result of a direct action on target mast cells. Moreover, a plausible mechanism of such a mode of action has been put forward; which involves the by-passing of the two-stage IgE antibody triggering mechanism and direct action of the offending drug on the so-called second "receptor".

Despite this progress in understanding of the mechanism of pseudo-allergic reactions, it is still necessary to explain why only a very small number of patients respond adversely to exposure to these various pharmaceutical agents. This aspect presents the next challenge to those interested in solving this troublesome problem; and will eventually lead, hopefully, to the devising of methods of anticipating the likelihood of a patient responding adversely to a particular pharmaceutical (or other foreign) agent in such a manner.

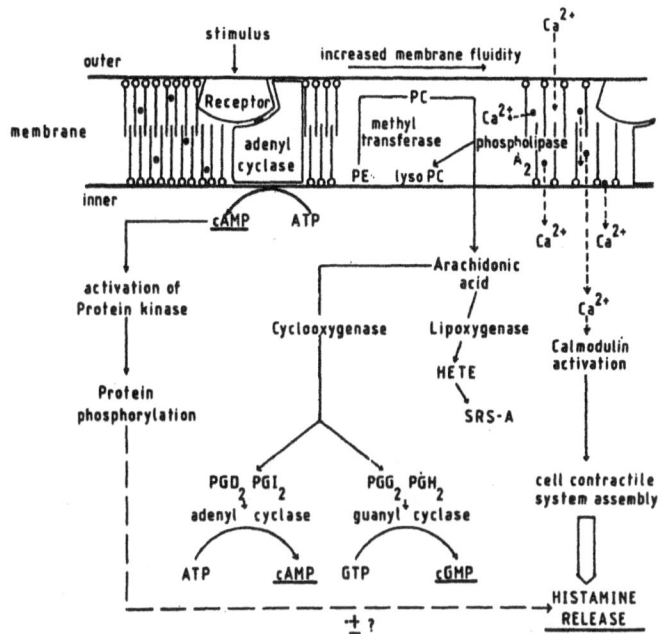

1. Diagrammatic depiction of the major biochemical events thought to be associated with the immunological triggering of mast cells. (Courtesy of Dr. D.S. Burt).

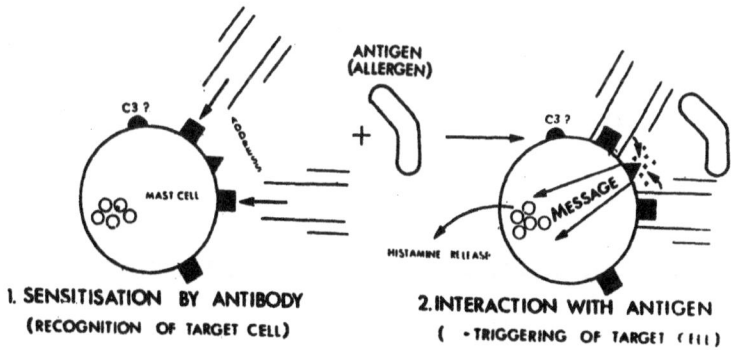

POSTULATED MECHANISM OF
IMMUNOLOGICAL TRIGGERING
OF MAST CELLS.

2. Postulated manner in which the cross-linking by antigen (allergen) elicits a conformational change in mast cell bound IgE antibody, with the formation of a direct trigger site within the Fc region.

ϵ-CHAIN PEPTIDE   Lys-Thr-Lys-Gly-Ser-Gly-Phe-Phe-Val-Phe

SUBSTANCE P   Arg-pro-Lys-Pro-Gln-Gln-Phe-Phe-Gly-Leu-Met-

3. Comparison of the primary sequences of a synthetic histamine releasing decapeptide comprising a sequence within the human $C_\epsilon 4$ domain and the histamine releasing neuropeptide substance P.

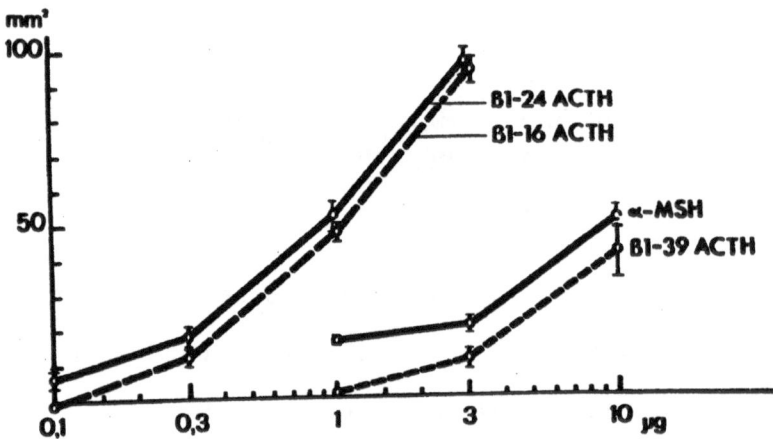

4. Vascular permeability inducing activity in guinea pigs; following intracutaneous injection subsequent to i.v. injection of Pontamine Sky Blue (Reproduced from Jaques R. Int. Archs. Allergy 1965, <u>28</u>, 221).

<u>ACTH</u>

1   16
NH_2-Ser-Tyr-Ser-Met-Glu-His-Phe-Arg-Trp-Gly-Lys-Pro-Val-Gly-Lys-Lys-

17   24
Arg-Arg-Pro-Val-Lys-Val-Tyr-Pro-

25   39
Asp-Gly-Ala-Glu-Asp-Glu-Leu-Ala-Glu-Ala-Phe-Pro-Leu-Glu-Phe-COOH

5. Primary sequence of porcine ACTH. Note the relatively high basicity of the 1-24 region, comprising the synthetic peptide hormone Synacthen; and the predominance of acidic amino acid residues in the rest of the molecule.

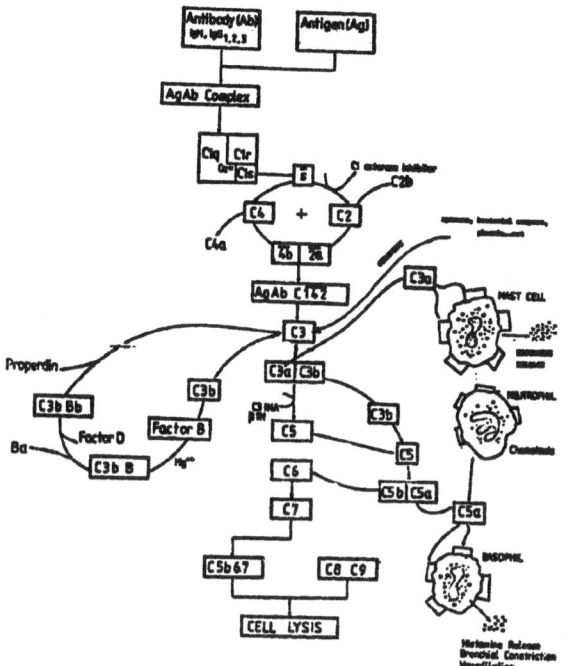

6. Outline of the main steps in the activation of the classical and alternative complement pathways.

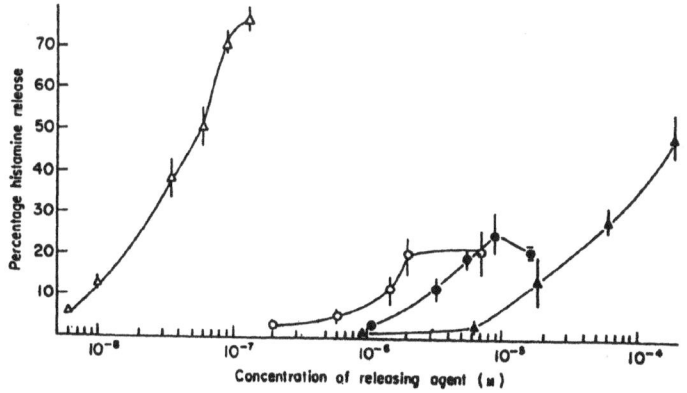

7. Mast cell histamine releasing activity (in vitro) of human anaphylatoxin fragments C3a(●) and C5a (○); compared with the activities of compound 48/80 (△) and bradykinin (▲). (Reproduced from Johnson A.R. et. al. Immunology 28, 1067).

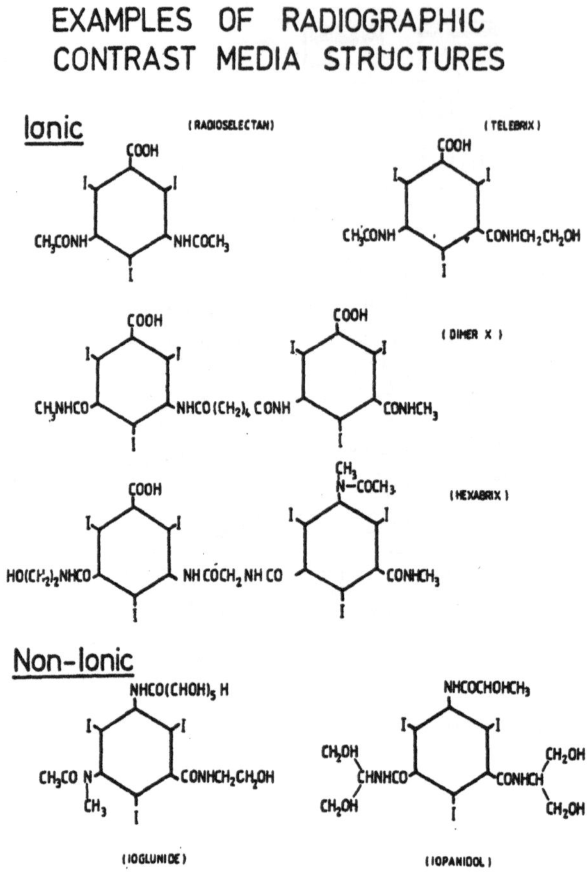

438

EXAMPLES OF RADIOGRAPHIC
CONTRAST MEDIA STRUCTURES

Ionic

(RADIOSELECTAN)

(TELEBRIX)

(DIMER X)

(HEXABRIX)

Non-Ionic

(IOGLUNIDE)

(IOPANIDOL)

8. Structures of some commonly used radio-graphic contrast
   media.

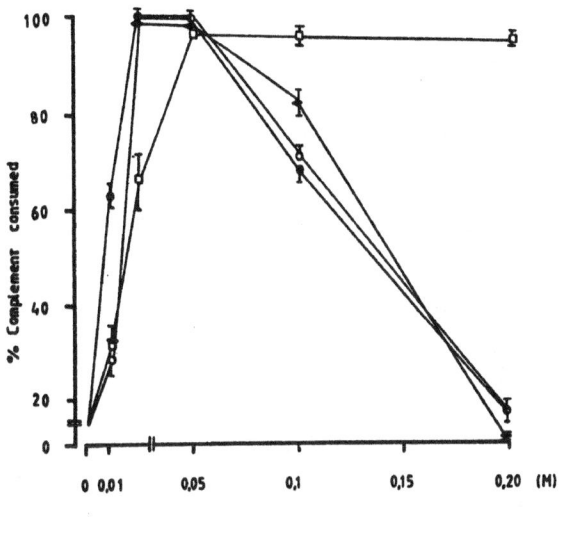

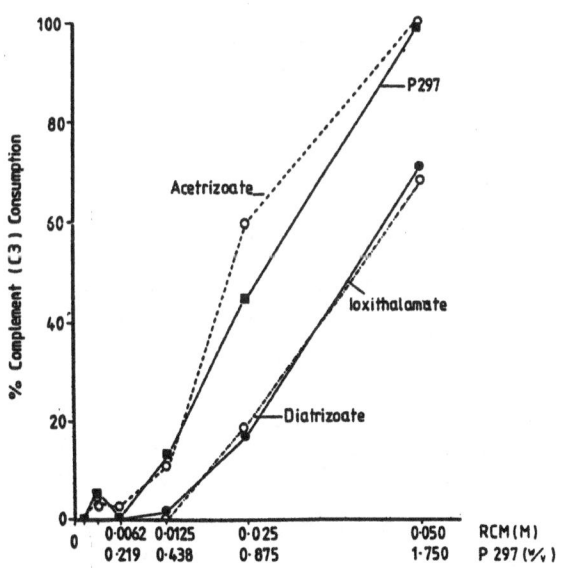

Demonstration of the complement (C3) reactivity of four
radio-graphic contrast media: methyl glucamine
acetrizoate (●);   methyl glucamine diatrizoate (◆);
methyl glucamine ioxithalamate (○);   and ioglunide (□), "P.297"

REFERENCES

Al-Ani W.S., Burt D.S. & Stanworth D.R. (1984) Results of in vitro investigations into the possible mechanisms of adverse clinical reactivity to radio-graphic contrast media (RCM). In preparation.

Barandun S., Kistler P., Jeune T.F. & Isliker H. (1962) Intravenous administration of human gamma globulin. Vox Sang. 7, 157.

Dewdney J.M. (1980) Pseudo-allergic reactions to antibiotics. in "Pseudo Allergic Reactions: Involvement of Drugs and chemicals. eds. Dukor P. et al. Vol. 1, 273. (Karger, Basel).

Dufton M.J., Cherry R.J., Colement J.W. & Stanworth D.R. (1984) The capacity of basic peptides to trigger exocytosis from mast cells correlated with their capacity to immobilise band 3 proteins in erythrocyte membranes. Biochem J. In Press.

Embling P.H., Evans H., Gutterz C., Holborrow E.J., Johns P., Johnson P.M., Papamichail M. & Stanworth D.R. (1978). The structural requirements for immunoglobulin aggregates to localise in germinal centres. Immunology, 34, 781.

Glen J.B., Davies G.E., Thompson D.S., Scarth & Thompson A.V. (1979) An animal model for the investigation of adverse responses to i.V. anaesthetic agents and their solvents. Br. J. Anaesth. 51, 819.

Hasselbacher P. & Hahn J. (1980) In vitro effects of radiographic contrast media on the complement system. J. Allergy Clin. Immunol. 66, 217.

Janeway C.A., Merler E., Rosen F.S., Salmon S. & Crain J.D. (1968) Intravenous gamma globulin metabolism of gamma globulin fragments in normal and agammaglobulinaemia persons. New England J. Med. 278, 919.

Jasani B., Mackler B., Kreil G., & Stanworth D.R. (1973) Studies on the mast cell triggering action of certain histamine liberators.Int.Arch Allergy 45,74-81.

Jasani B., Kreil G., Mackler B.F. & Stanworth D.R. (1979) Further studies on the structure requirements for poly-peptide-mediated histamine release from rat mast cells. Biochem J. 181, 623-632.

Lasser E.C., Lang J.H., Lyon S.G. and Hamblin A.E. (1979) Complement and contrast mediator reactors. J. Allergy Clin. Immunol. 64, 105.

Lorenz W., Doenicke A., Schonig B. & Neugebauer E. (1981) The role of histamine in adverse reactions to intravenous agents in "Adverse Reactions of Anaesthetic Drugs". ed. Thoronton (Elsevier /North Holland Biomedical Press). 69-238.

Lorenz W. & Doenicke A. (1978) Anaphylactoid reactions and histamine release by intravenous drugs used in surgergy and anesthesia in "Adverse Response to Intravenous Drugs" eds. Watkins and Ward (Academic Press) p. 83.

McLaughlan P., Stanworth D.R., Webster A.D.B. & Asherson G.L. (1974) Serum IgE in immune deficiency disorders. Clin.exp. Immunol. 16, 375.

Messmer K., Ljunstrom K-G., Gruber U-F. & Hedin H. (1980) Prevention of dextran-induced anaphylactoid reactions by hapten inhibition. The Lancet i, 975.

Riches D.W.H. & Stanworth D.R. (1980) Primary amines induced selective release of lysosomal enzymes from mouse macrophages. Biochem J. 188, 933.

Riches D.W.H. & Stanworth D.R. (1981) Studies on the possible involvment of complement component C3 in the initiation of acid hydrolase secretion by macrophages. I. Correlation between enzyme-releasing and complement-activating capacities of several secretagogues. Immunology 44, 29-39.

Richter A.W. & Hedin H.I. (1982) Dextran hypersensitivity. Immunology Today 3, 132-38.

Stanworth D.R., Humphrey J.H., Bennuch H. & Johansson S.G.O (1968) Inhibition of Prausnitz-Kustner reaction by proteolytic cleavage fragments of a human myeloma protein of immunoglogulin class E. The Lancet 17-18.

Stanworth D.R. (1973) Immediate Hypersensitivity: the Molecular Basis of the Allergic Response. North Holland Research Monographs Frontiers of Biology. Vol 28.

Stanworth D.R. (1980A) Oligo-peptide-induced release of histamine in "Pseudo-Allergic Reactions: 1. Genetic Aspects and Anaphylactoid Reactions" - (eds. P. Dukor, P. Kallos, H.D. Schlumberger and G.B. West) p. 56-1o7, Karger.

Stanworth D.R. (1980B) Contribution of complement. receptors to the triggering of mast cells and basophils. Proc. of Symp. on "Triggering of Phagocytic Cells". Szekesferervar (Kulltura, Budapest) 217-233.

Stanworth D.R. (1983A) Mechanisms of hypersensitivity. In "Immunotoxicology" Proc. 1st International Congress of Immunotoxicology, Surre 1982. Eds. Gibson, G.G. et al. (Academic Press) 1983, 71-85.

Stanworth D.R. (1984) The role of immunoreceptors. Proc. of the 25th Congress of the European Society of Toxicology, Budapest, June 1984.

Stanworth D.R., Coleman J.W. & Khan Z. (1984) Essential structural requirements for triggering of mast cells by a synthetic peptide comprising a sequence in the C 4 domain of human IgE. Molecular Immunology 21, 243-247.

Voohres A.B., Baker J. & Pulaski E.J. (1951) Reactions of Albino rats to injections of dextran (18453). Proc.Soc.Exp.Biol.Med. 76,254.

Watkins J. (1979) Anaphylactoid reactions to i.v. substances. Br. J. Anaesth. 51, 51.

West G.B. (1977) Anaphylactoid responses in rats. Int. Archs. Allergy appl. Immunol. 55, 542.

Witten D.M. (1975) Reactions to urographic contrast media. J. American Med. Assoc. 321, 974-7.

Witten D.M., Hirsch F.D. & Hartman G.W. (1973) Acute reactions to urographic contrast medium: incidence, clinical characteristics and relationship to history of hypersensitivity states. Amer. J. Roentgenol. 119, 832.

PROSPECTIVE MODELING FOR DELAYED CONTACT HYPERSENSITIVITY

E.V. Buehler

Hill Top Research, Inc.,
Research and Development Department,
Cincinnati, OH 45242, U.S.A.

It is an important precept that, prior to the introduction of new chemicals or products into commerce, they be evaluated for their potential to produce adverse effects. Thus, the art and science of toxicology has been evolving and will continue to evolve in order to detect and define the biologic effects of the chemicals in our environment. For this purpose an impressive array of animal tests and procedures have been described and formalized that attempt to simulate the conditions of human exposure so that adverse effects might be identified and thus avoided. At the same time, many of these same animal models are further utilized to define and describe the mechanism of action of these chemicals. The protocols for a safety program can, therefore, be many and varied, but the hallmarks of design and planning are the selection of relevant routes of exposure in order to investigate acute, subchronic and chronic effects. In all cases, the intent of the toxicologist is to provide a measure of exaggeration in order to assure an adverse effect and then to describe a dose-response relationship and a no-effect level. If the process is successful and the relevant exposure parameters are known, it is often possible to formulate a risk assessment for human exposures.

For materials that are intended for topical application to skin, even those that have only casual contact, it is important to describe their primary irritant and allergenic properties. If chemicals have allergenic potential, it is their ability to produce allergic contact dermatitis in the sensitized host that needs to be assessed. Clinically, in the human, allergic contact dermatitis is an eczematous disease and is differentiated from other eczemas as being due to a cell-mediated hypersensitivity. The dermatologist will base his diagnosis on a detailed case history of recent exposures to compounds and formulations and on a series of patch tests to identify a causative agent or agents(1). What is not generally recognized, is that patch test positivity is not necessarily indicative of clinical relevance. For example, Prystowski et al (2), found patch test positive skin reactions to common sensitizers in normal subjects, who had never experienced eczematous skin disease. Kligman (3) also reported a substantial incidence of positive skin reactions to poison ivy resins in subjets who were unaware of their susceptibility.

According to dogma, the pathogenesis of allergic contact dermatitis requires an initial exposure to a biologically active chemical of low molecular weight that alerts the immune system and produces a specific proliferation of T-lymphocytes that will eventually mediate the adverse reaction(s). The pathogenic magnification of this response to produce the diseased state, then occurs after subsequent exposures to the same chemical. For the most part these specific chemicals are presented to the skin in differing formulations and vehicles. Table 1 lists some properties that are necessary for a chemical to be a hapten and to initiate the delayed response that can eventually result in allergic contact dermatitis. It is essential that chemicals have this property of substantivity to skin and that their oil/water partition coefficient favors the skin over vehicle. Theoretically then, these chemicals penetrate into the skin and combine with epidermal and/or dermal protein to form complete antigens. It is important to remember that the skin presents a complex array of both soluble and insoluble proteins, all of which have the potential to combine and form antigens. It is likely that intermediate and xenobiotic metabolism is also an important factor in immunoregulation, when haptens are introduced by this route. The specificity of these antigens will, therefore, be at least partially and perhaps primarily directed towards native protein. It them becomes apparent that the physical nature of the antigen will be fundamental to the type of immune response that occurs. For example, it could be that soluble antigens from the skin are more likely to produce circulating antibody centrally, while insoluble antigens fixed to the site may preferentially enhance the T-cell response in the periphery.

Nevertheless, once these antigens are formed, the next step in the sequence is that of antigen processing by the macrophage. These two phases, antigen formation and antigen processing, are the most critical for the development of a proper model (Table 2). The diffusion gradient, that will determine distribution of antigen in skin, will primarily be affected by both hapten concentration and the qualities of the particular vehicle. In skin, antigen processingis performed by a specialized, fixed macrophage designated as the Langerhan cell (4). Although it might be expected that other macrophages could also be involved in antigen processing, particularly if a non-specific inflammatory reaction were to occur, it would be expected that the Langerhan cell is the more important cell for antigen recognition, processing and presentation to the appropriate lymophocytes. While it is relatively certain that the T-cell population of lymphocytes is solely responsible for the cell-mediated response, it is not so certain in the case of delayed contact hypersensitivity, whether or not the process occurs centrally or peripherally (5). It seems logical to assume, depending on many quantitative and qualitative aspects, that both might occur. From a practical standpoint, where small quantities of chemicals are involved and considering the reservoir effect of skin, it could be expected that peripheral sensitization is the predominant mode for the development of contact dermatitis.

Subsequent to the activation of the T-cells, the complex interactions and specific proliferation of thse cells then results in a specific allergic state that can be astivated on subsequent contact to produce the pathologic condition recognized as delayed contact hypersensitivity. The phenomenon itself is probably due to the inflammatory reactions induced by lymphokines released by non-specific lymphocytes that have been recruited to the area by the sensitized cells.

There have been many approaches suggested for the prospective analysis of chemicals for their ability to sensitize experimental animals, including topical application (6), injection of chemicals in salin (7), injection in Freund's Complete Adjuvant (8), and application under occlusive dressing (9). I will discuss the use of Freund's Complete Adjuvant (FCA) in some detail and then suggest that the use of the occlusive patch is more appropriate and is the superior approach.

It is a primary requisite of any animal model that the results of its use be relevant to the human situation. Table 3 reviews some undesirable qualities of injection techniques. The injection of chemicals alone, or with FCA, into the dermis bypasses the barrier properties of skin and nullifies those very chemical and physical properties of the chemical that determine its substantivity and penetrating capabilities. These qualities of the test material are perhaps most critical for clinical sensitization, particularly for those who assume that all chemicals have allergenic potential. In addition, injection negates the possibility of forming epidermal antigen that may also be important for the development of contact allergy. Finally, the granuloma formed after injection of an adjuvant is a foreign body response. This produces an influx of cells from the circulation that not only causes tissue destruction but also alters the character of the final response. In fact it is well known that Type II adjuvants, such as FCA, cause an enhanced IgG response in the guinea pig, and these kinds of antibody can play a regulatoryu role. From this standpoint it is also well to keep in mind that an adjuvant mediated expression of the immune response has been described (10). Similarly, although the blocking of tolerance has been suggested (10) as a possible mechanism of adjuvanticity, the production of tolerance is also a likely outcome following the use of adjuvants.

As examples, Ritz, <u>et al</u>. (11) showed two effects of adjuvant that could influence safety assessment. They were studying the structureactivity relationship of a homologous series of sultones. The first observation was that the order of antigenicity could change depending upon the concentration of the intradermally injected dose (Table 4). At a higher inducing dose (7.1 nmol) the C_{12} and C_{14} unsaturated sultones appeared to be more potent than the C_{10} and C_{16} counterparts. At a lower dose (0.23 nmol) the relative potencies appeared to be $C_{16} > C_{14} > C_{12} > C_{10}$. The results were attributed to the tolerogenic properties of the haptens that were more pronounced at the higher concentrations.

This phenomenon of tolerance via intradermal injection in adjuvant is the second effect reported by Ritz and is illustrated in the table 5. The results after injection are directly compared to results obtained when the C_{12} and C_{16} saturated sultones were tested by occlusive epicutaneous exposure. It is obvious that both homologues express their tolerogenicity, in adjuvant, but not when applied to the skin under occlusive patch. Furthermore, under occlusivity, the relative potencies of the two materials are much more obvious and have practical applicability. The lack of allergenicity of 1-hexadecene-1,3-sultone is most probably due to its lower rate of penetration. This reordering of sensitizers, as well as reports that several protein antigens (20) are contact allergens after injection in adjuvant are a serious detriment to the use of injection as a method for prospective testing.

Occlusion, on the other hand, is an effective way to exaggerate the normal mode of exposure and to mimic the induction and elicitation of the human disease (Table 6). It is a well accepted theory that occlusion increases the penetration of materials through the skin by inhibiting evaporation and by effectively hydrating the skin. It is also possible that the slight increase in temperature under the patch could effectively enhance penetration. More recently it has been shown that occlusion enhances the immune response by intensifying the density of Langerhan cells at the epidermal/dermal junction (12). It is these primary and essential characteristics, as well as the other considerations listed in the table, that make the occlusive patch the primary diagnostic tool for the dermatologist to differentiate among the various clinical eczemas, and to provide the means for identifying responsible etiologic agents. Furthermore, the use of the occlusive patch has been found to be the only successful mode for hapten presentation when humans are used for prophetic testing.

By developing a restrainer for guinea pigs it was possible to utilize this approach in an experimental model that has been used successfully for several years(9). Recently a more complete description has been provided that fully explains the mechanics and process of testing (13) and is essential reading for those attempting to utilize the technique. There are several considerations that are critical to the successful use of this procedure. It is, for example, critical that the test material be presented at the highest possible concentration in an optimizing vehicle. We generally recommend 80% ethanol/water for induction and acetone for challenge, although water and surfactant vehicles can also be appropriate. Since most test materials are inherently irritating subsequent to penetration, we use this biologic property to determine the highest non-irritating doses. For induction, moderate degrees of primary irritation are acceptable, but challenges should be performed at levels that produce no more than a spotty erythema in a minority of animals. These levels are easily determined by conducting pilot studies in small groups of animals. It is an important consideration that the irritation produced by this approach is due to the inherent biological properties of the molecule and is not comparable to the artifactual foreign body response to CFA. For conducting the test it is essential that occlusivity be maintained. Our experience indicates that restraint is necessary and that wrapping alone provides <u>inadequate</u> occlusion in most instances and can result in unacceptable stress when effectively carried out (14). The occlusive method can be standardized and validated by using 0.3% dinitrochlorobenzene (DNCB) to induce, and 0.2% and 0.02% DNCB to challenge. Almost all test animals should then respond to 0.2 % and about half of them to 0.02%

Challenge reaction (Table 7) are graded on individual animals according to the degree of erythema. Patchy erythema is given a score of 0.5, while mild, moderate and severe erythema are scored 1 through 3, respectively, The scores are recorded at 24 and 48 hours and are then averaged for both time periods. The incidence of positive responders, as well as their average reactivities at the two scoring perios, when compared to a group of naive test animals, gives a quantitative measure of the relative allergenic reactivity of the material. Although it is tempting at this point to identify the test material with regard to its potency, there are many other considerations besides incidence and severity that are equally important for hazard assessment (Table 8). Some of these are use concentration, vehicle, total dose, area of exposure, numbers of exposures, etc. Many of these factors can be evaluated in the guinea pig and are emphasized in table 8. The approaches that have been used and their results have been presented elsewhere and will not be discussed in detail (15, 16). However, it must be emphasized that the final assessment, by necessity, is accomplished in man. Therefore, whenever possible, it is recommended that controlled and closely monitored studies be completed on humans, prior to widespread consumer use of new materials. The more conservative policy is to conduct prophetic testing in man prior to any ad libitum use of the new material or formulation.

The one remaining aspect of experimental models that I would like to discuss is that of sensitivity. When the occlusive patch method was first introduced, it was presented as a method for detecting moderate to severe sensitizers in order to avoid exposing humans to these same materials in a repeated insult patch test (9). This was followed by the introduction of a complex method that included the injection of chemical in FCA as a means to "maximize" the potential to sensitize. This was proposed as a way to detect weak sensitizers and is known as the Magnusson/Kligman technique (8). The proposal is based on a supposition that all materials are potentially sensitizing and those that produced no reactions or very few reactions were considered to be "weak". This designation not only ignores the severity of response in sensitized animals, but is established without regard to the concentration of test materials. Without trying to define a weak sensitizer other than one that causes only minor clinical problems, whether in reference to incidence or severity, we propose that by the use occlusive patches it is possible to detect materials that can be defined as "weak." Since the suggestion by Magnusson & Kligman (8) that Complete Freund's Adjuvant maximizes the guinea pig's response to allergens, many modifications for testing have been introduced (20-23) and several authors have evaluated the various approaches (22,24,25). It seems to be a constant criticism that the use of an occlusive patch technique will not identify weak sensitizers (25). We have responded to one of these (14) by pointing out that the use of a wrapping procedure to replace restraint was inadequate, and failed to provide true occlusion.

Most recently a group of French investigators (24) compared seven methods using six putative sensitizers of varying potency. All but one of the methods utilized intradermal injection with / or without CFA in varying sequences with topical applications. Induction doses were arbitrarily selected but were constant among the various procedures. The occlusive patch methodology was apparently excluded because of its presumed lack of sensitivity. Three of the test materials tested by these authors were phenylenediamine, formalin, and benzocaine (Table 9). These three materials were evaluated in our laboratories during the process of validating the occlusive methodology and were reported in 1965 (9). The classification of these materials, as provided by these authors, was that phenylenediamine is a very strong sensitizer, formalin is a strong sensitizer and that benzocaine ia a weak sensitizer. The occlusive patch technique very clearly provides data for a comparable conclusion. The other test materials in the table were reported at the same time and are presented here to reinforce the perception of a wide range of reactivities. The seven methods reported in the French paper showed the most variation in their responses to benzocaine, the weakest sensitizer tested, and could perhaps be due to uncontrollable variables in the tests (e.g., depth of injections and occlusion).

Table 10 provides a summary of data collected over the years, and represents the basis for our comparative immunotoxicology screening program. It is based on the fact that chemicals with the potential to be contact allergens are currently part of our everyday environment and their current use provides a standard for the assumption of acceptable risk.

Dinitrochlorobenzene. This is the standard positive control in our program. The test conditions indicated on the slide are used to monitor our guinea pig populations to assure their continuing responsiveness, but also to assure us that the technical aspects of the procedure are being correctly followed.

Formaldehyde.This is another positive control material and not only represents a water soluble sensitizer but is also the standard for the comparison of new preservatives (16).

Tetrachlorosalicylanilide (TCSA).This is an interesting antimicrobial compound with a long standing and substantial reputation as a strong sensitizer and photo-allergen. The data illustrate its ability to allergenize without photoactivation.

LES 13-2035.This is the designation provided for alkyl ether sulfate, a nonionic surfactant, that produced a severe epidemic of contact dermatitis in

Scandanavia in 1966. Eventually it was determined by Ritz, Connor and their co-workers (34), that sultones, present as impurities, were the sensitizers responsible for the epidemic. The sultones had formed because of a change in the manufacturing process for this specific batch. By setting the proper standards, it was possible to reduce the sultones to levels that were not problematic. It is informative that both the Magnusson/Kligman and the Buehler methodologies were used and displayed comparable sensitivites (26,27). It is also instructive that this particular batch of surfactant is reported to have contained 30 ppm of sultone when these tests were being conducted (34). This means that the 5% challenge dose on the slide contained 1.5 ppm of sultone. We have continued to use the occlusive method for screening new non-ionic surfactants and have further substantiated the very fine sensitivity of this method.

Hydroxycitronella. This is a perfume ingredient with a long history of use. It certainly must be considered to be a weak sensitizer. Marzulli and Maguire reported that it was negative when tested by occlusion (25), but we believe they failed because of inappropriate technique (14). We continue to conduct a modest amount of screening of perfumes for allergenic potential and have successfully used the procedure to detect allergenic mixtures. It has been possible in many instances to substitute acceptable ingredients for the stronger sensitizers.

Benzoyl peroxide. This was detected in the guinea pig as a potential sensitizer when tested as a dermal pharmaceutical formulation (28). Not only can one consider this material to be a relatively weak sensitizer, but testing it in a formulation represents a valuable asset to this approach that is not available to those who recommend injection in adjuvant. It is also an instance where the incidence of guinea pig reactivity was identical to the reactivity of humans in a prospective repeated-patch test for hypersensitivity (28).

Dansyl chloride. This is a fluorescing material that has been used to label skin for various kinds of investigative programs. Friedlaender & Baer (30) have reported it to be a tolerogen/non-sensitizer when tested by open epicutaneous exposure, but a strong allergen by injection. When we examined the material, while considering it for use as a skin marker in a human clinical, it proved to be allergenic. For this reason, it was not used. Although a high concentration was used to induce sensitization, the reactivity seen at relatively low challenge levels (0.5%) would suggest that this material should not necessarily be considered as a weak sensitizer.

Table 11 summarizes another set of data produced by several authors (31-33) and provides still another instance of the sensitivity of the occlusive method. These quinazoline dyes are almost identical mixtures of materials and differ only in that the D&C Yellow 10 dye is the sulfated salt and this changes its solubility. In this case a weakly sensitizing material was differentiated from a non-sensitizing material that is chemically and functionally similar. Both guinea pig and human data were comparable. These kinds of data can often be used to find satisfactory substitutes for materials that could have the potential to produce adverse effects.

More recently, we have had occasion to exploit this same methodology in the investigation of the photoallergic potential of musk ambrette. Musk ambrette is one of two perfume raw materials that have been suspected of producing clinically relevant photoallergy in humans. It was first implicated when it was used as an ingredient at relatively high levels in an after-shave lotion. Attempts to sensitize humans with an empirically designed test were negative (17). Subsequently, more suspect cases have been reported. The first reports to appear, utilizing the guinea pig, stated that it was necessary to destroy the barrier (18) or to utilize Freud's Complete Adjuvant (19) along with intense irradiation, in order to produce any evidence of photoallergy. For this reason, it has been suggested that abrasion (during shaving) followed by sunlight exposure are necessary conditions for the induction of photoallergy.

The procedure that we used for the study of photoallergy uses only the occlusive patch for the introduction of materials into the guinea pig's skin. We observed that the combination of repeated shaving, depilation, stripping of skin by removal of the patch and intense irradiation produced severe reactions in the skin surrounding the patch site. We, therefore, modified a Hill Top Chamber(R) so that tape stripping did not occur in the patch site or adjacent to it. Another modification that was required was related to the light source. In order to test a significant number of animals, the most useful source of UV irradiation is that supplied by fluorescent bulbs. Since these are tubular, there is a variation in intensity along the length of the source that is determined by the inverse square of the distance from the source. Since we could not anticipate the specific wavelengths that would be most critical to producing photoallergy, we designed a system that would accommodate any combination of light sources that might prove to be effective. For this purpose we built a rotating circular light source. By utilizing yokes and eye guards and rotating the wheel at 8 revolutions/minute we were able to produce a constant and reproducible light exposure for each animal.

Table 12 summarizes the results with two test materials, musk ambrette, a putative photoallergen, and 8-methoxypsoralen, a known phototoxin. The experimental format was to expose each animal to the respective test agent, under occlusive dressing at the indicated concentration, for 4 hours on Monday, Wednesday and Friday, for three consecutive weeks. Each application was followed by an irradiation of the animals for an additional two hours by a bank of 12 blacklights that produced light almost exclusively in the range of 320-400 microns (UVA) at an intensity of 490-550 $\mu W/cm^2$. During the fifth week each animal was challenged using the same experimental conditions. The results show the incidence of animals responding in a manner that would be considered typical for delayed hypersensitivity. The pattern of reactivity of test and control animals in the groups treated with musk ambrette clearly show the property of photoallergenicity, with no propensity to sentitize without the added irradiation, or to produce a phototoxic effect. 8-Methoxypsoralin, on the other hand, showed reactivity whenever the test site was irradiated, irrespective of the induction conditions. These reactions were interpreted to be phototoxic with no indication of an ability to sensitize.

In conclusion, we have successfully used the occlusive patch method in guinea pigs as a screen for potential sensitizers. We no longer feel constrained to claim the detection of only moderate to strong sensitizers. By optimizing the test conditions, by testing at high concentration and selecting appropriate vehicles, we have consistently identified materials that could be considered as weak sensitizers in humans. The data presented here support this conclusion. Since this approach is more realistic and does not introduce the artifacts of adjuvant injection, I propose that it is a superior system.

TABLE 1

PROPERTIES OF A HAPTEN

SUBSTANTIVITY
PENETRATION
    EFFECT OF VEHICLE
    DIFFUSION GRADIENT
    RATE
REACTION WITH PROTEIN - SHARED SPECIFICITY
    SOLUBLE (SYSTEMIC?)
    INSOLUBLE (FIXED)

TABLE 2

KINETICS OF ANTIGEN PRESENTATION

DIFFUSION GRADIENT
    HAPTEN CONCENTRATION
    VEHICLE
ANTIGEN PROCESSING
    LANGERHANS CELL
    CIRCULATING MACROPHAGE (PRIMARY IRRITATION)
CENTRAL OR PERIPHERAL STIMULATION
PROLIFERATION
ELICITATION
    PROLIFERATION
    RECRUITMENT OF NON-SPECIFIC LYMPHOCYTES

TABLE 3

UNDESIRABLE QUALITIES OF INJECTION TECHNIQUES

BYPASS BARRIER
OBVIATE SOLUBILITY AND VEHICLE EFFECTS
DERMAL ANTIGENS ONLY
FOREIGN BODY RESPONSE (GRANULOMA)
NECROTIZING EFFECTS
QUALITATIVE CHANGE IN IMMUNE RESPONSE
    TOLERANCE (ADJUVANT MEDIATED DEPRESSION)
    RE-ORDERING OF SENSITIZERS
    FALSE POSITIVES (PROTEINS)
INDUCTION DOSE (CONCENTRATION) - ARBITRARY

TABLE 4

PRIMARY SENSITATION OF GUINEA PIGS

TO SELECTED LEVELS OF UNSATURATED SULTONES

SENSITIZER	CHALLENGE DOSE HMa DOSE (NMOL)	INDUCTION DOSE (NMOL)[1]	
		0.23	7.1
C_{10}	200	2/15	15/15
	20	0/15	15/15
	2	0/15	5/15
C_{12}	200	3/13	15/15
	20	1/13	15/15
	2	2/13	12/15
C_{14}	200	10/15	15/15
	20	5/15	15/15
	2	2/15	13/15
C_{16}	200	14/15	15/15
	20	9/15	14/15
	2	8/15	6/15

[1] NO. SENSITIZED/TOTAL TESTED.

TABLE 5

INDUCTION OF SENSITIZATION IN GUINEA PIGS WITH UNSATURATED
SULTONES BY INTRADERMAL AND EPICUTAENOUS ROUTES

ROUTE	INDUCTION DOSE (NMOL)	INDUCTION COMPOUND[a]	
		DDS	HDS
INTRADERMAL	7.1	15/15[b]	14/15
	71	11/14	13/15
	710	7/15	0/15
EPICUTANEOUS	71	4/15	0/14
	710	8/15	0/15
	7100	10/14	1/15

[a] DDS = 1-DODECENE-1,3-SULTONE; HSD = 1-HEXADECENE-1,3-SULTONE.

[b] NUMBER OF ANIMALS RESPONDING TO EPICUTANEOUS CHALLENGE

WITH 10 NMOL OF HOMOLOGOUS SULTONE OUT OF THE NUMBER TESTED

TABLE 6

THE UTILITY OF OCCLUSION IN A PROPHETIC TEST
FOR DELAYED CONTACT HYPERSENSITIVITY

INCREASES PRENETRATION
    PRECLUDES EVAPORATION
    HYDRATES THE SKIN
    RAISES TEMPERATURE
MOBILIZES LANGERHANS CELLS
EXAMINATION OF VEHICLE EFFECTS
    SOLUBILITY
    PENETRATION
    PHYSICOCHEMICAL KINETICS
DETERMINE INDUCTION DOSE RESPONSES
CORRALATES WITH HUMAN PROPHETIC TESTS

TABLE 7

EXAMPLE: PRIMARY SENSITIZATION RESULTS

EXPERIMENTAL GROUP		RESPONSE GRADE 0	0.5	1	2	3	INCIDENCE	SEVERITY
TEST GROUP	(24 HR)	6	2	7	4	1	12/20	1.0-0.8
	(48 HR)	8	2	6	4	0		
CONTROL GROUP	(24 HR)	7	3	0	0	0	0/10	0.2-0.1
	(48 HR)	9	1	0	0	0		

TABLE 8

SUPPLEMENTAL INFORMATION AFTER PRIMARY CHALLANGE

1.   CONFIRMATION OF ALLERGENIC POTENTIAL
    A) RECHALLENGE AT   CONCENTRATION
    B) DOSE RESPONSE AND NO EFFECTS LEVEL
2.   IDENTIFY COMPONENT (MIXTURES) OR IMPURITY
3.   INDUCTION DOSE RESPONSE
4.   VEHICLE (FORMULATION) EFFECT
5.   CROSS REACTIVITIES
    A) STRUCTURE ACTIVITY RELATIONSHIP
6.   OTHER VARIABLES
    AREA, TIME, NUMBER OF DOSES, ETC.

TABLE 9

CLOSED PATCH STUDIES WITH COMMON SENSITIZERS IN THE GUINEA PIG[a]

SENSITIZER		INCIDENCE OF SENSITIZATION[b]
1.0%	TETRACHLOROSALICYLANILIDE	8/10
0.75%	ALLYL ISOTHIOCYANATE	3/10
5.0%	MONOBENZYL ETHER OF HYDROQUINONE	3/5
14.0%	THIOGLYCEROL	6/10
2.0%	p-PHENYLENEDIAMINE HC1	10/10
50%	BENZOCAINE	2/10
5.0%	FORMALIN	3/10
1.0%	POTASSIUM CHROMATE	1/10

[a]BUEHLER, E.V. (1965). ARCH. DERMATOL. 91, 171-177.
[b]NO. SENSITIZED/NO. TESTED

TABLE 10

A VARIETY OF SENSITIZERS IDENTIFIED

BY USING OCCLUSIVE PATCH TESTING

TEST MATERIAL CONC.		CHALLENGE CONC. (%)	RESULTS INCIDENCE	REFERENCE
0.3%	DINITROCHLOROBENZENE	0.02; 0.2	5/10; 10/10	14
0.9%	FORMALDEHYDE	30	0/20	16
1.9%	FORMALDEHYDE	30	5/20	16
1.0%	TETRACHLOROSALICYL-ANILIDE	0.1	0/10	—
1.0%	TETRACHLOROSALICYL-ANILIDE	1.0	8/10	9
25%	LES 13-2035	5; 10; 20	1/20; 5/20; 12/20	27
30%	HYDROXYCITRONELLAL	3; 10	1/8; 2/8	14
10%	HYDROXYCITRONELLAL	10	0/8	14
10%	BENZOYL PEROXIDE	10	8/19	28
40%	DANSYL CHLORIDE	0.05; 0.5; 5.0	0/10; 2/10; 9/10	—

— Not published.

TABLE 11

COMPARATIVE SENSITIZATION RATES DURING PROPHETIC
TEST WITH TWO COSMETIC DYES

SPECIES TESTED	TEST MATERIAL CONC.	CALLENCE COCNC.(%)	RESULTS
GUINIA PIG[1]	40% D&C YELLOW 11	10; 3; 1	9/13; 4/ 13; 1/13
GUINIA PIG	50% D&C YELLOW 10	10	0/ 15
HAMAN[2]	20% D&C YELLOW 11	20	14/ 56
HAMAN[3]	20% D&C YELLOW 10	20	0/105

[1]LAMSON, ET AL. (1982). CONTACT DERMATITIS 8, 200.
[2]RAPAPORT (1980). CONTACT DERMATITIS 6, 364.
[3]AUST & MAIBACH (1981). CONTACT DERMATITIS 7, 257.

TABLE 12

A SUMMARY OF RESULTS: PHOTOALLERGY

INDUCTION CONDITIONS	CHALLENGE CONDITIONS	INCIDENCE
10% MA[1] + UVA[3]	10% MA + UVA	8/10
10% MA + UVA	10% MA	0/10
10% MA	10% MA + UVA	0/10
10% MA	10% MA	0/10
----	10% MA + UVA	0/5
----	10% MA	0/5
0.01% MOP[2] + UVA	0.01% MOP + UVA	10/10
0.01% MOP + UVA	0.01% MOP	0/10
0.01% MOP	0.01% MOP + UVA	7/10
0.01% MOP	0.01% MOP	0/10
----	0.01% MOP + UVA	9/10
----	0.01% MOP	0/10

[1]MA   – MUSK AMBRETTE
[2]MOP   – 8 METHOXYPSORALEN
[3]UVA   – ULTRAVIOLET LIGHT (320–400 NM)

REFERENCES

1. North American Contact Dermatitis Group (1975). The frequency of contact sensitivity in North America 1972-74. Contact Dermatitis 1, 277-280.

2. Prystowski, S.D., Allen, A.M., Smith, R.W., Nomomura, J.H., Odom, R.B. and Akers, W.A. (1979). Allergic contact hypersensitivity to nickel, neomycin, ethylenediamine and benzocaine. Arch. Dermatol. 115, 959-962.

3. Kligman, A.M. (1958). Poison ivy (Rhus) dermatitis. Arch. Dermatol. 77, 149-180.

4. Silberberg, I., Baer, R.L. and Rosenthal, S.A. (1976). The role of the Langerhans cell in allergic contact hypersensitivity. A review of findings in man and guinea pig. J. Invest. Dermatol. 66, 210-217.

5. Polak, L. (1980). Immunologic Aspects of Contact Sensitivity .S.Karger, NY, NY.

6. Klecak, G. (1977). Identification of contact allergens. In Dermatotoxicology and Dermatopharmacology, eds. Marzulli, F. and Maibach, H.I., Halstead Press, NY, NY.

7. Draize, J.H. (1959). Dermal toxicity. In Appraisal of the Safety of Chemicals in Foods, Drugs and Cosmetics. Published by the Association of Food & Drug Officials of the United States. Texas State Department of Health, Austin, Texas.

8. Magnusson, B. & Kligman, A.M. (1970). The identification of contact allergens by animal assay. The guinea pig maximization test. J. Invest. Derumatol. 52, 268-276.

9. Buehler, E.V. (1965). Delayed hypersensitivity in the guinea pig. Arch. Dermatol. 91, 171-177.

10. Asherson, G.L. and Allwood, G.G. (1969). Immunological adjuvants In The Biologic Basis of Medicine, 4, eds. Bittar, E.E. & Bittar, N., Academic Press, NY, NY.

11. Ritz, H. L., Connor, D. E. & Sauter, E. D. (1975). Contact sensitization of guinea pigs with unsaturated and halogenated sultones. Contact Dermatitis 1, 349-358.

12. Rieger, M. M. (1983). The Langerhans cell. Cosmetics & Toiletries 98, 46-50.

13. Ritz, H.L. & Buehler, E. V. (1980) Planning, conduct and interpretation of guinea pig sensitization patch tests. In Current Concepts in Cutaneous Toxicity, eds. Drill, V. A. & Lazar, P., Academic Press, NY, NY.

14. Buehler, E. V. (1982a). Comment on guinea pig test methods. Fd. Cosmet. Toxicol. 20, 494-495.

458

15. Buehler, E. V. (1983). *Experimental contact sensitivity*. In Immunotoxicology, eds. Gibson, G. G., Hubbard, R. & Parke, D. W., Academic Press, NY, NY.

16. Buehler, E.V. (1982b). *A prospective approach for evaluating experimental sensitizers*. The Toxicology Forum 1982 Annual Summer Meeting, Given Institute of Pathobiology, Aspen, CO.

17. Kaidbey, K. H. & Kligman, A. M. (1980). *Photomaximization test for identifying photoallergic contact sensitizers*. Contact Dermatitis 6, 161-169.

18. Kochever, I.E., Zalar, G.L., Einbinder, J. & Harber, L. C. (1979). *Assay of contact photosensitivity to musk ambrette on guinea pigs*. J. Invest. Dermatol. 73, 144-146.

19. Ichikawa, H., Armstrong, R. B. & Harber, L. C. (1981). *Photoallergic contact dermatitis in guinea pigs: improved induction technique using Freund's Complete Adjuvant*. J. Invest. Dermatol. 76, 498-501.

20. Maguire, H. C., Jr. (1973). *The bioassay of contact allergens in the guinea pig*. J. Soc. Cosmet. Chem. 24, 151-162.

21. Maurer, T., Thomann, P., Weinch, E. G. & Hess. R. (1975). *The optimization test in the guinea pig*. Toxicology 15, 163-171.

22. Klecak, G., Geleick, H. & Frey, J.R. (1977). *Screening of fragrance materials for allergenicity in the guinea pig. I. Comparison of four testing methods*. J. Soc. Cosmet Chem. 28, 53-64.

23. Brulos, M. F., Guillot, J. P., Martini, M. C. & Cotte, J. (1977). *The influence of perfumes on the sensitizing potential of cosmetic bases*. J. Soc. Cosmet. Chem. 20, 357.

24. Guillot, J. P., Gonnet, J. F., Clement, C. & Faccini, J. M. (1983). *Comparative study of methods chosen by the Association Francaise De Normalisation (AFNOR) for evaluating sensitizing potential in the guinea pig*. Fd. Cosmet. Toxicol. 21, 795-805.

25. Marzulli, F. N. & Maguire, H. C., Jr. (1982). *Usefulness and limitations of various guinea pig methods in detecting human sensitizers*. Fd. Cosmet. Toxicol. 20, 67-77.

26. Lindup, W. E. & Nowell, P. T. (1978). *Role of sultone contaminants in an outbreak of allergic contact dermatitis caused by alkyl ethoxy sulfates: A review*. Fd. Cosmet. Toxicol. 16, 59-62.

27. Walker, A. P., Ashforth, G. K., Davies, R. E., Newmann, E. A., & Ritz, H. L. (1973). Some characteristics of the sensitizer in alkyl ethoxy sulfate. Acta Dermatovener (Stockholm) 53, 141-144.

28. Poole, R. L., Griffith, J. F. & McMillan, F. S. K. (1970). Experimental contact sensitization with benzoyl peroxide. Arch. Dermatol. 102, 635-639.

29. Cunliffe, W. J. & Burke, B. (1982). Benzoyl peroxide: Lack of sensitization. Acta Dermatovener (Stockholm) 62, 458-459.

30. Friedlaender, M. H. & Baer, H. (1972). The role of the regional lymph node in sensitization and tolerance to simple chemicals. J. Immunol. 109, 1122-1130.

31. Lamson, S. A., Kong, B.M., & DeSalva, S. J. (1982). D&C Yellow Nos. 10 & 11: Delayed contact hypersensitivity in the guinea pig. Contact Dermatitis 8, 200-203.

32. Rapaport, M. J. (1980). Allergy to D&C Yellow No. 11. Contact Dermatitis 6, 364-365.

33. Aust, L. B. & Maibach, H. I. (1981). Modified Draize sensitization test with D&C Yellow No. 10 in combination dye systems. Contact Dermatitis 7, 357.

34. Connor, D. S., Ritz, H. L., Ampulski, R. S., Kowollik, H. G., Lim, P., Thomas, J. W. & Parkhurst, R. (1975). Identification of certain sultones as the sensitizers in an alkyl ethoxy sulfate. Fette Seifen Anstrich. 77, 25-29.

ALLERGIC DRUG REACTIONS

Amos, H.E.

International Medical Affairs Dept
ICI Pharmaceuticals Division
Mereside
Alderkey Park Macclesfield SK10 4TG
Cheshire

INTRODUCTION

In the past the immunotoxicologist has gained considerable comfort from the belief that drug hypersensitivity is an idiosyncratic response, therefore attempting to predict a potential hypersensitivity hazard from pre-clinical compound evaluation is futile. Although agreeing with the sentiment, it is not true to say that information gained in pre-clinical evaluation has no predictive value. The aim of this presentation will be to discuss immunochemical studies which may aid the identification of chemicals/drugs likely to form immunogens.

The basic immunological tenet for a drug immunogen is that drugs must be co-valently bound to macromolecules before they can initiate a primary antibody response. This constitutes the basis for the hapten hypothesis. The term hapten was coined to describe a substance which is not immunogenic per se but will induce a specific immunological response if conjugated to a macromolecular carrier. The hypothesis was formulated as a result of immunochemical studies on chemical contact sensitivity in which the formation of stable co-valent bonds with proteins was shown to be essential to establish the allergic state (1,2). Confirmation of this concept came during the 1960's from several groups working on penicillin allergy (3,5), who demonstrated that antibodies of the M or G type with specificity for the penicilloyl conjugate were readily formed. The absolute requirement for co-valent linkage has been challenged in experimental systems (6), but there is no good evidence to challenge its requirement for the production of clinically overt allergic drug reactions. The formation of conjugates between drugs and autologous macromolecules is thus, a central event in the induction of a drug hypersensitivity reaction, and it is important to establish mechanisms by which drugs are able to conjugate co-valently to proteins and to determine factors which may influence the process.

DIRECT PROTEIN REACTIVITY

From the work on penicillin it is now recognised that the ability of low molecular weight organic chemicals to stimulate an antibody response can be a direct function of their reactivity with nucleophilic groups on proteins or other macromolecules.

Penicillin, for example, has a reactive structure, the Beta lactam ring, which will form co-valent conjugates with proteins by reaction with nucleophilic amino, hydroxy, mercapto and histidiene groups. The major determinant formed, the penicilloyl conjugate, is formed between the Beta lactam carbonyl and -amino groups of lysine residues in proteins (3,4). Initially it was thought that the penicilloyl-protein conjugates were formed principally via the penicillenate rearrangement but subsequent studies have indicated that direct aminolysis is equally important (7). Further degradation of the penicilloyl determinant may give rise to other isomeric forms, which are clinically related more to reaginic antibody formation.

Most drugs do not possess direct protein reactivity, and this is to be expected since lipophilic drugs that react indicriminately with mammalian macromolecular structures are likely to be revealed as either mutagens or carcinogens in preclinical safety evaluation studies and are not developed as therapeutic compounds.

METABOLIC CONVERSION

The majority of drugs undergo metabolic conversion in the body mainly by a mixed function oxygenase system located within the microsomal organells. Phase I reactions introduce into the drug a suitable reactive centre which may then undergo conjugation with amio acids, glucuronic acid or sulphonic acid. Compounds that are well absorbed from the intestinal tract are in general lipophilic and hence need to be rendered more water soluble to facilitate excretion.

Reactive metabolites possess electro deficient active groups and are thus highly electrophilic. This allows them to react with nucleophilic sites which are abundant in large molecules such as proteins. There are data demonstrating a relationship between metabolism and toxicity of compounds such as paracetamol(8) 4-ipomeatol(9), aromatic amines and aromatic hydrocarbons (10), but data implicating reactive metabolites as haptens is sparse. There are however, three distinct types of reaction which involve metabolic process in the elicitation of drug hypersensitivity.

a) Metabolic Status and Auto Allergy

It has been known for some time, that a genetic polymorphism of acetylation exists in man and that rapid and slow acetylator phenotypes exist for the drugs hydralazine, isoniazid, procainamide and sulphamethazine. The status depends on the expression of N-acetyltransferase, and it has been estimated from population studies that approximately 53 % of all Europeans are slow acetylators. The clinical significance of slow acetylation is that patients are more likely to develop a form of lupus erythematosus when treated with the above mentioned drugs (11). There is no indication that in this type of reaction the drug acts as a hapten and induces a specific antibody response, but the correlation between metabolic status and diseases is well established.

b) Metabolites Acting on Haptens

Metabolites functioning as haptens was more clearly demonstrated by the investigation on adverse reaction induced by the Beta-receptor blocking drug practolol. Using an in-vitro microsomal mixed function oxygenase to metabolise practolol, antibodies could be detected to generated reactive species. The specificity of the metabolite antigenic determinants were not defined but a displacement assay with model compounds based on the practolol structure showed that an intact isopropanolamine side chain was important to the determinant. These studies did not demonstrate that the metabolite antigen-antibody interaction contributed to the clinical adverse effect. In fact, the data relating to the clinical correlation was inconclusive (12).

c) Metabolite-tissue Interaction

Involvement of metabolites in liver necrosis following exposure to halothane has been claimed. The mechanism does not require a halothane metabolite to function as a hapten, but to interact with liver cell membranes which then become altered and induce a cytotoxic auto antibody (13). The reactive metabolite is formed via the major oxidative pathway and is thus formed in the majority of individuals undergoing anaesthesia with halothane. It is not yet clear why such a readily formed metabolite which should react with hepatocytes in most individuals, induces an adverse reaction only in a very small number of subjects.

It is not known to what extent drug metabolites feature in allergic drug reaction, mainly because reactive species are difficult to identify and utilise in immunological assay systems. Further work exploring the applicability of the in-vitro metabolising system as used for practolol might produce more information.

CHEMICAL INTERACTIONS

The proposition that functional groups capable of co-valent bond formation can be generated in chemicals by interaction with environmental agents, is yet to be explored.

Chlorine, for example, is a relatively ubiquitous molecule, and it is widely used in domestic water supplies for purification. there is sufficient, albeit sparse literature, on N-chloramido compounds, to indicate that almost any compound carrying an imidic residue X-NH-Y will yield the corresponding chloramide X-NC1-Y on contact with elemental chlorine or the hypochlorite. Whether such interaction, which should encourage co-valent linkages with nucleophilic groups on proteins, will be of any significance in the formation of hapten protein conjugates, remains to be established.

CLINICAL SIGNIFICANCE OF CONJUGATES FORMED BETWEEN SMALL MOLECULAR WEIGHT CHEMICALS AND PROTEINS

The most important consequence of conjugate formation is activation of the immunological system, but it must be remembered that conjugation with endogenous compounds is a normal process in excretion, and many small molecules are rapidly cleared without recourse to antibody formation.

There are also many additional factors which operate to convert a co-valently bound complex into an immunogen.

1) Conjugate Stability

Triggering the immunological system takes a finite time, and the integrity of the antigenic determinant must be maintained for the duration. Thiol reactive drugs such as captopril which form disulphide linkages with plasma proteins, would be expected to stimulate antibodies. It has been shown that three hours after an intravenous administration of radiolabelled captopril to rats, 35% of total radioactivity in plasma was co-valently bound to plasma proteins. Such complexes however, are rapidly broken down in the presence of endogenous thiols such as glutathione and cysteine with the concomitant excretion of captopril mixed disulphides (14). Immunochemical studies in rabbits failed to demonstrate any antibodies with captopril specificity, inferring that the captopril-plasma protein conjugates were too labile to stimulate an antibody response, (Yeung and Park, 1984. Unpublished observations).

2) Epitope Density

There is an undoubted correlation between the degree of hapten substitution on the carrier molecule and immunogenic potency. For example, a conjugate which contains 11 penicilloyl residues per bovine serum albumen molecule will induce antibody formation in mice after a single injection, but if the ratio is less than one no antibodies can be detected even after three injections (15). It is worth noting that epitope density may influence the non-immune excretion of drug macromolecular conjugates. Using dinitrophenylated protein conjugates, it has been shown that following intravenous injection with epitope densities of 10-20 there was a marked increase in uptake of conjugate into the liver Kupfer cells (16,17). Subsequent degradation by liver lysosomal enzymes releases N-acetyldinitrophenyl lysine into the bile for excretion.

3) Nature of the carrier molecule

Little attention has been paid to the influence of the carrier molecule on antibody responses to haptens, but there are data to show that the influence may be considerable. In an elegant study using intra lymphatic infusion of various dinitrophenylated conjugates (18,19) for contact sensitivity it was shown that a cell mediated response was induced by

<u>in-vivo</u> conjugated afferent lymph node cells. Conjugation to
serum albumen or globulin failed to create en effective
immunogen.

Conjugation of haptens to immunoglobulin may lead to a state
of immunological tolerance rather than a specific hapten
immune response. Haptenated immunoglobulins are more
effective B cell tolerogens than haptenated non-immunoglobulin
proteins which suggest that the carrier portion of a drug
protein conjugate can contribute to its tolerogenicity as well
as to its immunogenicity.

4) Drug induced auto allergy

A difficult safety evaluation question which must be addressed
is the toxicological significance of auto antibodies induced
by drug administration. There is no doubt that auto
antibodies are found in systemic disease, eg, thyroiditis and
membranous nephritis, but auto antibodies arising in response
to a specific drug stimulus may occur without any concomitant
sign of an underlying pathological process. Moreover, the
antibodies are transient - their presence depending on the
continued initiating stimulus.

It is axiomatic that under normal conditions antibodies are
not produced against self tissue, but in normal individuals
there are auto-reactive B cells held under some form of
constraint which may be multifactorial, eg, colonal deletions,
suppressor cell activity or malfunction of antigen presenting
cells (20). The main constraint, however, on auto reactive B
cell clone activitation is suppression of T inducer cells.
This suppression can be bypassed if self determinants are
connected with a new carrier for which T induces are not
tolerant (20,21,22). The new carrier determinants can be
provided by a number of agents of which drugs may be one.
Production of auto antibodies by this mechnism will not
invariably lead to a disease state. There is an inbuilt
ability to dampdown auto antibody production through T
suppressor interactions; a mechanism which contributes to the
transient nature of the response.

An interesting suggestion but as yet unproven, is that certain
drugs may derepress gene coding for class II antigens (HL-D).
This would allow their expression in the plasma membrane and
create neodeterminants. It is not certain what the
consequences of such a mechanism would be, this would depend
on the stability of derepressed genes (23).

Auto antibodies, of course, may be an indication of direct
tissue toxicity, although conclusive evidence is difficult to
find. It was thought at the time that methyldopa could
interfere with the integrity of red blood cell membranes
leading to auto antibodies with specificity for the Rh antigen
system (24). There is some doubt, however, whether this is
the whole story as it has subsequently been shown that
methyldopa has an effect on the suppressor arc of the immune
response (25).

It is unlikely that these mechanisms comprehensively account for the production of auto antibodies but each of them may require a different toxicological interpretation. It is difficult, however, to decide which mechanism of auto antibody production is operating, when faced with the demonstration of auto antibodies without clinical signs of an untoward effect.

CONCLUSION

The study of drug allergies is a complex toxicological problem which outstrips the limited horizons of academic immunology. Being able to predict potential immunogens is a priority for the immunotoxicologist, but much more understanding is needed on the immunochemistry of immunogen formation before suitable test systems can be contemplated.

It is certainly an achievable aim to define the criteria necessary for a small molecular weight compound to switch on the immunological systems, but is this a toxic event? Clearly hypersensitivity can ensue, but the normal sequence of events may be that antibody formation is an adaptive response of the individual's normal biological activity. Certainly it is known that many individuals have antibodies to the pencilloyl conjugate of penicillin without experiencing clinical hypersensitivity (7). To what extent antibodies are found against other drugs during an uneventful therapeutic regime is not exactly known and it is doubtful if such a survey would ever be carried out.

Thus, although it may be possible to define a drug immunogen, it is not possible for pre-clinical evaluation studies to predict the incidence of hypersensitivity responses. It could be debated whether this objective would ever be reached, but as these date are necessary for patient protection, perhaps the emphasis should move from pre-clinical studies to the clinical monitory phase. This would entail specific monitoring of the immune response, utilising immunochemical data in immunological assays.

REFERENCES

1) Landsteiner K. (1945) The specificity of serological reactions. Harvard University Press, Cambridge

2) Eisen H.N., Orris L., Belman S. (1952) Elicitation of delayed allergic skin reactions with haptens. The dependence of elicitation on hapten combination with protein. J. Exp. Med. 95. 473-487

3) Batchelor F.R., Dewdney J.M., Cazzard D. (1965) Penicillin allergy: the formation of penicilloyl determinant. Nature (London). 206. 362-364

4) Parker C.W., de Weck A.K., Kern M., Eisen H.N. (1962) The preparation and some properties of penicillenic acid derivatives relevant to penicillin hypersensitivity. J. Exp. Med. 115.803-819

5) Levine B. B. (1965) Immunochemical mechanisms involved
    in penicillin hypersensitivity in experimental animals
    and in human beings. Fed. Proc. 24. 45-50

6) Plescia O. J., Braun W., & Palczuk N.C. (1964) Produc-
    tion of antibodies to denatured desoxyribonucleic acid.
    Prod. nat. Acad. Sci. (Wash.), 52. 279

7) Parker C.W. (1982) Allergic reactions in man. Pharma-
    cological Reviews 34. 84-104

8) Gillette J. R. (1981) An integrated approach to the
    study of chemically reactive metabolites of
    acetaminophen. Intern. Med. 141. 375-379

9) Boyd M R. (1977) Evidence for the Clara cell as a site
    of cytochrome P450-dependent mixed function oxidase
    activity in th lung. Nature 269. 713-715

10) Miller J.A. (1970) Carcinogenesis of chemicals: an
    overview. Cancer Res. 30. 559-576

11) Perry H.M. J., Tane M. & Camody S. (1970) Relationship
    of acetyl transferase activity to antinuclear antibodies
    and toxic symptoms in hypertensive patients treted with
    hydralazine J. Lab. clin. Med. 76. 114-125

12) Amos H. E. (1980) Immunologically mediated toxicity.
    Ciba. Symp. 76. Environmental Chemicals Enzyme Func-
    tion and Human Disease. Pub. Exceptor Medica,
    Amsterdam. 245-255

13) Vergani D., Mieli Vergani G., Alberti A., Neuberger J.M.,
    Eddleston A. L.W. F., David M. & Williams R. (1980)
    Antibodies on the surface of halothane altered rabbit
    hepatocytes in patients with severe halothane associated
    hepatitis. N.Eng. J. Med. 303. 66-71

14) Yeung J.H.K., Breckenridge A.M. & Park B.K. (1983) Drug
    protein conjugates VI. Role of glutathione in the
    metabolism of captopril and captopril protein conjugates.
    Biochem. Pharmac. 32. 3619-3625.

15) Kristofferson A., Ahlstedt S., & Svard P. O. (1977)
    Antigens in Penicillin Allergy III. The influence of the
    number of penicilloyl residues on the antigenicity of
    macromolecules as determined by radioimmunoassay (RIA),
    passive cutaneous anaphylaxis (PCA) and antibody
    induction. Int. Arch. Allergy App. Immunol. 55.
    23-28

16) Kitterringham N. R., Maggs J.K., Newby S. & Park B. K.
    (1984) Drug Protein Conjugates VIII. The metabolis fate
    of the dinitrophenyl residue conjugated to albumin.
    Biochem. Parmac. In press.

17) Buys C. H. C. M., De Jong A. S. H., Bouna J. M. N. & Gruber M. (1972) Rapid uptake by liver sinusoidal cells of serum, albumin modified with retention of its compact conformation. Biochemica et. Biophysica Acta. 392. 95-100

18) Soeberg B., Summerska T., Binns R.M. Balfour B. M. (1978a) Contact sensitivity in the pig II. Induction by intralymphatic infusion of DNP conjugated cells. Int. Arch. Allergy apl. Immun. 57. 114-125

19) Soeberg B., Summerska T., Binns R. M. Balfour B.M. (1978b) Contact sensitivity in the pig III. Induction by intralymphatic infusion of DNP-conjugated cell membranes and soluble proteins, free DNFB and small molecular weight derivatives. Int. Archs. Allergy appl. Immun. 57. 481-487

20) Weigle W.O. (1971) Recent observations and concepts in immunological unresponsiveness and autoimmunity. Clin. Exp. Immunol. 9. 437-444

21) Allison A. C., Denman A. M. & Barnes R. D. (1971) Co-operating and controlling functions of thymus-derived lymphocytes in relation to autoimmunity. Lancet 2. 135-136

22) Cooke A. & Lydyard P. M. (1981) The role of T cells in autoimmune disease. Path. & Res. Pract. 171. 173-175

23) Cooke A., Lydyard P. M. & Roitt I.M. Mechanisms of autoimmunity: a role for cross reactive idiotypes. Immunology Today 4. 170-175

24) Carstairs K. C., Breckenridge A., Dollery C. Y. & Worlledge S. M. (1966) Incidence of a positive direct Coombs' test in patients treated with alpha-methyldopa. Lancet, ii, 133

25) Worlledge S. M., Carstairs K. C. & Dacie J. V. (1966) Auto-immune haemolytic anaemia associated with alpha-methyldopa therapy. Lancet, ii, 135

CONTACT HYPERSENSITIVITY TO ENVIRONMENTAL CHEMICALS

H. Maibach

University of California Hospital,
U.C. Medical Centre,
San Francisco, CA 94/43
U.S.A.

DEFINITION

Allergic contact dermatitis has been defined in many ways:
the classical statement in toxicology texts states that it
occurs after multiple (rather than first) exposures, is
immunologic (cell mediated), and that it can be reproduced by
patch testing at low levels of antigen. In recent years this
definition has proven inadequate and it has led to incorrect
classification of several dermatitis producing chemicals. For
this reason, an operational, rather than a purely mechanistic
definition, has proven more useful. This operational definition includes not only patch test results, but verification
(retesting) and provocative use tests, to rule out the Excited
Skin Syndrome (see below).

It is not clear whether delayed hypersensitivity in the guinea
pig and man are identical in reference to allergic contact
dermatitis.   An important difference is that allergic contact
dermatitis can be passively transferred readily with immunogenic cells in the guinea pig, but not reliably in man.
Whether this is a technical or mechanistic difference is not
known.   Its practical ramification is that allergic contact
dermatitis in the guinea pig can be definitively defined in a
mechanistic sense by utilising passive transfer of immunogenic
cells; this opportunity is denied to us in human studies, and
argues for an operational rather than purely mechanistic
definition.

It is important to separate delayed hypersensitivity <u>per se</u>
from clinical allergic contact dermatitis. The latter clearly
implies a clinically demonstrable lesion. Many patients have
patch test hyperreactivity on a presumed hypersensitivity
basis without a clear history of clinical allergic contact
dermititis.   Others with patch test hyperrreactivity will not
respond to a provocative-use test with environmental agents
containing the antigen, thus other factors such as dose
pharmacokinetics, method of use, and other unidentified
factors must be involved.

TELEOLOGY OF HUMAN ALLERGIC CONTACT DERMATITIS

Why does man develop allergic contact dermatitis?   Patients
suffering from this clinical entity certainly ask this
question. In a teleological sense delayed hypersensitivity is
often protective, i.e., in resistance to microbial infection.
However, in advanced carcinomatosis, allergic contact dermatitis' and delayed hypersensitivity are diminished. Did man,
in fact, develop allergic contact dermatitis for some useful

function, or is it in fact a totally negative development for man? The answer should help decide the ultimate need and adviseability of the removing allergens from the human environment.

DIAGNOSTIC TECHNIQUES

The patch test was developed in 1896. Yet, it has only been in recent years, largely through the leadership of the International Contact Dermatitis Research Group, that any aspects ot this bioassay have been standardized. In spite of the many advances, much remains to be accomplished. Recently, Torkel Fisher (Uppsala) has identified many additional potential improvements: these includes identifying an extraordinary lack of homogenity in the standard commercial antigen preparations, and the importance of correct loading of patch test chambers. Unfortunately, even with the great improvement in our practical techniques in the last decade, no commercial practical patch test diagnostic kit exists suitable for use in much of the world where there is limited dermatological supervision. The development of stable, homogenous, easily applied preparations for the 100-200 most common allergens would greatly improve this aspect of health in the developed and under developed countries.

EPIDEMIOLOGY

Our knowledge of the epidemiology of allergic contact dermatitis has improved significantly - largely under the aegis of the International Contact Dermatitis Research Group. Unfortunately available data tell us only about the frequency of contact allergy in populations that have access to sophisticated dermatoallergy clinics. Even here, much of the data interpretation is clouded by the fact that only a few studies have been performed in which patch test respondees have been thoroughly evaluated - utilizing the operational techniques described above to ascertain the likelihood of a truly clinically relevant allergy. The importance of such follow-ups is that almost half of all positives in battery testing may be non specific (non-allergic) - due to the Excited Skin Syndrome, and not due to true allergy. Only when follow up studies of this type become generally available will we have a better view of the number of patients who have allergic contact dermatitis in this special clinical environment. The only available data,and that for a few chemicals, on the frequency of allergic contact dermatitis comes from the general population,i.e. from so called "normal" volunteers, who are not usually seen in the context of a dermatitis clinic. This type of data is urgently needed to validate the relevance of animal and human toxicologic assays for clinical allergic contact dermatitis in the general population.

TOXICOLOGIC ASSAYS

Guinea pig

The guinea pig assay has been vigorously exploited by many investigators since it was initiated by Landsteiner and Chase (1). The volume of data and the number of available methods are sufficiently large that a text book summarizing this aspect alone will shortly be published. It is clear that methods vary in their advantages and disadvantages. The tests are no better than the competence and experience of the investigator planning the study and the skills of the technician performing the tests. It is unfortunate that this task is often relegated to the most junior person in the laboratory, when, in fact, the complexity of design, performance, reading, and interpretation requires extensive training, experience and judgement. It is not until there are more laboratories fulfilling these latter criteria that public health will be served in this important area.

studies in humans.

In Europe there is considerable controversy over the appropriateness of performing human allergic contact dermatitis assays. In the United States the general experience has been that appropriately planned and supervised, the risk to the volunteer is minimal and the information gained invaluable for the general population The basic issue then is whether it is appropriate to apply new chemicals to an informed small population of volunteers under carefull supervision or if it is better to allow millions of consumers to unknowingly use the chemicals. It is my judgement that the former is preferable, ethical, and highly effective, in terms of public health.

Dose-Response Relationships

Whether dealing with experiments on the guinea pig or human or clinical allergic contact dermatitis in man, there has been considerable controversy over-dose response relationships. Some knowledgeable investigators have insisted that they do not exist. Industrial policy has sometimes taken the same approach. Fortunately current experimental data in the guinea pig and man indicates that there is a dose-response relationship and that much benefit can be obtained by determining the Minimum Threshhold Level for Induction and the Minimal Threshhold Level for Elicitation in such experiments (2). This allows one to begin to consider developing so called safety factors that are invaluable in making judgements of risk for intended use.

Structure-Activity Relationship (SAR)

Although guinea pig and human studies can identify contact allergens, the synthetis chemist needs quicker more efficient techniques to ascertain if he is likely to be developing a contact allergen. Dupuis and Benezra have summarized the data on what physico-chemical properties are involved in the proclivity of a chemical to induce allergic contact dermatitis (3).

This work is currently being extended in a cooperative venture between C. Benezra (Strasbourg), C.Sigman and T. Helmes (Menlo Park, California), and myself (4). All publications on guinea pig and human sensitization are being entered into the SRI computer with notation for the chemical structure, its physico-chemical properties, and quantification and qualification of the biological data. It is hoped that this SAR approach will lead to more approapriate prediction of sensitization proclivity from chemical structure.

PERCUTANEOUS PENETRATION

No matter what technique is used, i.e., SAR or assay systems in a guinea pig and/or man, there will be many situations in which the data will require sophisticated interpretation in terms of actual usage. Many chemicals (formalin, benzoyl peroxide, etc.) are potent sensitizers in these models. Human experience has indicated that they can be safely handled by the vast majority of human beings if the appropriate concentrations and circumstances are employed. Judgements about risk evaluation are facilitated if appropriate data on percutaneous penetration is available. Percutaneous penetration is a multi step procedure: several of these are quantifiable (5). When a chemical does not cross the skin and reach the appropriate immunogenic cells, there will be no allergy. Thus obtaining penetration and substantivety data is an efficent aid in interpreting the sensitization assays.

COMMENT

In summary, the last decades have been highly productive in the field of allergic contact dermatitis. However much of the information is clinically available only in limited centres. The next decade should see the training of more people who can bring this information to the remainder of the world and to improve upon the methodologies currently being used to diagnose and prevent allergic contact dermatitis.

REFERENCES

(1) Anderdersen, K. & Maibach, H. : Allergic Contact Dermatitis Assays in the Guinea Pig, in press, Karger, Basel.

(2) Marzulli, F. & Maibach, H. : Dermatotoxicology, 3rd. ed., Hemisphere Press, Washington, D.C. + McGraw Hill, New York, in press.

(3) Dupuis, & Benezra, C. : Allergic Contact Dermatitis: A Molecular Approach, Marcel Dekker, New York, 1983.

(4) Benezra, C., Sigman, C., Helmes, T. & Maibach, H. : Allergic Contact Dermatitis: A Structure Activity Approach, submitted for publication, 1984.

(5) Bronaugh, R. & Maibach, H. : Percutaneous Penetration: Principles and Practices, Marcel Dekker, New York, in press, 1985.

LUNG REACTIONS TO ENVIRONMENTAL CHEMICALS

J. MORLEY

Switzerland

EXPOSURE OF THE LUNG TO ENVIRONMENTAL CHEMICALS

The high metabolic requirements of human tissue necessitate regular inspiration and expiration to maintain adequate levels of tissue oxygen. Hence, exposure of airway epithelia to the environment is in essence constant. This circumstance can be presumed to account for the development and retention of certain anatomical and physiological features of the respiratory tract in mammalian species. For instance, respiration via the nares causes air to traverse a series of chambers,which serve to limit ingress of particles and of water-soluble noxi into the airways. A similar function is subserved by the branching of large airways within the lung, which favours deposition of particles by impaction. A physiological counterpart to these anatomical adaptations is provided by bronchoconstrictor responses to stimuli (such as particles of aerosols) which, together with the cough and sneeze reflexes, protect lung epithelium from exposure to noxi (1). Normally, the surface of airway epithelium is coated by plaques of mucus which can form a continuous layer. As in the stomach, this material may provide a barrier to noxi, including micro-organisms which may be precluded thereby from contact and attachment to epithelial cells. The mucus layer also facilitates removal of inhaled material, for the gel layer of this mucus blanket is transported in an adoral direction by ciliated cells which line tracheal and bronchial surfaces (2). It is likely that the response to certain noxi includes changes in the composition and volume of bronchial mucus secretion so as to facilitate removal by mucociliary transport, although quantitative description of such events is difficult to achieve. Finally, within the airways there is a sustained migration of haematogenous cells into the eipithelial surface. Cells of the granulocyte lineage may serve to assist in destruction of invading parasites; whilst activation of mononuclear cells to macrophages provides a mechanism for phagocytosis of particulate material, hence macrophages are the predominant cell type in samples of bronchial secretion or broncho-alveolar lavage. Lymphocytes are also represented in lung, not only as circulating cells, but as constituents of organised lymphoid tissue, which serves to respond to allergen exposure by local secretion of immmunoglobulin (IgA) into bronchial fluid, as well as by formation of immonoglobulins which enter the circulation (IgG and IgE) and by initiation of T-cell-dependent immune responses (3).

It is apparent, therefore, that the lung exhibits a number of features which combine to minimise the effects of noxious environmental chemicals. However, certain of these endogenous processes, particularly those involving cellular activation, may serve to induce tissue damage following exposure to noxious chemicals. Such processes can be considered to represent an excessive, or inappropriate, response to the inciting agent, alternatively responses may represent a manifestation of hypersensitivity to allergen.

Endogenous inflammatory reactions in lung

Even when an environmental chemical is directly cytotoxic, endogenous processes predominate in the tissue reaction, as is evidenced by a common pattern of inflammation, irrespective of the inciting agency (4). Inflammatory responses have been most extensively analysed in skin, but it is reasonable to presume that corresponding changes occur in lung. Lung tissue can respond to noxious stimuli by the expression of plasma protein extravasation indicative of increased vascular permeability. This can be visualised directly in the bronchi of experimental animals following intravenous injection of Evans blue dye prior to sacrifiece; whilst in man erythema and oedema of bronchial mucosa have been observed to be acute sequelae of antigen application during bronchoscopy (5). The erythematous element of the inflammatory response has not been measured in lungs of intact animals, but the extravasation can be quantitated conveniently by use of radiolabelled dye. In the isolated, perfused lung, agents such as histamine cause an increased resistance to perfusion, from which it may be inferred that exudation in responses to this and other permeability factors may include an element of increased bulk flow resulting from the increased hydrostatic pressure across capillary walls (6).

The endogenous agencies which induce increased vessel wall permeability in the lung are not dissimilar from those that are effective in skin; thus, amines such as histamine, peptides such as bradykinin, and phospholipids such as Paf-acether, are potent permeability factors. In skin, vasodilator materials strongly enhance the plasma protein extravasation which follows permeability factor injection or release. It is not known if such processes are operative in lung. In skin, the vascular action may cause an increase in the vessel wall area that has been affected by the permeability factor (7) and/or an increase in hydrostatic pressure at the site of increased vessel wall porosity. Extrapolation of this scheme to pulmonary tissue may not be warranted if the increased perfusion pressure is of primary importance in causing extravasation. Yet, there are indications that potentiation may be a feature of prostaglandin effects, on lung tissue. For example, PGF_2 alpha is a most potent expectorant by inhalation (8), even though in vitro it has only modest effects on mucus secretion, or on ciliary activity. Similarly, PGE_2, which relaxes airway smooth muscle in normal aninmals and has proved to be bronchoconstrictor in the majority of asthmatics and causes retrosternal pain following inhalation (9).

In terms of acute inflammatory reactions to environmental chemicals, there are several points of resemblance between the lung and the skin. Thus, in addition to the vascular manifestations that characterise inflammation, there is also an infiltration of haematogenous cells, with a preponderance of polymorphonuclear leucocytes during the acute response that can predispose to mononuclear cell accumulation. Such responses are commonly self-limiting and reflect progression of an endogenous inflammatory process. However, more persistent changes may follow stimuli to the lung, where by exposure is effectively constant (e.g. atmospheric pollution by oxides of nitrogen or sulphur, repeated inhalation of tobacco smoke, or alveolar deposition of silica or asbestos fibres). In such circumstances,there may be persisting cellular infiltration with secondary changes of pulmonary tissue. These secondary changes can include bronchial smooth muscle hypertrophy, mucus gland hypertrophy and hyperplasia, and activation of fibroblasts (10). The biochemical basis of these processes remains poorly understood, even though they represent the major determinants of lung pathology in prevalent diseases such as asthma, bronchitis, emphysema and carcinoma of the bronchus.

Platelet activating factor

Since inflammatory reactions conform to a common pattern, it is reasonable to attempt to relate persisting pathology to the release or generation of inflammatory mediators. However, until recently, the inflammatory stimulus provided by those mediators that have been characterised chemically have proved insufficient to account for the sustained pathology of cellular inflammation. A noteworthy exception is PAF (platelet activating factor) which can be referred to as Paf-acether, AGEPC or ARPL (11). PAF was described originally as a product of allergen activation of IgE-sensitised rabbit basophils. With an appreciation of the chemical structure of PAF, it has become evident that production of PAF is not restricted to the basophil and there is now evidence that PAF is also generated by neutrophils, macrophages, eosinophils and platelets; moreover, it is apparent that stimuli to PAF formation include both non-allergic and allergic agencies (11). In the context of lung pathology, it is noteworthy that PAF is produced in significant quantities by lung macrophages, as might be anticipated for a cell-type in which arachidonic acid comprises the major polyunsaturated acid constituent of membrane fatty acids and in which there is an abundance of phospholipase A_2 in the outer cell membrane (12). It is possible that there may be preferential formation of PAF by alveolar macrophages in certain forms of lung pathology, for it is known that different patterns of arachidonic acid metabolism are observed when cells collected by broncho-alveolar lavage from patients with asthma and bronchitis are cultured in vitro. Moreover, in asthma, it has been reported that alveolar macrophages produce significant quantities of PAF in circumstances in which normal cells are ineffectual (13). Thus, existing evidence favours a conclusion that PAF formation by lung tissue represents a common response during inhalation of noxious chemicals. It remains to be established whether the quantities of PAF so generated are sufficient to induce pathological effects; there is no convenient metabolic indicator of PAF formation, since lyso-PAF, the precursor and degradation product of PAF, exists in relatively high concen-

trations that would not be noticeably affected by PAF
metabolism. However, it is known that endogenous generation
of PAF results in impaired reactivity of circulating platelets
to PAF activation without loss of reactivity to other stimuli.
Such an effect can be achieved by inhalation of antigen
(14,15) or in acute severe astham (14). It is reasonable to
assume, therefore, that PAF can be formed in the lung in
amounts sufficient to cause substantial biological effects.

Both the nomenclature and much original research have emphasised the effect of PAF upon platelets. However, it is now
apparent that low concentrations of PAF can produce biological
effects, not only as a consequence of effects upon platelets,
but also by directly affecting other cell types (11). Hence,
during inflammation, both platelet-independent and
platelet-dependent effects can be anticipated. Thus, PAF
produces pronounced increased vascular permeability in animals
that have been depleted of circulating platelets, or in
animals in which platelet activation has been suppressed by
use of drugs (11); more direct evidence of
platelet-independent processes is provided by the observation
that PAF produces increased vascular permeability in isolated
perfused lungs (11). On the other hand, cell accumulation at
sites of PAF application only becomes evident in animals when
platelets are responsive to PAF. Thus, platelet accumulation
precedes the accumulation of granulocytes and the more persistent accumulation of mononuclear cells that is evident in
response to PAF in guinea-pig skin (11,16), but these effects
are not evident in the rat, whose platelets are unresponsive
to PAF. In the lung, such cellular inflammatory responses to
PAF inhalation are both pronounced and persistent, such that,
after single exposure of the rabbit lung to PAF, inflammatory
changes remain evident for up to a month (17).

Bronchoconstrictor responses to PAF are also platelet- dependent and, hence, are not evident in animals from which platelets have been depleted. The acute bronchoconstrictor response to intravenous PAF is impressive because of the potency of
this material; perhaps of greater biological relevance
however, is the more sustained response to inhalation of PAF,
which becomes evident over several hours. This response is
reminiscent, in both time-course and histopathology, of the
response to allergen inhalation in IgE-sensitised animals
(18). It is now known that increased bronchial
hyper-reactivity is a consequence of allergen inhalation in
such experimental animals, as is also evident in allergic
asthmatics; hence, it may be presumed that the response to
PAF may be succeeded by increased hyper-reactivity, especially
as responses both to PAF (18) and allergen (18) are sensitive
to inhibition by DSCG. Should this prediction be fulfilled,
then effects of PAF as a bronchoconstrictor agent will be
determined by two processes: firstly, by acting as an acute
constrictor agent and, secondly, by serving as an agency which
sensitises the lung to other agents. This latter effect is of
considerable interest because of the theoretical and practical
consequences that arise. At an academic level, the subordina-
tion of mast cells to macrophages in schemes of asthmatic

pathology represents a major shift of emphasis; the practical consequence lies in the prospect of identifying appropriate therapy for airway hyper-reactivity and, more particularly, for prophylaxis against the intensification of airway hyper-reactivity that may be a consequence of ingestion or inhalation of environmental chemicals. It must be emphasised that generation of PAF to produce adverse effects in the lung need not necessarily depend upon exposure to chemical agents by inhalation. Oral ingestion of materials can also activate platelets by generating PAF systematically, as during release of entreric endotoxin into the circulation. In this later category may be included not only food allergens, but also chemial toxins or food additives, which may be ingested in amounts sufficient to cause pseudo-allergic reactions (19).

Therapeutic implications

Acute severe inflammatory reactions to inhaled chemicals may necessitate anti-inflammatory therapy, in which circumstances steroids are pre-eminent. In these circumstances and for other less severe consequences of adverse reactions to inhaled or ingested chemicals, it is conventional to advocate avoidance of the inciting chemical. Thus prevention of future occurrences of tissue injury can be achieved by elimination or enclosure of the offending chemical. For environmental chemicals that are rarely encountered and can be unequivocally identified, such advice is of undisputed benefit. However because of the many possible responses of lung tissue, such an approach may be inappropriate. Thus, when pseudo-allergic reactions to drugs or food are identified, it is usual to instigate avoidance measures. However, such advice may be difficult to adhere to, since the inciting agent or agencies may be ubiquitous in distribution or even difficult to identify. Moreover, exposure may be inherent in the environment of an individual, such as with an occupational allergy, when avoidance would mean long-term, premature, unemployment. Understandably, such advice is unwelcome to an affected individual. Furthermore, although it is widely accepted that avoidance is unquestionably beneficial, such an assumption may be unwarranted. For example, in analgesic hypersensitivity, the exquisite sensitivity of certain individuals may be overcome by regular exposure to an analgesic such as aspirin; conversely, such subjects become highly sensitive to aspirin following aspirin avoidance (20). This type of phenomenon may account for the mixed fortunes of avoidance therapy and raise questions as to the benefit of indiscriminate use of this therapeutic strategy for ubiquitous chemicals to which individuals have become hypersensitive.

On the other hand, many hypersensitivity reactions are due to antibody-mediated allergic responses. Individuals who develop high titers of IgE to a specific allergen can respond to inhalation of such substances by severe and sustained inflammatory reations (21). Such allergic asthamatics benefit from allergen avoidance although benefit only becomes clearly evident over a period of months. Individuals showing such hypersensitivity may, in practice, be unable to avoid common allergens for a sufficient period for reversal of pathological changes in lung to become evident. An analogous problem may be posed by highly reactive industrial chemicals which enter the environment, for whilst such substances are not toxic per se, they may induce toxic reactions by systemic effects which change the responsivity of a subject, as is well illustrated by toluene di-isocyanate (23).

It is of interest to consider what proportion of the population may have been adversely affected by chemicals to an extent that they have significant airway pathology. There is a high prevalence of respiratory disease in Western society which, in part, may be attributed to regular exposure to viral infection of the airways and to regular inhalation of tobacco smoke. However, there is also evidence that children commonly experience wheezing in early life and this impression is confirmed from estimates of the incidence of children with increased reactivity to bronchial provocation (e.g. histamine inhalation), when values between 10 and 20% have been cited. Such children may be classified as asthmatic or may be considered as predisposed to subsequent expression of clinical asthma. Participation of genetic and infective fctors cannot be precluded (24), but it seems inescapable that environmental chemicals contribute to this abnormality in a substantial proportion of affected individuals. Asthma death is relatively uncommon, so that mortality does not provide a satisfactory estimate of asthma incidence. However, it is noticeable that death rates seem little affected by a progressive improvement of therapeutics in this disease, which may warrant suspicion of an increase in the incidence and severity of asthma.

Thus, a pattern emerges in which the tendency to persistent airway dysfunction, either as asthma or bronchitis, is increased by the exposure to environmental chemicals of natural (allergen and toxins) or synthetic (haptens, pseudo-allergens and toxins) origin. Persisting airway dysfunction may possibly reverse as a consequence of endogenous influence (i.e. puberty or pregnancy); however, more commonly it continues as a sub-clinical state which can be manifest as asthma in circumstances involving further inflammatory events. It is suggested that the events which determine this intensification of symptomatology involve PAF formation and consequent neutrophil activation (18). Hence, changes which impair this succession of events will be prophylactic for expression of asthma and possibly exacerbation of bronchitis. Drugs which have been shown to be effective inhibitors of PAF-induced pathology include DSCG, ketotifen, theophylline and steroids. DSCGH impairs PAF-induced pathological events in the lung by a mechanism yet to be identified. Ketotifen and theophylline, on the other hand, have been shown to impair platelet-dependent secretion, both in vitro and in vivo at therapeutic concentrations. In addition to inhibiting platelet-dependent secretion, other sites, are affected which may be presumed to include leucocyte activation and recruitment (i.e. anti-flammatory effects). Low concentrations of ketotifen suffice to inhibit the secretory effect of platelet activation without impairing the thrombotic function of these organelles and there is a noteworthy absence of long-term toxicity both from this drug and from theophylline. Consideration should therefore be given to the identification of compounds of low toxicity whose use in prophylaxis could preempt progression into asthma and possibly bronchitis in subjects who are unavoidably exposed to environmental chemicals that induce astham or bronchitis in predisposed individuals.

480

REFERENCES

1. J.G. Widdicombe, Re gulation of tracheobronchial smooth muscle, Physiol. Rev., 43 (1963) 1-37.

2. A Wanner, Clinical Aspects of mucociliary transport, Am. Rev. Resp. Dis., 116 (1977) 73-125.

3. P. cole, Immunology of Respiratory Diseases. In `Immunology in Medicine' (Eds) E.J. Holborrow and W.G. Reeves, Academic Press, London, 1977.

4. H. florey (d), General Pathology, W.B. Saunders Compagny, Philadelphia, 1958.

5. B.J. Hutchcroft, Cited in discussion, In 'Asthma: Physiology, Immunopharmacology and Treatment' (Eds) L.M. Lichtenstein and K.F. Austen, Academic Press Inc, New York, 1977.

6. A.C. Guyton (ed), Textbook of Medical Phsiology, W.B. Saunders Company, Philadelphia, 1971.

7. T.J. Williams, prostaglandin E2, Prostaglandin I2 and the vascular changes of inflammation, Brit. J. Pharmacol., 65 (1979) 517-527.

8. M.T. Lopez-Vidriero, I. Das, R.Picot, A.P. Smith & L. Reid, Bronchial secretion from normal human airways after inhalation of prostaglandin F 2 alpha, acetylcholine, histamine and citric acid, Thorax, 32 (1977) 734-739.

9. C.W. Parker, Aspirin sensitive asthma. In 'Asthma: Physiology, Immunopharmacology and Treatment' (Eds) L.M. Lichtenstein and K.F. Austen, Academic Press, London (1977) pp. 301-315.

10. E.D. Bateman, R.J. Emerson & P.J. Cole, Mechanisms of fibrogenesis. In 'Occupational Lung Diseases: Research, Approaches and Methods' (Eds) H. Weill and M. Turner-Warwick, Marcell Dekker, New York, 1981.

11. C.P. Page, W. Paul, C.B. Archer, D.M. MacDonald & J. Morley, Paf-acether, a mediator of acute and persisting inflammation to non-allergic and allergic stimuli. In 'Platelet Activating Factor' (Eds) J. Benveniste and B. Arnoux, Elsevier Science Publishers B.V. (1983) pp. 354-366.

12. R. Roubin, M. Tence, J.M. Mencia-Huerta, B. Arnoux, E. Ninio & J. Benveniste, A chemically defined monokine-macrophage derived platelet activating factor. In 'Lymphokines' (Ed) E. Pick, Academic Press, New York, In press.

13. B. Arnoux, A. Grimfeld, P. Duroux & A. Denjean, Alveolar macrophages/Paf-acether. A new association in the pathogenesis of human asthma. In 'Platelet Activating Factor' (Eds) J. Benvensite and B. Arnoux, Elsevier Science Publishers B.V. (1983) pp. 335-341.

14. P.J. Thompson, J.M. Havas, H. Bilani, M. Turner-Warwick & J. Morley, Platelets, platelet activating factor and asthma, am. Rev. Resp. Dis., 129 (1984) A3.

15. H.J. Beer, Wirkungen des 'Platelet activating Factor' (PAF) auf die Thrombozyten des Menschen, Thesis, University of Zurich (1984).

16. A. Dewar, C.B. Archer, W. Paul, C.P. Page, D.M. MacDonald & J. Morley, Cutaneous and pulmonary histopathological responses to Platelet activating Factor (Paf-acether) in the guinea-pig, J. path., 144 (1984) 25-31.

17. G. Camussi, I. Pawlowski, C. Tetta, C. Roffinello, M. Alberton, J. Brentjens & G. Andres, Acute lung inflammation induced in the rabbit by local instillation of 1-o-octadenyl-2-acetyl-sn-glyceryl-3-phosphorylcholine or of native platelet activating facor, Am. J. Path., 112 (1983) 78-88.

18. J. Morley, S. Sanjar & C.P. Page, Platelet activation as a basis for asthma exacerbation, Lancet, In Press.

19. P. Dukor, P. Kalllers, H.D. Schlumberger & G.B. West (Eds), Pseudo-Allergic Reactions: Volume 1, Genetic Aspect, and Anaphylactic Reactions, Karger Press, Basel, 1980.

20. S. Bianco, M. Robuschi, G. Petrini & L. Allegra, Respiratory effects due to aspirin (ASA); ASA induced tolerance in ASA-asthmatic patients, Bull. Eur. Physiopath. Resp. 13 (1977) 123.

21. J. Pepys, Immunopathology of allergic lung diseases, Clin. Allergy, 3 (1973) 1-22.

22. E.R. Tomy, M.D. Chapman & T.A.E. Platts-Mills, Mite faeces are a major source of home dust allergens, Nature 289 (1981) 592-593.

23. R.J. Davies & A.D. Blainey, Occupational Asthma, In 'Asthma' 2nd Edition (Eds) T.J.H. Clark and S. Godfrey, Chapman and Hall Medical, London (1983) 202-242.

24. R. Townley, R. Hopp, R. Coleman & A. Bewtra, Methacoline (M) inhalation challenge as a potential genetic marker, Respiration 46 (1984) 62.

LIST OF PARTICIPANTS

ACKERMANN M.
MEDICAL COLLEGE OF PENNSYLVANIA,
DEPARTMENT OF MICROBIOLOGY/IMMUNOLOGY,
3300 Henry Avenue
U.S.A. - PHILADELPHIA PA 19129

ADORINI L.
LABORATORIO DI PATOLOGIA,
ENEA-CRE,
Casaccia - C.P.2400
I-00100 ROMA

AMOS H. E.
ICI PLC, PHARM. DIVISION
Mereside, Alderley Park
UK-MACCLESFIELD, CHESHIRE

ANDERSEN K. E.
DEPARTMENT OF DERMATOLOGY,
GENTOFTE HOSPITAL
Niels Andersenvej 65
DK-2900 HELLERUP

APPLEFORD D. J. A.
LIFE SCIENCE RESEARCH LTD.
EYE
UK-SUFFOLK IP23 7PX

ARANYI C.
IIT RESEARCH INSTITUTE
10 West 35th Street
U.S.A. - CHICAGO IL 60616

d'ARGY R.
UNIVERSITY OF UPPSALA,
BIOMEDICAL CENTRE,
DEPARTMENT OF TOXICOLOGY
Biomedicium BOX 594
S-75124 UPPSALA

ASHERSON G. L.
DIV. OF IMMUNOLOGICAL MEDICINE
CLINICAL RESEARCH CENTRE
Watford Road
UK-HARROW HA1 3VJ

BABABUNMI E. A.
DEPARTMENT OF BIOCHEMISTRY,
UNIVERSITY OF IBADAN,
COLLEGE OF MEDICINE
NIGERIA-IBADAN

BALAZS T.
FOOD AND DRUG ADMINISTRATION,
DIVISION DRUG BIOLOGY HFD 414
200 C Street SW
U.S.A. - WASHINGTON DC 20204

BASSI L.
R.B.M.
I-IVREA (TO)

BEKESI J. G.
NEOPLACTIC DISEASES, MOUNT SINAI
HOSPITAL & SCHOOL OF MEDICINE
One Gustave L. Levy Place
U.S.A -NEW YORK NY 10029

BENNETT A. E.
COMMISSION OF THE EUROPEAN COMMUNITIES,
HEALTH AND SAFETY DIRECTORATE
Bâtiment Jean Monnet
Rue Alcide de Gasperi
L-2920 LUXEMBOURG

BERG N.
NOVO INDUSTRIES LIMITED
Novo Alle
DK-2880 BAGSVAERD

BERLIN A.
COMMISSION OF THE EUROPEAN COMMUNITIES,
HEALTH AND SAFETY DIRECTORATE
Bâtiment Jean Monnet
Rue Alcide de Gasperi
L-2920 LUXEMBOURG

BERNARD A.
UNIVERSITE CATHOLIQUE DE LOUVAIN
FACULTE DE MEDECINE
Clos Chapelle aux Champs 30
B-1200 BRUXELLES

BERNIER J.
DEPARTMENT OF BIOLOGICAL SCIENCES,
UNIVERSITY OF QUEBEC, MONTREAL
CP.8888
CANADA-MONTREAL SUC. A H3C3P8

BERODE
INST. UNIVERSITAIRE DE MEDECINE
DU TRAVAIL D'HYGIENE INDUSTRIEL.
Route de la Clochatte
CH-1052 LE MONT SUR LAUSANNE

BETZ A.
LABORATOIRE NATIONAL DE SANTE
42 Rue du Laboratoire
B.P.1102
L-1011 LUXEMBOURG

BLANE G.
LABORATOIRES FOURNIER
50 Rue de Dijon
F-21121 FONTAINE LES DIJON

BONTINCK W. J.
ECETOC
250 Avenue Louise Bt 63
B-1050 BRUXELLES

BOOTMAN J.
HEAD OF SHORT STUDIES
LIFE SCIENCE RESEARCH
EYE
UK-SUFFOLK IP23 7PX

BRADLEY W. A.
CIBA-GEIGY PHARMACEUTICALS
Stamford Lodge, Altrincham Road
UK-WILMSLOW, CHESHIRE SK9 4LY

BRAUN D. G.
CIBA-GEIGY Limited
K-125.15.16
CH-4002 BASEL

BROCADES ZAALBERG O.
MEDICAL BIOLOGICAL LABORATORY TNO
Lange Kleiweg 139 PO.BOX 45
NL-2280 AA RIJSWIJK

BROOKS B.
IMMUNOTOXICOLOGIST,
INTERNATIONAL BUSINESS MACHINES
CORPORATION (IBM)
750 Sumner
U.S.A. - LONGMONT CO

BUEHLER E. V.
HILL TOP RESEARCH, INC.,
RESEARCH & DEVELOPMENT DEPARTMENT
P.O. BOX 42501
U.S.A. CINCINNATI OH 45242

CAILLARD L.
RHONE POULENC INTER SERVICE RP/DSE
Les Miroirs,
18 Avenue d'Alsace Cedex 29
F-92097 PARIS LA DEFENSE 3

BICK P.
DEPARTMENT OF MICROBIOLOGY AND
IMMUNOLOGY,
MEDICAL COLLEGE OF VIRGINIA
U.S.A. - RICHMOND VA 23298

BOGAIEVSKY Y.
LABORATOIRES FOURNIER
50 Rue de Dijon
F-21121 FONTAINE LES DIJON

BOOTHMAN R.
DEPARTMENT OF HEALTH
Custom House
IRL-DUBLIN 1

BOTHAM P. A.
ICI CENTRAL TOXICOLOGY LAB.
Alderley Park
UK-MACCLESFIELD,CHESHIRE SK104TJ

BRAMAN S.
24 Chemin Briquet
CH-1209 GENEVA

BREMMER J.
SHELL INTERNATIONAL PETROLEUM
COMPANY LIMITED HSEL/228
York Road
UK-LONDON SE1 7NA

BROGREN C. H.
ARBEIJDSTILSYNET-
ARBEJSMILJØINSTITUTET
Baunegaardsvej 73
DK-2900 HELLERUP

BRUAUX P.
INST.D'HYGIENE & D'EPIDEMIOLOGIE
14 Rue J. Wytsman
B-1040 BRUXELLES

BYE S.
ICS/EHE DIVISION,
WORLD HEALTH ORGANIZATION
CH-1211 GENEVA 27

CAREMI I.
ZAMBELETTI S.p.A.
Via Zambeletti
I-20021 BARANZATE

CARPY S.
SANDOZ., AGRO-TOXICOLOGY
Postfach
CH-4002 BASEL

CHARBONNIER C.
INSTITUT MERIEUX,
DEPARTEMENT OF DEVELOP. & REC.
17, Rue Bourgelat
F-69002 LYON

CLARK B.
FISONS PCL, PHARMACEUTICAL DISISION S+T
LABORATORIES
Bakewell Road
UK-LOUGHBOROUGH, LEICS LE110RH

DALL V.
NOVO INDUSTRI A/S
Novo Alle
DK-2880 BAGSVAERD

DAWSON W.
LILLY RESEARCH CENTRE LTD.
Erl Wood Manor
UK-WINDLESHAM, SURREY

DAY J. H.
DIVISION OF ALLERGY & IMMUNOLOGY
DEPARTMENT OF MEDICINE
Queens University
CANADA-CDN KINGSTON, ONTARIO

DE PLAEN P.
INST. D'HYGIENE & D'EPIDEMIOLOGIE
14 Rue J. Wytsman
B-1040 BRUXELLES

DE RUSSIS R.
ISTITUTO MEDICINE DEL LAVORO
I-BARI

DEAN J. H.
CHEMICAL INDUSTRY,
INSTITUTE OF TOXICOLOGY
P.O. BOX 12137
RESEARCH TRIANGLE PARK NC27709
U.S.A.

DELTOUR G.
CENTRE INTERNAT. DE TOXICOLOGIE
BP.563
F-27005 EVREUX CEDEX

DENCKER L.
UNIVERSITY OF UPSALA,
BIOMEDICAL CENTRE,
DEPARTMENT OF TOXICOLOGY,
Biomedicium BOX 594
S-751 24 UPPSALA

DESCOTES G.
CLINICAL MIDY RESEARCH CENTER
F-34082 MONTPELLIER

DESCOTES J.
IMMUNOTOXICOLOGY UNIT,
LABORATORY PHARMACOLOGY,
FACULTY MEDICINE A. CARREL
Rue G. Paradin
F-69008 LYON

DESI I.
INST. OF HYGIENE & EPIDEMIOLOGY
UNIVERSITY MEDICAL SCHOOL
Dom tér 10
H-6720 SZEGED

DEWDNEY J. M.
BEECHAM PHARMACEUTICALS
RESEARCH DIVISION
Yewtree Bottom Road
UK-EPSOM, SURREY KT185XQ

DOLAN M. A.
BEECHAM PRODUCTS RES. DEPART.
ST. Georges Avenue
UK-WEYBRIDGE, SURREY KT13 ODE

DONAUBAUER H-H.
HOECHST AG,
DEPARTMENT OF TOXICOLOGY
P.O. BOX 800320
D-6230 FRANKFURT/M-80

DOSSOU G.
L'OREAL,
LABO. DE RECHERCHE FONDAMENTALE
1 Avenue de Saint-Germain BP.22
F-93601 AULNAY SOUS BOIS CEDEX

DRAPER M.
WORLD HEALTH ORGANISATION,
I.L.O. - U.N.E.P.
CH-1211 GENEVA 27

DUPRAT P.
M.S.D.,
CHIBRET RESEARCH LABORATORIES
Route de Marsat
F-63200 RIOM

DYWICKI O.
LABORATOIRE CASSENNE
BP.31
F-95521 CERGY-PONTOISE CEDEX

DZIEDZIC D.
GENERAL MOTORS RESEARCH LAB.,
GM TECHNICAL CENTER
U.S.A. - WARREN MI 48090

EBBON G. P.
CONCAWE BABYLON
Kantoren A
NL-2595 AA DEN HAAG

EPSTEIN I.
DIRECTOR,
DEPARTMENT OF LABORATORIES,
MINISTRY OF HEALTH
P.O. BOX 6115
ISRAEL-91060 JERUSALEM

EXON J. H.
SCHOOL OF VETERINARY MEDICINE,
UNIVERSITY OF IDAHO
U.S.A. - MOSCOW ID 83843

FARINE J-C.
LABORATOIRE OM S.A.,
DEPARTMENT OF RESEARCH
22 Rue du Bois-du-Lan
CH-1217 MAYRIN/GE

FIELDER
MEDICAL DIVISION C4,
HEALTH & SAFETY EXECUTIVE
Baynards House
1 Chepstow Place
UK-LONDON W2 4NF

FLINT O. P.
ICI PHARMACEUTICALS DIVISION
Mereside Alderley Park
UK-MACCLESFIELD, CHES. SK10 4TG

FOURNIER E.
HOPITAL FERNAND WIDAL
200 Rue du Faubourg St. Denis
F-75475 PARIS CEDEX

FOURNIER M.
DEPARTMENT OF BIOLOGICAL SCIENCES,
UNIVERSITY OF QUEBEC, MONTREAL
CP.8888
CANADA-MONTREAL SUC. A H3C3P8

GOING H.
FEDERAL MINISTRY OF YOUTH,
FAMILY AND HEALTH
Kennedy Allee
D-5300 BONN 2

GALIHER N. G.
ZOECON CORPORATION,
PALO ALTO
U.S.A. - CALIFORNIA

GARDNER D. E.
NORTHROP SERVICES INC.,
TOXICOLOGY
P.O. BOX 12313
RESEARCH TRIANGLE PARK NC27709
U.S.A.

GATENBY P. A.
DEPARTMENT CLINICAL IMMUNOLOGY,
ROYAL PRINCE ALFRED HOSPITAL
Missenden Road
AUS-CAMPERDOWN NSW 2050

GLASER U.
FRAUENHOFER INSTITUT
D-5848 SCHMALLENBERG

GLEICHMANN E.
MEDIZINISCHES INSTITUT FUR
UMWELTHYGIENE
Auf'm Hennekamp 50
D-4000 DUSSELDORF

GLEICHMANN H.
DIABETES FORSCHUNGSINSTITUT,
UNIVERSITY OF DUSSELDORF
Auf'm Hennekamp 65
D-4000 DUSSELDORF

GOVAERTS M.
CENTRE BELGE ANTI-POISONS
1 Rue Joseph Stallaert bte 15
B-1060 BRUXELLES

GRAEPEL P.
CIBA-GEIBY AG
R-1030, 1.01 Postfach
CH-4002 BASEL

GRANJEAN P.
ODENSE UNIVERSITY
J.B. Winslowvej 19
DK-5000 ODENSE

GRONDEL J. L.
AGRICULTURAL UNIVERSITY,
DEPARTMENT OF EXPERIMENTAL
ANIMAL MORPHOLOGY AND CELL BIOLOGY
P.O. BOX 338
NL-6700 AH WAGENINGEN

GUNNARSSON K.
A.B. LEO
P.O. BOX 941
S-251 09 HELSINGBORG

HALL J.
DEPARTMENT OF TUMOUR IMMUNOLOGY,
INSTITUTE OF CANCER RESEARCH
UK-SUTTON, SURREY

HEWETT C.
A. EXP. PATHOLOGIE UND TOXIKOLOGIE,
BOEHRINGER INGELHEIM
D-6507 INGELHEIM

HOFFMAN M.
4000 MASSACHUSETTS Avenue, N.W.
U.S.A. - WASHINGTON D.C. 20016

GOMEZ-REINO J.
MINISTERIO DE SANIDAD Y CONSUMO,
INSTITUTO NATIONAL DE LA SALUD,
HOSPITAL "I° DE OCTUBRE",
SECTION RHEUMATOLOGY
E-MADRID

GRAA K.
DANISH OCCUPATIONAL INSTITUTE, KTA
Ryesgade 113
DK-2100 COPENHAGEN Ø

GRAHAM J. A.
U.S. ENVIRONMENTAL PROTECTION AGENCY,
HEALTH EFFECTS RESEARCH LABORATORY,
TOXICOLOGY BRANCH (MD-82)
RESEARCH TRIANGLE PARK NC27711
U.S.A.

GREENLEE W. F.
DEPARTMENT OF CELL BIOLOGY,
CHEMICAL INDUST. INSTITUTE TOXICOLOGY
P.O. BOX 12137
RESEARCH TRIANGLE PARK NC277009
U.S.A.

GUENCHEVA G. P.
INSITUTE FOR STATE CONTROL OF DRUGS
26 Bul Vl Zaimov
BG-SOFIA

HADDEN J. W.
IMMUNOPHARMACOLOGY PROGRAM,
UNIVERSITY OF S. FLORIDA,
COLLEGE OF MEDICINE
12901 North 30th Street
U.S.A. - TAMPA FL 33612

HEIMANN K-G.
BAYER AG,
INSTITUT FUR TOXIKOLOGIE
Friederich-Ebert-Strasse 217
D-5600 WUPPERTAL 1

HILDEBRAND B.
BASF AKTIENGESELLSCHAFT - TOXIKOLOGIE
D-6700 LUDWIGSHAFEN

HOFMANN A.
INSTITUTE OF TOXICOLOGY E. MERCK
Postfach 4779
D-6100 DARMSTADT

HORAKOVA Z.
FOOD SAFETY AND INSPECTION SERVICE,
U.S. DEPARTMENT OF AGRICULTURE
5508 Oakmont Avenue
U.S.A. - BETHESDA MD 20817

HUETER G.
U.S. ENVIRONMENTAL PROTECTION AGENCY,
HEALTH EFFECTS RESEARCH LABORATORY
(MD-51)
P.O. BOX 12313
RESEARCH TRIANGLE PARK NC27711
U.S.A.

HUGO P.
DEPARTMENT OF BIOLOGICAL SCIENCES,
UNIVERSITY OF QUEBEC, MONTREAL,
CP.8888
CANADA-MONTREAL SUC. A H3C3P8

HULON W. C.
ETHYL CORPORATION
451 Florida Boulevard
U.S.A. - BATON ROUGE LA 70801

HUNTER W.
COMMISSION OF THE EUROPEAN
COMMUNITIES,
HEALTH AND SAFETY DIRECTORATE
Bâtiment Jean Monnet
Rue Alcide de Gasperi
L-2920 LUXEMBOURG

HURTENBACH U.
INSTITUT FUR UMWELTHYGIENE
Auf'm Hennekamp 50
D-4000 DUSSELDORF

JEAN P.
CENTRE DE TOXICOLOGIE MEDICALE,
CENTRE ANTI-POISONS,
HOPITAL SALVADOR
249 Boulevard Sainte-Marguerite
F-13274 MARSEILLE CEDEX 9

JOHANSSON H-E.
KABIVITRUM AB
S-112 87 STOCKHOLM

JOOSTEN H.
ORGANON INTITUTE B.V.,
DRUG SAFETY RESEARCH & DEVELOPMENT
LABORATORIES
P.O. BOX 20
NL-5340 BH OSS

KALLAND T.
LUNDS UNIVERSITET INSTITUTE OF
ANATOMY
Biskopsgatan 7
S-223 62 LUND

KAMMUELLER M. E.
UNIVERSITY OF UTRECHT
Biltstraat 172 3572 BP
NL-UTRECHT

KEMPER F. H.
INSTITUT FUR PHARMAKOLOGIE UND
TOXIKOLOGIE DER UNIVERSITAT MUNSTER
Domagkstrasse 12
D-4400 MUNSTER/W.

KERKVLIET N. I.
OREGON STATE UNIVERSITY,
COLLEGE OF VETERINARY MEDICINE
U.S.A. - CORWALLIS OR 97331

KIMBER I.
ICI CENTRAL TOXICOLOGY LABORATORY
Alderley Park
UK-MACCLESFIELD, CHESHIRE SK104TJ

KLECAK
HOFFMANN-LAROCHE
Grenzacherstrasse 264
CH-4002 BASEL

KODAT V.
MINISTRY OF HEALTH OF CZECH SOC.REP.
DEPARTMENT HYGIENE & EPIDEMIOLOGY
CZECHOSLOVAKIA-PRAGUE

KOOPMAN T. S. M.
DUPHAR B.V.,
DEPARTMENT OF TOXICOLOGY
c.j. van Houtenlaan 36
P.O. BOX 2
NL-1380 AA WEESP

KRISTOFFERSON A.
ASTRA LAKEMEDEL AB,
RESEARCH & DEVELOPMENT LABORATORIES
BIOCHEMICAL NEUROPHARMACOLOGY,
IMMUNOLOGY
S-15185 SODERTALJE

KRZYSTYNIAK K.
DEPART.DES SCIENCES BIOLOGIQUES,
UNIVERSITE DE QUEBEC
C.P.8888, SUCC. "A"
CANADA-MONTREAL, P.QUEBEC H3C3P8

KUPER C. F.
CIVO - TNO
P.O. BOX 360
NL-3700 AJ ZEIST

LAFONTAINE A.
INST. OF HYGIENE AND EPIDEMIOLOGY
95 Boulevard Brand Whitlock
B-1200 BRUXELLES

LAMBERT P.
DEPARTMENT OF PATHOLOGY,
CENTRE MEDICAL UNIVERSITAIRE
CH-1211 GENEVA 4

LANGE P.
DEPT. PHARMACOLOGY & TOXICOLOGY
UNIVERSITY OF ROSTOCK
Leninallee 70
D.D.R. - 25 ROSTOCK

LAWRENCE D. A.
DEPARTMENT OF MICROBIOLOGY/IMMUNOLOGY
ALBANY MEDICAL COLLEGE
47 New Scotland Avenue
U.S.A. - ALBANY NY 12208

LEACH C.
IIT RESEARCH INSTITUTE
10 West 35th Street
U.S.A. - CHICAGO, ILLINOIS 60616

LEVIN R. A.
NORWICH-EATON PHARMACEUTICALS
P.O. BOX 191
U.S.A. - NORWICH NY 13815

LEWALTER J.
BAYER AG
Ruettersweg 130
D-5090 LEVERKUSEN

LILLIEHOOK B.
NATIONAL DEFENCE RESEARCH INSTITUTE,
ABC RESEARCH DEPARTMENT (FOA 4)
Cementvägen 20
S-90182 UMEA

LORENZ J.
BUNDESANSTALT FUR ARBEITSSCHUTZ
Vogelpothsweg 50-52
D-4600 DORTMUND

LUINI W.
ISTITUTO MARIO NEGRI
Via Eritrea 62
I-20157 MILANO

LUSTER M. I.
IMMUNOTOXICOLOGY SECTION,
NIEHS/NIH
P.O. BOX 12233
RESEARCH TRIANGLE PARK NC27709
U.S.A.

MADSEN C.
INSTITUTE OF TOXICOLOGY,
NATIONAL FOOD INSTITUTE
MØRKHØJ Bygade 19
DK-2860 SØBORG

MAIBACH H. I.
UNIVERSITY OF CALIFORNIA HOSPITAL,
U.C. MEDICAL CENTER
U.S.A. - SAN FRANCISCO CA 94143

MARAVELIAS C.
DEPARTMENT OF FORENSIC MEDICINE &
TOXICOLOGY,
UNIVERSITY OF ATHENS,
MEDICAL SCHOOL
GR-ATHENS

MARTENS M.
MINISTERE DE LA SANTE PUBLIQUE ET
DE LA FAMILLE,
INST. D'HYGIENE & D'EPIDEMIOLOGIE
14 Rue Juliette Wytsman
B-1050 BRUXELLES

MASEK K.
INSTITUTE OF PHARMACOLOGY
CZECHOSLOVAK ACADEMY OF SCIENCES
Albertov 4
CS-128 00 PRAGUE 2

MATTIELLO G.
LABORATORIO D'IGIENE & PROFILASSI
Campo della Lane 601
I-30125 VENEZIA

MAYR W.
ASTA AG
Artur Ladebeckstrasse 128-152
D-4800 BIELEFELD

MERCIER M.
INTERNATIONAL PROGRAMME ON CHEMICAL
SAFETY,
W.H.O.
CH- 1211 GENEVE 27

MIHICH E.
GRACE CANCER DRUG CENTER,
ROSWELL PARK MEMORIAL INSTITUTE,
DEPARTMENT OF HEALTH
666 Elm Street
U.S.A. - BUFFALO NY 14263

MORIN A.
INSTITUT PASTEUR,
IMMUNOTHERAPIE EXPERIMENTALE
28 Rue du Docteur Roux
F-75724 PARIS CEDEX 15

MOULONGUET D.
ROUSSEL UCLAF,
DIRECTION MEDICALE
102-111 Route de Noisy
F-92230 ROMAINVILLE

MUNSON A. E.
DEPARTMENT OF PHARMACOLOGY,
MEDICAL COLLEGE OF VIRGINIA
U.S.A. - RICHMOND VA 23298

NAVA A.
FARMITALIA CARLO ERBA,
RSB/TOSSICOLOGIA
Via Imbonati 24
I-20159 MILANO

ODERMATT P.
FEDERAL OFFICE OF PUBLIC HEALTH
P.O. BOX 2644
CH-3001 BERNE

MAURER T.
CIBA-GEIGY AG
CH-4002 BASEL

MELCION C.
RHONE-POULENC SANTE
13 Quai Jules Guesde
F-94403 VITRY SUR SEINE CEDEX

METALLINOS
INSTITUTE OF TOXICOLOGY E. MERCK,
Postfach 4779
D-6100 DARMSTADT

MILLER K.
BIBRA
Wood Mansterne Road
UK-CARSHALTON, SURREY

MORROD R. S.
RESEARCH TOXICOLOGY MANAGER,
IMPERIAL CHEMICAL INDUSTRIES, LTD.,
CENTRAL TOXICOLOGY LABORATORY
Alderley Park
UK- Nr. MACCLESFIELD SK10 4TJ

MOUSTAFA L. A.
WORLD HEALTH ORGANIZATION,
IPCS INTERREGIONAL RESEARCH UNIT,
A206 - BOX 12233
RESEARCH TRIANGLE PARK NC27709
U.S.A.

NARDI E.
UNIVERSITA DI ROMA,
ISTITUTO DI SEMIOTICA,
PATOLOGIA E CLINICA MEDICA
I-ROMA

NEVEU P. J.
U.E.R. DE MEDECINE,
GROUPE DE RECHERCHE DE BIOCHEMIE
HERMATOLOGIE
34 Rue du Jardin des Plantes
F-86034 POITIERS

OHSAWA M.
DEPARTMENT ENVIRONMENTAL TOXICOLOGY,
FACULTY PHARMACEUTICAL SCIENCES,
TEIKYO UNIVERSITY
Sagamiko
J-KANAGAWA 199-01

OLKOWSKI Z. L.
N.E. EMORY UNIVERSITY CLINIC,
LABORATORY OF TUMOR BIO & CLINIC
IMMUNOLOGY
1365 Clifton Road
U.S.A. - ATLANTA GA 30322

ORBACH S.
INSTITUT DE CANCEROLOGIE ET
D'IMMUNOGENIQUE,
HOPITAL PAUL BROUSSE
12/16 Avenue P. Vaillant Couturier
F-94800 VILLEJUIF

PAGE C.
PRECLINICAL RESEARCH,
SANDOZ LTD.
CH-4002 BASEL

PAINE A.
DHSS, DEPARTMENT OF TOXICOLOGY,
ST. BARTHOLOMEW HOSPITAL,
MEDICAL COLLEGE
Dominion House 59
Bartholomew Close
UK-LONDON EC1 7ED

PAL T. M.
ENKA b.v. BEDR. GENEESK. DIENST
Ie Bokslootweg 17 Pb. 8
NL-7800 AA EMMEN

PARK B. K.
DEPARTMENT OF PHARMACOLOGY &
THERAPEUTICS,
LIVERPOOL UNIVERSITY
P.O. BOX 147
UK-LIVERPOOL L69 3BX

PARODI A-L.
ECOLE NATION. VETERIN. D'ALFORT,
CHAIRE D'ANATOMIE PATHOLOGIQUE
7 Avenue Général de Gaulle
F-94704 MAISONS-ALFORT CEDEX

PASCAL M.
LABORATOIRES FOURNIER,
CENTRE DE RECHERCHE
50 Rue de Dijon
F-21121 FONTAINE LES DIJON

PASQUET J.
RHONE-POULENC SANTE
13 Quai Jules Guesde
F-94403 VITRY SUR SEINE CEDEX

PAUWELS R.
ACADEMIC HOSPITAL
De Pintelaan 185
B-9000 GENT

PELIKAN Z.
Wouter Berthoutlaan 62
NL-4871 AK ETTEN-LEUR (NB)

PENN I.
DEPARTMENT OD SURGERY,
UNIVERSITY OF CINCINNATI,
MEDICAL CENTER
231 Bethesda Avenue (558)
U.S.A. - CINCINNATI OH 45267

PENNINKS A. H.
PATHOLOGY-TOXICOLOGY INSTITUT,
DEPARTMENT OF EXPERIENCE,
STATE UNIVERSITY UTRECHT
Bilstraat 172
NL-3572 BP UTRECHT

PETERSON L. B.
MERCK SHARP & DOHME RESEARCH
LABORATORIES
P.O. BOX 2000
U.S.A. - RAHWAY NJ

POLLITT F.
TOXIC SUBSTANCES DIVISION,
DEPARTMENT OF THE ENVIRONMENT
Romney House, 43 Marsham Street
UK-LONDON SWIP 3EB

POLMAR S. H.
WASHINGTON UNIVERSITY SCHOOL OF
MEDICINE,
DEPARTMENT OF PEDIATRICS,
IMMUNOLOGY & MICROBIOLOGY
P.O. BOX 14871
U.S.A. - ST. LOUIS MO 63178

POSTE G.
SMITH KLINE & FRENCH LABORATORIES
1500 Spring Garden Street POB 7929
U.S.A. - PHILADELPHIA PA 19101

RAMET J.
DEPARTMENT OF PEDIATRICS INTENSIVE
CARE,
AKADEMISCH ZIEKENHUIS,
VRIJE UNIVERSITEIT BRUSSEL
Laarbeeklaan 101
B-1090 BRUSSEL

RILEY A. J.
OCCUPATIONAL HEALTH CENTRE,
BRITISH PETROLEUM,
BP RESEARCH CENTRE
Chertsey Road
UK-SUNBURY ON THAMES, MIDDX
TW16 7LN

ROOK A. H.
NATIONAL INSTITUTES OF HEALTH
Buildings 10, Room 11b-13
U.S.A. - BETHESDA MD 20205

ROTOLO V. S.
UNIVERSIDAD NATIONAL DE ROSARIO
Santa Fe 3100
ARGENTINA-ROSARIO 2000

SCHMIDT W.
BAYER A.G.
Aprather Weg
D-5600 WUPPERTAL

SCHNEIDER P.
DOKTOR KARL THOMAE Gmbh
D-7950 BIBERACH an der RISS

SELGRADE M. J.
HERL, U.S. ENVIRONMENTAL PROTECTION
AGENCY
M.D. 82
RESEARCH TRIANGLE PARK NC27711
U.S.A.

SHOHAM J.
DEPARTMENT OF LIVE SCIENCES,
BAR ILAN UNIVERSITY
ISRAEL-52100 RAMAT GAN

PRIGENZY L. S.
DEPARTMENT OF CLINICAL PATHOLOGY,
STATE UNIVERSITY OF CAMINAS,
SCHOOL OF MEDICINE
Caixa Postal 1170
BR-13100 CAMPINAS

RIETHMULLER G.
INSTITUTE OF IMMUNOLOGY,
UNIVERSITAET MUENCHEN
Schillerstrasse
D-8000 MUENCHEN

ROBINS A.
UNIVERSITY OF NOTTINGHAM,
CANCER RESEARCH CAMPAIGN
LABORATORIES,
University Park
UK-NOTTINGHAM NG7 20D

ROSENFELD
INSERM-HOSPITAL PAUL BROUSSE
F-94800 VILLEJUIF

SCHLEUSENER A.
MAX VON PETTENKOFER-
INSTITUT DES BUNDESGESUNDHEITSAMT
ABT. TOXIKOLOGIE DER LEBENSMITTEL UND
BEDARFSGEGENSTAENDE
Postfach 330013
D-1000 BERLIN 13

SCHMUTZLER W.
ABTEILUNG PHARM MED FAK DER RWTH
AACHEN, MED-THEORESTISCHE INSTITUT
Schneeberweg
D-5100 AACHEN

SEINEN W.
UNIVERSITY OF UTRECHT
Bilstraat 172 3572 BP
NL-UTRECHT

SHANKAR R.
INDUSTRIAL TOXICOLOGY RESEARCH CENTRE
P.O. BOX 80
IND-226001 LUCKNOW (UP)

SIBLEY P.
GLAXO GROUP RESEARCH LIMITED
GB-WARE, HERTS SG12 0DJ

SIEGMUND
SCHERING AG -
VORKLINISCHE ENTWICKLUNG
EXP. TOXIKOLOGIE
Müllerstrasse 170 Postfach 650311
D-1000 BERLIN

SIRONI M.
ISTITUTO MARIO NEGRI
Via Eritrea 62
I-20157 MILANO

SMITH E.
INTERNATIONAL PROGRAMME ON
CHEMICAL SAFETY,
WORLD HEALTH ORGANIZATION
CH-1211 GENEVE 27

SNOEIJ N.
UNIVERSITY OF UTRECHT
Bilstraat 172 3572 BP
NL-UTRECHT

SORS A. I.
COMMISSION OF THE EUROPEAN
COMMUNITIES
ENV. RESEARCH PROGRAMME, XII/G,
200 Rue de la Loi
B-1049 BRUXELLES

SPURLING NW.
GLAXO GROUP RESEARCH LIMITED
UK-WARE, HERTS SG12 ODJ

STANWORTH D. R.
RHEUMATOLOGY AND ALLERGY RESEARCH
UNIT,
DEPARTMENT OF IMMUNOLOGY,
UNIVERSITY OF BIRMINGHAM
Edgebaston
UK-BIRMINGHAM

STEJSKAL V.
ASTRA PHARMACEUTICALS AB,
TOXICOLOGY LABORATORIES
S-15185 SODERTALJE

TEELMAN K.
HOFFMANN-LA ROCHE
CH-4002 BASEL

SILICE C.
RHONE POULENC AGRONOMIE
14-20 Rue Pierre Baizet
F-69623 LYON CEDEX 09

SMITH C.
SANDOZ CORPORATION BUILDING 404,
ROOM 448
Route 10
U.S.A. - EAST HANOVER NJ 07936

SMITH I. K.
IMPERIAL CHEMICAL INDUSTRIES PLC,
PHARACEUTICALS DIVISION,
Mereside Alderley Park
UK-MACCLESFIELD, CHES. SK10 4TG

SOLIMAN S. A.
DEPARTMENT PESTICIDE CHEM.,
FACULTY OF AGRICULTURE,
UNIVERSITY OF ALEXANDRIA
EGYPT-ALEXANDRIA

SPREAFICO F.
ISTITUTO DI RICERCHE FARMACOLOGICHE
"MARIO NEGRI"
Via Eritrea 62
I-20157 MILANO

STAALHANDSKE T.
AB LEO RESEARCH LABORATORIES
BOX 941
S-251 09 HELSINBORG

STEEN M.
STATE POLLUTION CONTROL AUTHORITY
P.O. BOX 8100
N-OSLO 1

TACHON P.
HAZLETON - I.F.T.,
INSTITUT FRANCAIS DE TOXICOLOGIE
BP. 109
F-69210 L'ARBRESLE

TEIRLINCK O.
P. HEYMANS INSTITUT - RUG -
ACADEMISCHE ZIEKENHUIS
De Pintelaan 135
B-9000 GENT

THOMAS P. T.
IIT RESEARCH INSTITUTE,
LIFE SCIENCE RESEARCH DIVISION
10 West 35th Street
U.S.A. - CHICAGO ILL 60616

TOURAINE J. L.
INSERM U-80
HOPITAL E. HERRIOT, PAVILLON P.
4 Place D'Arsonval
F-69374 LYON CEDEX 2

TRYPHONAS H.
HEALTH AND WELFARE
Tunney's Pasture
CDN-OTTAWA, ONTARIO K1A OL2

TUBARO E.
WELLCOME ITALIA S.P.A.
Via del Mare 36
I-00040 POMEZIA

VAN DER VENNE M-T.
COMMISSION OF THE EUROPEAN
COMMUNITIES,
HEALTH AND SAFETY DIRECTORATE
Bâtiment Jean Monnet
Rue Alcide de Gasperi
L-2920 LUXEMBOURG

VAN ESSCHE R.
SCIENT. TRAVENOL
130 Chaussée de la Hulpe
B-1050 BRUXELLES

VAN LOVEREN H.
RIJKS INSTITUUT VOOR DE
VOLKSGEZONDHEID
Antonie van Leeuwentoelaan 9
NL-BILTHOVEN

VAN SITTERT N. J.
SHELL INTERNATIONALE PETROLEUM Mij
b.v.
Postbus 162
NL-2501 AN DEN HAAG

VECCHI A.
ISTITUTO DI RICERCHE FARMACOLOGICHE
MARIO NEGRI
Via Eritrea 62
I-20157 MILANO

VERBOVEN M.
DEPARTMENT OF PEDIATRICS,
ACADEMIC HOSPITAL,
VRIJE UNIVERSITEIT BRUSSEL
Laarbeeklaan 101
B-1090 BRUSSEL

VERLINDEN
FEDERATION INDUSTRIES CHIMIQUES,
BELGIQUE
Square Marie Louise 49
B-1040 BRUXELLES

VICARI G.
DEPARTMENT OF IMMUNOLOGY,
ISTITUTO SUPERIORE DI SANITA
Viale Regina Elena 299
I-00161 ROMA

VOS J. G.
NATIONAL INSTITUTE OF PUBLIC HEALTH
AND ENVIRONMENTAL HYGIENE
Antonie van Leeuwenhoeklaan 9
NL-3720 BILTHOVEN

VU-NGOC-HUYEN D.
L.E.R. SYNTHELABO
23-25 Avenue Morane-Saulnier
F-92360 MEUDON-LA-FORET

WEISSE
INSTITUTE OF TOXICOLOGY E. MERCK
Postfach 4779
D-6100 DARMSTADT

WETZIG H.
A. NATTERMANN ET Cie Gmbh
Nattermann-Allee
D-5000 KOLN 30

WHITE H.
GENERAL MOTORS RESEARCH LAB.
GM Tech. Center
U.S.A. - WARREN 48090 -9058

WOOD S.
DEPARTMENT OF LABOUR
Mespil Road
IRL-DUBLIN 2

ZARATZIAN V.
U.S.D.A.
300-12th St. S.W. Room 510
U.S.A. - WASHINGTON DC 20250

ZAYKOV C.
INSTITUTE OF HYGIENE AND
OCCUPATIONAL HEALTH,
MEDICAL ACADEMY
Boulevard Dimitar Nestorov 15
BULGARIA-SOFIA 31

ZBINDEN G.
FEDERAL INSTITUTE OF TECHNOLOGY,
E.T.H., UNIVERSITY OF ZURICH
Schorenstrasse 16
CH-8603 SCHWERZENBACH, ZURICH